HANDBOOK OF RESEARCH METHODS IN HEALTH PSYCHOLOGY

T0386351

In this comprehensive handbook, Ragin and Keenan present an all-encompassing analysis of the variety of different methods used in health psychology research.

Featuring interdisciplinary collaborations from leading academics, this meticulously written volume is a guide to conducting cutting-edge research using tested and vetted best practices. It explains important research techniques, why they are selected, and how they are conducted. The book critically examines both cutting-edge methods, such as those used in NextGen genetics, nudge theory, and the brain's vulnerability to addiction, as well as the classic methods, including cortisol measurement, survey, and environmental studies. The topics of the book span the gamut of the health psychology field, from neuroimaging and statistical analysis to socioeconomic issues such as the policies used to address diseases in Africa, anti-vaxers, and the disproportionate impact of climate change on impoverished people.

With each section featuring examples of best research practices, recommendations for study samples, accurate use of instrumentation, analytical techniques, and advanced-level data analysis, this book will be an essential text for both emerging student researchers and experts in the field and an indispensable resource in health psychology programs.

Deborah Fish Ragin is Professor Emeritus, Montclair State University. She also served as an American Psychological Association Representative to the United Nations, focusing on the psychosocial impact of HIV/AIDS, and currently serves as a representative to the United Nations for the Non-Governmental Organization (NGO), Society for the Psychological Study of Social Issues. She is the author of *Health Psychology: An Interdisciplinary Approach* (3rd Ed., Routledge/Taylor & Francis).

Julian Paul Keenan is a Professor in the Department of Biology and the Director of the Cognitive Neuroimaging Laboratory at Montclair State University. He previously served on the faculty at Harvard Medical School and is the Founding Editor of *Social Neuroscience*. He has published in *Science*, *Nature*, and *Proceedings of the Academy of Sciences*.

HANDBOOK OF RESEARCH METHODS IN HEALTH PSYCHOLOGY

Edited by Deborah Fish Ragin and Julian Paul Keenan

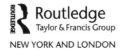

NEW YORK AND LONDON

First published 2021
by Routledge
52 Vanderbilt Avenue, New York, NY 10017

and by Routledge
2 Park Square, Milton Park, Abingdon, Oxon, OX14 4RN

Routledge is an imprint of the Taylor & Francis Group, an informa business

Library of Congress Cataloging-in-Publication Data
A catalog record for this book has been requested

ISBN: 978-1-138-59534-7 (hbk)
ISBN: 978-1-138-59533-0 (pbk)
ISBN: 978-0-429-48832-0 (ebk)

Typeset in Bembo
By Apex CoVantage, LLC

CONTENTS

Contents

Contents

ABOUT THE EDITORS

Deborah Fish Ragin and
Julian Paul Keenan

Deborah Fish Ragin is a professor emeritus of psychology at Montclair State University. She earned her AB in psychology and Hispanic studies from Vassar College and her MA and PhD in psychology from Harvard University. She has been a member of the faculties of Hunter College at the City University of New York and Mount Sinai School of Medicine's (now Ichan School of Medicine) Department of Emergency Medicine (New York City). Her professional work in health includes her service for five years as an American Psychological Association (APA) Representative to the United Nations, where she focused on global efforts to address the psychosocial impact of HIV/AIDS; a three-year term as president of the APA's Society for the Study of Peace, Conflict, and Violence (Division 48, Peace Psychology); a member of the Health Research Council of the Health Psychology Division (Division 38) of the American Psychological Association; and a member of the UN Non-Governmental Organization (NGO) team representing the Society for the Psychological Study of Social Issues. Dr. Ragin's research focuses on health systems and healthy policy, examining disparities in health care. She has authored articles on HIV/AIDS, domestic violence, health care disparities, healthy communities, and research ethics, and is also the author of a leading textbook entitled *Health Psychology: An Interdisciplinary Approach*, published by Routledge/Taylor & Francis Group, now in its third edition. In the international market, *Health Psychology* has been translated into Chinese and is used in universities in Australia, Canada, and New Zealand. Dr. Ragin also serves as a reviewer on several international and national journals, including *Social Science and Medicine*, *American Journal of Nursing*, and the *Journal of Interpersonal Violence*.

Julian Keenan is a professor of biology at Montclair State University and a former professor of psychology at Montclair State University. His previous position was in the Department of Neurology at Harvard Medical School, and he regularly collaborates both nationally and internationally. He has his PhD from the University at Albany in Biopsychology. He has published on concussions, depression, depersonalization, and other clinical conditions (he co-edited a book on clinical conditions of consciousness: *The Lost Self*, Oxford), but his focus is on cognition and the brain incorporating neuroimaging and evolution with genetics. He has authored and edited numerous books, including volumes for Cambridge, MIT, and Harper Collins Ecco. His books have been translated into German and Japanese, and he has edited a book published in Japan. Dr. Keenan has published articles in *Science, Nature*, and the *Proceedings of the National Academy of Science*. Dr. Keenan cofounded the Taylor & Francis journal *Social Neuroscience*, which is now in its eleventh year. He is often in the popular press (e.g., Hulu, FoxNews, RadioLab) and has hundreds of media appearances.

ABOUT THE CONTRIBUTORS

Matthew L. Aardema, PhD, received his PhD in ecology and evolutionary biology from Princeton University. He is currently an assistant professor in the Biology Department at Montclair State University and a visiting scientist at the Sackler Institute for Comparative Genomics at the American Museum of Natural History in New York City. His current research focuses on comparative genomics in relation to blood feeding and wing loss in arthropod disease vectors and the phylogenomics of *Culex* mosquitoes. Recent publications include peer-reviewed articles in the *Journal of Clinical Microbiology* and *Genome Biology and Evolution*.

Daniel Malik Achala, MPhil, is a researcher and the programmes officer at the African Health Economics and Policy Association (AfHEA). Daniel has an MPhil in economics from the Kwame Nkrumah University of Science and Technology, Kumasi, Ghana. He has previously taught undergraduate economics courses at the University of Ghana Distance Education Programme at Workers College, Tamale, and the Jayee University College, Accra. His current research interests include child and maternal health, health financing, social determinants of health, development economics, and international economics. He has some publications in these areas.

John Ele-Ojo Ataguba, PhD, is an associate professor and director of the Health Economics Unit, University of Cape Town. John has a PhD in economics from the University of Cape Town. He is the interim South African Research Leader (chair) in Health and Wealth and serves in the leadership of a number of other boards and committees, including deputy executive director for the African Health Economics and Policy Association (AfHEA), member of the board of directors for the International Health Economics Association (iHEA), member of the World Economic Forum's Global Future Council for Health and Healthcare, research fellow for the Partnership for Economic Policy (PEP) network, and was a Mellon Mandela Fellow at Harvard University, Cambridge. He is the recipient of several prestigious awards. His research interests include health economics methodology design, health financing, health inequality, equity in health and health care, social determinants of health, and the economics of aging.

Chris Atim, PhD is a senior program director at the Results for Development Institute (R4D) based in Accra, Ghana. He received his PhD (1993) in economics from the University of Sussex, UK, and postdoctoral training in epidemiology and health economics in London and York. He has more than 25 years' experience working on, teaching, and researching health economics and financing in Africa and providing technical assistance and advice on health financing, economics, and policy to governments, NGOs, and regional institutions in over two dozen African countries. Chris is the founding executive director of the African Health Economics and Policy Association (AfHEA), dedicated to strengthening the capacities of African health economists and policy experts and promoting the application of tools of health economics, financing, and policy in health-sector decision-making in Africa. At the invitation of the Ghanaian president, he chaired the Presidential National Health Insurance Scheme (NHIS) technical committee from 2015 to 2016, to make the NHIS more sustainable, efficient, equitable, accountable, and responsive to users.

Jelani Awai, is a student at Montclair State University, majoring in psychology. His research interests include the mind and human behavior. He is currently pursuing an interest in industrial/organizational psychology examining motivation and human behavior in the workplace.

Shaun Bhatia, MS, earned a Master of Science in epidemiology from the University of Illinois at Urbana-Champaign. After serving as a researcher with violence prevention initiatives at the University of Illinois at Chicago, Shaun joined the Center for Community Research at DePaul University, also in Chicago. He is currently a PhD candidate in community psychology at DePaul University. His research interests include crime prevention, education equity, statistical methodology, and spatial data science. Shaun also serves as a statistical consultant for NGOs.

Alexander Dean Bracken, BA, received his BA in psychology from Montclair State University. Currently, he is a graduate student in the Department of Psychology Master's of Psychological Sciences Program. Alexander has conducted research in health psychology and cognitive science as both an undergraduate and graduate student, using various techniques ranging from human experimentation to qualitative analysis. Building on his work and interest in how people think, make decisions, and react in social and physical environments, Alex plans to continue his studies in health psychology at the doctoral level.

Janet Brenya is a student at Montclair State University and works in the Cognitive Neuroimaging Laboratory in the Department of Biology at the university. She specializes in frontal lobe investigations, using transcranial magnetic stimulation, and has investigated self-deception and the prefrontal cortex. Janet also specializes in other facets of neuroscience, including addiction, alcoholism and nicotine via vaping/e-cigarettes.

S. Chandrashekara, MD, a pioneer in the research field of rheumatology and immunology in India, is presently serving as the managing director of ChanRe Rheumatology Immunology Center and Research, Bengaluru, India. He received his MD in general medicine from Mysore Medical College, Karnataka, and his DM in clinical immunology from Sanjay Gandhi Postgraduate Institute of Medical Sciences, Lucknow, India. He is a renowned rheumatologist and immunologist with over 20 years of consultant-grade experience and expertise. He has published more than 90 articles in international and national journals and has penned 14 reference books in rheumatology and 9 patient education books and authored a chapter in the fifth edition of *Manual of Rheumatology*. He is presently serving as the vice president of the Indian Rheumatology Association and is a principal investigator for several clinical trials on rheumatoid arthritis (RA), systemic lupus erythematosus (SLE), gout, fibromyalgia, and osteoarthritis and is the recipient of several prestigious awards.

Katherine Chavarria is a student at Montclair State University and a research assistant in the Cognitive Neuroimaging Laboratory in the Department of Biology at the university. Katherine's research focuses on the use of transcranial magnetic stimulation (TMS). She is a co-author on several papers on the medial prefrontal cortex and deception detection.

Christo P. Cilliers, PhD received his PhD in communication and media studies from the University of South Africa (UNISA), Master of Arts in communication management from the University of Pretoria, and Honors Degree in communication (specializing in marketing communication), also from UNISA. He is an associate professor in the Department of Communication Science at UNISA, where he supervises masters and doctoral students and teaches in the media studies stream. His main research interests lie in visual studies, gender studies, popular culture, and health communication.

Joseph Cotler, PhD, received his PhD in social psychology from the University of Birmingham. He is a project director at the Center for Community Research at DePaul University, Chicago. His current research interests are the assessments of cytokine biomarkers for chronic fatigue syndrome (CFS) and myalgic encephalomyelitis (ME), the reduction of stigma among ME/CFS patients, and changes in the economic behavior of recovery-home residents. Additionally, previous publications include a large community-based prevalence study of ME/CFS in pediatrics and an algorithmic assessment of different chronic illnesses with post-exertional malaise. He has worked in the field of community psychology since February 2018.

Curtis R. Coughlin II, MS, MBe, CGC, is an associate professor of pediatrics and associate faculty at the Center for Bioethics and Humanities at the University of Colorado, Anschutz Medical Campus. He trained in genetics at Arcadia University and bioethics at the University of Pennsylvania. He is a clinical ethicist at the Children's Hospital, Colorado, and a current member of the Clinical Genetics Resource's (ClinGen) Consent and Disclosure Recommendation Committee. He previously served as the chair of the ethics advisory group for the National Society of Genetic Counselors and the ethics content expert for the Colorado Department of Public Health and Environment's Newborn Screening Program. His research interest includes return of results and secondary findings identified through genomic sequencing and the impact of genomic medicine on vulnerable populations.

Maya Crawford is a student at Montclair State University. She conducts research at the Cognitive Neuroimaging Laboratory in the Department of Biology at the university, focusing on finding areas of the brain that relate to specific functions using TMS. Going forward, she will also continue her work as an intern at New York University Langone Cardiothoracic Surgery Center.

Matthew J. Criscione, BS, holds a Bachelor of Science in biology from Montclair State University and is currently enrolled in the Louisiana State University School of Veterinary Medicine, where he will obtain his Doctor of Veterinary Medicine (DVM) degree. He has worked in the Cognitive Neuroimaging Laboratory, as well as the Marine Ecosystem Laboratory, researching the effects of disease ecology, and at the Laboratory Animal Vivarium at Montclair State University. Matthew's research interests include the neural structure of human/nonhuman intelligence via the evolutionary roots of social neuroscience.

Constanza de Dios, PhD, obtained her doctorate in psychology from the University of South Florida, where she studied the influence of reward salience on attention selection using psychophysiological techniques. As a postdoctoral research fellow, at the Center for Neurobehavioral Research, she applies data science approaches to clinical research on addiction at the University of Texas Health Science Center in Houston.

Jessica Devine, BS, is a graduate of the Purdue University Department of Health and Kinesiology. She engaged in research with Dr. Eicher-Miller and the Purdue University Department of Nutrition Science throughout her undergraduate study. Jessica's interest and experience include nutrition epidemiology and analysis of complex survey data. Her current project analyzes data from the National Health and Nutrition Examination Survey (NHANES) collected by the Centers for Disease Control and Prevention.

Heather A. Eicher-Miller, PhD, earned her PhD in nutrition science from Purdue University. She is an associate professor in nutrition science at Purdue University. She is also the director of Indiana's Emergency Food Resource Network, an online source of nutrition education for emergency food providers in Indiana. Her research focuses on improving food insecurity, which affected 11% of U.S. households in 2018 and creates uncertainty regarding the availability of nutritionally adequate and safe foods. Her efforts to evaluate and create evidence-based interventions, programs, and policies have reduced food insecurity and improved access to resources, which enhance health.

Ama Pokuaa Fenny, PhD, has a PhD in health economics from the Department of Public Health, Aarhus University, Denmark, and an MSc in health, population and society from the London School of Economics & Political Science (UK). She is a research fellow with the Institute of Statistical, Social and Economics Research (ISSER) at the University of Ghana. Since 2005, she has researched and published in the area of developmental issues in health financing, health service delivery, and social protection. Her current research areas include finding synergies to integrate governmental policies into service delivery systems in Africa.

Alessia Fichera is a student at Montclair State University, majoring in psychology and criminal justice. Her research focuses on addressing the psychological and emotional issues of motivation and the impact of the justice system on people's health and the health of the community.

Brandon G. Fico, MS, received his Master of Science in exercise physiology from Florida Atlantic University. He is now a doctoral candidate in the Department of Kinesiology and Health Education at the University of Texas at Austin. He recently published in the *Journal of Human Hypertension* and the *American Journal of Hypertension*. Current research interests include how the autonomic nervous system influences vascular function.

Elana M. Gloger, MS, received her BS from Ohio University, where she majored in biology and psychology. She is currently a PhD student studying clinical health psychology at the University of Kentucky. She is mentored by Dr. Suzanne C. Segerstrom in the Department of Psychology. Her research interests include psychoneuroimmunology, self-regulation, and stress throughout the lifespan.

Brooks B. Gump, PhD, MPH, received his doctorate in experimental psychology with concentrations in health psychology and an MPH in epidemiology. He is the Falk Family Endowed Professor of Public Health in the Department of Public Health in the David B. Falk College of Sport and Human Dynamics at Syracuse University. His program of research considers the biopsychosocial contributors to cardiovascular disease risk in children, with a focus on environmental toxicants.

Roy H. Hamilton, MD, MS, obtained his bachelor's degree in psychology from Harvard University, his MD and a master's degree in health sciences technology from Harvard Medical School and the Massachusetts Institute of Technology (MIT), respectively. He is an associate professor in the departments of Neurology and Physical Medicine and Rehabilitation at the University of

Pennsylvania (Penn) and directs Penn's Laboratory for Cognition and Neural Stimulation and the Penn Brain Science, Translation, Innovation, and Modulation (brainSTIM) Center. His research employs a multidisciplinary approach that combines noninvasive brain stimulation, behavioral measures, and neuroimaging to explore a range of topics, including language ability, cognitive control, visuospatial processing, semantic memory, and creativity. He has received numerous prestigious awards recognizing his contributions as a clinician, scientist, and educator. He is an assistant dean of Diversity and Inclusion at the Perelman School of Medicine and the inaugural vice chair of Diversity and Inclusion in the Department of Neurology at Penn, and one of the associate editors for equity, diversity, and inclusion for the journal *Neurology* and the associated journals of the American Academy of Neurology.

Jessica L. Hoffman, PhD, earned her doctorate in psychology with an emphasis on behavioral neuroscience at the University of South Florida. Her research focuses primarily on alcohol addiction and encompasses the investigation of neural mechanisms that regulate the positive reinforcing properties of alcohol. She is currently a postdoctoral research fellow at the Bowles Center for Alcohol Studies at the University of North Carolina-Chapel Hill.

Bryce Hruska, PhD, earned his doctorate in experimental psychology with concentrations in health psychology and quantitative methods. He is an assistant professor in the Department of Public Health in the David B. Falk College of Sport and Human Dynamics at Syracuse University. His program of research considers risk and resilience factors associated with mental health outcomes following trauma exposure in occupational and medical populations.

Chun-Jung "Phil" Huang, PhD, earned his PhD degree in rehabilitation and movement science at Virginia Commonwealth University with an exercise physiology emphasis. Dr. Huang has recently been named a fellow of the American College of Sports Medicine through the research path. His primary research focuses on exercise, obesity, and inflammation. Specifically, he examines the underlying effects of obesity and stress-induced inflammatory mechanisms and how exercise may reduce chronic stress-associated negative impacts on cardiovascular disease and other obesity-associated chronic inflammatory problems.

Michael R. Hulsizer, PhD, graduated from Kent State University with a degree in experimental psychology. He is a professor and chairperson of the Department of Psychology and a fellow in the Institute for Human Rights and Humanitarian Studies at Webster University in St. Louis, Missouri. Michael teaches a variety of statistics and methodology courses (e.g., statistics, advanced statistics, research methods, and science/pseudoscience), as well as applied psychology classes (e.g., social, motivation and emotion, prejudice and discrimination, physiological psychology). He has written about various topics related to the teaching of psychology, research methods, peace psychology, social justice, hate groups, and genocide. Michael is co-author with Linda M. Woolf of *A Guide to Teaching Statistics: Innovations and Best Practices*.

Yasmin M. Hussein, BA, BS, graduated from Montclair State University earning a BA in psychology and a BS in mathematics. She is currently a PhD candidate at Fordham University in New York City, studying psychometrics and quantitative psychology. Her current research focuses on the phenomena of algorithm aversion and how to incorporate algorithmic advice into decision-making. More specifically, she is interested in how the amount of transparency of algorithmic models affects individuals' willingness to follow the algorithm's advice.

Leonard A. Jason, PhD, earned his PhD from the University of Rochester. He is a professor of psychology and director of the Center for Community Research at DePaul University, Chicago. He has been actively involved in efforts to reduce stigma for those with CFS and ME. Leonard has been involved in community-based epidemiologic research for both youth and adult samples. His other current research interests are in public policy, community building, evaluating recovery homes for those with substance use disorders, and preventing violence among urban youth.

Veronica Julien is a student at Montclair State University and a psychology major. Her research interests include the mental health of young adolescents, specifically examining how therapeutic sessions assist adolescents through difficult situations. She currently works in the Infant Development Lab at Montclair examining eye-tracking behaviors of infants.

Andy V. Khamoui, PhD, is an assistant professor in the Department of Exercise Science and Health Promotion at Florida Atlantic University. He completed doctoral work in exercise physiology at Florida State University and postdoctoral training in the Division of Respiratory and Critical Care Physiology and Medicine at Los Angeles Biomedical Research Institute at Harbor-UCLA Medical Center. He has a broad background in exercise physiology, skeletal muscle biology, and mitochondrial function in health and disease. Dr. Khamoui's current research addresses the tissue-specific mechanisms linking mitochondrial metabolism to cancer cachexia, a life-threatening complication of cancer characterized by unintended weight loss, skeletal muscle dysfunction, and physical frailty. This work seeks to improve supportive care and treatment options for the millions of patients fighting cancer.

Ayesha Khan, PhD, earned her PhD in behavioral neuroendocrinology and is an associate professor in the Faculty of Science at McMaster University, Ontario, Canada, where she also holds the position of associate director of curriculum and pedagogy at the School of Interdisciplinary Science. As part of a multi-institutional Canadian initiative, she designs research questions around student mental health with publications in journals that focus on the scholarship of teaching and learning.

Rachel Kramer, PhD, is clinical faculty in the Behavioral Medicine and Clinical Psychology Department at Cincinnati Children's Hospital Medical Center in Cincinnati, Ohio. She earned her bachelor's degree in psychology from Montclair State University, her master's in psychology from American University, and her PhD in clinical psychology from the University of North Dakota. Dr. Kramer specializes in and provides evidence-based eating disorders treatment to youth. Her research interests include neural correlates of self-awareness; risk for post-traumatic stress disorder (PTSD) development among adolescents; and the association between yoga practice, self-compassion, and mindfulness on eating disorder symptoms and body image. She has recently published in the *Journal of Treatment and Prevention*. She is currently involved in research projects evaluating factors affecting family-based treatment outcome.

Tae Kyoung Lee, PhD, is a lead research analyst in the department of Public Health Sciences at the University of Miami, Miller School of Medicine. Dr. Lee received his PhD in human development and family studies from the University of Georgia. His research focuses on quantitative methods and developmental psychopathology in adolescence. He has authored and co-authored over 50 publications in journals such as the *American Journal of Public Health*, *Child Development*, *Health Psychology*, *Development and Psychopathology*, and *Structural Equation Modeling*. He co-authored *Higher-Order Growth Curves and Mixture Modeling with Mplus: A Practical Guide*, published by Routledge Press (2016).

Krystal Lynch, PhD, MPH, earned her PhD in human nutrition from the Bloomberg School of Public Health, Johns Hopkins University in Baltimore, Maryland. She is an assistant professor in nutrition and dietetics at Eastern Illinois University. She also provides expertise on research and evaluation efforts to the Purdue University Extension Nutrition Education Program, which implements the Supplemental Nutrition Assistance Program-Education (SNAP-Ed) and the Expanded Food and Nutrition Education Programs (EFNEP) for the state of Indiana. Her research focuses on the implementation and evaluation of community nutrition programs targeting resource-limited populations in the United States.

Alan Marshall, PhD, is a senior lecturer in quantitative methods at the University of Edinburgh, Edinburgh, UK. He earned his PhD from the University of Manchester and is a social statistician by training with both substantive and methodological research interests. His substantive research has drawn on longitudinal data from social surveys in the UK and overseas to better understand the social and biological determinants of inequalities observed in health and well-being in later life. He has made methodological research contributions around the development of local estimates and projections of populations and of populations in poor health in collaboration with the UK's national statistical agencies and local authorities.

Sabihah Moola, PhD, is a senior lecturer at the University of South Africa (UNISA), where she specializes in health communication. She earned her PhD in sociological health communication from UNISA. Her areas of specialization include health communication, health care provider–patient relationships, public health care, diabetes, HIV/AIDS (among other illnesses), health care ethics, health care teamwork issues, decolonization of health care, social and cultural aspects related to health care, patient-centered care, health promotion, and edutainment. She also lectures in the field of media studies. She holds a National Research Foundation (NRF)–Thuthuka grant, which was awarded for her PhD degree. She has published in the field of media studies, including health communication and health promotion.

Marceleen M. Mosher, MA, is an adjunct instructor in the Department of Communication Studies at Augsburg University in Minneapolis, Minnesota. She earned her master of arts degree in communication studies from Sam Houston State University. Much of her academic work centers on the intersection of nature, technology, and power. Marceleen is a co-contributor to *Eco Culture: Disaster, Narrative, Discourse* and regularly presents at regional, national, and international conferences on topics such as fracking, climate science, and catastrophe.

Catherine Walker O'Neal, PhD, is an assistant research scientist in the Department of Human Development and Family Science at the University of Georgia. Dr. O'Neal received her PhD in child and family development from the University of Georgia. Her research focuses on informing evidence-based outreach efforts through increased understanding of the interplay of risk and resilience among families facing acute or chronic stressors. Her research utilizes advances quantitative methods in evaluating contextual and ecological effects on individual and family outcomes, particularly their mental health, physical health, and relational well-being. She co-authored *Higher-Order Growth Curves and Mixture Modeling with Mplus: A Practical Guide* (Routledge Press, 2016) and regularly publishes her research in well-respected family science journals, including *Journal of Family Psychology*, *Family Process*, *Journal of Marriage and Family*, and *American Journal of Community Psychology*.

Jordanne Nelson, BS, is a recent graduate of Montclair State University, attaining a Bachelor of Science degree in public health, with a concentration in community health education. At Montclair she worked in the Cognitive Neuroimaging Laboratory and assisted with gene annotations/sequencing of an isolated SEA-PHAGE in the Department of Biology at Montclair State University. Currently, she is employed as a patient registry associate at the Life Raft Group, a local cancer research facility.

Joy E. Obayemi, MD, is a general surgery resident in the Department of Surgery at the University of Michigan. She obtained her bachelor's degree in sociology from Stanford University and as a Fulbright Scholar in France completed a master's 1 degree program in interdisciplinary social sciences at École Normale Supérieure (ENS) and École des Hautes Études en Sciences Sociales (EHESS). Dr. Obayemi then obtained her MD from the Perelman School of Medicine at the University of Pennsylvania, where she continued to engage in research at the intersection of public health and social sciences. She has presented her research at a variety of conferences. She has also published her global surgery research in peer-reviewed journals and received National Institutes of Health (NIH) funding for short-term research on disparities in transplant pharmacogenomics.

Sukhvinder S. Obhi, PhD, is a professor of psychology, neuroscience, and behavior and director of the Neurosociety Lab and the Social Brain, Body and Action Lab at McMaster University in Canada. Dr. Obhi earned his PhD from University College London in the UK and was a visiting graduate fellow at Harvard Medical School. His research is supported by multiple federal grants, and he has a strong history of industry research collaboration. He is known for his work on the psychology and neuroscience of power, self–other processing, and the sense of agency. Academic contributions include over 70 articles, three books, and membership on multiple editorial boards for psychology and neuroscience journals.

Kheyyon Parker, BS, a recent graduate of Montclair State University, received his Bachelor of Science in nutrition and food science with a concentration in dietetics. Kheyyon is a food entrepreneur whose business partnership, "Business Solo's Food," won second place in the MSU Pitch contest, earning him start-up money and professional support. Kheyyon aspires to become a nutrition researcher specializing in weight management, aging, and human performance.

Jennifer A. Reich, PhD, is a professor of sociology at the University of Colorado, Denver. She earned her PhD in sociology from the University of California, Davis. Her research examines how individuals and families weigh information and strategize their interactions with the state and service providers in the context of public policy, particularly as they relate to health care and welfare. She is author of two award-winning books, *Fixing Families: Parents, Power, and the Child Welfare System* and *Calling the Shots: Why Parents Reject Vaccines*; co-editor of the book, *Reproduction and Society*; and has written more than 35 articles and book chapters that explore childhood vaccinations, reproductive health, welfare, multiracial families, public assistance, and recovery after disaster.

Kathy Sanders-Phillips, PhD, is a pediatric/developmental psychologist who completed her PhD at Johns Hopkins University. She is a professor emerita of pediatrics and child health at the Howard University College of Medicine. Her work focuses on the social determinants of health, as well as the interface between psychological and biological functioning in children and youth. At Howard University, she founded and directed the Research Program in the Epidemiology and Prevention of Drug Abuse and AIDS (PEPDAA)—a National Institutes of Health-funded transdisciplinary research training program—and was director of research for the DC-Baltimore Research Center on Child Health Disparities from 2002 to 2012. Dr. Sanders-Phillips has provided technical assistance to the National Institute of Drug Abuse (NIDA), as well as the Medical Research Council in South Africa on increasing the number of minorities in health disparities research and served as a member of the National Advisory Council for NIDA.

Dennis A. Savaiano, PhD, is the Virginia Claypool Meredith Professor of Nutrition Policy at Purdue University. He is also director of the Community Health Partnerships/Indiana State Department of Health Coalition Development Program. He received his PhD in nutrition from the University of California, Davis. He has published on school community interventions focused on improving the diets of youth (particularly young women), the effectiveness of community health coalitions, and developed and led many successful efforts focused on health promotion as dean of the Purdue University College of Consumer and Family Sciences.

Liliia Savitska is a student at Montclair State University, majoring in biology. She also works in the Cognitive Neuroimaging Laboratory in the Department of Biology at the university. Her research focuses on relationship conditions, menstrual cycles, and the effect on frontal lobe investigations.

Kelly Ann Schmidtke, PhD, earned her doctorate in experimental psychology from Auburn University, Auburn, Alabama. She currently works as an assistant professor at the University of Warwick's Medical School in Coventry, UK. She is also a member of the Behavioral Science Group at Warwick Business School. Her research explores the application of psychological principles to experimental philosophy and real-world interventions. The contributions to experimental philosophy have been largely dedicated to understanding lay people's concepts of perceptible properties and epistemology. The contributions to applied psychology aim to change the health, wealth, and well-being of people using light-touch and low-cost mechanisms, also known as nudges.

Suzanne C. Segerstrom, PhD, MPH, is a professor of psychology at University of Kentucky. Dr. Segerstrom has a BA in psychology and music from Lewis and Clark College, a PhD from the University of California, Los Angeles, and her MPH in biostatistics from the University of Kentucky. Her research focuses on the relationships among personality, well-being, and health. Funded projects include investigations of the relationship between self-regulation and immunological aging in midlife and older adults. She has a number of prestigious awards for her research at the university.

Valeria Skafida, PhD, is a senior lecturer in social policy at the University of Edinburgh, Edinburgh, UK. She earned her PhD in social policy from the University of Edinburgh. Her research interests and expertise lie across the disciplines of social policy, sociology, and public health. Most of her research to date has involved using longitudinal data to understand how young children's health and well-being outcomes are socially stratified, examining how early experiences or events relate to subsequent outcomes, especially in relation to breastfeeding, infant and child nutrition, and the eating habits of children and families.

Aaron L. Slusher, PhD, is a broadly trained stress physiologist and current postdoctoral research fellow within the School of Kinesiology at the University of Michigan, Ann Arbor, Michigan. He earned a PhD in exercise physiology at Virginia Commonwealth University, Richmond, Virginia. Most recently, his research examines the capacity of acute and chronic exercise to positively regulate telomere length in various metabolically active tissue and cell types. In addition, he conducts basic science research investigating the differential regulation of telomere length maintenance mechanisms in stem and cancer cells. His research has contributed towards the development of effective exercise intervention strategies and the identification of molecular targets that regulate telomere lengths and increase the health span of an aging population.

Gregory T. Smith, PhD, is a professor and chair of psychology at the University of Kentucky. He earned his BA in psychology at Kalamazoo College and his PhD in clinical psychology at Wayne State University. His research has three foci: psychometric theory and validity theory; relationships among personality, psychosocial learning, and addictive behaviors, including substance use and disordered eating; and reciprocal models of predictive risk among dysfunctional behaviors and personal characteristics. He is the recipient of numerous awards for research and mentorship.

Heather E. Soder, PhD, earned her doctorate in psychology at the University of South Florida. She is currently a research fellow at the Center for Neurobehavioral Research on Addiction at the University of Texas Health Science Center at Houston. She primarily employs human electrophysiological methods to study the underlying neural mechanisms of motivation, reward and punishment sensitivity, and reward learning and how these processes contribute to addiction.

Stephanie Spero, BA, is a recent graduate of Montclair State University, where she majored in family science and human development, also earning a double minor in psychology and public health. Currently, Stephanie is working toward her certification as a child life specialist and is employed at a New Jersey–based hospital.

Madison Sunnquist, MA, is a graduate student in clinical-community psychology at DePaul University, Chicago, Illinois. She joined the Center for Community Research in April 2012, where she has participated in research focused on understanding the lived experiences of individuals with ME and CFS. Most recently, Madison worked on a community-based epidemiological study of pediatric ME and CFS.

Diana M. Thomas, PhD, received her BS from the University of Montana and her doctorate in mathematics from the Georgia Institute of Technology. After completing a National Research Council postdoctoral fellowship at the United States Military Academy and the Army Research Laboratory, she taught at Montclair State University, serving also as the director of the Center for Quantitative Obesity Research. Currently she is a professor of mathematical sciences at the United States Military Academy at West Point, with joint research appointments at the Columbia University Obesity Research Center and the Pennington Biomedical Research Center. She has published over 140 peer-reviewed articles in exercise, fitness, nutrition, and body weight regulation and serves on the editorial board for the *European Journal of Clinical Nutrition*, *PLOS One*, and *Nutrition and Diabetes*. Her work has been reported in a number of leading periodicals, including the *New York Times* and *Wall Street Journal*, as well as CBS News and ABC News. She is also the recipient of several prestigious awards.

Joseph E. Trimble, PhD, earned his doctorate from the University of Oklahoma, Institute of Group Relations, in social psychology and is retired and lives in Bellingham, Washington. He has over 50 years of experience conducting social and behavioral research with ethnic populations, primarily American Indians and Alaska Natives; he has played significant roles in leadership within the multicultural communities and within psychology. He generated over 150 publications on cross-cultural and ethnic topics in psychology, including 22 edited, co-edited, and co-authored books including *Working Culturally and Competently with Persons of African, Asian, Latino, and Native Descent: The Culturally Adaptive Responsive Model of Counseling*; *Counseling Across Cultures*; and *Diversity and Leadership*, among others. He is the recipient of numerous prestigious teaching and research awards.

Ivo Vlaev, DPhil, is a professor of behavioral science at the Warwick Business School, University of Warwick. Ivo received a DPhil (PhD) in experimental psychology from the University of Oxford, St. John's College. He was a research fellow at University College London and senior lecturer at Imperial College London. Ivo's research focuses on developing an integrated theory of behavior change, which combines principles from psychology, neuroscience, and economics. Testing the theory involves developing and evaluating behavior change interventions in various domains such as health, finance, education, and environment. He has an extensive record of research in decision science (behavioral economics) and behavior change, which is published in peer-reviewed academic journals, book chapters, and government reports. Ivo is also a co-author of the famous UK Cabinet

Office MINDSPACE report, which provides a framework for designing effective policy utilizing the latest insights from behavioral sciences (also known as nudge theory).

Melinda R. Weathers, PhD, earned her doctorate from George Mason University and is an associate professor in the Department of Communication Studies at Sam Houston State University in Huntsville, Texas. Her scholarly interests include intercultural communication, gender and women's health issues, climate change and public health, and new communication technologies. Dr. Weathers' research has encompassed a range of topics addressing issues related to messages within relational, institutional, societal, and health contexts. Specifically, she has explored communication-related issues between doctors and patients, Hispanic caregivers and older adults, heterosexual dating partners, and climate change and public health messaging. She has published widely in professional journals, including *Howard Journal of Communications, Communication Quarterly, Journal of Women and Social Work, Communication Studies, Patient Education and Counseling, Environmental Communication*, and *Communication Education*.

Troy A. Webber, PhD, earned his doctorate in clinical psychology at the University of South Florida and is currently a clinical neuropsychologist at the Michael E. DeBakey VA Medical Center. His research background includes behavior genetics, externalizing behavior (to include substance use), longitudinal data analysis, and clinical neuropsychological assessment.

J. Kenneth Wickiser, PhD, was awarded his Bachelor of Science in engineering physics and nuclear engineering from the United States Military Academy, West Point, New York, and then served as a military intelligence aviation officer in the army. After service, he earned a Master of Science in mechanical engineering from the University of Alabama, Tuscaloosa, Alabama, and a PhD in molecular biophysics and biochemistry from Yale University. Following his postdoctoral work in the Laboratory of Molecular Neuro-Oncology at the Rockefeller University, he joined the faculty of the Department of Chemistry and Life Science at West Point in 2007. Currently, he is a professor of biochemistry and now serves as the associate dean for research at West Point. He is the principal investigator and clinical biochemist for human research studies involving injury, illness, and human performance at West Point.

Kandauda A. S. Wickrama, PhD, is a professor in the Department of Human Development and Family Science at the University of Georgia. Dr. Wickrama received his PhD in sociology from Iowa State University. His research focuses on life course social epidemiology, international health, and quantitative research methods. He has investigated how socioeconomic context and individual life experiences influence individual mental and physical health over the life course. He has published widely in professional journals and has co-authored numerous chapters in edited volumes. He has also authored or edited several books, including *Higher-Order Growth Curves and Mixture Modeling with Mplus: A Practical Guide* published by Routledge Press. He is the recipient of numerous prestigious awards.

Linda M. Woolf, PhD, earned her PhD in applied-experimental psychology from Saint Louis University. Currently, she is a professor of psychology and international human rights at Webster University in St. Louis, Missouri, where she teaches a variety of courses related to the Holocaust, genocide, human rights, ethics, and peace psychology. Recent articles and book chapters focus on peace, social justice, hate groups, torture, LGBT and women's rights, psychosocial roots of genocide, and research diversity issues. She is co-author with Michael R. Hulsizer of *A Guide to Teaching Statistics: Innovations and Best Practices*.

Saeed Yasin, BS, is a recent graduate of Montclair State University, receiving a bachelor of science in biology with a minor in chemistry. He will be attending New York Institute of Technology's College of Osteopathic Medicine in fall 2020, in hopes of attaining a DO/PhD. Saeed has been a part of the Cognitive Neuroimaging Lab for the past four years, becoming head laboratory assistant in his final year. As a laboratory assistant of the Cognitive Neuroimaging Lab, Saeed has achieved many accomplishments, producing many publications and becoming a recipient of the Wehner Student Research Grant.

Amel Youssef, BS, received her undergraduate degree in biological sciences from Montclair State University's Honors Program. While there, she worked under the mentorship of Dr. Julian P. Keenan as a lab coordinator in the Neurocognitive Imaging Lab. She continues to further her knowledge and is pursuing a career in the medical field.

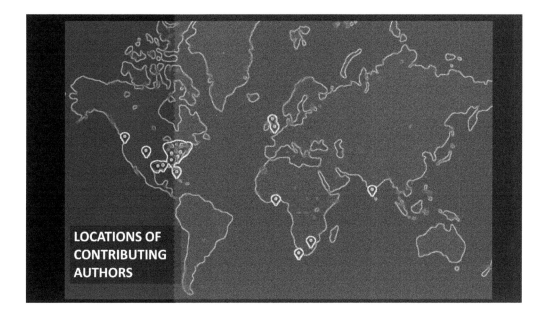

LOCATIONS OF CONTRIBUTING AUTHORS

PREFACE

Julian Paul Keenan and Deborah Fish Ragin

We are in strange times to be sure. It is 2020 and most of us are in our homes, wearing masks and thinking about antibodies. This is the year graduates stay home and schools close.

Comparing today with the most similar event, one concludes that the severe acute respiratory syndrome (SARS) outbreak of 2003 is generally a footnote or an afterthought. Those who remember an almost empty Toronto or the Rolling Stones concert that followed probably do not remember much more or think of it often. The deaths were in the hundreds and the cases in the thousands. People may recall the Canadian or Chinese connection (the two main epicenters), but by 2005, this version of the virus disappeared. While some people saw this as Act I, others saw this as a flop or overhype, a blizzard that did not arrive or an all-bark dog.

It is unlikely that the SARS-2/COVID-19 outbreak of 2020 will be a footnote in history. The final edits of this book are being performed in the midst of the sequel to the previous SARS outbreaks, which turn out to be the "Empire" to the original "Star Wars"; more epic and almost assuredly more memorable. The deaths and the cases are counted in the millions, not the thousands or the hundreds. The job loses similarly are in the millions. The coronavirus pandemic is now mentioned with the Spanish flu and HIV in terms of worldwide impact. Books will be written, and responses analyzed; however, let us point this out immediately:

The 2020 coronavirus crisis is/was a crisis of health psychology.

The psychology in which people dealt with the disease is why we have this book that is now in your hands. From researching governmental responses to investigating the underlying post-traumatic stress disorder (PTSD) that is emerging, it is critical that this never happens again. The eventual response is going to involve diagnosing and treatment via genetics, but such a response is futile if only the upper socioeconomic strata (SES) gets attended to. The lesson of 2020 is that we need to think bigger as health psychologists. Here we hope to provide a foundation for such big thinking.

Thinking big means that within the first three chapters the book highlights statistical methods AND shamanism. While this may *seem* disjointed, it is not. All the great scientists that we have learned from tend to have a knack of being well-rounded. That is to say they test their hypotheses from whatever angle fits best. A well-versed molecular biologist knows when to concentrate on behavior or what is being indicated by the fossil record. The statistical tools highlighted by Michael R. Hulsizer and Linda M. Woolf are those that any health psychologist should know. These are meant for those that already have a basic knowledge of stats, but with a basic knowledge, even "scary" techniques like meta-analysis in structural equational modeling are made easy here. Trimble's chapter on healing techniques among indigenous populations follows and could not be more different from the previous chapter. Examining "soft" research, Chapter 3 takes a very different view of health psychology, one typically not encountered in a Western university. We encourage all to read this—even the most hard-core quantitative researcher. Ragin frames the overview with a summary of selected theories in health psychology, demonstrating progression in the field from theories that focused on individual-level health determinants to current theories that advocate a more ecological view of factors that shape health outcomes.

The Genetics Studies and Health section gives an overview of addiction and genetics. These are two critical topics. Health psychology is built upon understanding and solving problems, and this section is "the wheelhouse" of understanding, investigating, and ultimately delivering quality and important research. Genetics confounds many people that are new to it. First, there are the myths that perpetuate in the field, such as its difficulty or elusiveness. Second, there are the promises that it is "the future". There is also a "scary" factor about gene manipulations, stealing genomes, and a re-emergence of eugenics.

What we have discovered is there are a few simple tips for the genetics researcher. First, know both the past and the present. Both the history and innovation influence every study. From Thomas Morgan to NextGen sequencing, each plays off the other. We would not have human trials in CRISPR (clustered regularly interspaced short palindromic repeats) today if we didn't have twin studies. Knowing a little about today's techniques and yesterday's bolsters the researcher immensely. We see that here with Youssef et al.'s chapter (Chapter 4) on techniques that range from breeding to CRISPR itself. However, this is only the beginning. Aardema's chapter (Chapter 7) about next-generation sequencing is quite current. If one is interested in being involved in today's best techniques, Aardema provides a user-friendly introduction. However, genetics is rarely a "one-trick pony," so applying both genetics methods chapters will make one a well-rounded investigator. Chapter 8, which is Coughlin's take on the ethics of genetics, is a wonderful read. If anyone were to pose research with more ethical questions than those raised by genetics, we would love to know what that is. From privacy to patents, from mosquito extinction to selective abortion, from race to pet cloning, genetics has it all. But even the subtle issues like some of those that Coughlin highlights are fascinating, including genetic disclosure. Telling a person she has a gene that might make her more likely to have alcohol abuse tendencies could have the most unintended consequences.

Chapters 5 and 6 walk us through methods used to study addiction and alcoholism. Crawford et al. examine some of the many methods in Chapter 5. Like genetics, we are reminded that just because a method is 'old' doesn't mean it is outdated. For example, human twin studies give us information that cannot be obtained using any other method. If one needs to know the genetics of a behavior that only exists in humans (e.g., alcohol's influence on Broca's aphasia), human twin studies remain the primary technique. Soder et al. (Chapter 6) provide an exciting and powerful look at methods to study addiction. Again, knowledge of older techniques (even classical conditioning) are relevant to the application of modern addictions such as fentanyl. However, event-related potentials are now being used in ways previously undiscovered, and here we get introduced to them.

The editors of this volume have taught (and were taught) that the health psychologist must have many tools in his or her pocket. This is now a literal statement, as the emergence of the smartphone has changed everything. The ability to collect data at all times from so many people without having to invest in any hardware has changed the field drastically. Chapter 9 (Criscione et al.) highlights but one use of the smartphone. The overall theme of the chapter is that physiological techniques are now more inexpensive and simpler to use than ever. From smartphones to cortisol sampling, any lab can now obtain impressive physiological data. Thomas and Wickiser (Chapter 12) take this theme one step further, examining innovative uses of devices that measure energy intake in real time. No more waiting or relying on personal logs or diaries. They illustrate the advantages of this cutting-edge technology for studies of obesity and nutrition. We hope the reader finds encouragement in all of the chapters to pursue physiological research. Physiometrics and biomarkers are highlighted by Gloger et al. in Chapter 10. Cortisol, which is arguably the most important physiological measure, makes another appearance here as well as other biomarkers, and the inflammatory discussion is extremely engaging.

Huang et al. (Chapter 11) and Kramer (Chapter 13) also tell us something about stress. Kramer is a practicing clinical psychologist dealing with the everyday struggles of her clients. Kramer's chapter focuses on depression and includes social networking and details such as recall bias. Huang and colleagues take a much more medical/biological approach and clearly define the relationship between tests like the Stroop and arterial pressure. Kahn and Obhi conclude the stress discussion in Chapter 14. This excellent discussion includes great work on hormones as well as ways to induce stress in laboratory settings. It is greatly appreciated that the authors include a method that works for neuroimaging, as assessing behavior in the 'scanner' is not so easy.

Parts IV and V serve, on the one hand, as the application to "the real world" and, on the other, to balance the work on genetics and individual-level factors determining health. Part IV examines health research with different populations. Ragin et al. lead this section, examining the important contributions and the conundrums involved when using neighborhood data to make inferences about individual health outcomes, specifically for adolescents. Marshall and Skafida (Chapter 16) broaden the examination into multilevel factors of health through their re-examination of the acclaimed work on the "social gradient" in health. At the other end of the spectrum, Moola and Cilliers (Chapter 18) take us on a tour of giving voice through research. The theme of participatory research permeates this chapter on gender and aging and demonstrates wonderful uses of this approach, especially in postcolonial countries. Lee et al. (Chapter 19) write the chapter we wish we had in graduate school. Taking us on a tour of statistics in an understandable manner, we see how esoteric terms really get applied to the study of socioeconomic factors influencing adolescent health behaviors. Finally, Jason et al. (Chapter 17) take a disease-centered approach. From stigma to frequency, this chapter demonstrates methods in elucidating disorders while talking about often-overlooked issues such as stigma. It also reminds us of the problems inherent in research when concepts or issues are ill defined.

The next section on the environment starts with Hussein et al. (Chapter 20) looking at an overview of the field with classic methodology, but more importantly, explaining why natural and manmade disasters force researchers to use less-favored research techniques. Reich's chapter on vaccines highlights where animal studies can no longer help us. On paper, in a test tube, or in a controlled setting, it is difficult to predict what actually happens when, for example, resistance to proven health-protecting strategies emerge: a very topical chapter to be sure. Reich's chapter (Chapter 21) begins with the scary data of vaccine compliance, and it ends with a subtle warning of what noncompliance means. In Chapter 22, Sanders-Phillips gives us research that is critical to the field of heath psychology. She takes us through the various measures of violence, how to achieve effective results, and reminds us of sobering facts such as homicide being the leading cause of death in African American adolescents. After reading Chapter 23, one will be a lead research expert. From half-lives to extraction to application, Hruska and Gump educate and inform the reader about the intricacies of lead research. Obayemi and Hamilton present a wonderful and powerful series of studies that highlight the impact of economic geography on health. From food deserts to twin studies, Chapter 24 provides insightful critique and insight on how to perform quality research in the local economic environment. How does one measure the impact of climate change on health? Weather and Mosher in Chapter 25 fill us in. While the entire chapter is excellent, we hope everyone will pay attention to the questions used in the surveys analyzed, as well as extended research beyond surveys. There is much to be gained by doing so.

The final section, Part VI, starts with Devine et al. (Chapter 26) Chapter 26 where they discuss health policy and outcomes. For those on the outside, this seemingly daunting research is broken down step by step. Can policy make children eat their vegetables? The authors describe how one might answer that very question. Atim et al. take us from Ghana to Brazil in Chapter 27 and let us not forget Zambia or Uganda or Tanzania, taking a look at health economics research with surprising findings and implications for health policy. Even to the outside researcher with no plans on doing research on health coverage, this chapter is gripping, informative, and succinct. Speculation about the future (and the present yet fully examined) is what Chapter 28 looks at in terms of genetics. Is it possible that one day, very soon, one will cough on their iPhone and Siri will deliver not only a diagnosis but the exact bar code of one's gut microbiome? Yasin and Keenan let us know what exists now that will get us to that place. Chapter 29 covers the classic topic of psychoneuroimmunology. Chandrashekara breaks down the research, including the basics of cellular mechanisms in terms of immune response but also sets up the reader for advanced concepts that are at the current, cutting edge of the field and suggest future research possibilities. In the final chapter on nudge theory, Schmidtke and Vlaev remind us that nudge theory works not just on individuals but as governmental policy as well. From organ donation to salience, we are given a wonderful tour of this newer, but to some controversial, idea in health psychology.

ACKNOWLEDGMENTS

If it takes a village to raise a child, it takes almost as many people to produce a book, especially one of this scope. The editors are grateful for the assistance, support, and contributions of everyone who helped develop this project. First, a heartfelt thanks to Lucy Kennedy and Charlotte (Lottie) Mapp at Taylor & Francis for their guidance, advice, and support at every step of this project. Everyone should be lucky enough to have such a great editorial team! A special thanks to Cloe Holland for sorting through the volumes of permissions and agreement documents and for finding the perfect cover image. Our sincerest thanks also to the outstanding production team at Taylor & Francis, led by the Production Editor, Kris Siosyte, and assisted by the Project Manager, Christopher Matthews and his team at Apex CoVantage, whose expertise translated our work into an excellent end product. We must also thank Christine Chronister and Julie Toich at Rutledge/New York for their support and assistance with the beginning stages of this project.

The editors are extremely grateful to all the contributing authors who volunteered their expertise, time, and considerable effort to produce outstanding chapters that illustrate quite clearly the inter-disciplinary and global nature of health research. Through their research and these chapters, these experts in the fields of biology, business, communication sciences, health economics, health policy, medicine, public health, psychology, and sociology tutored the editors in cutting-edge research theories and methodologies applicable to health in general and more specifically to health psychology. They have provided outstanding chapters that collectively provide the best road map for the future of research in health psychology. We thank them for this invaluable education.

Often, people who contributed 'behind the scenes' are overlooked, but not so here. The editors are only too aware of the crucial contributions of Alexander Dean Bracken, Yasmin M. Hussein, Raina Glover, and Molly Trimble. We thank them for their extensive editorial assistance and support, and perhaps most of all for their patience!

Deborah Fish Ragin also thanks her colleagues at Montclair State University for their support and encouragement and former colleagues at Mount Sinai School of Medicine, Department of Emergency Medicine, for their assistance in research which shaped her current perspective on health care. Lastly, she cannot thank enough her family—husband Luther M. Ragin Jr., her parents and children—for the decades of support, encouragement, patience, and love they showered on her over the years. This work is the fruits of their labors, too, and it is dedicated to them with love.

Julian Paul Keenan would like to thank all of his colleagues at Montclair State University, across the country and abroad. All have made him smarter and all have pushed him to be a better scientist. Each collaboration is a story he gets to tell years later in his classes as he emphasizes that science moves to a sweeter song when you work with friends. Some of the colleagues he has known for many decades now. He loves them and they are his family.

The bees, chickens, cats, guinea pig, birds, dog, and worms on the compost pile are all thanked. In the age of quarantine, it is amazing that a small group of animals can keep one sane. He looks forward to the days of cows and horses and goats. Likewise, the great writers, artists, and musicians that are the background to this book are thanked. Stevie Ray, Hank Mobley, Rush, Keith Jarrett, Pat Metheny, and Bill Frisell are inspirations.

His students make all the difference in the world. Without them, there would be nothing. His lab is a place where disbelief (in oneself) turns to belief. This is a group that eats, researches, eats some more, and has a great time while learning. They are graduates and high school students and all in between, and each 'kid' keeps him young with their energy, humor, insight, and passion for truth.

His wife Ilene and daughter Harper are thanked. He loves them both and looks forward to each day when he gets to see Harper become a young adult, an academic, a sports star, an animal lover, and a pretty cool companion. Thank you both, and all the love.

PART I

Theories and Methodologies

1

APPLYING THEORIES IN HEALTH PSYCHOLOGY

Deborah Fish Ragin, Yasmin M. Hussein, Alessia Fichera, and Jelani Awai

Overview

New developments in science and medicine, changes to health policies and health systems, an expanding list of determinants that influence health status, and cultural differences in the definition of and treatments for health all advance our understanding of health outcomes.

At the same time, these developments present challenges to existing theories of health behaviors, pushing the field to adopt a more interdisciplinary approach. Many researchers now agree that health is best understood when using diverse perspectives, considering both the intrinsic (i.e., biological, human behavior/lifestyle) and extrinsic (i.e., social and physical environments, health systems, health policy, and health economic) factors that shape outcomes. The roles of the individual and cognition in shaping health behaviors remain important pieces of the equation. But they are just that: *pieces* of the puzzle. People do not exist in a vacuum. We are embedded, to greater and lesser extents, in multiple networks. We are influenced by and respond to multiple environments (e.g., neighborhoods, schools, workplaces, communities, and larger societal milieus).

The notion of multiple influences on health behaviors and outcomes is not new to health psychology. In 1980, Matarazzo (1980) redefined the field of **health psychology**, incorporating aspects of the newly developed field of behavioral health. Thus, he defined the emerging field of *health psychology* as:

> the aggregate of the specific educational, scientific, and professional contributions of the discipline of psychology to the promotion and maintenance of health, the prevention and treatment of illnesses, and the identification of etiologic and diagnostic correlates of health, illness and related dysfunction, and to the analysis and improvements of the health care system and health policy formation.
>
> *(p. 815)*

Matarazzo's definition brings us closer to an ecological view of health psychology, one that considers the interrelations between organisms and their environment (Glanz, Rimer, & Viswanath, 2008). Uniquely, ecological models allow us to examine how environmental and policy variables affect health. In addition, the ecological view incorporates the psychological, social, and organizational factors typically included in other models, such as the cognitive-based (also called individual-level) models.

In this chapter, we review select cognitive-based and ecological models of health. We begin with a brief overview of both types of models and further examine three commonly used cognitive-based models in health psychology research: the Theory of Planned Behavior, the Health Belief Model, and the Biopsychosocial Model. Consistent with the chronological development of models in the field, we then explore two ecological models—the Social Ecological Model and the Behavioral Ecological Model.

While reading this chapter, it is important to remember that many of the models and theories were (and still *are*) tested primarily, if not exclusively, in Western cultures. As the authors of several chapters in this handbook remind us, some theories and research methodologies favored in Western cultures are either unsupported or inappropriate when examining global health behaviors and outcomes. The theories may fail to explain behaviors in non-Western cultures because they impose a set of assumptions, beliefs, or values about behaviors that are inconsistent with the examined culture (see Trimble, Chapter 3). Similarly, the measures employed to test these theories may be ill-suited for use in other cultures, or outright rejected, due to their emanation from colonizing countries with troubled histories with non-Western cultures (see Moola & Cilliers, Chapter 18). We will explore some of these critiques in later chapters.

Cognitive-Based vs. Ecological Models

Cognitive-based models (sometimes referred to as individual-level theories or models, Crosby, Kegler, & DiClemente, 2002) focus on the individual as the principal determinant of health outcomes. The popularity of these models appears to be rooted in a number of assumptions about individuals, as well as some inherent strengths and limitations of the research that supports them. Specifically, these theories assume that: 1) individuals place a high value on good health serving as a motivator for behavior or behavior change (Bosworth, Horner, Edwards, & Matcher, 2000; Foster, Frijters, & Johnson, 2012; Ng, Ntoumanis, & Thogersen-Ntoumanis, 2012); 2) individuals also possess sufficient agency and self-efficacy to initiate and sustain behavioral change (Velicer, Prochaska, & Redding, 2006); and 3) that an individual's behavior is volitional (Leventhal, Rubin, Leventhal, & Burns, 2001; Schwarzer, 2008). Yet the literature on health behavior change is rife with studies that challenge each of these assumptions (Sheeran, 2002; van Helvoort-Postulart, Dirksen, Kessels, vanEngelshoren, & Huunink, 2009 Vermaire, vanExel, van Loveren & Brouwer, 2012).

Cognitive-based models also lend themselves to analytical designs such as controlled trials or interventions that are empirical and can lead to strong statistical findings (Crosby, et al., 2002). These designs are often the preferred methodologies of psychologists (the field of study of most of this chapter's authors; hence, no disparagement). It is not surprising, therefore, to find a number of controlled trial or intervention studies in the psychological literature to test the effectiveness of **cognitive-based models** of health behavior change.

By comparison, **ecological models** of health build on an interdisciplinary approach, studying the relationship between an organization and its environment (Stokols, 1996). Bronfenbrenner (1979) adapted this model to explain child development, suggesting that the child is influenced by *and* influences the social environment (McLeroy, Bibeau, Steckler, & Glanz, 1988). McLeroy, and colleagues (1988), Stokols (1992), and Stokols, Grzywacz, McMahan, and Phillips (2003) and others later adapted this concept of mutually influencing agents to explain health behaviors. Their newer models divide the environment into smaller analytic levels, and espouse multilevel influences on behaviors, including intrapersonal (biological, psychological, lifestyle choices), interpersonal (social, cultural), and environmental factors (organizations, the physical environment, and policy determinants).

Current ecological health researchers expand McLeroy et al.'s and others' concept of multilevel influences, identifying four principles common to most such models. First, consistent with the core concept, they contend there are multiple influences on specific health behaviors. Second, these multiple influences interact across different levels. Third, notwithstanding this interaction, *ecological models* of health should focus on specific behaviors and isolate the primary influences at each level. Finally, the most effective interventions for changing behaviors should be multilevel, consistent with the influences (Sallis, Owen, & Fisher, 2008).

Both *cognitive-based* and *ecological models* enjoy robust support from health researchers. Which model researchers choose to test or support may depend largely on their own beliefs about behavior change. What is clear, however, is that ecological models of health behavior represent a paradigm shift away from earlier models that focused on the individual as the primary agent of change to one that sees the individual acting within and reacting to a complex system of factors that drive change (Crosby, et al., 2002).

Research in Practice

The Theory of Planned Behavior

The **Theory of Planned Behavior (TPB)**, introduced by social psychologist Ajzen (1985), was an extension of the **Theory of Reason Action (TRA)** proposed by Ajzen and Fishbein (1980). It was intended to address noted shortcomings in the original *TRA*. Thus, a brief overview of *TRA* is needed to provide a foundation for the later theory.

Theory of Reasoned Action

A core tenet of the *TRA* is that people are "rational actors" (Montano & Kasprzyk, 2008), a belief which some contend is not shared by other theories or models (more on this in just a moment; van der Pligt, de Vries, Manstead, & van Harreveld, 2000). According to the *TRA*, an individual's behavior is determined by his or her intentions, conceivably, the most important factor determining whether a behavior is performed. These intentions are, in turn, determined by related **attitudes** (about the behavior) and **subjective norms**, here meaning what other people—specifically those in one's social, professional, or family network—would think about the behavior (Ajzen & Fishbein, 1980). Attitudes and subjective norms may not influence each other, but they do independently influence behavioral intent and thus the behavior itself.

Studies have uncovered a significant limitation to this theory, however. Most researchers would support that *TRA* does indeed predict intention to act, as in the intention of African American men to obtain information about prostate cancer (Ross, Kohler, Grimley, & Anderson-Lewis, 2007) or the intention of teachers and students to accept each other's friend request on Facebook (Sheldon, 2016). On the other hand, most also acknowledge that this theory only predicts *volitional behaviors*, or the behaviors over which the individual exerts significant control (Montano & Kasprzyk, 2008). That is to say, it is not able to predict unintentional, spontaneous, or even habitual behaviors. If, according to *TRA*, intentions determine behavior, then this theory cannot explain unintentional acts. Considering the frequent occurrence of addictive, habitual, and involuntary behaviors on the part of individuals, this is a glaring omission and a likely justification for the theory's revision.

Additionally, critics of the theory suggest that assumptions about the individuals' rational decision-making processes may be erroneous. Conner and Norman (2005a) contend that while individuals may "calculate" the probability of performing a behavior and its likely outcomes, that tells us nothing about the decision-making process itself. For example, the proposition that a person's belief about the perceived risk of contracting an illness will affect his or her likelihood of engaging in a specific preventive behavior is debatable. According to Conner and Norman (2005b), while perceived risk may have an impact on earlier stages of a behavior, the effect is unlikely sustained more proximal to the time of the risk. Earlier research by Walter, Vaughan, Ragin, and Cohall (1994) suggests just that. After students in select New York City high schools received an eight-week lesson on HIV-AIDS—its etiology, transmission routes, risk assessment, and prevention strategies—they rated themselves high in, among other things, their ability to use HIV/AIDS prevention strategies. However, they rated themselves low in the ability to use risk-prevention strategies in real time at parties or other venues where substance use might prohibit them from implementing their newly acquired skills (i.e., proximal to risk). Later studies also identify this dilemma, calling it the "intention-behavior gap" (Sheeran, 2002). Consequently, it is a major limitation of this theory (Downing-Matibag & Geisinger, 2009; Luszczynska, Sobczyk, & Abraham, 2007).

The *TPB* is largely a revised version of the *TRA*. It introduces the concept of ***perceived behavioral control***, defined as an individual's perception of the ease or difficulty of performing a behavior. This new concept redresses nonvolitional actions, which do not require prior thought (Ajzen, 1985).

Testing the Theory of Planned Behavior

Like its predecessor, the *TPB* is a cognitive-based model that makes assumptions about the rationality of the actor and the internal factors that influence one's intention to engage in a specific behavior (Ajzen, 1985). The **Theory of Planned Behavior** states that one's *attitudes towards the behavior*, one's *subjective norms*, and one's beliefs about the difficulty of completing the behavior, called ***perceived behavioral control***, collectively determine the probability of the actor performing the behavior. Interestingly, this last concept bears a striking resemblance to Albert Bandura's (1977) construct ***self-efficacy***, which he describes as the notion that a person is more likely to engage in a specific behavior if that person believes they have the skills or abilities to perform the behavior.

Guo, Hermanson, Berkshire, and Fulton's (2019) study of healthcare management's intention to use evidence-based management (EBMgt) in the US health system offers one test of the TPB and its components. As the name implies, EBMgt is the practice of making management and personnel decisions using the best available evidence obtained from four principal sources: the best available scientific research findings, organizational data, professional experience and judgment, and stakeholders' values and concerns. Originally employed in research on medical care systems, it is now widely used in other industries.

Using the 2014 American Hospital Guide, Guo, and colleagues (2019) identified the chief executive officers (CEOs) of 6,400 hospitals and health systems using pre-existing criteria. Then the researchers employed a two-stage cluster random sampling procedure. During Stage 1, they selected regions/states in each of the 14 states. In Stage 2, they selected specific hospital/health systems within each region/ state. A total of 1,210 surveys were distributed via Qualtrics, an online survey system, and through mailed surveys. Approximately 13% ($n = 154$) of the targeted sample completed and returned the surveys.

Consistent with the *TPB* model, Guo, and colleagues' (2019) questionnaire explored the effect of CEOs' *attitudes toward the behavior* (interest in learning EBMgt principles or if EBMgt improves the quality of management decision-making), *subjective norms* (intention to use EBMgt), *perceived behavioral control* (academic capability, social acceptance, physical appearance), and demographic factors (age, education, gender, years of experience) on intention to use the management tool. The study revealed that *attitudes toward the behavior* were the strongest predictor influencing healthcare administrators' use of EBMgt. This supports the view that a positive attitude about the behavior and its intended outcomes—here being improved quality of patient care and better decision-making—influences intention to use. Conversely, *subjective norms*, the second *TPB* factor, was not predictive of intention to use EBMgt. This suggests that administrators were not influenced by other healthcare administrators' (i.e., their peers) use of the technique. They might listen to their peers' or colleagues' opinions, but it was not dispositive. Finally, and perhaps not surprisingly, Guo and colleagues found that the third factor, *perceived behavioral control*, was a stronger predictor of intention to use EBMgt. What is more, the authors suggest that factors that comprise one's *perceived behavior control* include not only an individual's perceived abilities but may also include behaviors not entirely under the actor's control. For example, one's physical appearance or social acceptance, lack of access to EBMgt resources, or lack of knowledge and skills to evaluate the evidence for EBMgt could also influence an individual's *perceived behavioral control*.

This study poses an interesting challenge to *TPB*. By suggesting that *perceived behavioral control* can be influenced by both internal and external factors (e.g., lack of access to EBMgt resources), these findings may demonstrate the need for an ecological model even when the concepts tested are presumed to be individual-level factors only. Further testing is warranted, however, as one noted limitation of this study is its nonexperimental methodology.

The Health Belief Model

The **Health Belief Model (HBM)**, developed in the early 1950s by US Public Health Services social psychologist Rosenstock, is a behavior change model initially intended to explain why people refused free, early-detection mechanisms (e.g., disease preventive or screening tests) for largely asymptomatic illnesses like tuberculosis or cervical cancer (Rosenstock, 1974). The model was expanded (Rosenstock, Strecher, & Becker, 1988) later to examine an individual's responses to symptoms of illness or disease (Kirscht, 1974). Since its inception, the *HBM* has been employed as a conceptual model in health behavior research, a model to explain health behavior change, and a mechanism to support intervention programs to change health behaviors or maintain new ones (Champion & Skinner, 2008; Carpenter, 2010; Deshpande, Basil, & Basil, 2009; Jallian, Motlagh, Solhi, & Gharibnavaz, 2014; see also Jones, Smith, & Llewellyn, 2014 for critique of HBM).

Rosenstock, Strecher, and Becker (1988) proposed five key constructs to explain people's willingness or reluctance to seek preventive health measures: **perceived susceptibility, perceived severity, perceived benefits, perceived barriers, and cues to action**. According to their model, in order for a person to seek preventive treatment or screening, a person would have to believe that he or she is personally at risk or **susceptible** to the disease. Second, the individual must perceive that the **severity** of the disease would pose serious medical and/or clinical consequences, potentially affecting social, familial, or work obligations. Third, regardless of susceptibility and severity, action would also depend on the perception of potential benefits from the actions. The individual then weighs his or her **perceived benefits** of such action. These benefits could accrue to the individual as well as others potentially affected by the illness. Finally, regardless of benefits, if barriers such as monetary cost, convenience, pain, or even stigma outweigh the positive outcomes, these **perceived barriers** may lead to what Rosenstock (1974) coined "conflicting motives of avoidance" (p. 331). Such events could negate any potential benefit of the behavior.

For example, a person may consider testing to determine their HIV/AIDS status. However, if testing could result in stigma against the individual, a person might forgo testing. This was the situation encountered by healthcare workers in southern Africa in the early 2000s, who believed that residents of remote villages would welcome the arrival of mobile HIV/AIDS testing units. They proposed that mobile testing units reduce or eliminate distance, travel cost, and time barriers to testing, giving villagers the ability to receive an HIV diagnosis and possible counseling in a region of the world afflicted with rising HIV prevalence rates. Instead, they found villagers often stigmatized those tested, regardless of the test results. In some instances, even family members ostracized the tested, fearing that the village would also stigmatize the family (Pendry, 2001). Similarly, studies using the HBM to examine rates of HIV/AIDS testing have reported opposition to testing by HIV-positive gay and bisexual men, heterosexual African men and women in England, and HIV-positive women in the United States (Abel, 2007; Dodds, 2006). The researchers cite stigma as a reason for refusal.

The fifth concept in Rosenstock, Strecher, and Becker' (1988) original *HBM*, **cue to action**, refers to the trigger(s) that lead an individual to seek treatment. *Cues* has received little research focus, in part because of the challenges in defining and measuring this variable. Hochbaum (1958) proposed that *cues* could be either internal triggers, such as pain, or external factors, such as advice from a family member or friend. In addition, these variables range from being easily identifiable to subtle or imperceptible. Consequently, *cues* prove to be difficult to isolate and test (Champion & Skinner, 2008).

The concept of **self-efficacy**, defined as an individual's confidence that they can complete a desired health behavior, was not included in the original *HBM* because the model focused on whether a person *would* perform a behavior, not on whether they *perceived they could* engage in the task. Nevertheless, Rosenstock, Strecher, and Becker (1988) added the construct in 1988, possibly due to studies demonstrating the strength of models that include *self-efficacy*. It has been widely cited in tests of the *HBM* model as the strongest predictor of behaviors (Bulgar, White, & Robinson, 2010; James, Pobee, Oxidine, Brown, & Joshi, 2012; Yue, Li, Wellin, & Bin, 2015). Interestingly, researchers have also incorporated *self-efficacy* in other theories as an important predictor of behavioral intent (Gerend & Shepherd, 2012; Lippke, Wiedemann, Ziegelman, Reuter, & Schwarzer, 2009; Sheeran, Maki, Montanaro, Avishai-Yikshak, Bryan, & Klein, 2016).

Testing the Health Belief Model

Many studies have tested this model, making it one of the most widely used frameworks in health psychology (Champion & Skinner, 2008). In the only comprehensive review of 29 studies testing the explanatory power of the *HBM*, Janz and Becker (1984) found strong evidence to support three of the four principal constructs of the model. *Perceived barriers* was the strongest of the four constructs in explaining preventive health behaviors and "sick role behaviors," here meaning behaviors of people diagnosed with an illness and who either seek or adhere to medical advice. *Perceived susceptibility* explained only preventive health behaviors, and *perceived benefits* explained only sick role behaviors. *Perceived severity* explained little in the way of behaviors.

Current studies testing the *HBM* yield largely similar results with a few "twists." For example, recently Babazadeh, Ghaffari-Fam, Oliaee, Sarbazi, Shirdel, Mostafa-Gharabeghi, et al. (2019) tested the *HBM's* ability to predict Pap smear screening behaviors among more than 200 women in rural Iran. Employing a cross-sectional, two-stage, random cluster sampling technique, they randomly selected two (out of five) rural clinics (Stage 1) and 220 women from the two clinics (Stage 2) to participate in the study. After obtaining standard demographic information (i.e., age, level of education, family socioeconomic status, and personal history of urinary tract infection), the researchers orally administered an *HBM* questionnaire. This questionnaire assessed women's perceived susceptibility, severity, benefits, and barriers to Pap smears, as well as their perceived self-efficacy. Results show that perceived benefits of Pap smears (i.e., "having a Pap smear will increase chances of early diagnosis of a possible tumor in the cervix," p. 3), perceived self-efficacy, and age of the participant were the strongest predictors of cervical cancer screenings. Generally, women with prior Pap histories, minor genital infections, or familial histories of cervical cancer were more prone to perceive the benefits of the procedure. They also expressed the greatest self-efficacy. Conversely, younger women were less likely to present themselves for screenings.

Babazadeh, et al. (2019) note, however, that while their study detected no impact of socioeconomic status on likely screening behavior (perhaps due to their sampling from a low-socioeconomic-status, rural population with little economic variability), other studies do. Research by Datta, Blair, Sylvestre, Gauvin, Drouin, and Mayrand (2018) cite extrinsic factors, including immigrant status, lower educational attainment, and lack of access to healthcare, as reasons why women never obtained or did not seek cervical cancer screening. Similarly, Domingo, Noviani, Noor, Ngelangel,

Limpaphayom, Thuan, et al. (2008) note the negative impact of insufficient healthcare infrastructure and sociocultural, political, and economic upheaval in South Asia (Indonesia, Malaysia, the Philippines, Thailand, and Vietnam) on screening behaviors.

This issue of extrinsic factors returns us to a critique of *HBM* first raised by Becker (1974). He noted the need to examine the role of socio-behavioral factors in influencing health behaviors. For example, he pointed to the potential influence of modifying factors such as patient–provider relationship, patient–provider communication, and continuity of care by the same physician as potential determinants of health behaviors. Taken together, these critiques suggest that, like in the case of the *TPB*, the role of additional external factors must be addressed.

The *HBM's* original purpose was to focus on prevention rather than treatment of disease (Rosenstock, 1974). To that end, it has been used to develop intervention programs aimed at teaching beneficial health behaviors or facilitating behavioral change. Nevertheless, there are limitations. The *HBM* relies on the assumption that health is a primary concern for individuals, hence a motivator to act, and that *cues to action* in one's environment will trigger behavioral change. *Cues to action* may reduce the "intention–behavior" gap, a problem with the *TPB*, but it is not clear whether a goal of good health is a strong enough motivator for behavior change. Finally, two methodological issues continue to plague the model. First, researchers note that measuring the *HBM* constructs is difficult, in part, due to inconsistent definitions. The difficulty defining and measuring *cues to action* is one example. There are a plethora of possible cues to prompt behavior, some overt, and others subtle. Linking the correct cues with the health issue and its associated behavior is a methodological challenge. Second, measures used to assess health behaviors cannot be standardized across health issues (Champion & Skinner, 2008). For example, the assessment tool for evaluating barriers to colonoscopies are not equally useful when assessing barriers for Pap smear screenings, raising the need to develop discrete assessment tools for a variety of illnesses. In spite of these methodological challenges, the *HBM* remains a compelling theory.

The Biopsychosocial Model

The **Biopsychosocial Model (BPS)** weighs the role of biological (*bio*), psychological (*psycho*), and social (*social*) factors on individuals' health outcomes. Developed by Engel (1977a), it was an alternative to the widely used Biomedical Model. To Engel, the Biomedical Model—which he characterized as Western society's folk model of disease—assumed that all diseases were primarily the result of measurable biological microorganisms or entities. It ignored the social (e.g., familial, cultural, community), psychological (e.g., emotional or personality traits), and behavioral factors that also contribute to health (Engel, 1977b). Engel proposed the BPS to take the missing determinants of health in the Biomedical Model into account and to redefine the tasks of medical practitioners (Engel, 1980), encouraging them to view medicine as a human discipline by bringing more empathy and compassion into their practices (Borrell-Carrió, Suchman, & Epstein, 2004).

Engel's perspective incorporates earlier views of health. He included views espoused by noted philosophers in ancient Greece, like Hippocrates (Kleisiaris, Sfakianakis, & Papathanasiou, 2014), and of some traditional medicine cultures like those of Native Americans who hold a holistic view of health.

The *BPS* model also derived, in part, from its precursor, the diathesis-stress (D-S) model. According to this model, the biological, genetic, or psychological characteristics of a person may increase the chances of a person developing a disorder (Banks & Kerns, 1996). Thus, a person with a predisposition to depression is more likely to display that disorder in response to an environmental trigger (stress) than someone who is not predisposed as a function of preexisting characteristics (e.g., genetics, neurochemical imbalance).

Engel (1977b) claims his model expounds upon the D-S model by encompassing additional and essential determinants of health in order to address needs, key of which are the patient, their social context, systems developed by society to address illness, the physician's role, and a healthcare system. To accomplish this goal, Engel's *BPS* model proposes three principal components that contribute to an individual's condition: biological, psychological, and social. **Biological factors** refer to the patient's genes, physiological composition, and even microorganisms, acknowledging the important role of genetic and biological factors in many health outcomes. **Psychological factors** include emotions, personality traits, and psychosocial variables, as well as a person's health beliefs. Finally, **social factors** include variables such as socioeconomic status (SES), interpersonal relationships, familial, and cultural influences.

Testing the Biopsychosocial Model

Over the past several decades, a number of studies have documented a relationship between psychological and biological factors. Take, for instance, the immune system. Classic studies by Cohen (2005) demonstrated a relationship between stress and hormone production. Similarly, work by Schulz, Martire, Beach, and Scheier (2005) established an indirect relationship between stress and increased mortality. Moscowitz, Epel, and Acree (2008) also documented the relationship between positive affect and decreased mortality rates. In addition, recent studies in the field of psychoneuroimmunology continue to suggest relationships between psychological states and immune system functions (see Ragin, 2018 for a more complete review).

Research on the role of *social factors* also suggests a relationship with health. Adams, Hurd, McFadden, Merrill, and Ribeiro's (2003) study on the relationship between health and wealth among older adults reports an association between SES and the gradual onset of negative health status, including mental health or degenerative and chronic health conditions. Likewise, Smith's (2007) longitudinal study suggests that family income may be a significant predictor of adult health status even when prior health issues are controlled. Finally, Clougherty, Souza, and Cullen (2010) showed that job title was linked to health outcomes, reinforcing their earlier findings that a "better" job does indeed correlate with better health outcomes.

Perhaps one of the strongest recent studies in support of the *BPS* is Wijenberg, Slapert, Kohler, and Bol's (2016) study examining fatigue in patients with **multiple sclerosis (MS)**, a persistent neurological disease that entails chronic inflammation of the central nervous system and damage to the nerve fibers, which disrupts the body's normal neurological functions. *MS* causes a number of symptoms, including fatigue, headaches, lightheadedness, soreness, and blurred vision. The most common of these symptoms, and the one rated the most debilitating among patients, is fatigue (Minden, Frankel, Hadden, Perloff, Srinath, & Hoaglin, 2006).

Wijenberg, et al. (2016) developed a *BPS* to cross-validate previous findings demonstrating that fatigue in *MS* patients could be explained by physical symptoms (disease severity, fatigue) and psychological symptoms (depression, catastrophizing about fatigue—here meaning a fearful interpretation of fatigue, such as extreme negative reactions or perceived helplessness; Wijenberg, et al., 2016).

This study, conducted in the Netherlands, included 226 clinically diagnosed *MS* patients from 18 to 65 years of age who were recruited from the Neurology Department of a Netherlands hospital. In addition to basic demographic information (age, gender, highest level of education attained, marital status, and use of psychopharmacological drugs), participants were assessed on two physical dimensions (physical disability and disease severity) and four psychological dimensions (fear avoidance, catastrophizing, fatigue, and depression). To assess physical disability, the researchers employed a Dutch translation of the physical dimension subsection of the Short Form Health Survey (SF-36). This self-report survey assesses a patient's health on eight subscales, including general health, physical functioning, role limitations due to physical health problems, social functioning, and mental health, among others. Examples of questions from the SF-36 include General Health: "I seem to get sick a little easier than other people" and Pain: "How much bodily pain have you had in the last 4 weeks"; (McHorney, Ware, Lu, & Sherbourne, 1994, p. 45). Participants were scored on each subsection using a standardized score ranging from 0 to 100. A perfect score of 400 suggested no physical disabilities, an optimal score.

Disease severity was determined from the Expanded Disability Status Scale (EDSS), a rating scale completed by healthcare providers to measure the disability status of people with *MS* by quantifying their functionality on eight systems (e.g., cerebellar, brainstem, mental, and bowel and bladder, among others), yielding a functional systems score (FSS). Scores ranging in the scale from 1 to 4.5 (using increments of .5) generally describe people with normal ambulatory functions (e.g., 2.0 = "minimal disability in one functional system" or 3.5 = "fully ambulatory with but with moderate disability in one functional system"; Kurtzke, 1983, p. 1451). Scores 5 through 9.5 describe decreasing levels of functional and ambulatory ability (e.g., 7.0 = "unable to walk beyond approximately 5 meters even with assistance" or 8.5 = "essentially restricted to bed much of the day"; p. 1451).

To assess psychosocial factors, Wijenberg, et al. (2016) used four self-report measures. The first, the Tampa Scale for Kinesiophobia (TSK) by Vlaeyen, Kole-Snijders, Rotteveel, Ruesink, and Heuts (1995), was adapted to assess fatigue-related fear and avoidance behavior. The higher the score, the higher the level of fear-avoidance behaviors. Included also in Wijenberg, et al.'s study was the Michielsen, De Vries, and Van Heck's (2003) Fatigue Catastrophizing Scale (FCS), a 10-item scale that obtains self-reported data on the frequency of catastrophizing thoughts about pain. The third scale, the Abbreviated Fatigue Questionnaire (AFQ; Alberts, Smets, Vercoulen, Garssen, & Bleijenber, 1997), is a four-item scale that measured a patient's self-expression of fatigue on a 7-point Likert scale. Scores ranged from 4 to 28, with the higher scores representing increased severity of physical fatigue. Finally, a subscale of the Hospital Anxiety and Depression Scale (HADS) measured the patient's intensity of depression. Seven questions, rated on a 4-point scale (0–3), assessed *MS* patients' current expressions of depression (Snaith, 2003). Scores greater than 11 indicate probable depression.

Wijenberg, et al. (2016) report that, collectively, these measures validate their adjusted *BPS*, showing that catastrophizing, depression, disease severity, physical disability, and fear avoidance directly or indirectly contribute to fatigue in persons with diagnosed cases of *MS*. Specifically, depression and physical disability were both directly associated with fatigue. The authors report that this integrated fatigue model adapts and strongly supports a *BPS* for explaining the fatigue in *MS* patients.

The numerous studies testing the *BPS* model suggest that it has made a significant contribution to the field of psychology as well as medicine. Medical researchers and practitioners who understood Engel's efforts to encourage physicians to treat the whole person and not just the symptom have embraced this model (Chervenak, McCullough, & Brent, 2011; Drossman, 1998; Saraga, Fuks, & Boudreau, 2014). Nevertheless, it is not immune to criticism.

Armstrong (2002) finds that this model is still too rooted in medicine and a biomedical approach. He contends that the core of the model is solidly biomedical with psychological and sociological "bits" appended. Ghaemi (2009) criticizes the vagueness of the model, comparing it to a list of ingredients rather than a recipe. Missing, according to him, is the level of impact each of the three components have on an individual's state. The *BPS* model fails to provide guidelines on how to prioritize the influence of each component. Consequently, the application of the model is left to the user's discretion, relying on the user to vote his or her preference (Ghaemi, 2009). Such variability will predictably yield a range of conflicting study outcomes.

Engel's vision of a more expansive physician role appears to be another weakness of the model. He suggests the physician's role be "remade" to address the sociological, psychological, and biological needs of patients. Yet the sociological components that affect health are vast. They include physical, structural, and social environments; health systems; and health and economic policy. Subsuming all of these variables into a broad category of "sociological factors" strains the capabilities of any professional and of this model.

Ecological Models

Albert Bandura is credited by some as an early pioneer of ecological models. His concept, ***reciprocal determinism***, notes that behaviors must be viewed in the context of environmental events (E), personal factors (P), and behaviors (B) that influence outcomes (Kohler, Grimley, & Reynolds, 1999). Each of these elements interact—significantly and simultaneously—with the other two. Thus, environmental events influence personal factors, and likewise, personal factors can and do reciprocally influence environmental events. Similarly, personal factors influence behaviors, and behaviors reciprocally influence personal factors (Ragin, 2018). The same type of relationship exists between behaviors and environmental events.

Yet as researchers note (e.g., Ragin, 2018), it is almost impossible to test this concept of reciprocal determinism. The proposed simultaneous interaction of all three variables makes it impossible to isolate one of the variables in order to test the remaining two. The Social Ecological and Behavioral Ecological Models also view behaviors as the product of the relationship between an organization and its environment and may share this limitation.

The Social Ecological Model

In the ***Social Ecological Model (SEM)***, health and overall well-being are determined by physiological, psychological, social, and emotional factors, in addition to a host of ecological factors (McLeroy, et al., 1988), including physical environmental determinants (e.g., water or air pollution; McDaniel, 2018). The *SEM* is rooted in a number of core ecological themes that explore the relationship among environmental conditions, human behavior, and overall well-being (Stokols, 1996). It borrows from the transdisciplinary study of ***systems theory***, a field that seeks to explain the behavior of a host of complex, organized systems (Whitchurch & Constantine, 2009). Thus, *SEM* recognizes and credits the many contributions of biology and individual behavior—including lifestyle choices, sociocultural, and environmental factors—on overall well-being. Yet it contends that it is both the separate *and* combined impact of these factors that best accounts for overall well-being. In sum, it suggests that the dynamic interaction between these multiple levels offers the best explanation of health outcomes (Stokols, 1996).

There are, however, points of divergence among *SEM* theorists. A full review of the variations in *SEM* theory is beyond the scope of this chapter, but one example is worth noting. According to Stokols (1996), specific environmental health events, like air pollution, may affect people differently based, in part, on the individual's physiological, physical, psychological, and emotional well-being, and, in part, on the dynamic relationship between people and their environment. Borrowing from systems theory, the *SEM* concludes that there is a mutual influence between people and their environment, which may result in interdependence, negative feedback, or homeostasis. Likewise, mutual influences also exist in the sociocultural and organizational roles of individuals and health. For example, one's professional role as a manager or supervisor may suggest behaviors that entail high levels of monitoring and oversight of employees, role behaviors that could increase stress levels and substantially influence the well-being of the manager.

McLeroy, and colleagues (1988), however, suggest a more finely delineated model, posing five levels of behavioral influence: ***intrapersonal, interpersonal, organizational, community, and policy***. In their version of the *SEM*, the ***intrapersonal*** consists of personal characteristics that influence behavior (e.g., beliefs, or attitudes about the behavior). *Interpersonal* is a person's social networks, such as family and friends, that contribute to that person's identity development. ***Organizational*** includes the more formal structures such as schools, churches, or other institutions that promote specific, sometimes role-defining, behaviors. **Community** refers to the broader sociocultural networks or societal environments that define an individual's socially accepted, normative behaviors. Finally, **public policy** is, as the name suggests, the rules or laws established by local, regional, or federal agencies that regulate health behaviors (McLeroy, et al., 1988; King, Merten, & Wong, 2018).

Testing the Social Ecological Model

Perhaps the strongest endorsement of the *SEM* comes from the Centers for Disease Control and Prevention (CDC). The CDC (2019) recently adopted an *SEM* framework for the prevention of suicide. They advocate a four-level *SEM* model to understand violence and the effect of prevention strategies: individual, relationships, communities, and societies.

Langhinrichsen-Rohling, Snerr, Slep, Heyman, and Foran (2011) employ the CDC's model to examine its effectiveness in predicting the risk of suicidal ideation in active military personnel. Their study of approximately 53,000 US Air Force troops (approximately 80% males and 80% non-Hispanic white) employed 19 measures assessing the role of four ecological factors—individual, family, workplace, and community constructs—likely to predict suicidal ideation.

Briefly, active-duty Air Force members were invited by email to complete a self-administered survey online. The survey included seven individual-level scales (e.g., depressive symptoms, Center for Epidemiological Studies Depression Scale [CES-D]; financial stress [Chance in Canada Survey]; physical health, [SF-36]). Five measures assessed family constructs, including the Quality of Marriage Index, an intimate partner violence (IPV) victimization scale to assess experiences of physical assault, and spouse preparedness for deployment. Five measures assessed workplace constructs, including the participant's satisfaction with the Air Force, workgroup cohesion, and workplace relationship satisfaction. Finally, four measures assessed community constructs: an established 1989 Army soldier and family survey, community safety scale, and community resources (See Langhinrichsen-Rohling, et al., 2011).

Results of the study identified significant predictors of suicidal ideation at each of the four assessed ecological levels. Depressive symptoms and alcohol problems (individual level), relationship satisfaction and victimization (family level), hours worked (workplace level), and social support (community level) all predicted suicidal ideation in the past 12 months.

A second study by Goebert, Chang, Chung-Do, Else, Hamagami, Helm, et al. (2012) examining the social ecological determinants of youth violence among Asian and Pacific Islander high school students similarly tests the ability of an ecological model to explain physical or emotional violence, violence perpetration, or victimization. Their study employed the CDC's Compendium of Assessment Tools and the Relational Aggression and Prosocial Behaviors scales in addition to measures developed by the Asian/Pacific Islander Youth Prevention Center to assess violence and victimization outcomes. Their findings illustrate the advantage of using the ecological model to obtain a comprehensive understanding of youth experience. Specifically, their findings challenge the belief that peers have the greatest impact on adolescents. Rather, analysis using the ecological model framework suggests that the school environment mediates peer exposure. What is more, their findings suggest that family factors contribute to peer exposure and to the community's and adolescent's risk/protection of violence (Goebert, et al., 2012).

These fascinating results notwithstanding, the *SEM* does have limitations. The first issue with the *SEM* is its comprehensiveness, which is both an advantage and a burden. As both Langhinrichsen-Rohling, et al. (2011) and Goebert, et al. (2012) show, including multilevel factors provides a more complex picture of behaviors. Nevertheless, testing multiple levels in the same study is challenging and may omit useful information. Boehmer, Lovegreen, Haire-Joshu, and Brownson (2006) illustrate the difficulties in their study of obesity and the built environment. Their inability to account for important social, interpersonal, and biological factors due to the large number of variables assessed limited their ability to correlate obesity and the built environment.

Similar to Ghaemi's (2009) critique of the *BPS* model, the *SEM* lacks specific guidelines on how to prioritize the influence of each component or level. Finally, *ecological models* and their focus on complex interactions across levels present challenges to experimental designs that aim to identify and isolate distinct causal or contributory factors (Sallis, Owen, & Fisher, 2008). Such designs might be possible with large sample sizes, posing yet another constraint on research employing ecological models.

Behavioral Ecological Model

A second *ecological model* proposed to address health behaviors is the ***Behavioral Ecological Model (BEM)***. Similar to the *SEM*, the *BEM* posits that behaviors are influenced by multilevel factors that include sociological, cultural, economic, and other environmental determinants. Yet there are distinctions between these two.

The *BEM* is rooted within learning theory, specifically the principles of operant conditioning. According to this theory, all behaviors are learned through an interaction with physical, social, and cultural environments (Hovell, Roussos, Hill, Johnson, Squire, & Gyenes, 2004). As Hovell, Wahlgren, and Gehrman (2002) suggest, behavior is an outcome whose explanation can be found in the environment. More specifically, behavior is shaped by the environment. Cultures select and reinforce behaviors as a function of the consequences produced by the behaviors. But in order for behaviors to change or be sustained in a culture, the behaviors must be reinforced and practiced by a sizable number of the population. For instance, if everyone in a cultural group prays before eating a meal, the chances that a person in that group will do likewise is quite high.

Thus, using a learning theories and ecological approach, the *BEM* proposes that behavior will be shaped and controlled through physical and social reinforcements. A change in a person's physical environment can lead to modifications in a person's health behaviors or risks, mediated through changes in the social responses to such environmental alterations (Hovell, et al., 2002). For example, schools providing free lunch programs for low-income children have often found their efforts to provide nutritious meals thwarted by the stigma that accompanies such offerings. Instead, providing free school lunches to *all* elementary children, regardless of ability to pay, thereby erasing the stigma, may encourage lower-income students to obtain the free lunch rather than forego eating. It may also encourage other students to take the free meals. Eliminating the stigma of free lunch may change behaviors, leading to improved nutrition for all students, including the target group. This example also illustrates the bidirectional nature of this model, one that allows for social influences to shape behavior and vice versa (Dresler-Hawke & Whitehead, 2009).

A more current example, but too current to be tested in published research, is the effect of wearing surgical or other protective masks in the midst of a global viral pandemic, such as the 2020 coronavirus (COVID-19) pandemic. Anecdotally, New York City residents commented on news feeds from China in which the majority of people depicted wore a face mask during the height of the outbreak in Hubei province. Perhaps some thought it an overreaction and an unlikely method of preventing the spread of the disease. Fast-forward just a few weeks later and increasing numbers of New York City residents were themselves voluntarily wearing masks. In fact, the behavior spread from just a few observers to the majority, especially in retail establishments.

Testing the Behavioral Ecological Model

Ayers, Hofstetter, Hughes, Park, Paik, Irvin, et al.'s (2010) study tests the *BEM*, although it does not specifically mention the *BEM* as the theoretical foundation for the study. They examined the home smoking restrictions of South Koreans living in Seoul with the same ethnic group living in California. Telephone interviews with 500 Koreans in Seoul and approximately 2,800 Korean Americans in California revealed that Koreans in Seoul were significantly less likely to experience home smoking bans or smoking restrictions. And, predictably, home smoking restrictions reduced participants' exposure to second-hand smoke. This unique comparison of the same ethnic group in different cultural environments supports the premise espoused in *BEM*, namely that physical environments together with cultural or social environments can and do reinforce behaviors. Additionally, in this case the cultural views that impact smoking restrictions hold direct implications for health outcomes. Thus, more than just an ecological explanation of outcomes, this study implies behavioral shaping and reinforcement, based on environmental and cultural contexts, can be critical determinants of health behaviors.

As with *SEMs*, *BEMs* are both comprehensive and complex. They emphasize the importance of environmental contingencies on health behaviors and outcomes, something that has been underrepresented in earlier theories. Acknowledging the importance of these factors, however, entails more work on how best to measure and prioritize their influences.

Conclusion

Health outcome studies that focused on individual-level factors did so for good reason. Some researchers suggest that these individual-level factors account for 40% of preventable deaths (Reid, 2010/2011). But a growing body of current research suggests that these behavioral factors are influenced as much by the social context of the individual as by their own individual risk factors (Reis, 2010/2011; Institute of Medicine, 2003). This begs the question, what factors contribute to the social context, which, in turn, influence the behavioral factors leading to poorer health outcomes? The evolution in health psychology theories from *cognitive based* to *ecological* and other emerging models may provide a mechanism to examine individuals and their health outcomes in context, here meaning the multilevel systems proposed in the *SEM* and *BEM*.

As the Langhinrichsen-Rohling, et al. (2011), Goebert, et al. (2012), and Ayers, and colleagues (2010) studies show, there are multiple environmental influences on an individual and they exist on multiple levels. What is more, according to Stokols (1996, 2003) and others who embrace the systems-level theories of health outcomes, these factors interact within and across levels simultaneously. The multiple interactions within and across levels, however, also pose problems for these theories. As suggested by Ghaemi (2009) regarding the *BPS* model, for instance, when employing ecological models, how do researchers prioritize the factors to be identified and tested? This is indeed a methodological challenge to anyone considering these models. Yet the potential to provide a fuller explanation of an individual's health outcomes while accounting for their environmental triggers may be worth the challenge.

References

Abel, E. (2007). Women with HIV and stigma. *Family & Community Health*, *30*, S104–S106. http://dx.doi.org.ezproxy.montclair.edu:2048/10.1097/00003727-200701001-00013

Adams, P., Hurd, M. D., McFadden, D., Merrill, A., & Ribeiro, T. (2003). Healthy, wealthy, and wise? Test for direct causal pathways between health & socioeconomic status. *Journal of Econometrics*, *112*(1), 3–56. https://doi.org/10.1016/S0304-4076(02)00145-8

Ajzen, I. (1985). From intentions to actions: A theory of planned behavior. In K. Kuhl & J. Beckman (Eds.), *Action control: From cognitions to behavior* (pp. 11–39). Heidelberg, Germany: Springer-Verlag.

Ajzen, I., & Fishbein, M. (1980). *Understanding attitudes and predicting social behavior*. Englewood Cliffs, NJ: Prentice-Hall.

Alberts, M., Smets, E. M., Vercoulen, J. H., Garssen, B., & Bleijenberg, G. (1997). "Abbreviated fatigue questionnaire": A practical tool in the classification of fatigue. *Netherlands Tijaschrift voor Geneeskunde, 141*(31), 1526–1530.

Armstrong, D. (2002). Theoretical tensions in biopsychosocial medicine. *The Health Psychology Reader, 4*, 66–78. https://doi.org/10.1016/0277-9536(87)90368-6

Ayers, J. W., Hofstetter, R. C., Hughes, S. C., Park, H., Paik, H.-Y., Irvin, V. L., et al. (2010). Smoking on both sides of the Pacific: Home smoking restrictions and secondhand Smoke exposure among Korean adults and children in Seoul and California. *Nicotine & Tobacco Research, 12*(11), 1142–1150. https://doi.org/10.1093/ntr/ntq164

Babazadeh, T., Ghaffari-Fam, S., Oliaee, S., Sarbazi, E., Shirdel, A., Mostafa-Gharabeghi, P., et al. (2019). Predictors of Pap smear screening behavior among rural women in Tabriz, Iran: An application of Health Belief Model. *International Journal of Cancer Management, 12*(5), e87246. doi:10.5812/ijcm.87246

Bandura, A. (1977). Self-efficacy: Towards a unifying theory of behavioral change. *Psychological Review, 84*(2), 191–215. http://dx.doi.org.ezproxy.montclair.edu:2048/10.1037/0033-295X.84.2.191

Banks, S. M., & Kerns, R. D. (1996). Explaining high rates of depression in chronic pain: A diathesis-stress framework. *Psychological Bulletin, 119*(1), 95–110. https://doi.org/10.1037/0033-2909.119.1.95

Becker, M. H. (1974). The Health Belief Model & sick role behaviors. *Health Education & Behaviors, 2*(4), 409–419. https://doi.org/10.1177/109019817400200407

Boehmer, T. K., Lovegreen, S. L., Haire-Joshu, D., & Brownson, R. C. (2006). What constitutes an obesogenic environment in rural communities? *American Journal of Health Promotion, 20*(6), 411–421. https://doi.org/10.4278%2F0890-1171-20.6.411

Borrell-Carrió, F., Suchman, A. L., & Epstein, R. M. (2004). The biopsychosocial model 25 years later: Principles, practice, and scientific inquiry. *The Annals of Family Medicine, 2*(6), 576–582. https://doi.org/10.1370/afm.245

Bosworth, H. B., Horner, D. R., Edwards, L. J., & Matcher, D. B. (2000). Depression & other determinants of value placed on current health status by stroke patients. *Stroke, 31*, 2063–2069. https://doi.org/10.1161/01.STR.31.11.2603

Bronfenbrenner, U. (1979). *The ecology of human development*. Cambridge, MA: Harvard University Press.

Bulgar, M. E., White, K. M., & Robinson, N. G. (2010). The role of self-efficacy in dental patients' brushing and flossing: Testing an extended Health Belief Model. *Patient Education & Counseling, 78*(2), 269–272. https://doi.org/10.1016/j.pec.2009.06.014

Carpenter, C. J. (2010). A meta-analysis of the effectiveness of Health Belief Model variables in predicting behavior. *Health Communication, 25*(8), 661–669. https://doi.org/10.1080/10410236.2010.521906

Centers for Disease Control and Prevention. (2019). The social-ecological model: A framework for prevention. *Violence Prevention*. Retrieved from www.cdc.gov/violenceprevention/publichealthissue/social-ecologicalmodel.html?CDC_AA_refVal=https%3A%2F%2Fwww.cdc.gov%2Fviolenceprevention%2Foverview%2Fsocial-ecologicalmodel.html

Champion, V. L., & Skinner, C. S. (2008). The Health Belief Model. In K. Glanz, B. K. Rimer, & K. Viswanath (Eds.), *Health behavior and health education: Theory research and practice* (pp. 45–66). San Francisco, CA: Jossey-Bass.

Chervenak, F. A., McCullough, L. B., & Brent, R. L. (2011). The professional responsibility model of obstetrical ethics: Avoiding the perils of clashing rights. *American Journal of Obstetrics & Gynecology, 205*(2), 315. https://doi.org/10.1016/j.ajog.2011.06.006

Clougherty, J. E., Souza, K., & Cullen, M. R. (2010). Work & its role in shaping the social gradient in health. *Annals of the New York Academy of Science, 1186*, 102–124. doi:10.1111/j.1749-6632.2009.05338.x

Cohen, S. (2005). Keynote presentation at the eighth international congress of behavioral medicine: The Pittsburgh common cold studies: Psychosocial predictors of susceptibility to respiratory infectious illness. *International Journal of Behavioral Medicine, 12*(3), 55–79. https://doi.org/10.1207/s15327558ijbm1203_1

Conner, M., & Norman, P. (2005a). Predicting health behaviors: A social cognition approach. In M. Conner & P. Norman (Eds.), *Predicting health behaviors* (pp. 1–18). Berkshire, UK: Open University Press.

Conner, M., & Norman, P. (2005b). Predicting health behaviors: Future directions. In M. Conner & P. Normal (Eds.), *Predicting health behaviors* (pp. 324–372). Berkshire, UK: Open University Press.

Crosby, R. A., Kegler, M. C., & DiClemente, R. J. (2002). Understanding and applying theory in health promotion practice and research. In R. DiClemente, R. A. Crosby, & M. C. Kegler (Eds.), *Emerging theories in health promotion, practice and research* (pp. 1–16). San Francisco, CA: Jossey-Bass.

Datta, G. D., Blair, A., Sylvestre, M. P., Gauvin, L., Drouin, M., & Mayrand, M. H. (2018). Cervical cancer screening in Montreal: Building evidence to support primary care and policy interventions. *Preventive Medicine, 11*, 265–271. https://doi.org/10.1016/j.ypmed.2018.02.037

Deshpande, S., Basil, M. D., & Basil, D. Z. (2009). Factors influencing health eating habits among college students: An application of the Health Belief Model. *Health Marketing Quarterly*, *26*(2), 145–164. https://doi.org/10.1080/07359680802619834

Dodds, C. (2006). HIV-related stigma in England: Experiences of gay men & heterosexual African immigrants living with HIV. *Journal of Community & Applied Social Psychology*, *16*(6), 472–480. https://doi.org/10.1002/casp.895

Domingo, E. J., Noviani, R., Noor, M. R., Ngelangel, C. A., Limpaphayom, K. K., Thuan, T. V., et al. (2008). Epidemiology & prevention of cervical cancer in Indonesia, Malaysia, the Philippines, Thailand & Vietnam. *Vaccine*, *26*(Suppl. 12), M71–79. https://doi.org/10.1016/j.vaccine.2008.05.039

Downing-Matibag, T. M., & Geisinger, B. (2009). Hooking up & sexual risk taking among college students: A Health Belief Model perspective. *Qualitative Health Research*, *19*(9), 1196–1209. https://doi.org/10.1177%2F1049732309344206

Dresler-Hawke, E., & Whitehead, D. (2009, June 25). The behavioral ecological model as a framework For school-based anti-bullying health promotion intervention. *Journal of School Nursing*, *3*, 195. https://doi.org/10.1177%2F1059840509334364

Drossman, D. A. (1998). Gastrointestinal illness & the biopsychosocial model: Presidential address. *Psychosomatic Medicine*, *60*(3), 258–267.

Engel, G. L. (1977a). The need for a new medical model: A challenge for biomedicine. *Holistic Medicine*, *4*(1), 37–53. doi:10.3109/13561828909043606

Engel, G. L. (1977b). The need for a new medical model: A challenge for biomedicine. *Science*, *196*(4286), 129–139. https://psycnet.apa.org/doi/10.1037/h0089260

Engel, G. L. (1980). The clinical application of the biopsychosocial model. *American Journal of Psychiatry*, *137*(5), 535–544.

Foster, G., Frijters, P., & Johnson, D. W. (2012). The triumph of hope over disappointment: A note on the utility value of good health expectations. *Journal of Economic Psychology*, *33*(1), 206–214. https://doi.org/10.1016/j.joep.2011.09.010

Gerend, M. A., & Shepherd, J. E. (2012). Predicting human papillomavirus vaccine uptake in young adult women: Comparing the Health Belief Model & Theory of Planned Behavior. *Annals of Behavioral Medicine*, *44*(2), 171–180. https://doi.org/10.1007/s12160-012-9366-5

Ghaemi, S. (2009). The rise and fall of the biopsychosocial model. *British Journal of Psychiatry*, *195*(1), 3–4. https://doi.org/10.1192/bjp.bp.109.063859

Glanz, K., Rimer, B. K., & Viswanath, K. (2008). *Health behavior and health education: Theory, research, and practice* (4th ed.). San Francisco, CA: Jossey-Bass.

Goebert, D., Chang, J. Y., Chung-Do, J., Else, I. R. N., Hamagami, F., Helm, S., et al. (2012). Social ecological determinants of youth violence among ethnically diverse Asian and Pacific Islander students. *Maternal & Child Health Journal*, *16*, 188–196. https://doi.org/10.1007/s10995-010-0726-0

Guo, R., Hermanson, P. M., Berkshire, S. D., & Fulton, L. V. (2019). Predicting intention to use evidence-based management among U.S. healthcare administrators: Application of the theory of planned behavior and structural equation modeling. *International Journal of Healthcare Management*, *12*(1), 25–32. https://doi.org/10.1080/20479700.2017.1336856

Hochbaum, G.M. (1958). *Public participation in medical screening programs: A socio-psychological study*. Washington, DC: U.S. Department of Health, Education, and Welfare, Public Health Service.

Hovell, M. F., Roussos, S., Hill, L., Johnson, N. W., Squire, C., & Gyenes, M. (2004). Engineering clinical leadership & success in tobacco control: Recommendations for policy & practice in Hungary & Central Europe. *European Journal of Dental Education*, *8*, 51–60. https://doi.org/10.1111/j.1399-5863.2004.00324.x

Hovell, M. F., Wahlgren, D. R., & Gehrman, C. A. (2002). The behavioral ecological model: Integrating public health. In R. J. DiClemente, R. A. Crosby, & M. C. Kegler (Eds.), *Emerging theories in health promotion practice & research: Strategies for improving public health* (pp. 347–385). San Francisco, CA: Jossey Bass.

Institute of Medicine. (2003). *Unequal treatment: Confronting racial and ethnic disparities in health care*. Washington, DC: The National Academies Press.

Jallian, F., Motlagh, F. Z., Solhi, M., & Gharibnavaz, H. (2014). Effectiveness of self-management promotion education programs among diabetic patients based on Health Belief Model. *Journal of Education Health Promotion*, *3*(14), 75–79. https://dx.doi.org/10.4103%2F2277-9531.127580

James, D. C. S., Pobee, J. W., Oxidine, D. L., Brown, L., & Joshi, G. (2012). Using the Health Belief Model to develop culturally appropriate weight-management material for African-American women. *Journal of the Academy of Nutrition & Dietetics*, *112*(5), 664–670. https://doi.org/10.1016/j.jand.2012.02.003

Janz, N. K., & Becker, M. H. (1984). The Health Belief Model: A decade later. *Health Education Quarterly*, *11*(1), 1–47. https://doi.org/10.1177%2F109019818401100101

Jones, C. J., Smith, H., & Llewellyn, C. (2014). Evaluating the effectiveness of Health Belief Model interventions in improving adherence: A systematic review. *Health Psychology Review, 8*(3), 253–269. https://doi.org/10.1080/17437199.2013.802623

King, J. L., Merten, J. W., & Wong, T.-J. (2018). Applying a socio-ecological framework to factors related to nicotine replacement therapy for adolescent smoking cessation. *American Journal of Health Promotion, 32*(5), 1291–1303.

Kirscht, J. P. (1974). The Health Belief Model and illness behavior. *Health Education Monographs, 2,* 2387–2408. https://doi.org/10.1177%2F109019817400200406

Kleisiaris, C. F., Sfakianakis, C., & Papathanasiou, I. V. (2014). Health care practices in ancient Greece: The Hippocratic ideal. *Journal of Medical Ethics and History of Medicine, 7,* 6. Retrieved from www.ncbi.nlm.nih.gov/pmc/articles/pmc4263393/

Kohler, C. L., Grimley, D., & Reynolds, K. (1999). Theoretical approaches guiding the development & implementation of health promotion programs. In J. M. Raczynski & R. J. DiClemente (Eds.), *Handbook of health promotion & disease prevention: The Springer series in behavioral psychophysiology & medicine* (pp. 23–49). Boston, MA: Springer.

Kurtzke, J. F. (1983). Rating neurological impairment in multiple sclerosis: An expanded disability status scale (EDSS). *Neurology, 33*(11), 1444–1452.

Langhinrichsen-Rohling, J., Snerr, J. D., Slep, A. M. S., Heyman, R. E., & Foran, H. M. (2011). Risk for suicidal ideation in the U.S. Air Force: An ecological perspective. *Journal of Consulting & Clinical Psychology, 79*(5), 600–612. https://psycnet.apa.org/doi/10.1037/a0024631

Leventhal, H., Rubin, C., Leventhal, E. A., & Burns, E. (2001). Health risk behaviors & aging. In J. E. Birren & K. W. Schaire (Eds.), *Handbook of the psychology of aging* (5th ed., pp. 186–214). San Diego, CA: Academic Press.

Lippke, S., Wiedemann, A. U., Ziegelman, J. P., Reuter, T., & Schwarzer, R. (2009). Self-efficacy moderates the mediation of intentions into behavior via plan. *American Journal of Health Behavior, 33*(5), 521–529. https://doi.org/10.5993/AJHB.33.5.5

Luszczynska, A., Sobczyk, A., & Abraham, C. (2007). Planning to lose weight: Randomized Controlled trial of an implementation intention prompt to enhance weight reduction among overweight & obese women. *Health Psychology, 26*(4), 507–512. https://psycnet.apa.org/doi/10.1037/0278-6133.26.4.507

McDaniel, J. T. (2018). Prevalence of chronic obstructive pulmonary disease: County-level risk factors based on the Social Ecological Model. *Perspectives in Public Health, 138*(4), 200. https://doi.org/10.1177%2F1757913918772598

McHorney, C. A., Ware, Jr., J. E., Lu, J. F. R., & Sherbourne, C. D. (1994). The MOS 36-item short-form health survey (SF-36). III: Test of data quality, scaling assumptions, and reliability across diverse patient groups. *Medical Care, 32*(1), 40–66.

McLeroy, K., Bibeau, D., Steckler, A., & Glanz, K. (1988). An ecological perspective on health promotion programs. *Health Education and Behavior, 15*(4), 351–377. https://doi.org/10.1177%2F109019818801500401

Matarazzo, J. D. (1980). Behavioral health and behavioral medicine: Frontiers for a new health psychology. *American Psychologist, 35,* 807–817. https://psycnet.apa.org/doi/10.1037/0003-066X.35.9.807

Michielsen, H. J., De Vries, J., & Van Heck, G. L. (2003). Psychometric qualities of a brief self-rated fatigue measure the fatigue assessment scale. *Journal of Psychosomatic Research, 54,* 345–352. https://doi.org/10.1016/S0022-3999(02)00392-6

Minden, S. L., Frankel, D., Hadden, L., Perloff, J., Srinath, K. P., & Hoaglin, D. C. (2006). The Sonya Slifka longitudinal multiple sclerosis study: Methods and sample characteristics. *Multiple Sclerosis, 12,* 24–38. https://doi.org/10.1191%2F135248506ms1262oa

Montano, D. E., & Kasprzyk, D. (2008). Theory of Reasoned Action, theory of planned behavior, and the integrated behavioral model. In K. Glanz, B. K. Rimer, & K. Viswanath (Eds.), *Health behavior and health education: Theory, research, and practice* (4th ed., pp. 67–92). San Francisco, CA: Jossey-Bass.

Moscowitz, J. T., Epel, E. S., & Acree, M. (2008). Positive affect uniquely predicts lower risk of mortality in people with diabetes. *Health Psychology, 27*(Suppl. 1), S73–82. https://psycnet.apa.org/doi/10.1037/0278-6133.27.1.S73

Ng, J. Y. Y., Ntoumanis, N., &Thogersen-Ntoumanis, E. (2012). Self-determination theory applied to health context: A meta-analysis. *Perspectives on Psychosocial Science, 7*(4), 325–340. https://doi.org/10.1177%2F1745691612447309

Pendry, B. (2001, June). *Stigma and HIV/AIDS in South Africa.* Presentation at the 21st United Nations General Assembly, Special Session on HIV/AIDS, New York, NY.

Ragin, D. F. (2018). *Health psychology: An interdisciplinary approach* (3rd ed.). New York, NY: Routledge/Taylor & Francis Group.

Reid, C. (2010/2011). Building communities and improving health: Finding new solutions to an old problem. *Community Investments: Health and Community Development, 22*(3), 2–10.

Rosenstock, I. M. (1974). Historical origins of the Health Belief Model. *Health Education Monographs*, *2*(4), 328–335. https://doi.org/10.1177%2F109019817400200403

Rosenstock, I. M., Strecher, V. J., & Becker, M. H. (1988). Social learning theory and the Health Belief Model. *Health Education Quarterly*, *15*(2), 175–183. https://doi.org/10.1177%2F109019818801500203

Ross, L., Kohler, C. L., Grimley, D. M., & Anderson-Lewis, C. (2007). The theory of reasoned action and intention to seek cancer information. *American Journal of Health Behavior*, *3*(2), 123–134. https://doi.org/10.5993/AJHB.31.2.2

Sallis, J. F., Owen, N., & Fisher, E. B. (2008). Ecological models of health behaviors. In K. Glanz, B. K. Rimer, & K. Viswanath (Eds.), *Health behavior and health education: Theory, research and practice* (4th ed., pp. 485–482). San Francisco: Jossey-Bass Publishers.

Saraga, M., Fuks, A., & Boudreau, J. D. (2014). George Engel's epistemology of clinical practice. *Perspectives in Biology & Medicine*, *57*(4), 482–494. https://doi.org/10.1353/pbm.2014.0038

Schulz, R., Martire, L. M., Beach, S. R., & Scheier, M. F. (2005). Depression and mortality in the elderly. *Current Directions in Health Psychology*, *9*(6), 204–208. https://doi.org/10.1111%2F1467-8721.00095

Schwarzer, R. (2008). Modeling health behavior change: How to predict and modify the adoption & maintenance of health behaviors. *Applied Psychology*, *57*(1), 1–29. https://doi.org/10.1111/j.1464-0597.2007.00325.x

Sheeran, P. (2002). Intention-behavior relations: A conceptual & empirical review. *European Review of Social Psychology*, *12*, 1–36. https://doi.org/10.1080/14792772143000003

Sheeran, P., Maki, A., Montanaro, E., Avishai-Yikshak, A., Bryan, A., & Klein, W. M. P. (2016). The impact of changing, attitudes, norms and self-efficacy on health-related intentions and behaviors. *Health Psychology*, *35*(1), 1178–1188.

Sheldon, P. (2016). Facebook friend request: Applying the Theory of Reasoned Action to student-teacher relationships on Facebook. *Journal of Broadcasting and Electronic Media*, *60*(2), 269–285. https://doi.org/10.1080/08838151.2016.1164167

Smith, J. P. (2007). Impact of socioeconomic status on health over the life-course. *Journal of Human Resources*, *42*, 739–764. doi:10.3368/jhr.XLII.4.739

Snaith, R. P. (2003). The hospital anxiety & depression scale. *Health & Quality of Life Outcome*, *1*, 29–32. https://doi.org/10.1186/1477-7525-1-29

Stokols, D. (1992). Establishing and maintaining healthy environments: Towards a social ecology of health promotion. *American Psychologist*, *47*, 6–22. https://psycnet.apa.org/doi/10.1037/0003-066X.47.1.6

Stokols, D. (1996). Translating social ecological theory into guidelines for community health promotion. *American Journal of Health Promotion*, *10*(4), 282–298. https://doi.org/10.4278%2F0890-1171-10.4.282

Stokols, D., Grzywacz, J. G., McMahan, S., & Phillips, K. (2003). Increasing the health promotive capacity of human environments. *American Journal of Health Promotion*, *18*, 4–13. https://doi.org/10.4278%2F0890-1171-18.1.4

van der Pligt, J., de Vries, N. K., Manstead, A. S. R., & van Harreveld, F. (2000). The importance of being selective: Weighing the role of attribute importance in attitudinal judgement. *Advances in Experimental Social Psychology*, *32*, 135–200. https://doi.org/10.1016/S0065-2601(00)80005-2

Van Helvoort-Postulart, D., Dirksen, C. D., Kessels, A. G. H., vanEngelshoren, J. M. A., & Huunink, M. G. M. (2009). A comparison between willingness to pay & willingness to give up time. *European Journal of Health Economics*, *10*, 81–91. https://doi.org/10.1007/s10198-008-0105-6

Velicer, W. F., Prochaska, J. D., & Redding, C. A. (2006). Tailored communications for smoking cessation: Past successes & future directions. *Drug & Alcohol Review*, *25*, 47–55. https://doi.org/10.1080/09595230500459511

Vermaire, J. H., vanExel, N. J. A., van Loveren, C., & Brouwer, W. B. F. (2012). Putting your money where your mouth is: Parent's valuation of good oral health of their children. *Social Science & Medicine*, *75*(12), 2200–2206. https://doi.org/10.1016/j.socscimed.2012.08.018

Vlaeyen, J., Kole-Snijders, A. M. J., Rotteveel, A. M., Ruesink, R., & Heuts, P. H. T. G. (1995). The role of fear of movement/(re)movement in pain disability. *Journal of Occupational Rehabilitation*, *5*(4), 235–252. https://doi.org/10.1007/BF02109988

Walter, H. J., Vaughan, R., Ragin, D. F., & Cohall, A. (1994). Prevalence and correlates of AIDS-related behavioral intentions among urban minority high school students. *AIDS Education and Prevention*, *6*, 339–350.

Whitchurch, G. G., & Constantine, L. L. (2009). Systems theory. In P. Boss, W. J. Doherty, R. LaRossa, W. R. Schumm, & S. K. Steinmetz (Eds.), *Sourcebook of family theories & methods* (pp. 325–355). Boston, MA: Springer.

Wijenberg, M. L. M., Slapert, S. Z., Kohler, S., & Bol, Y. (2016). Explaining fatigue in multiple sclerosis: Cross-validation of a biopsychosocial model. *Journal of Behavioral Medicine*, *39*, 815–522. https://doi.org/10.1007/s10865-016-9749-3

Yue, Z., Li, C., Wellin, Q., & Bin, W. (2015). Application of the Health Belief Model to improve the understanding of antihypertensive medication adherence among Chinese patients. *Patient Education & Counseling*, *98*(5), 669–673. https://doi.org/10.1016/j.pec.2015.02.007

2
STATISTICAL TOOLBOX OF PSYCHOLOGY

Michael R. Hulsizer and Linda M. Woolf

Overview

Over the past 40 years, the field of health psychology has expanded across a range of domains such as clinical health psychology (Sandhu & Patel, 2013; Smith, Williams, & Ruiz, 2016), rehabilitation psychology (Brenner, 2019), and occupational health psychology (Graham, Howard, & Dougall, 2012). Concomitant with the growth of health psychology as a field of practice has been the growth of the discipline within academic psychology (Kaplan, 2009). Empirical research in the field examining the biological, psychological, and social aspects of health and illness have flourished, and the journal *Health Psychology* remains one of the top journals for empirical research in the field with a five-year impact factor of over 4.4 (American Psychological Association: APA, 2020).

With the growth of health psychology, there has been an expanding need to connect theory to practice as well as interventions to long-term behavior change (Hilton & Johnston, 2017). As such, researchers are increasingly moving away from primary reliance on traditional research designs comparing groups on specific variables within a clinical or laboratory setting. Although traditional designs are useful in establishing internal validity—cause and effect—such designs do not reflect the complexity and individuality of human health behaviors and needs. Additionally, these designs typically are limited in terms of external validity—the ability to generalize to contexts outside the clinical/laboratory settings to the home or community. Relatedly, many of these studies may also fail to reflect the diversity of populations—persons and peoples—across a range of health-related dimensions and the development of culturally appropriate interventions.

This chapter focuses on five emerging alternative research models that researchers can use to study health behaviors and interventions: idiographic designs, ecological momentary assessment, survival analysis, meta-analytic structural equational modeling, and Bayesian statistics. Each section of this chapter includes an explanation of the method, an illustrative case example, and information relevant to additional resources on the topic. It should be noted that researchers are continuing to explore new techniques and methods to advance health psychology and as such, this chapter is not a definitive guide to all new developing designs and statistical tools in the field.

Research in Practice

Within-Person Idiographic Designs (e.g., n-of-1 Studies)

The traditional approach to determining whether an intervention or treatment is effective is to employ a between-subjects **randomized controlled trial (RCT)** in which one group of participants is exposed to the intervention and another group is given a placebo or placed in the control condition. Significant differences in mean responses are then noted, and conclusions are made with the assumption that the results will apply to most individuals. The problem with this approach, as noted by Kwasnicka and Naughton (2020), is that it is not a true person-centered approach. That is, the resultant intervention or treatment approaches advocated by the researchers might work for the average person, but most likely will not be effective for all individuals—and might in fact be harmful.

In order to develop a person-centered approach, the researcher needs to investigate what will work for specific persons, families, or institutions. Kwasnicka and Naughton (2020) report that **within-person idiographic designs** such as case reports and **n-of-1** studies can enable the researcher to better examine the pattern of responses over time, explore the relationship between the predictor and outcome variables, and determine if the treatment is effective for the target audience. Kwasnicka, Inauen, Nieuwenboom, Nurmi, Schneider, Short, and colleagues (2019) provide an overview of the *n-of-1* research design, including a discussion of the challenges and potential solutions inherent within it.

There are two basic types of *within-person idiographic designs*—observational and experimental. **Observational idiographic designs** tend to be exploratory in nature. Measures such as surveys, diaries, medical records, and physiological data may be collected but are primarily used to further illustrate the phenomenon being investigated or better understand the nature of cognitive or behavioral processes occurring within the individual. Studies of this sort are extremely helpful in identifying variables of interest and in the development of hypotheses for use in experimental designs. For example, Kwasnicka, Dombrowski, White, and Sniehotta (2017) used *observational idiographic* methods to study weight loss management.

Experimental idiopathic designs include *n-of-1* studies using an AB, ABA, or ABABA design. Researchers have asserted that *n-of-1 RCTs*, in which the participant serves as their own control group, is the ideal standard for *experimental idiopathic designs* (Kwasnicka & Naughton, 2020). Nonetheless, there are always concerns about the statistical power associated with *n-of-1 designs*. Researchers can address the issue of power by developing studies that have several repeated observations over time. With any time-series design, researchers need to be cognizant of data autocorrelation, in which errors from different times of measurement are correlated, thus leading to potentially faulty models or conclusions. To see the range of health behavior research studies, researchers may wish to examine McDonald, Quinn, Vieira, O'Brien, White, Johnston, and colleagues' (2017) systematic review of almost 40 *n-of-1* studies.

Sniehotta, Presseau, Hobbs, and Araújo-Soares (2012) conducted an excellent factorial *RCT* to test the effect of **behavior change techniques (BCTs)** designed to increase physical activity among healthy adults using an *n-of-1 design*. The *BCTs* used by the researchers were based on self-regulation theory and included goal setting and self-monitoring (Carver & Scheier, 1982). The researchers conducted a 2 (goal setting vs. active control) × 2 (self-monitoring vs. active control) factorial *RCT* using the *n-of-1 design* with ten healthy adult participants. The participants were randomly placed in either the intervention or control condition over the course of two months for both goal setting and self-monitoring (30 days for each condition). The dependent variable was the number of steps taken each day as measured by an electronic pedometer—a device that records each step a person takes by noting the motion of the person's hands (which typically move in concert with a step). Previous research indicated that the researchers would have sufficient power (80%) to conduct statistical analyses.

According to Vieira, McDonald, Araújo-Soares, Sniehotta, and Henderson (2017), there is a lack of consensus on the best approach for analyzing *n-of-1* data. In fact, many *n-of-1* studies are not statistically analyzed or are examined using less powerful statistical techniques. When determining how to analyze data from *n-of-1* studies, researchers need to recognize that data has a time-series structure which, due to the lack of independent observations, may be prone to autocorrelation.

The process of pre-whitening can be used to remedy the presence of autocorrelation within each data series. Conceptually, **pre-whitening** is an operation that transforms a time series by making data behave statistically like white noise—thus eliminating the autocorrelation. The data transformation (i.e., whitening) occurs prior to primary planned analyses (hence the 'pre' in *pre-whitening*). Thus, the process of *pre-whitening* strengthens the analyses and provides more confidence in the results (see Hobbs, Dixon, Johnston, & Howie, 2013 for the complete description of this process). Sniehotta, and colleagues (2012) examined the presence of autocorrelation in steps data series and determined that they did not need to conduct *pre-whitening* before the implementation of parametric statistical approaches.

In addition to descriptive statistics, Sniehotta, et al. (2012) conducted single-case ordinary least squares regressions on each participant to determine whether goal setting and self-monitoring were effective approaches for each participant. The results of the overall analyses revealed that self-monitoring led to increased step counts and that goal setting approached significance. Single-case analyses also revealed significant results for specific individuals.

The results of Sniehotta, et al. (2012) suggest that researchers can conduct *idiographic designs* such as *n-of-1* studies to experimentally address complicated questions within the field of health psychology. However, the *n-of-1* methodology has several limitations. First, researchers need to select variables that are less likely to carry over from one setting to another. Researchers also need to be cognizant of power when designing an *n-of-1* study. In these studies, statistical power is a function of the number of data points collected from one individual. The more data points, the greater the power. As indicated earlier, there is no consensus on the type of analysis most appropriate in *n-of-1* studies. However, Vieira, et al. (2017) encouraged researchers to consider using dynamic models to analyze the data due to the fact that these models can adjust for many of the issues (e.g., autocorrelation, time-varying covariates, time lag) associated with *n-of-1* studies. Dynamic models such as **autoregressive distributed lag (ARDL)** models work well in this situation because they allow the researcher to describe changes occurring over time. Distributed lag models are used to examine situations in which the effect of a regressor *x* on *y* occurs over time rather than all at once. There are many different lag models (e.g., polynomial, geometric), but the *ARDL* model addresses the distributed lag problem more efficiently than these other models. In addition, *ARDL* models enable researchers to investigate the effect of the past and future through the inclusion of lagged variables. Most importantly, *ARDL* models adjust for the presence of autocorrelation.

Ecological Momentary Assessment

Advancements in technology have enhanced our ability to conduct psychological research in a fashion that maximizes internal validity. New approaches to analyzing data have furthered our confidence in research results. However, there has been a growing chorus of researchers who have focused on the fact that these advances have sometimes come at the expense of external validity. Although we may find significance and can replicate findings in the lab environment, the results may not reflect what is happening outside the walls of the artificial lab environment. Health psychology researchers have used written data diaries to collect longitudinal data, but this method is limited—diaries are relatively intrusive and often not completed in real time but rather, after the fact. **Ecological momentary assessment (EMA)** is the merger of technology and data diaries in which participants are prompted throughout the day to indicate their current state. Over time, the mechanism for recording data has gone from paper and pencil measures and audio recorders to the use of small handheld computers and **personal digital assistant devices (PDAs** such as a Palm Pilot). Currently, many researchers engage participants by sending text messages, having participants complete data survey applications (e.g., Qualtrics) on smart phones, and/or wearing various medical monitors that record and send ongoing health data (e.g., heart rate) back to the researcher.

Examples of *EMA* studies began to appear in psychological research in the early 1990s. A special section of *Health Psychology* devoted to *EMA* began with Shiffman and Stone's (1998) introduction of the technique and continued with Schwartz and Stone's (1998) assessment of the most appropriate statistical approaches for examining the rich data obtained when using *EMA*. Several research articles using the technique rounded out the special section. Researchers interested in a comprehensive overview of *EMA* should read Shiffman, Stone, and Hufford (2008).

An excellent example of a research article using *EMA* in the field of health psychology was conducted by Nock, Prinstein, and Sterba (2009). In this study, the researchers examined the incidence of **self-injurious thoughts and behaviors (SITBs)** among adolescents and young adults. This type of research question provides an excellent example of the benefits of *EMA*. Researchers argued that most general theories focusing on why people engaged in *SITBs* was based on laboratory research as opposed to field research. Although existing research was high in internal validity, these studies were understandably lacking in external validity due to the fact that this kind of behavior was unlikely to appear in the laboratory environment—the prior research was retrospective and produced limited generalizability.

The development of *EMA* techniques enabled the researchers to examine *SITBs* as they occurred in real time. To do so, the researchers had participants carry a *PDA* over the course of 14 days. At the time, these devices (e.g., Palm Pilot) were popular and similar in size to the average smart phone carried by people today.

At the beginning of the study, participants provided informed consent (including parents for those under 18), completed a questionnaire which assessed their history of *SITBs*, and received instruction in how the *PDAs* worked. Researchers also assessed the participant's current psychiatric diagnoses during a baseline session. Throughout the ensuing 14 days, participants were prompted to complete an entry twice a day (midday and end of day) as well as whenever they experienced any *SITBs*. The researchers monitored the submissions to ensure that participants were compliant and assess if professional intervention was warranted to protect the health and well-being of the participants. The presence of *SITBs* prompted follow-up questions regarding the context in which the *SITBs* occurred and how long the participant engaged in these thoughts and/or behaviors. Questions were also asked if the participant chose an alternative behavior. This approach resulted in the collection of data on 1,262 thought and behavior episodes for the 30 participants.

The data analysis approach taken by Nock, and colleagues (2009) was consistent with the best practices detailed by Schwartz and Stone (1998). Specifically, after reporting basic descriptive statistics, the researchers used **generalized hierarchical linear modeling (HLM)** to examine this data. One important decision in *HLM* is establishing the nesting structure of the model. Models are nested if one model contains all the terms of the other and at least one additional term. After selecting the appropriate nesting structure, the researchers checked for **seriality** (e.g., the extent to which autocorrelation exists, given the observations are so close together in time), **cyclicity** (e.g., the extent to which observations occurred at night versus during the daytime), and **trend** (e.g., included a time-within-day predictor) to determine the appropriate functional form of change over time. Finally, Level 1 and Level 2 predictors were added to the resultant model.

The data analysis revealed that participants reported an average of 5.0 thoughts of **nonsuicidal self-injury (NSSI)** and 1.6 actual episodes of *NSSI* per week. Suicidal thoughts were less frequent (1.1 per week) and generally did not lead to actual suicide attempts. However, suicidal thoughts were of longer duration than *NSSI* thoughts. Of particular concern, *NSSI* thoughts did co-occur with thoughts of alcohol/drug use and binging/purging 15% to 20% of the time.

A main strength of this study was the ability to collect data happening in real time in a real-world setting without the limitations associated with retrospective studies. However, there were some weaknesses—most notably, the sample size was relatively small (30 participants) and less diverse than needed to generalize to the general population. In addition, although carrying a *PDA* was relatively common when the study was conducted, it was not normal to be pinged to respond to a survey (although today it is somewhat more common for a smart phone to demand your attention using pings). With this type of study, there also are concerns about noncompliance (Ram, Brinberg, Pincus, & Conroy, 2017) or participants simply falsifying data (Litt, Cooney, & Morse, 1998). Although the former can be addressed by the careful development of unobtrusive technology (e.g., smart phone apps), the latter can be difficult to tease out. Lastly, there are also concerns (Ram, et al., 2017) regarding the implementation of multilevel models such as *HLM*. For example, Richardson, Fuller-Tyszkiewicz, O'Donnell, Ling, and Staiger (2017) have encouraged researchers to use *regression tree modeling (RTM)* as an alternative to multilevel modeling. *RTM* automates the search for interactions, makes it easier to identify similar subgroups, and most importantly allows for the creation of decision trees that summarize the results in an easy-to-digest visual fashion. Despite these advantages, Richardson and colleagues acknowledge some limitations (e.g., generalization). Other researchers, such as Modecki and Mazza (2017), have expressed some concerns regarding this approach.

Survival Analysis

In the late 1980s, Gardner and Griffin (Gardner & Griffin, 1989; Griffin & Gardner, 1989) introduced *survival analysis* (also known as *hazard regression*) to the field of psychology. Prior to the introduction of this statistical technique, the analysis was primarily used by medical professionals to examine the time it took for an event to occur—typically death or systems failure. *Survival analysis* can be quite simple, requiring only two variables—the presence or absence of an event and the time it took for the event to occur. More complex versions of *survival analysis* examine the role several factors play in the timing of an event. Connell (2012) provides a comprehensive overview of survival statistics in prevention and intervention studies.

Of course, most psychological studies are not investigating a terminal life event, but rather may be interested in how much time it takes to get to a particular event. Examples include exploring the transition from casual drug use to injecting drugs such as opiates (Young & Havens, 2011), determining the likelihood of engaging in drug use (Henry, Thornberry, & Huizinga, 2009), examining the impact of health events on resilience (Morin, Galatzer-Levy, Maccallum, & Bonanno, 2017), and investigating the predictors of teenage motherhood (Meade, Kershaw, & Ickovics, 2008). When survival data is collected in these cases, it is often referred to as *time-to-event* data. Inherently, some individuals will reach the event (e.g., death, drug use), whereas other participants might continue past the point at which the final event data is collected (e.g., do not die, remain sober). In these situations, we do not know if or when they will reach the event in question. Consequently, data is incomplete and thus censored for those specific individuals.

Landau (2002) examined several 'conventional' statistical techniques used to examine *time-to-event* data (e.g., multiple regression, logistic regression, t-test, Mann-Whitney U). Each of the approaches was inappropriate due to the fact *time-to-event* data is typically positively skewed and, more importantly, these conventional analyses cannot handle censored data. According to Landau, the only means to properly examine censored data is by conducting a *survival analysis*.

In an excellent study, Armitage (2005) used *survival analysis* to examine whether the Theory of Planned Behavior (Ajzen, 1991) can be employed to predict the maintenance of physical activity. In addition, the study allowed Armitage to evaluate the cumulative effects of past behavior on future behavior with objective measures of behavior (versus self-reports). Armitage included variables from the Theory of Planned Behavior such as attitude, subjective norm, perceived behavioral control, and behavioral intention. All were measured on a 7-point scale at baseline and three months later at follow-up.

To examine this data, Armitage (2005) used descriptive statistics, univariate, and multivariate analyses. He also examined the uniformity of the attendance distribution using the ***Kolmogorov-Smirnov***

(K-S) statistic. This nonparametric measure is designed to compare a sample distribution against a flat (uniform) reference probability distribution. A statistically significant *K-S* statistic suggests that the observed pattern deviates from uniformity. To investigate the impact of past behavior on future behavior, Armitage employed a repeated measures analysis of variance with **Helmert contrasts**. The use of these specific contrasts enables the researcher to examine the mean of each categorical variable (e.g., current attendance) as compared to succeeding variables (e.g., subsequent attendance). However, the *survival analysis* he conducted is the primary focus for this chapter.

Armitage (2005) first calculated a **Kaplan–Meier survival curve** to demonstrate a reduction in survival rate over time (i.e., failure to continue the exercise program). The *Kaplan-Meier curve* is a visual representation of the probability of survival at a certain time plotted over a specific time period. Armitage found that a significant minority of people had their data censored, meaning they maintained their attendance over the full three-month study period. Armitage used Cox's (1972) **proportional hazard technique** to determine whether the planned behavior variables predicted survival rates. This technique allows the researcher to simultaneously examine the effect of several factors on the rate (i.e., hazard rate) of an event, such as survival, at a specific point in time. Armitage found that an increase in perceived behavioral control was associated with a significant reduction in the hazard rate (32%). Although not significant, an increase in behavioral intention also reduced the hazard rate (10%).

One limitation of the traditional *survival analysis* is the assumption that once an event is censored, it cannot happen again. This conclusion makes sense if the event is terminal (e.g., death) but might not reflect reality if the event is defined as, for example, a lapse in the exercise regimen—people often start and stop their exercise routine due to life's natural intrusions. To account for this possibility, Armitage (2005) conducted a repeatable events *survival analysis* by pooling observations so that each person had one censored interval but could also have a variety of uncensored intervals. This data manipulation allowed for the analysis of the planned behavior variables with a traditional Cox (1972) *proportional hazards model*. The analysis revealed that, similar to the traditional *survival analysis* results discussed earlier, increases in perceived behavioral intention significantly reduced the hazard rate by 29%. Although not statistically significant, an increase in behavioral intention reduced the hazard rate by 6%.

Armitage (2005) was one of the first researchers to examine the ability of the Theory of Planned Behavior to predict the maintenance of health behavior. The use of a *survival analysis* enabled Armitage to properly deal with the skewed nature of the data and, most importantly, the presence of censored events. Interestingly, Armitage was one of the first researchers to utilize a **repeatable events survival analysis** to examine health psychology data. To examine this data, Armitage pooled the recurrent observations and used the Cox (1972) *proportional hazard model*.

There is some uncertainty in the literature regarding the best approach to analyzing recurrent data within a *survival analysis*. Some researchers have continued to employ the *Cox proportional hazard model*. Others, like Thenmozhi, Jeyaseelan, Jeyaseelan, Isaac, and Vedantam (2019), have asserted that researchers using the *Cox proportional hazard model* with recurrent data are ignoring issues of autocorrelation—the assumption that recurrent events are correlated. Thenmozhi and colleagues examined the various methods for modeling recurrent event data. One model that stood out was the **Prentice-Williams-Peterson Counting Process Model** (**PWP CP**; Prentice, Williams, & Peterson, 1981). This approach analyzes recurrent data stratified by events by initially placing all at-risk participants in the first stratum, but only including those with an actual event in subsequent analyses. Not only was the *PWP CP* model statistically superior, it was also the right choice for their research question. This led Thenmozhi and colleagues to conclude that "the choice of an appropriate method for analyzing the recurrent event data should not be decided only on statistical basis but also based on the research question" (p. 253). However, the use of the *PWP CP* model has not been universally adopted.

Meta-Analytic Structural Equational Modeling

Separately, ***meta-analysis (MA)*** and ***structural equation modeling (SEM)*** have been used in psychological research for over 40 years (Card, 2017). Each of these statistical techniques has been influential in expanding our knowledge base in health psychology. Yet each of these techniques were also limited by methodological constraints. Recently, advances in computing power and the availability of more powerful statistical software platforms have made the merger of these two techniques possible. As a result, researchers are now able to better test more sophisticated models that match the complexity of health psychology behavior apparent in our everyday lives (Card, 2017).

The primary challenge in combining *MA* and *SEM* is the fact that each technique was built on a different foundation—distributions of correlations and covariance matrices, respectively (Cheung & Chan, 2005). Attempts to combine these statistical approaches began in the late 1980s and early 1990s, but were hampered by the lack of a uniformly accepted approach and limitations inherent in the statistical software available at the time (Schulze, 2007). Currently, the ***two-stage structural equation modeling*** (***TSSEM***; Cheung & Chan, 2005) approach to combining *MA* and *SEM* is the most well-accepted path to conducting *meta-analytic structural equational modeling* (*MASEM*). This approach provides a solid foundation for the analysis and addresses many of the issues associated with earlier attempts to marry these statistical techniques. See Cheung (2015a) for an overview of *MASEM*.

The first stage of the analysis involves the application of meta-analytic procedures to create correlation matrices associated with each construct from the model to be tested and then transforming this data into a pooled correlation matrix accounting for fixed or random effects. Most meta-analyses cast a large net to capture a wide variety of studies using different measures and, as such, the random effects model is typically used. Researchers typically report the homogeneity of the correlation matrices. In the second stage, the researcher uses the pooled correlation matrix and its asymptotic covariance matrix as an observed covariance matrix to determine if the data fits the proposed model using *SEM*. Cheung and Hong (2017) note that it is critical that the models to be tested are conducted a priori so that the analysis is a theory-driven approach (versus data driven). A ***weighted least squares (WLS)*** estimation method is then used to fit *structural equation models*. The *WLS* approach, also known as the asymptotically distribution free estimation method, allows the researcher to fit *structural equation models* with non-normal data (Cheung & Hong, 2017). After fitting the models, ***goodness-of-fit indices*** can be used to evaluate the degree to which the data fits the proposed model. These indices estimate the degree to which the hypothesized model can reproduce the data (usually the variance-covariance matrix). A model with a high degree of fit is one that is reasonably consistent with the data.

The free statistical package **R** is often used in *MASEM analyses*. This open-source statistical environment is built on a true computer language, which better enables users to customize *R* to meet needs as elementary as a *t*-test or complex as *MASEM* analyses. The *MASEM* package in *R* (Cheung, 2015b) has made it relatively simple to conduct the analysis. ***Macros*** are available to conduct the analysis in **SPSS**. Custom *macros* are 'mini-programs' created by statisticians to enable researchers to conduct specific analyses by simply adding the code to the normal syntax of SPSS. Unfortunately, most of the *MASEM macros* rely on univariate methods, which are less desirable in this analysis (Jak, 2015).

An excellent example of *MASEM* was conducted by Zhang, Zhang, Schwarzer, and Hagger (2019). They conducted a *MASEM* study to examine past studies which used the ***health action process approach*** (***HAPA***; Schwarzer, 2008) involving self-efficacy, intention, planning, and behavior. The *HAPA* approach to health behavior uses a social-cognitive model to identify the motivational and volitional determinants associated with healthy choices. The study examined the degree to which past studies fit the *HAPA* model; tested specific model predictions; explored the impact of past behavior; and tested moderators such as behavior type, sample type, measurement lag, and study quality.

Zhang, and colleagues (2019) preregistered the meta-analysis on the ***PROSPERO*** database of systematic reviews. *PROSPERO* is an international database in which researchers can prospectively (i.e., at inception) register their systematic reviews to promote transparency and avoid unplanned duplication. After registering the inclusion criteria, the researchers conducted the literature review using electronic databases and manual searches. The final set of 95 studies was then coded by type of behavior, sample type, lag between measures of *HAPA* constructs and health behavior, and study quality.

As is the case with most *MASEM* studies, analyses are typically conducted using the two-stage approach discussed earlier (Cheung & Chan, 2005). The authors also examined the potential effect of selective reporting bias using the ***precision effect test (PET)*** and the ***precision effect estimate with standard error (PEESE) estimator***. The *PET* test determines whether there is a nonzero true effect once publication bias is accounted for and corrected. The *PEESE* estimator provides a better estimate of the empirical effect when corrected for publication bias. Given the *PET* test demonstrated that effect sizes were statistically significant, the *PEESE* estimate was taken as the bias-adjusted effect size. This approach did not alter conclusions with respect to overall effect sizes.

Zhang, et al. (2019) tested two models (original and truncated) using *MASEM*. The results revealed that action self-efficacy had the biggest impact on health behavior via intentions and maintenance self-efficacy. Action planning and coping planning predicted health behavior and mediated the effects of intentions and maintenance self-efficacy on behavior. That said, the direct effect of intentions and maintenance self-efficacy on health behavior were very pronounced. Researchers discovered that the inclusion of past behavior weakened the relationship between intention and health behavior.

The study also investigated the impact of moderators such as cognition and behavior type, sample type, and measurement lag on health behaviors. The results revealed that the effects of action self-efficacy on intentions and behavior were more pronounced when physical activity was the target health behavior. Volitional self-efficacy had a bigger effect in samples focusing on dietary behavior. The other moderators did not lead to any appreciable effects.

Overall, results suggested that self-efficacy is an influential correlate of intentions and health behavior—although the effect itself is modest. The authors did note some caveats and suggestions for future work. Most notably, Zhang, et al. (2019) called for more experimental research using factorial designs examining *HAPA*. In addition, the researchers suggested that future studies should adopt statistical techniques (e.g., ***cross-lagged panel designs***), which would allow for the testing of specific directional and reciprocal effects among study variables.

MASEM can enable the researcher to investigate complex models within the field of health psychology. The processes and statistical tools to use this technique are now accessible—although *R* itself can take some time to master. There are still some areas which can be improved within *MASEM*. For example, Cheung and Hong (2017) note that employing analysis of covariance matrices in *MASEM* is more desirable than analysis of correlation matrices. However, covariation matrices do require that the measurement of study variables be identical in all studies used in the meta-analysis. This is rarely the case, although future studies may be able to develop a means to overcome this limitation. There has also been discussion on how to incorporate effect size heterogeneity into *MASEM*. This technique, labeled ***full information meta-analytical structural equation modeling*** (**FIMASEM**; Yu, Downes, Carter, & O'Boyle, 2016), has some advantages but also some limitations (Cheung, 2018; Yu, Downes, Carter, & O'Boyle, 2018).

Bayesian Statistics

Frequentist statistics have long dominated research in psychology. This approach involves establishing a null and alternative hypothesis, setting the significance level, analyzing the data using parametric statistics, determining the *p*-value, and then comparing the *p*-value to an agreed-upon minimum level for reporting purposes (Beard & West, 2017). However, a recent review of the literature found that the proportion of psychological articles using Bayesian analyses has steadily grown since 1990 (van de Schoot, Winter, Ryan, Zondervan-Zwijnenburg, & Depaoli, 2017). That said, many of the articles cited in van de Shoot and colleagues' analysis were either introducing the concept of Bayes-ian statistics or were simulation studies investigating the application of this approach under various conditions (e.g., different populations, missing data).

So, what are **Bayesian statistics**? For a complete discussion of Bayesian methods, see Feinberg and Gonzalez (2012), Hoff (2009), and Kaplan and Depaoli (2013). Essentially, much of the difference between the *frequentist* and *Bayesian* approach comes down to probability. The *frequentist* approach treats probability as the likelihood an event will happen under the same identical circumstances. Whereas Bayes's theorem states that probability is, in and of itself, a form of scientific knowledge that is based on previous knowledge and current experience. Consequently, *Bayesian statistics* allows for expert knowl-edge that exists prior to the observation of the data to be converted into what is referred to as a **prior probability distribution**. A *Bayesian* analysis works by combining this *prior probability distribution* with the results of contemporaneous data (collected in the current experiment) to create a revised probability distribution (**posterior probability**). Interestingly, the creation of the *posterior probability distribution* mirrors how subjective belief changes when someone encounters new data (Austin, Brunner, & Hux, 2002). Accordingly, this *posterior probability distribution* can be used as prior information in subsequent studies.

Researchers turn to *Bayesian* analyses for a variety of reasons. In their review of the use of *Bayes-ian statistics* in psychological research, van de Schoot, and colleagues (2017) found that researchers utilize this approach due to design limitations, computational problems with *WLS* estimation, or a desire for more accurate parameter estimates. Some researchers using regression analyses incorporate *Bayesian statistics* because they found it appealing to incorporate prior knowledge into the estimation process. Many researchers rely on *Bayesian* analyses to improve performance when they have small sample sizes.

Unfortunately, despite the benefits, there are relatively few empirical studies in the field of health psychology that use *Bayesian statistics* (Beard & West, 2017). To encourage more research using this technique, health psychology journals have been publishing articles designed to explain Bayesian methods in simple terms, provide simulation studies to walk researchers through the steps associated with *Bayesian* analyses, and offer statistical guides to conduct analyses (e.g., Depaoli, Rus, Clifton, van de Schoot, & Tiemensma, 2017).

An excellent recent study by Blashill, Goshe, Robbins, Mayer, and Safren (2014) published in *Health Psychology* used a **Bayesian approach to structural equation modeling (BSEM)** to investigate **body image disturbance (BID)** and health behaviors among sexual minority men living with the human immuno-deficiency virus (HIV). Blashill and colleagues noted that several factors influence the prevalence of *BID*. For example, there is evidence that **lipodystrophy**, in which the body is unable to produce and maintain healthy fat tissue, may contribute to *BID*. The degree to which individuals value the Western beauty ideal (i.e., appearance investment) may also perpetuate *BID*. The analysis was conducted to examine how *BID* affects **antiretroviral therapy (ART)** adherence and overall sexual health. According to Blashill and colleagues, some studies suggest depression may mediate the relationship between *BID* and poor adherence to *ART*. Other studies have noted that *BID* may affect condom use, resulting in risky sexual practices. The *BSEM* was designed to examine the relationship among these variables.

Participants were 106 sexual minority men living with HIV. All participants received a mea-sure of *BID* and *lipodystrophy* (Assessment of Body Change and Distress questionnaire–Short Form), appearance investment (Multidimensional Body–Self Relations Questionnaire), depression (Center for Epidemiological Studies–Depression), and condom use self-efficacy (Condom Use Self-Efficacy Scale). Participants were also given a questionnaire that assessed their *ART* adherence, HIV sexual transmission risk behavior, and body mass index.

The model was tested using *BSEM*. According to Muthén and Asparouhov (2012), this approach to *SEM* uses informative, small-variance *prior probability distributions* that reflect previous theories and the researcher's prior beliefs. As far as the output, the *BSEM* model produced two estimates of model adequacy—convergence (using the convergence statistic) and model fit (using the posterior predic-tive *p*-value). Effect size was calculated for each indirect effect.

The analyses revealed that the model tested using the *BSEM* approach fit this data well, with significance noted at each hypothesized pathway. Specifically, *lipodystrophy* and appearance investment were associated with elevated *BID*. *BID* predicted increased depressive symptoms and lowered condom use self-efficacy. Predictably, these mediators were associated with poor sexual health behaviors.

The study demonstrated the utility of applying Bayesian methods to complex statistical analyses such as *SEM*. Although the nature of the study precluded causal inferences, the authors thought, in some cases, it was plausible to assume directionality (e.g., *lipodystrophy* and appearance investment are more likely to be antecedents than consequences of *BID*). That said, a longitudinal design could be employed to address the possible confound of order and enable a conclusion of causality.

Overall Strengths and Limitations

Increasingly, technology has made it possible for researchers to investigate complex questions within the field of health psychology. For example, there has been a long history of researchers asking participants to record their thoughts, feelings, and/or behaviors at various times during the day using survey methods. However, these paper and pencil measures, which were the only options at the time, were not the most reliable measures. As technology has improved, researchers interested in using *EMA* within their research design have been able to upgrade from paper and pencil approaches to a smart phone, which coupled with various apps, can be used to collect biometric health data, deliver surveys, and record responses—all in real time. Plus, this data can often be remotely downloaded for later analysis.

Technological advancements in statistical software have greatly enhanced the ability of researchers to ask complex questions and employ the statistical techniques needed to address those questions. For example, statistical packages with a user-friendly, point-and-click interface such as *SPSS* and *SAS* have made it simple to run complex analyses such as **multivariate analysis of variance (MANOVA)** and **multivariate analysis of covariance (MANCOVA)**. Indeed, it is difficult to search for studies that employ these analyses, given these statistical techniques are no longer generally referenced in the abstract due to the ubiquity of these approaches—researchers only need to devise a proper design and collect enough participant data—*SPSS* will do the rest.

Several of the techniques discussed earlier in our discussion, such as *MASEM*, *survival analyses*, and *Bayesian statistics*, do require statistical packages that are more advanced. Fortunately, statistical software such as *R* is freely available and often the first choice among statisticians conducting research using these techniques. *R* is designed around a true computer language and allows users to define new functions. Consequently, statisticians interested in these more sophisticated analyses have been working together to develop statistical packages in *R* that can be used by any interested researcher. In addition, conferences (e.g., use*R*!) are available to assist researchers.

The increased use of *Bayesian statistics* is a welcome addition to the field of health psychology. Recently, the American Statistical Association (Wasserstein & Lazar, 2016) presented six principles for the proper use and interpretation of the *p*-value to reinforce good statistical practice and avoid practices such as '*p*-hacking' and 'data-dredging,' which involve reporting small *p*-values at the expense of scientific reasoning and replicability. Statisticians were encouraged to supplement or replace *p*-values with other approaches such as Bayesian methods.

Lastly, increased use of *n-of-1* studies allows researchers to explore whether an intervention or treatment approach would work for specific persons, families, or institutions. By using a person-centered approach, researchers can better understand how the relationship between the intervention, the treatment, and the person changes over time. If done properly, *n-of-1* designs can be as statistically and methodologically rigorous as your typical between-subjects *RCT*.

Although several notable strengths are associated with the implementation of these statistical approaches, there are some challenges. The biggest issue is the fact that many of the techniques discussed earlier are complicated. Adding to that issue is the fact that until recently there has not been a clear consensus as to the best approach for analyzing resultant data. As such, researchers need to spend time reading the literature and attending conference presentations and workshops devoted to these statistical techniques or packages (e.g., *R*). Fortunately, these resources are available and are cited throughout this chapter.

Another challenge is that some of the techniques discussed in the chapter are still not widely published in the field of health psychology (e.g., *Bayesian analyses*) or there is still some debate as to the proper approach for conducting the analysis (e.g., *n-of-1* studies). In addition, technology is rapidly advancing and as a result, equipment that was once cutting edge (e.g., *PDAs*) are now expensive paperweights. Researchers need to invest wisely and be prepared for the possibility that the equipment they are using will be obsolete in three to five years. Lastly, researchers must remember the fundamentals. Modecki and Mazza (2017) noted that although smart phones have made collecting *EMA* data relatively easy, it can still be a challenge to collect useful, reliable, and valid *EMA* data.

Recommendations for Future Research

Technological advances have increased our ability to conduct research in a manner that matches the complexity of the phenomena we are examining. Increased computing power, advances in statistical software (e.g., *R*), and the emergence of wearable technology to complement the ubiquity of smart phones has made collecting and analyzing data much easier. However, researchers still need to be cognizant that the data is only as good as the methods that were employed when the data was collected. Plus, the resultant conclusions might only be relevant to a small subsection of the population.

For example, Chang and Sue (2005) suggested that the current focus on achieving high internal validity, often at the expense of external validity, has introduced a bias in psychology. Specifically, the authors asserted that research in psychology has systematically excluded multicultural research. Fortunately, several of the statistical techniques discussed in this chapter can be used to increase external validity and highlight marginalized populations. For example, *n-of-1* studies and *Bayesian statistics* can make it easier for researchers to investigate small populations without feeling pressure to aggregate non-white populations to achieve internal validity.

Researchers also need to be aware of the hidden limitations associated with increased reliance on technology for data collection. For example, researchers can now harvest data from crowdsourcing websites (e.g., Amazon's Mechanical Turk), social media (e.g., Twitter), and web-based surveys (e.g., Social Psychology Network). Unfortunately, this data is often overly representative of participants from societies that are Western, educated, industrialized, rich, and democratic (WEIRD). In addition, according to Woolf and Hulsizer (2019), our focus on technological solutions to collecting data can leave out individuals who cannot participate due to limitations in literacy, language, socioeconomic status, and disability. We need to be careful how we use the technology at our disposal.

Undergraduate and graduate programs also need to increase student exposure to open-source statistical environments such as *R*. Although traditional statistical packages like *SPSS* and *SAS* may be appropriate for most statistical analyses, they are costly and are not as flexible as open-source programs such as *R*. Most importantly, many of the advanced statistical approaches discussed in this chapter are primarily conducted using *R*. That said, the main hurdle with *R* is the steep learning curve associated with working within the *R* environment. However, there are several free online resources (https://learningstatisticswithr.com/) and user conferences (use*R*!) that are very accessible.

Conclusion

The Biomedical Model of illness focuses on disease, infirmity, and treatment. Health psychology expands our understanding of well-being to include an emphasis on the whole person—physical, psychological, social—living within multicultural communities. This focus on not just treatment but also prevention and relevant interventions is key in meeting the demands of a changing world. In

2019, the United Nations estimated that one-fourth of the populations of both Europe and North America will be over the age of 65 by the year 2050—populations that can dramatically benefit from health psychology practice and interventions (United Nations, 2019). Additionally, increasing numbers of Americans are reporting rising levels of stress in their daily lives (APA, 2019). Moreover, the world continues to face the risk of potential pandemics due to diseases such as Ebola or novel viruses like COVID-19, which require behavior change of both those infected and exposed individuals and communities. Only through increased understanding of health-behavior interactions can we expect to meet the challenges of both today and tomorrow. Expanded research within health psychology is vital to the development of culturally appropriate, empirically valid interventions and treatments with both well and ill populations and communities.

References

Ajzen, I. (1991). The theory of planned behavior. *Organizational Behavior and Human Decision Processes*, *50*(2), 179–211. https://doi.org/10.1016/0749-5978(91)90020-T

American Psychological Association. (2019). *Stress in AmericaTM 2019*. Retrieved from www.apa.org/news/press/releases/stress/2019/stress-america-2019.pdf

American Psychological Association. (2020). *Health psychology*. Retrieved from www.apa.org/pubs/journals/hea/index?tab=3

Armitage, C. J. (2005). Can the theory of planned behavior predict the maintenance of physical activity? *Health Psychology*, *24*(3), 235–245. https://doi.org/10.1037/0278-6133.24.3.235

Austin, P. C., Brunner, L. J., & Hux, J. E. (2002). Bayeswatch: An overview of Bayesian statistics. *Journal of Evaluation in Clinical Practice*, *8*(2), 277–286. https://doi.org/10.1046/j.1365-2753.2002.00338.x

Beard, E., & West, R. (2017). Using Bayesian statistics in health psychology: A comment on Depaoli et al (2017). *Health Psychology Review*, *11*(3), 298–301. https://doi.org/10.1080/17437199.2017.1349544

Blashill, A. J., Goshe, B. M., Robbins, G. K., Mayer, K. H., & Safren, S. A. (2014). Body image disturbance and health behaviors among sexual minority men living with HIV. *Health Psychology*, *33*(7), 677–680. https://doi.org/10.1037/hea0000081

Brenner, L. A., Reid-Arndt, S. A., Elliott, T. R., Frank, R. G., & Caplan, B. (2019). *Handbook of rehabilitation psychology* (3rd ed., L. A. Brenner, S. A. Reid-Arndt, T. R. Elliott, R. G. Frank, & B. Caplan, Eds.). American Psychological Association. https://doi.org/10.1037/0000129-000

Card, N. A. (2017). Advances in meta-analysis methodologies contribute to advances in research accumulation: Comments on Cheung & Hong and Johnson et al. *Health Psychology Review*, *11*(3), 302–305. https://doi.org/10.1080/17437199.2017.1345646

Carver, C. S., & Scheier, M. F. (1982). Control theory: A useful conceptual framework for personality: Social, clinical, and health psychology. *Psychological Bulletin*, *92*(1), 111–135. https://doi.org/10.1037/0033-2909.92.1.111

Chang, J., & Sue, S. (2005). Culturally sensitive research: Where have we gone wrong and what do we need to do now? In M. G. Constantine & D. W. Sue (Eds.), *Strategies for building multicultural competence in mental health and educational settings* (pp. 229–246). Hoboken, NJ: John Wiley & Sons.

Cheung, M. W.-L. (2015a). *Meta-analysis: A structural equation modeling approach*. Wiley. https://doi.org/10.1002/9781118957813

Cheung, M. W.-L. (2015b). metaSEM: An R package for meta-analysis using structural equation modeling. *Frontiers in Psychology*, *5*, 1521. https://doi.org/10.3389/fpsyg.2014.01521

Cheung, M. W.-L. (2018). Issues in solving the problem of effect size heterogeneity in meta-analytic structural equation modeling: A commentary and simulation study on Yu, Downes, Carter, and O'Boyle (2016). *Journal of Applied Psychology*, *103*(7), 787–803. https://doi.org/10.1037/apl0000284

Cheung, M. W.-L., & Chan, W. (2005). Meta-analytic structural equation modeling: A two-stage approach. *Psychological Methods*, *10*(1), 40–64. https://doi.org/10.1037/1082-989X.10.1.40

Cheung, M. W.-L., & Hong, R. Y. (2017). Applications of meta-analytic structural equation modelling in health psychology: Examples, issues, and recommendations. *Health Psychology Review*, *11*(3), 265–279. https://doi.org/10.1080/17437199.2017.1343678

Connell, C. M. (2012). Survival analysis in prevention and intervention programs. In L. Jason & D. Glenwick (Eds.), *Methodological approaches to community-based research* (pp. 147–164). American Psychological Association. https://doi.org/10.1037/13492-009

Cox, D. R. (1972). Regression models and life tables. *Journal of the Royal Statistical Society: Series B, 34*, 187–202. https://doi.org/10.1111/j.2517-6161.1972.tb00899.x

Depaoli, S., Rus, H. M., Clifton, J. P., van de Schoot, R., & Tiemensma, J. (2017). An introduction to Bayesian statistics in health psychology. *Health Psychology Review, 11*(3), 248–264. https://doi.org/10.1080/1743719 9.2017.1343676

Feinberg, F. M., & Gonzalez, R. (2012). Bayesian modeling for psychologists: An applied approach. In *APA handbook of research methods in psychology. Vol 2: Research designs: Quantitative, qualitative, neuropsychological, and biological* (pp. 445–464). American Psychological Association. https://doi.org/10.1037/13620-024

Gardner, W., & Griffin, W. A. (1989). Methods for the analysis of parallel streams of continuously recorded social behaviors. *Psychological Bulletin, 105*(3), 446–455. https://doi.org/10.1037/0033-2909.105.3.446

Graham, H., Howard, K. J., & Dougall, A. L. (2012). The growth of occupational health psychology. In R. J. Gatchel & I. Z. Schultz (Eds.), *Handbook of occupational health and wellness* (pp. 39–59). Springer Science + Business Media. https://doi.org/10.1007/978-1-4614-4839-6_3

Griffin, W. A., & Gardner, W. (1989). Analysis of behavioral durations in observational studies of social interaction. *Psychological Bulletin, 106*(3), 497–502. https://doi.org/10.1037/0033-2909.106.3.497

Henry, K. L., Thornberry, T. P., & Huizinga, D. H. (2009). A discrete-time survival analysis of the relationship between truancy and the onset of marijuana use. *Journal of Studies on Alcohol and Drugs, 70*(1), 5–15. https://doi.org/10.15288/jsad.2009.70.5

Hilton, C. E., & Johnston, L. H. (2017). Health psychology: It's not what you do, it's the way that you do it. *Health Psychology Open, 4*(2). https://journals.sagepub.com/doi/10.1177/2055102917714910

Hobbs, N., Dixon, D., Johnston, M., & Howie, K. (2013). Can the theory of planned behaviour predict the physical activity behaviour of individuals? *Psychology & Health, 28*(3), 234–249. https://doi.org/10.1080/08 870446.2012.716838

Hoff, P. D. (2009). *A first course in Bayesian statistical methods.* Springer. https://doi.org/10.1111/j.1751-5823. 2010.00109_17.x

Jak, S. (2015). *Meta-analytic structural equation modeling.* Springer. https://doi.org/10.1007/978-3-319-27174-3

Kaplan, D., & Depaoli, S. (2013). Bayesian statistical methods. In T. D. Little (Ed.), *The Oxford handbook of quantitative methods (Vol. 1): Foundations* (pp. 407–437). Oxford, UK: Oxford University Press. https://doi.org/10.1093/oxfordhb/9780199934874.013.0020

Kaplan, R. M. (2009). Health psychology: Where are we and where do we go from here? *Mens Sana Monographs, 7*(1), 3–9. https://doi.org/10.4103/0973-1229.43584

Kwasnicka, D., Dombrowski, S. U., White, M., & Sniehotta, F. F. (2017). N-of-1 study of weight loss maintenance assessing predictors of physical activity, adherence to weight loss plan and weight change. *Psychology & Health, 32*(6), 686–708. https://doi.org/10.1080/08870446.2017.1293057

Kwasnicka, D., Inauen, J., Nieuwenboom, W., Nurmi, J., Schneider, A., Short, C. E., et al. (2019). Challenges and solutions for N-of-1 design studies in health psychology. *Health Psychology Review, 13*(2), 163–178. https://doi.org/10.1080/17437199.2018.1564627

Kwasnicka, D., & Naughton, F. (2020, March). N-of-1 methods: A practical guide to exploring trajectories of behaviour change and designing precision behaviour change interventions. *Psychology of Sport and Exercise, 47.* https://doi.org/10.1016/j.psychsport.2019.101570

Landau, S. (2002). Using survival analysis in psychology. *Understanding Statistics, 1*(4), 233–270. https://doi.org/10.1207/S15328031US0104_03

Litt, M. D., Cooney, N. L., & Morse, P. (1998). Ecological Momentary Assessment (EMA) with treated alcoholics: Methodological problems and potential solutions. *Health Psychology, 17*(1), 48–52. https://doi.org/10.1037/0278-6133.17.1.48

McDonald, S., Quinn, F., Vieira, R., O'Brien, N., White, M., Johnston, D. W., et al. (2017). The state of the art and future opportunities for using longitudinal n-of-1 methods in health behaviour research: A systematic literature overview. *Health Psychology Review, 11*(4), 307–323. https://doi.org/10.1080/17437199.2017.1316672

Meade, C. S., Kershaw, T. S., & Ickovics, J. R. (2008). The intergenerational cycle of teenage motherhood: An ecological approach. *Health Psychology, 27*(4), 419–429. https://doi.org/10.1037/0278-6133.27.4.419

Modecki, K. L., & Mazza, G. L. (2017). Are we making the most of ecological momentary assessment data? A comment on Richardson, Fuller-Tyszkiewicz, O'Donnell, Ling, & Staiger, 2017. *Health Psychology Review, 11*(3), 295–297. https://doi.org/10.1080/17437199.2017.1347513

Morin, R. T., Galatzer-Levy, I. R., Maccallum, F., & Bonanno, G. A. (2017). Do multiple health events reduce resilience when compared with single events? *Health Psychology, 36*(8), 721–728. https://doi.org/10.1037/hea0000481

Muthén, B., & Asparouhov, T. (2012). Bayesian structural equation modeling: A more flexible representation of substantive theory. *Psychological Methods, 17*(3), 313–335. https://doi.org/10.1037/a0026802

Nock, M. K., Prinstein, M. J., & Sterba, S. K. (2009). Revealing the form and function of self-injurious thoughts and behaviors: A real-time ecological assessment study among adolescents and young adults. *Psychology of Violence*, *1*(S), 36–52. https://doi.org/10.1037/2152-0828.1.S.36

Prentice, R. L., Williams, B. J., & Peterson, A. V. (1981). On the regression analysis of multivariate failure time data. *Biometrika*, *68*(2), 373–379. https://doi.org/10.1093/biomet/68.2.373

Ram, N., Brinberg, M., Pincus, A. L., & Conroy, D. E. (2017). The questionable ecological validity of ecological momentary assessment: Considerations for design and analysis. *Research in Human Development*, *14*(3), 253–270. https://doi.org/10.1080/15427609.2017.1340052

Richardson, B., Fuller-Tyszkiewicz, M., O'Donnell, R., Ling, M., & Staiger, P. K. (2017). Regression tree analysis of ecological momentary assessment data. *Health Psychology Review*, *11*(3), 235–241. https://doi.org/10.1080/17437199.2017.1343677

Sandhu, H., & Patel, S. (2013). The rapid growth of health psychology in medical schools and clinical practice. In M. Forshaw & D. Sheffield (Eds.), *Health psychology in action* (pp. 183–194). Wiley-Blackwell. https://doi.org/10.1002/9781119943280.ch17

Schulze, R. (2007). Current methods for meta-analysis: Approaches, issues, and developments. *Zeitschrift Für Psychologie/Journal of Psychology*, *215*(2), 90–103. https://doi.org/10.1027/0044-3409.215.2.90

Schwartz, J. E., & Stone, A. A. (1998). Strategies for analyzing ecological momentary assessment data. *Health Psychology*, *17*(1), 6–16. https://doi.org/10.1037/0278-6133.17.1.6

Schwarzer, R. (2008). Modeling health behavior change: How to predict and modify the adoption and maintenance of health behaviors. *Applied Psychology: An International Review*, *57*(1), 1–29. https://doi.org/10.1111/j.1464-0597.2007.00325.x

Shiffman, S., & Stone, A. A. (1998). Introduction to the special section: Ecological momentary assessment in health psychology. *Health Psychology*, *17*(1), 3–5. https://doi.org/10.1037/h0092706

Shiffman, S., Stone, A. A., & Hufford, M. R. (2008). Ecological momentary assessment. *Annual Review of Clinical Psychology*, *4*, 1–32. https://doi.org/10.1146/annurev.clinpsy.3.022806.091415

Smith, T. W., Williams, P. G., & Ruiz, J. M. (2016). Clinical health psychology. In J. C. Norcross, G. R. VandenBos, D. K. Freedheim, & M. M. Domenech Rodríguez (Eds.), *APA handbook of clinical psychology: Roots and branches* (Vol. 1, pp. 223–257). American Psychological Association. https://doi.org/10.1037/14772-012

Sniehotta, F. F., Presseau, J., Hobbs, N., & Araújo-Soares, V. (2012). Testing self-regulation interventions to increase walking using factorial randomized N-of-1 trials. *Health Psychology*, *31*(6), 733–737. https://doi.org/10.1037/a0027337

Thenmozhi, M., Jeyaseelan, V., Jeyaseelan, L., Isaac, R., & Vedantam, R. (2019). Survival analysis in longitudinal studies for recurrent events: Applications and challenges. *Clinical Epidemiology and Global Health*, *7*(2), 253–260. https://doi.org/10.1016/j.cegh.2019.01.013

United Nations. (2019). *Aging*. Retrieved from www.un.org/en/sections/issues-depth/ageing/

van de Schoot, R., Winter, S. D., Ryan, O., Zondervan-Zwijnenburg, M., & Depaoli, S. (2017). A systematic review of Bayesian articles in psychology: The last 25 years. *Psychological Methods*, *22*(2), 217–239. https://doi.org/10.1037/met0000100

Vieira, R., McDonald, S., Araújo-Soares, V., Sniehotta, F. F., & Henderson, R. (2017). Dynamic modelling of n-of-1 data: Powerful and flexible data analytics applied to individualised studies. *Health Psychology Review*, *11*(3), 222–234. https://doi.org/10.1080/17437199.2017.1343680

Wasserstein, R. L., & Lazar, N. A. (2016). The ASA statement on *p*-values: Context, process, and purpose. *The American Statistician*, *70*(2), 129–133. https://doi.org/10.1080/00031305.2016.1154108

Woolf, L. M., & Hulsizer, M. R. (2019). Infusing diversity into research methods = good science. In K. D. Keith (Ed.), *Cross-cultural psychology: Contemporary themes and perspectives* (2nd ed., pp. 107–127). Wiley-Blackwell. https://doi.org/10.1002/9781119519348.ch6

Young, A. M., & Havens, J. R. (2012). Transition from first illicit drug use to first injection drug use among rural Appalachian drug users: A cross-sectional comparison and retrospective survival analysis. *Addiction*, *107*(3), 587–596. https://doi.org/10.1111/j.1360-0443.2011.03635.x

Yu, J. (Joya), Downes, P. E., Carter, K. M., & O'Boyle, E. H. (2016). The problem of effect size heterogeneity in meta-analytic structural equation modeling. *Journal of Applied Psychology*, *101*(10), 1457–1473. https://doi.org/10.1037/apl0000141

Yu, J., Downes, P. E., Carter, K. M., & O'Boyle, E. H. (2018). The heterogeneity problem in meta-analytic structural equation modeling (MASEM) revisited: A reply to Cheung. *Journal of Applied Psychology*, *103*(7), 804–811. https://doi.org/10.1037/apl0000328

Zhang, C.-Q., Zhang, R., Schwarzer, R., & Hagger, M. S. (2019). A meta-analysis of the health action process approach. *Health Psychology*, *38*(7), 623–637. https://doi.org/10.1037/hea0000728

3

"THE CIRCLING SPIRITS CALL US HOME": MARGINAL METHODS, THE SHAMAN, AND RELATIONAL APPROACHES TO HEALING RESEARCH

Joseph E. Trimble

Overview

The title of this chapter, "The Circling Spirits Call Us Home," refers to the calling many social science researchers and traditional indigenous healers "hear" to follow their respective practices. Many researchers and traditional healers alike will tell you they felt called to their practices, and following very different paths, they answered their callings. Those scholars and researchers who are drawn to spend time with traditional healers in order to study their ways often find themselves struggling at the edge of their mainstream disciplines. To fulfill their research goals, they must quickly learn to understand and cope with life in the context of a cultural group living on the margins of the mainstream's lifeways and thoughtways. However, most conventional investigators will find the study of traditional healers within these settings stretches their tools and their credibility in ways they never anticipated.

Though the work is challenging, and unpredictable, numerous scientific discoveries and accomplishments come from curious researchers who place themselves at the edge of their fields of inquiry. Science cannot advance rapidly, or at all, with the monotonous repetition of conventional methods and wisdom. Science grows and prospers only when we afford investigators the opportunity to take a topic to the edge of existing knowledge. With this in mind, the following chapter will explore approaches, procedures, and methods that support research into the heart of the lifeways and thoughtways of indigenous people and their communities, with considerations for mainstream health researchers and providers.

The ways traditional indigenous people relate to life are often very different from those who hold Western worldviews. Traditional indigenous healers embrace and practice the deep meaning and influence of spirit, the sacred, and the meaning of place in all relationships. Knowledge of these traditional ways simply cannot be obtained through the scientific grid.

Primary among traditional indigenous communities is the belief that the sacred, the spirit, and spirituality are omniscient, omnipresent, and omnipotent; this belief is indisputable and unassailable. Yet these deeply held beliefs are not without those in the scientific community who criticize them for their seemingly animalistic qualities; their ethereal, mystical fundamentals; and their lack of demonstrable empirical evidence. Frequently hidden from the view of outsiders, traditional belief systems and practices are a prime source for explanations of various experiences ranging from the occurrence of natural phenomena to the cause and treatment of physical and psychological conditions.

To illustrate these points, let me present a personal story: Four decades ago three of my close American Indian friends and I, fresh with PhDs in our pockets and fully trained in the current Western ways to conduct mental health protocols with cross-cultural clients, spent a few days in a traditional lodge in a remote area of South Dakota. Two Native healers, holy men, accompanied us. The healers had extended us the invitation to be with them because they wanted us to hear their stories. We understood we were there to learn about their ways of healing, along with the traditions, ceremonies, and customs of their world. Through one story after another, the healers thoroughly engaged us in the deep mysteries of many traditional practices we had heard about over the years, but we had little knowledge of their deeper historical meaning. During the day, we walked the area outside the lodge alone or gathered in groups talking, reflecting, and deeply probing the wisdom unfolding in the stories we were hearing. With community members joining us on the chilly evenings, we prepared and cooked meals together in the lodge, a small fire always burning at its center.

On the morning of our last day together, the healers asked us to explain how we psychologists provided "healing" for those in need. The clinical psychologist in our group, who had considerable experience working in mental health settings focused on providing services for different multicultural clients, described the usual Western counseling methodology: how the client signed up for a session, some of what took place in the first and subsequent sessions, how the "counseling" unfolded, and what generally happened in each session. Another friend added a few features of the relationship between the mental health helper and the client. The healers listened intently, though often with puzzled expressions.

Following our detailed descriptions, the healers began to ask the following questions: Do you personally know the clients? Why do they have an appointment with you for an hour each week? Do they always show up? Why do you talk and talk with them and they with you? How do you know you helped or healed them? Do you ever see them again? Does the talking occur in a sacred place? Do you ask the spirits to help you as you talk with them? Do spirits sometimes come into the room where you are sitting? Why do you sit when the two of you talk? Why aren't others present when you talk with one another? Do you ask their ancestors to join you? Is the room where you are sitting clean and clear of evil spirits? Are both of you clean and clear of anything bad that may interfere with the talking and healing? Do the clients prepare for each meeting by sweating, praying, meditating, and fasting? Do counselors also prepare this way for each meeting with the client? Why do you take notes? What happens to the two of you after the client is healed?

We attempted to answer each of their surprising questions. With each response, we focused more on what we were saying to them and the possibility their questions were more profoundly meaningful and appropriate than we realized. On that day, we could not ignore that conventional counseling and psychotherapy were a very long way from including the spiritual, the sacred, or the meaning of place in their healing practices. We also began to consider the real possibility that centuries-old traditional healing practices were as powerful, maybe even more so, than contemporary approaches to physical and mental health.

Research in Practice

The Shaman's Place Today

While faith healers in one form or another can be found in nearly all cultures, their current status within indigenous groups captures considerable attention. Medicine men or women or, preferably, **shaman**, are a deep and integral part of contemporary indigenous cultures. People believe in their powers and generally will seek them out before the services of modern medicine. Similarly, many communities view their *shaman* as reservoirs of their ancestral ways, treat discussions about their practices and beliefs with utmost secrecy, and ward off attempts to exploit or research the holy person and their practice. Native people fear the *shaman's* wrath in the face of personal exploitation and injustices, and community members avoid the fact or appearance of either. So important is the *shaman's* presence that some communities view them as the organizational core of the community; they appear at and sometimes oversee the community's activities, festivals, ceremonies, and religious affairs.

Shamans provide a major function in indigenous communities. In the strict sense, they are not leaders politically or traditionally. And yet because of who they are and what they do, *shaman* serve to unify kinship relations, clans, and in some cases, entire villages. The power attributed to them usually surpasses that of the village council, local physicians, and other local aficionados. The *shaman's* gifts and power defy comprehension in conventional terms; their power is spiritually based and, hence, viewed with respect and awe by those they serve. Moreover, *shaman* firmly believe that everything is connected to everything else. Spiritual, physical, psychological, physiological, and health-related aspects of existence are seen as interconnected and inseparable (Rosensweig, 1992). The person and their situations are viewed through a holistic lens.

Marginality: At the Edge of Mainstream Norms

Shaman generally are viewed as "marginal" people by social scientists. Marginality is a term used to denote the effects of being excluded from the mainstream of a society on an individual or group level. In the words of Everett Stonequist (1937), marginal people are those whose "fate has condemned (them) to live in two societies and in two, not merely different, but antagonistic cultures" (p. 5). For most indigenous communities, *shaman* stand as symbols of their traditions and customs and yet are generally able to live and adjust to the demands of sociocultural change imposed by the dominant culture. The contemporary status of the *shaman* holds enduring fascination for many scholars. My particular interest is twofold, stemming from my long-term personal experiences and my recent interest in investigating the resilient social-psychological characteristics of *shaman* and shamanic practice. The former presents little or no problem simply because of its personal nature for me; the latter, quite the contrary, introduces and presents numerous challenges for social science researchers and our work.

Typically, social and clinical psychological studies of *shaman* are viewed as marginal by many mainstream social scientists. First, the investigator must rely on personal documents, personal testimonies, and other sources of biographic or autobiographic material in order to piece together a useful database. The more "hard-core" purists of the behavioral and social sciences view such techniques as biased, unverifiable, and suspect. Second, the investigator's efforts are often viewed as suspect not only by colleagues but also by the *shaman's* community and kinship network. The suspicion may be even more intense when the investigator is native to the community or of a recognizable indigenous background. And finally, there is the lens through which "outsiders" view the *shaman*, creating diagnoses such as anomic depressive, paranoid schizophrenic, or "crazy witch doctor" to characterize the *shaman* as an old indigenous person who lives in a dream world and practices magic. In short, shamanic studies may involve the use of marginal methods by investigators who are seen as marginal researchers of people who themselves maintain a marginal lifestyle.

Stonequist (1937) introduced the concept of "the marginal man" to the social science field some 80 years ago. Basically, he viewed the "marginal man" as a person caught between two somewhat incompatible sociocultural positions. As a result of being on the edge of both societies and not fully accepted by either, the "marginal" person may develop a distinct personality style. Descriptions of these marginal persons are hardly flattering, for they often are labeled as irrational, excessively concerned about racial identity, hostile towards others, and prone to psychological stress, including feelings of powerlessness, inferiority, and hopelessness. While Stonequist's characterizations predict a grim outcome for those who are bicultural, he offers a glimmer of optimism. He, and later Park (1950), argued that marginal people can emerge as social critics and often respond more creatively to social situations than persons from homogeneous backgrounds. In some instances, marginal people are at the forefront of social change, leading social movements designed to challenge the structure that led to their inferior status.

Studies of the "marginal man" concept have progressed slowly. Several tend to emphasize the negative characteristics of one's marginal status and the poor decision outcomes of people "caught between two conflicting reference groups" (Sherif & Sherif, 1956, p. 635). Summaries of several studies conclude biracial persons residing in predominantly racist societies do express different personality characteristics (cf. Starr & Roberts, 1982). Mann (1958), in particular, argues the negative characteristics postulated by the Stonequist–Park theory actually emerge from the individual being denied access to something that is an inalienable right to everyone else except them. However, simply being biracial, Mann goes on to add, is hardly sufficient cause for the negative characteristics to emerge.

A few researchers have explored the situations in which marginal persons occasionally find themselves. Goldberg (1941), for example, makes a distinction between "marginal cultures" and "personal marginality." He argues that a particular culture may have marginal status within a more dominant one, but the people may not develop the classic personality characteristics found by other researchers. Some indigenous communities are marginal cultures, meaning they have minority status, and yet community members can be healthy, fully functioning, competent people.

Few researchers picked up on Goldberg's promising thesis. A survey of the literature reveals much of the work in this area leans to the negative side of marginal experiences. That marginal people experience the struggle of adjusting to a bicultural world is fairly well documented, but there is another point to consider: One can instead view the marginality experience as a spectrum that includes the positive experiences of bicultural, marginal persons who manage to coexist effectively in a heterogeneous society.

Marginal Methods

Typically, studies of individuals are treated as biographies but can differ in terms of the approaches taken to explore a person's life. Analytic case studies and the ethogenic approach outlined by De Waele and Harré (1979) are certainly acceptable research procedures. Similarly, the classic work of Gordon Allport in 1940 on the use of personal documents stands as a valuable resource for biographic and assisted autobiographic research (Smith, Harre, & Van Langenhove, 1995). Whatever the procedure, however, the database produced by biographic research is viewed in psychology with a good deal of skepticism, largely because of its highly subjective nature. On the other hand, ethnobiographic research seems to carry a lot of credibility in other fields, particularly anthropology and history (Sodderqvist, 1991; Olney, 1980).

Historical Biographic Studies of Shaman

Over the years, biographic studies of *shaman* have been the province of anthropology and focused for the most part on the more prominent individuals among certain North American Indian groups. Most of the accounts are essentially descriptive life histories of the person as he or she lived it. Edward Sapir's (1921) work on *The Life of a Nootka Indian*, for instance, touches on the significant portions of a certain man's life. *Sun Chief*, an assisted autobiography by Leo Simmons (1942), traced the growth and development of a Hopi *shaman* but cast the portrayal as a symbol of the tribe's folkways.

Some anthropologists have taken on the added task of providing a detailed analysis of a *shaman's* character. Most notable is the classic work by Leighton and Leighton (1949) of Gregorio, a Navajo hand-trembler. In their work, they present a life chart showing not only sequences of Gregorio life but also the significant events surrounding the major changes in his life. They argue the validity of this research because the major concerns of the hand-trembler's life adequately represented those of other Navajos living in the same area of the reservation.

The anthropologist-historian Nancy Oestreich Lurie (1961) in her guided autobiography of the Winnebago Mountain Wolf Woman departed little from the conventional life history approach. Her slight departure from the method produced a good analysis of Winnebago sex role relationships and their attitudes towards non-Indians. She also provides a nice analysis of Mountain Wolf Woman's relationship with her brother Crashing Thunder, the subject of yet another life history by Paul Radin (1926).

In her biography of a Yaqui woman Jane Holden Kelley (1978) emphasizes the relationship between the individual and the forces of the changing sociocultural system. She blends together a description of the influential factors affecting the adaptive strategies used by Yaqui women, sparked with some interpretation and analysis.

Psychology emphasizes the study of affect, behavior, and cognition and promotes objectivity in that endeavor. Behavioral accounts of the life of *shaman* can be strictly objective descriptions, but then the meaning behind the *shaman's* actions lures investigators into some form of analysis. At this point, they depart from objectivity to subjectively assess a behavior's meaning, and in so doing become vulnerable to criticism from empiricists and supposedly objective purists.

Many, and I include myself here, maintain it is appropriate to explore the study of the *shaman's* behavior from a social psychological perspective. The following summary of a Pacific Northwest coast *shaman* places emphasis on the marginal nature of the research process when working under the special circumstances associated with marginal indigenous communities.

Ethnocultural Researchers

Critics of biographical research often stereotype researchers as "voyeurs," whose interest in the preoccupations of their subjects holds an enduring fascination above and beyond their hosts' mundane experiences of general living. In anthropology, many who have spent a good deal of their careers recording the life histories of their respondents are seen as reclusive, loners, impractical, and, yes, frustrated clinicians. Further, as Langness and Frank (1978) remind us, "the field worker may well come to the conclusion that attempting life histories is not worth the cost in time or in rapport" (p. 19). The price one has to pay for the sojourn in a seemingly exotic region of the world—New Guinea, for instance—may indeed outweigh the presumed professional and scientific gains one might achieve there.

The anthropologist Morris Freilich (1970) sees the field worker/biographer as a marginal native. He states, "regardless of time, place or people present, he almost invariably ('comes on') as marginal to society" (p. vii). Apart from the perceptions of family members and society in general, social science views the ethnographer as "an object of ambivalent feelings" whose theories are grounded more in descriptions of behaviors rather than quantifications of scaled responses or conventional measures of psychological constructs.

Freilich (1970) describes his experiences among the Mohawk Indian community in Brooklyn as indicative of his own "marginal status." In an effort to capture in-depth profiles of Mohawk steel workers, he actively participated in the rigors of Indian barroom drinking, weekend sojourns to reservations, etc., to establish the much-needed rapport with the community. He accomplished his goals, but not without the pains of feeling rejected, insulted, and generally abused.

Then there is the matter of a social psychologist taking on ethnographic biographical research. In some instances, ignorant of what is to come; one may choose the marginal status and thus endure the criticisms, suspicions, and doubt that can arise. An ethnographic research venture is not straight-forward, as it does not lend itself to the requirements of laboratory-controlled studies. Consequently, there are critics, the guardians of pure empiricism, and the skeptics who question the validity and reliability of the healer's stories and the testimonies of community members.

Conventional biographic methods typically produce "soft" data. It is this soft data that places investigators in a position for their research to be dismissed. However, advances in field-based and ethnographic studies and approaches have generated reliable procedures for conducting biographic and life history research (Denzin & Lincoln, 2018). Gordon Allport (1940) gave us a good start, but we need more than mere personal documents. In seeking alternative and perhaps more productive research techniques, we may find ourselves at the edge of the research enterprise. The ethogenic approach, or more colloquially the "Brussels Method" proposed by De Waele and Harré (1979), is a promising approach to biographic studies. It is complicated, time consuming, costly, and produces an enormous amount of data. According to Harré (1979, 1983) ethogenic psychology is a research approach where the significance of one's actions and their identities is linked to the larger structure of societal norms and cultural resources.

. . . And Now Shadow Walker

In defense of "soft" data, I include here an ethno-biographical research account of a collaboration I personally experienced with a local *shaman*. Years ago, a request was made of me to document the life and times of a local healer by his family. The respondent in this instance was a local traditional *shaman* I knew as Thomas, also known as Shadow Walker. My anthropologist friends strongly urged that I accept the request, while my psychologist acquaintances offered little more than caution. There also were the opinions of the local indigenous community to consider: "You shouldn't write about Shadow Walker's experiences and practices; the white man has no business knowing about our spiritual ways and our medicine men," one vocal kin of the healer's family told me. Another pointed out I had an obligation to keep silent about my personal experiences with the spirits and the spirit-bound ceremonies of the tribe because discussing the life of a traditional spirit healer could, the elder reminded me, bring evil upon my family and me. Add to these opinions and warnings the key family members of the *shaman* who, seemingly oblivious to the concerns of the others, kept asking when I was going to begin my project for them.

As a social psychological researcher in this context, I found myself in a uniquely marginal position. I recognized the value of the research I was being asked to do for its historical and anthropological contributions, but I wondered about the status of the work in the domain of multicultural psychology. Another concern centered on what kind of personal contribution I would be making to the regional community of Shadow Walker. A little background may clarify the nature of my dilemma.

Thomas was 81 years of age when I met him and had lived much of his life in the upper tier area of the Cascade Mountains in the Pacific Northwest of the United States. He spoke Spanish and the local tribal language and was considered by many local people to be the last "true" spirit healer. He had survived the rigors of immigration and resettlement and the harsh, abrupt changes imposed upon marginalized people of his age. In spite of these hardships, he remained a symbol of the past and present-day traditional spiritual practices.

Thomas's grandfather gave him the name Shadow Walker. According to family legend, at an early age Thomas often would stand or sit in the shadows of trees or large bushes. When the shadows faded or disappeared, Thomas would then tell stories about the plants and how they experienced their lives in the forests. He told his family and friends he could feel and know what the plants were feeling and knowing. Later in life, Thomas was able to stand in the shadows of people and feel as though he was one with them in body, soul, and spirit. If they were experiencing pain, sorrow, sadness, joy, happiness, or love, he would experience those emotions with them. He began to use the knowledge he gained from walking in others' shadows to heal them from discomfort and pain, whether physical or emotional.

There are not enough descriptors to adequately describe Thomas's character, but humility, generosity, kindness, empathy, strength, and integrity are a few. He was deeply spiritual; he believed, as most indigenous people do, in the omnipresence and omnipotence of the spirit world. As a *shaman*, through singing, dancing, and prayer Thomas was able to communicate with and harness the power of the spirit world and the supernatural. *Shaman*, according to the anthropologist Pamela Amoss (1978), "have the gift of the eye (and) are the only ones who can see the soul" (p. 46). When a person loses or fears loss of soul, which is believed to weaken the individual and leave them vulnerable to mental and physical illness, the *shaman* "examines" the person in an effort to determine if indeed soul loss has occurred and, if so, where the soul went. The *shaman* then works to bring the soul part back and reunite it with the individual, thereby creating an environment most conducive to the "patient's" physical or mental healing.

Some *shamans*, especially Thomas, not only are able to fend off soul loss but also can recover lost objects, effectively communicate with the dead, "cure" people with afflictions based on emotional disorders and relieve bodily pains and infections. On any given day, numbers of people could be found at his home on the mountain seeking help for a personal or spiritual problem. These requests are in no way small, for the healing procedures require the presence of a few drummers and singers and take hours to several days to complete. Drummers and singers are paid by the "patient," but Thomas himself received little in the way of monetary compensation. Instead, gifts of appreciation are traditional and were commonly given to him.

Like many *shamans*, Thomas would ask the person seeking his assistance to fast for a few days, pray, and avoid negative activities and people. On the day of the healing Thomas and his helpers would cleanse and smudge the small community lodge with herbs, the leaves and bark of sacred trees, dried and ground-up special plants known only to Thomas, and the resin incense of medicinal trees. Often Thomas would have the person seeking help and those supporting him or her drink an herbal tea. Thomas would then ask the person seeking help to sit in the center of the lodge. A colorful woolen blanket would be draped over his or her shoulders. Thomas then sat across from the person, and singers and drummers would surround them in a circle, their number varying depending on their availability. Family, friends, and invited guests would be seated outside this inner circle.

Following the singing and drumming, Thomas would go into a deep trance, during which silence was maintained in the lodge. While in the trance state, Thomas often quivered and shook for short periods. The length of his time in trance varied from client to client. He could be in a trance for several minutes to several hours. Once he regained consciousness, he would begin "working" on the client. He might very gently rub or wave his hands over their head, shoulders, back, hips, and legs. After "working" on the person for a time, he again would go into a trance state. This trance and rubdown routine might be cycled through several times during a healing session; in the course of a day Thomas could repeat the cycle as many as five or six times. If the day's healing practices did not bring a resolution for the person, Thomas would end the day with songs and prayers. The complete healing ceremony would begin again the following day. The ceremony eventually ended when Thomas declared the person "cured" or "healed." A celebratory meal would then follow, and expressions of gratitude shared with Thomas, the family, and the attendees, all of whom are vital to a successful healing. The spirits, too, would be generously praised and thanked for their presence and help.

As an observer, I found it difficult to maintain my "sense of objectivity" at these healing ceremonies, for they created a deeply affecting atmosphere. The drumming and singing resonated with me to the extent that I felt connected as one with the people and everything unfolding in the lodge. Other researchers who have collaborated with traditional healers and *shaman* recount similar experiences. The accuracy of one's later accounts of such events can be, and even likely are, compromised under these extraordinary circumstances, for they are difficult to put into words.

I was deeply impressed with Thomas's unusually high success rate in helping people with spiritual and health problems, finding lost objects or bodies, and more. So well-known was his fame and degree of success that many sought his assistance. Even a local physician, steeped in modern medicine and well connected within that arena, told me he received a cure from Thomas for a shoulder problem he had not been able to receive from other physicians.

Many of Thomas's family and community members thought of him as a loner. He loved to walk and would do so most days. Sometimes he invited others to accompany him and other times he took off by himself. He often wandered into the nearby forests and would stay in isolated places for days; on a few occasions, he was gone for over a month. On these ventures, he always brought along his walking stick; an old, highly honed knife; and his dog Curly, a mixed-breed mutt. Family and friends were concerned for his health and safety during these protracted wanderings, but he claimed these journeys brought him closer to nature, the creator, and the ancient wisdom that influenced the power of his relationships with people in need of his assistance.

In his later years, a family member or friend would secretly tail Thomas on his forays into the forest, for they grew understandably concerned about his ability to endure long stays outdoors without assistance. He had hip problems and his knees would sometimes buckle, but he never complained about these problems, nor let them stop him from his "walk-abouts." As for the "trackers," Thomas knew they were behind him and appreciated their concern for his health and safety.

Sometimes Thomas went alone into the small community lodge to sit in the center for hours. On cold nights, he would light a small fire in the pit and wrap himself in one of his many colorful woolen blankets. He prayed, chanted songs, and occasionally cried out for help and guidance. No one interfered during these occasions; however, a few stood in the background to keep a watchful eye on him. He deeply cherished these occasions, calling them his "time with the spirits."

I could spend a good deal more time describing and analyzing Thomas's many healing activities—-even ones involving whole villages—but what strikes me as most significant is the extent to which Shadow Walker symbolized and enacted a culturally grounded lifestyle. He and his community viewed healing as holistic, though they did not use that word. Their conception of healing encompassed every aspect of one's being, including the surroundings where the healings took place, for to them these elements are inseparable; Shadow Walker did not stray from these convictions and beliefs. In the words of anthropologist Margaret Mead (1959), the *shaman's* "position within that group is a perfect sample of the group-wide pattern on which he is acting" (p. 648). Thomas was a marginal person within a marginal culture who lived a full, productive life of a rich and unusual nature, belying the view of many who characterize these holy men as mystical outsiders.

But Is This Proper Science?

Just about everyone at one time or another has heard a story about a person cured by a faith healer. Such stories have a recurring theme: The main story line has a person suffering from a chronic, sometimes deadly, ailment. Every available form of conventional medical treatment produces little or no cure. As a last resort, the desperate patient seeks out the services of a faith-based or spiritual healer. Through some miraculous and mysterious process, the patient responds by recovering completely from their ailment. Variations on these recovery stories are fleshed out with personal testimonies and eyewitness accounts of the healing events. Though dubious characterizations of such healers (e.g., tricksters) and events are common, many stories persist and can be found in every culture, often defying the usual erosion effects brought on by the passing of time.

When researching *shaman* and their communities, the question becomes what do you do as a social scientist when what you are reporting seems overwhelmingly subjective, as the narrative demonstrates? Is the elaborate healing ceremony practiced among indigenous communities a magic show, or are spirits really there to heal the person? While a person who was ill seems to have become demonstrably, sometimes miraculously, well, was the ceremony simply a placebo that worked? On the other hand, was it the fasting, the drumming, the community support, the expectation of healing, or the absolute belief in the *shaman's* powers that effected a cure? Where is the proof that anything worked except a strong belief in unseen spirits and hallucinations? And, importantly, does Western scientific, by-the-numbers proof matter anyway? The person and the community became healthier. So, who cares? Is that science? Alternatively, is dismissing ethno-biographical research among these communities another way for skeptics with advanced degrees to say, "These people naively cling to beliefs in spirits and ghosts"?

Field Research Involves Collaborative Partnerships

Researchers who are given the opportunity and take on the task of conducting research with traditional healers are usually invited to spend time with the community, family, and those who have benefited from healings. At times, a challenging and daunting responsibility involving spending considerable time in the community, the venture begins with the principle that one's investigations and explorations are guided by authentic respect for the unique cultural lifeways and thoughtways of the ethnocultural community. Researchers must embrace the value that their research ventures are collaborations and partnerships (Trimble, 2010). Trickett and Espino (2004) summarized the emerging literature on community-based partnerships this way:

> It is time to place the collaboration concept in the center of inquiry and work out its importance for community research and intervention. Although some would see it as merely a tool or strategy for getting the 'real' work of behavioral science done, our strong preference is to view the research relationship in community research and intervention as a critical part of the 'real' work itself.
>
> *(p. 62)*

Without establishing and working through community partnerships, research ventures are doomed to failure at every stage of the process. This perspective and orientation add new research challenges, challenges best captured in the advice offered by Goodenough (1980) when he affirmed:

> Field workers have to honor the ethical principles of the host community in which they work as well as those of their home communities. They have to be honest about their research objectives and their sponsorship. They must not deceive the local people regarding their intent or the intended uses of their research. They must consider the impact of the conduct of the research on the people under study and do all they can to insure against what the people will regard as significant negative effects.
>
> *(p. 49)*

A core element in the scheme of the ***Ecology of Lives*** research approach developed by Trickett and Espino (2004) is the concept of principled cultural sensitivity. The concept was introduced to the field of community psychology by Trickett, Kelly, and Vincent (1985) and Trickett and Birman (1989) as a core component of the *Ecology of Lives* approach to field-based research collaboration. Principled cultural sensitivity is based on respect for whom the research and interventions are intended and would prohibit interventions that violate cultural norms. The main goal of *Ecology of Lives* research and intervention is community development wherein the project is constructed in such a way that it becomes a resource to the community. Unless one cares and is knowledgeable about how lives are led at the community level, such a goal would be difficult, if not impossible, to achieve. The approach further emphasizes the importance of culture as an historical and contemporary aspect of the framework within which individuals appraise their situation and their options. The research perspective emphasizes the community context as the stage upon which individual behavior occurs.

In the opening chapter of *The Straight Path*, clinical cross-cultural psychologist Richard Katz leads readers into his book through a brief conversation with Fijian healer Ratu Noa', who said

> Sometimes our story must be told by one of us—from the inside; sometimes by one of you—from the outside. Today, our story must be told by someone like you. And I am happy about that because you know our story. You look like one of them, but you're really one of us.
>
> *(Katz, 1993, p. 3)*

In his writings, Katz repeatedly points out that traveling along the straight path requires constant struggle and vigilance. The journey is not a clear and linear process, but rather one filled with ambiguity, confusion, and temptation, sometimes leading to wrong turns on the way to understanding. Specific behaviors may be necessary to travel a straight path. The straight path is a way of being and not so much an exact guide for the way life should be lived. Critical to this way of being are fundamental values and attitudes needed to find and stay on the path, typically including respect, humility, love, sharing, and service (Katz, 1993). Gene Hightower's interview with the traditional American Indian healer Beaver provides similar advice. Beaver pointed out that one must develop their spiritual nature and decide to live by principles. He also pointed out that one should maintain good principles and not to give up on them—and stay with them. And one should, he said, always believe what you are doing is the right thing to do (Hightower, 2019).

Katz (1982, 1993), in his beautifully written and dramatic descriptions of "boiling energy" among the Kalahari Kung and the "straight path" among Fijians, enlightens the mysteries of indigenous healing from the perspective of one who apprenticed himself to healers with the healers' and the community's permission. Katz, Biesele, and St. Denis (1997), in an enthralling book, *Healing Makes Our Hearts Happy*, recount the story of the Kalahari Jul'hoansi and the extraordinary power of spiritual energy that affirms the community's traditions and relationships. The authors maintain that

> Part of the story we have to tell involves the interplay in contemporary Jul'hoan (Kalahari) tradition expectation and observation of conservative ideology and creative symbolism. It is a story of history—both past and present—told by a "committee" of Jul'hoan people. The voice in the book is not one person but a medley of voices. A story where truth lies—if it exists—in verbal communication. It is a story of the dialogue and question and answer and how that dialogue may create a new understanding that is mutual and useful to the Jul'hoansi.
>
> *(p. 156)*

The eloquent words of Katz, and colleagues resonate profoundly with Joseph Gone's concluding observation. Specifically, Gone states

> Substantive community involvement and engagement in the formulation of integrative approaches exposes the particular interests of the dominant professional agenda even as it reformulates that agenda to its own ends (Gone, 2008). Consequently, it remains imperative that such initiatives in Indian country extend well beyond the creative achievements of a single individual—no matter how ingenious, poetic, or politic—to the collective energies and efforts of community members engaged in charting a sustainable and self-determined therapeutic praxis that reflects their own distinctive strategy for hurdling the colonial abyss.
>
> *(Gone, 2010, p. 225)*

Consequently, without firmly establishing a collaborative long-term relationship with communities, the likelihood of garnering an abiding partnership is slim (Trimble & Mohatt, 2006).

Relational Methodology

Relational methodology is "a process-centered approach nurturing a culturally sensitive and ethically responsible relationship. The process recognizes the human relationship of the researchers with research participants as a relationship of equals, as broader than the research project, and as characterized by genuine respect" (Trimble, Rivkin, & Allen, in press, p. 2). The establishment of trust and respect occurs through the nature and depth of relationships researchers create and sustain in their host communities. Relationships of this kind do not occur when one relies on a "safari approach," also referred to as "helicopter research," for data collection in which the researcher drops in for a short period of time to collect data and then leaves, and in some instances, is never to be heard from again.

Developing and nurturing relationships with community members and leaders take a considerable amount of time—maybe years. It means spending precious time visiting with people at social functions such as community gatherings, celebrations, ceremonies, local school events, and related activities. It means spending time with community leaders such as elected officials and elders, as well as visiting with parents of school-aged youth and the youth themselves. It means being willing to engage in long conversations that have nothing at all to do with one's research interests. If a researcher wishes to establish and nurture a relationship with the community, the commitment must be authentic and born of a deep abiding interest in the ways, customs, and thoughts of the people.

Community relationships can extend from the casual to those generated from the affectionate care that accompanies profound friendships. The nature of the relationship, in turn, can influence the quality of the information a researcher seeks to obtain in the course of the study or investigation. Thus, along with advocating the value and significance of six virtues, specifically trustworthiness, benevolence, capacity for awe, respect, awareness of one's limitations in the face of ambiguous and uncontrollable circumstances, and humility, researchers should seriously consider framing their field-based research around the formation and maintenance of responsible relationships; these form the major component of establishing community partnerships and collaborative arrangements. Relational methodology means that one takes the time to nurture relationships not merely for the sake of expediting the research and gaining acceptance and trust but because one should care about the welfare and dignity of all people.

Spirituality and Healing

Spiritual beliefs are at the core of the healing practices and ceremonies for indigenous people (King & Trimble, 2013). Indigenous spirituality is centered on the Creator and human beings' unique, personal relationship with the Creator. By definition, spirituality is everywhere, imbued in all life (earth's beings, rocks, trees, wind, etc.). While historically this view has been seen as primitive and animistic, when simply substituting the word spirit for energy, we have quantum physics' definition of energy/matter as constantly spinning and vibrating, each one radiating its own unique energy signature. Spirituality encompasses relationships with all beings. These sacred teachings come from oral traditions, some over 8,000 years old.

As contrasted with the dominant Western European view that humans are superior to the rest of creation, indigenous people see themselves as an integral part of creation. Many dimensions of spirituality (encompassing health, well-being, social responsibility, community development, etc.) embrace this idea. Thus, the central purpose in life is to take care of the earth and to serve others. Personal well-being cannot be separate from one's connectedness to this purpose. Peace and wholeness come through living in balance. The afterlife is a continuation of physical life on an energetic plane and includes a continual process of teaching and learning lessons (Fukuyama, Siahpoush, & Sevig, 2005). In many North American Indian tribes and Alaska Native villages, a spiritually connected way of life is often symbolized by a circle. The Diné emphasize harmony and beauty in relationships and connections with others and nature; the Apache call this *living in the pollen way*; for the Lakota, one can choose to follow the Red Road or the Black Road, each of which presents unique challenges for the proper way to live; for the Inupiat Eskimo, *ahregah*, or "well-being," is a state in which one experiences a healthy body, inner harmony, and "a good feeling within"; and for the Ojibwe, the Seven Council Fires of Life mark significant transitions through life stages. Locust (1985) points out,

> Native American Indians believe that each individual chooses to make himself well or to make himself unwell. If one stays in harmony, keeps all the tribal laws and the sacred laws, one's spirit will be so strong that negativity will be unable to affect it. Once harmony is broken, however, the spiritual self is weakened and one becomes vulnerable to physical illness, mental and /or emotional upsets, and the disharmony projected by others.
>
> *(p. 4)*

This "path" or "way of living" provides the individual with traditionally grounded directions and guidelines for living a life free of emotional turmoil, confusion, animosity, unhappiness, poor health, and conflict-ridden interpersonal and intergroup relations. The goal of traditional spiritual beliefs and practices is to provide assistance for the individual and/or community to once again find the "straight path" or way back to the circle and balance. This is illustrated by Diné distrust of Western medicine because it does not concern itself with whether the patient's life is in balance or whether their own life is in balance when they intervene with pills or surgery (Schwarz, 2008). Lori Alvord, the first female Navajo surgeon, put it this way, "Although a surgical procedure focuses on a single organ, I always tried to stay aware of the whole person—organs, mind, and spirit, the harmony of their entire being" (Alvord & Van Pelt, 1999, p. 111).

In the clinical psychologist Richard Katz's (1999) book, *The Straight Path of the Spirit: Ancestral Wisdom and Healing Traditions in Fiji*, Richard explains and elaborates on his firm belief that healing is a process of transition towards meaning, balance, wholeness, and connectedness, and these key elements are deeply rooted in the healing traditions and practices of countless traditional shamans and healers.

The essence of the healing relationship is nicely captured by the words of Joseph Eagle Elk, a 20th-century Lakota healer:

> The medicine man is not the only expert. Everyone has a purpose. Everyone is born to a family and a community for a reason. Like I explained about the tobacco, or the tree, or the animals. We are all alive, all have a purpose, and we all help each other. So, each of us must learn to pay attention to what we learn from our dreams, what the animals tell us, and what nature says.

Joseph Gone (2006) recounts the life and experiences of the Gros Ventre healer, Bull Lodge, and the influence he had on keeping their traditional healing methods and techniques alive within the context of the Gros Ventre worldview (cf. Horse Capture, 1992). The intent of his description is to demonstrate that "cultural divergences in subjectivity and experience are directly relevant for any comparison of therapeutic principles and practices" (Gone, 2006, p. 17). Gone's inspired description clearly demonstrates that Bull Lodge was connected to both the spirit world and everyday life in his community, providing him with the sacred healing knowledge necessary to effect recovery from suffering and hardship for his people.

In recent years, a handful of psychologists have given attention to the healing practices of indigenous "medicine people" that goes well beyond the use of an ethnographic participant-observer sojourn (O'Brien, 2008). These well-written and thoroughly researched life stories extend beyond written accounts of the healer's life and community. Rich descriptions are provided that reveal psychological profiles of the healer's sociocultural and psychosocial influences on their character and healing effectiveness. In an introspective, informative, and sensitively written autobiography, Gerald Mohatt and Joseph Eagle Elk (2000) related the life story of the practices, experiences, and career of a traditional Native American Indian healer. Cross-cultural clinical psychologist Mohatt added a unique perspective that enabled him to highlight the psychological dimensions and worth of Eagle Elk's healings by placing them in a cross-cultural context.

Establishing Culturally Resonant Relationships With Communities

One's deeds and actions are open to the assessment and evaluation of others, especially if one is a stranger to a community. In a fundamental sense, researchers who are new to a community are "other" to the community and the community is "other" to them. Truth, therefore, is sanctioned or foreclosed by the researcher. To know this, researchers must become aware of how they are being represented in the community. Whatever the researcher's intention and research needs, their presence and actions will be scrutinized and assessed by community members. Is the researcher willing to be open to others' close and continuous observations, comments, and questions about their actions and beliefs? The question is more than speculative, for it speaks to one's willingness to be scrutinized, along with granting community residents permission and corresponding authority to question one's values, beliefs, and actions. Moreover, the questions may not stop with the assessment of character, but focus, too, on the way the research is being conducted and why the researcher is resorting to the use of procedures and measures unfamiliar to residents and participants (Gone, 2019).

Universal acceptance of the researcher's virtues and principles can be debated from a relativist perspective. Respect and trust, for example, may have different meanings and expression across cultural groups. Their meaning for researchers may not coincide with their meaning within the worldview of a culture different and foreign to the outsider. Put in slightly different terms: Are there different meanings for what constitutes trust and respect? If there are differences in the meaning of the values, how does one earn trust and respect within the context of another culture? And, most important, how does one know they have earned and established trust and respect? Ibrahim (1996) and Vasquez (1996) remind us that all cultural groups have ethical standards, often embedded in their legends, traditions, and customs; these standards may not resonate with those of the researcher's cultural orientation (see Trickett & Espino, 2004). "To facilitate character and moral development in a multicultural system," maintains Ibrahim (1996), "we have to identify all the moral ideals that each (cultural) system subscribes to and find common ground" (p. 83). Learning the deep cultural meaning of what constitutes trust and respect therefore requires the researcher to spend time with the community. One will soon discover that community members will put the researcher through a sequence of "tests" to assess their level of commitment to working closely with them and to learn about their cultural ways (Trickett & Espino, 2004). Discovering the meaning of these virtues must occur long before the research enterprise is set in motion.

Conclusion

Ethical planning for scientific inquiry involving the changing patterns of ethnocultural diversity requires flexibility and sensitivity to the contextual challenges and concerns of each ethnic group and research problem (U.S. Office of the Surgeon General, 2001). The points for consideration raised in this chapter are not intended to serve as regulation, policy, or absolute prescriptions for research ethics practices. The purpose, rather, is to assist stakeholders—investigators, funding agencies and institutional review boards, research participants, and ethnocultural communities—in the responsible conduct of research, in identifying key ethical crossroads, and in developing culturally sensitive decision-making strategies.

Ethical planning must not be an afterthought or sidebar consideration in the framing and organization of a research venture; it must be an integral component of the entire process. To ensure its proper place, researchers and practitioners should be prepared to collaborate with the communities; share results that have practical value; and accept the conditions imposed by the community in gaining access to those in need of spiritual, psychological, or physiological assistance. In addition, research sojourners must be aware of the scientific, social, and political factors governing the rules of professional conduct embodied in federal regulations and professional codes. It is essential to know and follow professional research codes and ethics standards, as they provide complete guidance for identifying and resolving complex ethical challenges too often inherent in providing research services and applicable outcomes for all ethnocultural populations and their communities.

In closing out this chapter, the wisdom of James Skeen can provide direction for understanding the value and role of virtuous thoughts and actions in research settings. Skeen (2002) maintained,

> Virtuous behavior is a worthy objective for all of us. No one is perfect, or capable of being perfect, but each of us has a need-strength profile that makes the acquisition of certain virtuous traits difficult and others relatively easy. But just knowing that it is possible to err in two directions—excess and deficiency—is valuable information.
>
> *(p. 18)*

References

Allport, G. W. (1940). The psychologist's frame of reference. *Psychological Bulletin, 37*, 1–28. https://psycnet.apa.org/doi/10.1037/h0060064

Alvord, L. A., & Van Pelt, E. C. (1999). *The scalpel and the silver bear.* New York: Bantam.

Amoss, P. (1978). *Coast Salish spirit dancing: The survival of an ancestral religion.* Seattle: WA University of Washington Press.

Denzin, N. K., & Lincoln, Y. S. (Eds.). (2018). *The Sage handbook of qualitative research.* Thousand Oaks, CA: Sage Publications.

De Waele, J.-P. & Harré, R. (1979). Autobiography as a psychological method. In G. P. Ginsberg (Ed.), *Emerging strategies in social psychological research.* Chichester: John Wiley.

Freilich, M. (Ed.). (1970). *Marginal natives: Anthropologist at work.* New York: Harper & Row.

Fukuyama, M., Siahpoush, F., & Sevig, T. D. (2005). Religion and spirituality in a cultural context. In C. Cashwell & J. S. Young (Eds.), *Integrating spirituality and religion into counseling: A guide to competent practice* (pp. 123–142). Alexandria, VA: American Counseling Association.

Goldberg, M. M. (1941). A qualification of the marginal man theory. *American Sociological Review, 6*(1), 52–58.

Gone, J. P. (2006). "As if reviewing his life": Bull Lodge's narrative and the mediation of self-representation. *American Indian Culture and Research Journal, 30*(1), 67–86. https://doi.org/10.17953/aicr.30.1.m53n5t773126g05k

Gone, J. P. (2008). "So I can be like a Whiteman": The cultural psychology of space and place in American Indian mental health. *Culture & Psychology, 14*, 369–399. https://doi.org/10.1177%2F1354067X08092639

Gone, J. P. (2010). Psychotherapy and traditional healing for American Indians: Exploring the prospects for therapeutic integration. *The Counseling Psychologist, 38*, 166–235. https://doi.org/10.1177%2F0011000008330831

Gone, J. P. (2019). Considering Indigenous research methodologies: Critical reflections by an Indigenous knower. *Qualitative Inquiry, 25*(1), 45–56. https://doi.org/10.1177%2F1077800418787545

Goodenough, W. H. (1980). Ethnographic field techniques. In H. C. Triandis & J. W. Berry (Eds.), *Handbook of cross-cultural psychology: Methodology* (Vol. 2, pp. 39–55). Boston, MA: Allyn & Bacon.

Harré, R. (1979). *Social being: A theory for social psychology.* Oxford, UK: Basil Blackwell.

Harré, R. (1983). *Personal being: A theory for individual psychology.* Cambridge, MA: Harvard University Press.

Hightower, G. (2019). *Insights on counseling American Indians: Conversations with Beaver.* San Diego, CA: Cognella.

Horse Capture, G. P. (1992). *The seven visions of Bull Lodge: As told by his daughter, Garter Snake.* Lincoln, NE: University of Nebraska Press.

Ibrahim, F. A. (1996). A multicultural perspective on principle and virtue ethics. *The Counseling Psychologist, 24*(1), 78–85. https://doi.org/10.1177%2F0011000096241003

Katz, R. (1982). *Boiling energy: Community healing among the Kalahari Kung.* Cambridge, MA: Harvard University Press.

Katz, R. (1993). *The straight path: A story of healing and transformation in Fiji.* Reading, MA: Addison-Wesley.

Katz, R. (1999). *The straight path of the spirit: Ancestral wisdom and healing traditions in Fiji.* New York, NY: Simon & Schuster.

Katz, R., Biesele, M., & St. Denis, V. (1997). *Healing makes our hearts happy.* Rochester, VT: Inner Traditions.

Kelley, J. H. (1978). *Yaqui women: Contemporary life histories.* Lincoln, NE: University of Nebraska Press.

King, J., & Trimble, J. E. (2013). The spiritual and sacred among North American Indians and Alaska Natives: Synchronicity, wholeness, and connectedness in a relational world. In K. I. Pargement, J. Exline, J. Jones, A.

Mahoney, &E. Shafranske (Eds.), *Handbook of psychology, religion, and spirituality*. Washington, DC: American Psychological Association.

Langness, L. L., & Frank, G. (1978). Fact, fiction and the ethnographic novel. *Anthropology and Humanism Quarterly, 3*(1–2), 18–22. https://doi.org/10.1525/ahu.1978.3.1-2.18

Leighton, A. H., & Leighton, D. C. (1949). *Gregorio, the hand-trembler: A psycho-biographical personality study of a Navajo Indian*. Cambridge, MA: Harvard University Press.

Locust, C. (1985). Wounding the spirit: Discrimination and traditional American Indian belief systems. In G. Thomas (Ed.), *U.S. race relations in the 1980s and 1990s: Challenges and alternatives* (pp. 219–232). New York, NY: Hemisphere.

Lurie, N. O. (1961). *Mountain wolf woman, sister of Crashing Thunder: The autobiography of a winnebago woman*. Ann Arbor, MI: University of Michigan Press.

Mann, J. W. (1958). Group relations and the marginal personality. *Human Relations, 11*(1), 77–92.

Mead, M. (1959). *An anthropologist at work: Writings of Ruth Benedict*. Boston, MA: Houghton-Mifflin.

Mohatt, G., & Eagle Elk, J. (2000). *The price of a gift: A Lakota Healer's story*. Lincoln, NE: University of Nebraska Press.

O'Brien, S. J. C. (2008). *Religion and healing in Native America: Pathways for renewal*. Westport, CT: Praeger.

Olney, J. (1980). Autobiography and the cultural moment: A thematic, historical, and bibliographical introduction. In J. Olney (Ed.), *Autobiography: Essays theoretical and critical* (pp. 127–163). Princeton, NJ: Princeton University Press.

Park, R. E. (1950). *Race and culture*. Glencoe, IL: The Free Press.

Radin, P. (Ed.). (1926). *Crashing Thunder: The autobiography of an American Indian*. New York, NY: Appleton.

Rosensweig, M. R. (1992). Psychological science around the world. *American Psychologist, 39*, 877–884. https://psycnet.apa.org/doi/10.1037/0003-066X.47.6.718

Sapir, E. (1921). The life of a Nootka Indian. *Queens' Quarterly, 28*, 232–243.

Schwarz, M. T. (2008). "Lightening followed me:" Contemporary Navajo therapeutic strategies for cancer. In S. J. C. O'Brien (Ed.), *Religion and healing in Native America: Pathways for renewal* (pp. 19–42). Westport, CT: Praeger.

Sherif, M., & Sherif, C. W. (1956). *An outline of social psychology* (revised ed.). New York, NY: Harper & Row.

Simmons, L. W. (1942). *Sun chief: The autobiography of a Hopi Indian*. New Haven, CT: Yale University Press.

Skeen, J. W. (2002). Choice theory, virtue ethics, and the sixth need. *International Journal of Reality Therapy, 22*(1), 14–19.

Smith, J. A., Harre, R., & Van Langenhove, L. (1995). *Rethinking psychology*. London, UK: Sage Publications.

Sodderqvist, T. (1991). Biography or ethnobiography or both? Embodied reflexivity and the deconstruction of knowledge-power. In F. Steir (Ed.), *Research and reflexivity* (pp. 143–162). London, UK: Sage Publications.

Starr, P. D., & Roberts, A. E. (1982). Community structure and Vietnamese refugee adaptation: The significance of context. *The International Migration Review, 16*(3), 595–618. https://doi.org/10.1177%2F019791838201600303

Stonequist, E. V. (1937). *The marginal man*. New York, NY: Scribner.

Trickett, E. J., & Birman, D. (1989). Taking ecology seriously: A community development approach to individually-based interventions. In L. Bond & B. Compas (Eds.), *Primary prevention and promotion in the schools* (pp. 361–390). Newbury Park, CA: Sage Publications.

Trickett, E. J., & Espino, S. L. (2004). Collaboration and social inquiry: Multiple meanings of a construct and its role in creating useful and valid knowledge. *American Journal of Community Psychology, 34*, 1–71. https://doi.org/10.1023/B:AJCP.0000040146.32749.7d

Trickett, E. J., Kelly, J. G., & Vincent, T. A. (1985). The spirit of ecological inquiry in community research. In E. Susskind & D. Klein (Eds.), *Community research: Methods, paradigms, and applications*. New York, NY: Praeger.

Trimble, J. E. (2010). The virtues of cultural resonance, competence, and relational collaboration with Native American Indian communities: A synthesis of the counselling and psychotherapy literature. *The Counselling Psychologist, 38*(2), 243–256. https://doi.org/10.1177%2F0011000009344348

Trimble, J. E., & Mohatt, G. V. (2006). Coda: The virtuous and responsible researcher in another culture. In J. E. Trimble & C. B. Fisher (Eds.), *Handbook of ethical and responsible research with ethnocultural populations and communities* (pp. 325–334). Thousand Oaks, CA: Sage Publications.

Trimble, J. E., Rivkin, I., & Allen, J. (Eds.). (in press). *Relational methodology: Engaging connections and knowledge transformation through research with indigenous populations*. San Diego, CA: Cognella.

U.S. Office of the Surgeon General. (2001). *Mental health: Culture, race, and ethnicity*. Rockville, MD: Substance Abuse and Mental Health Services Administration. Retrieved from www.ncbi.nlm.nih.gov/books/NBK44243

Vasquez, M. L. (1996). Will virtue ethics improve ethical conduct in multicultural settings? *The Counseling Psychologist, 24*(1), 98–104. https://doi.org/10.1177%2F0011000096241006

PART II

Genetic Studies and Health

4

GENETICS RESEARCH METHODS

Amel Youssef, Matthew J. Criscione, and Julian Paul Keenan

Overview

It is impossible to know the precise future of health psychology, but it is certain that genetics will play an ever-increasing role. It is not a revelation that genetics are important to health and mental well-being. What may be surprising is that future is now. Current techniques that are both inexpensive and relatively easy are commonplace and within any researcher's capability. From establishing genomes to knocking out genes, any researcher can easily perform genetic research in humans. The central dogma (DNA makes RNA makes protein) tells us that DNA (deoxyribonucleic acid) is at the root of all things living. This includes the nervous system, and we acknowledge that genetics play not only a direct but also an indirect role in a person's health by influencing health decisions made by the brain. Along any part of this chain, most questions can be addressed, from the genetics of cancer to the gene expression in healthy diet choices. What we wish to emphasize here is that the barriers that used to exist are for the most part no longer present and that with very little investment, it is now possible to ask and answer genetic questions in health, psychology, and the integration of the two.

The myth that genetic techniques are too complex for the non-geneticist to implement must be dispelled. The dream of bringing genetics to the public is here, from *23andMe* and *Ancestry.com*, to the availability of bench testing at a reasonable cost. Obviously, many know of some big trends in genetics, as the past two decades were filled with lots of fanfare surrounding the Human Genome Project and cloning. However, these headline-grabbing articles and news bits have partially hidden the fact to many researchers that they, too, can join the genetic revolution at little cost in time or money.

Research in Practice

To 'do' genetics, a second myth should also be dispelled. There is a notion that there is no longer a need for traditional genetic research. The idea of breeding rats or recruiting monozygotic twins seems like an old idea that has little utility today. However, nothing could be further from the truth. Twin studies and breeding research remain critical and can address questions that molecular techniques cannot. Classic Mendelian concepts such as mating, strains, dominance, and expected ratios are often both the first and the last step in establishing phenotypic phenomena such as mental health. *Drosophila melanogaster* (fruit fly) has been used in auditory perception research mainly because the generational times are under a month, leading to the breeding of auditory processing differences with a year on the calendar. There is no way to get these breeding times in mammals. Further, in our case,

<50>51</50>

the flies were inexpensive, simple to manipulate, did not require Institutional Animal Care and Use Committee (IACUC) permission, and studies were done in both the larvae stages and adult stages such that we even could determine the genetics of the developmental timeline. Similar benefits exist for breeding in other organisms (see later).

Health is clearly a genetic issue. From expression of malicious DNA to virus invaders and cancers, all health researchers can theoretically gain mastery of some genetics whether they expressly perform research or just stay abreast of the current findings. It is hard to imagine any first-world health care system devoid of genetics in the next decade. From tracing the origin of bacterial outbreaks to devising Alzheimer's treatments, health is being reshaped by genetic progress today and tomorrow.

Health psychology is primed to be dominated by genetics. We consider one of the first neuroimaging studies employing molecular genetic genotyping in humans performed by Turhan Canli's group, where differences in genotype were correlated with reactivity to anxiety-provoking stimuli (Canli & Lesch, 2007). Canli found a role for the amygdala in processing the stimuli and that certain alleles (versions of a gene) lead to an amygdala that was more negatively prepared to deal with anxiety-producing stimuli. With causality established and the method of brain expression realized, it became potentially easier to diagnose and treat anxiety and depression. For example, treatment for a person suffering from major depressive disorder could be based on the presence or absence of the alleles in question.

No one among us has been able to obtain anything close to mastery of genetic techniques. With ever-changing technology and findings, it is clearly not feasible to stay ahead of the curve in terms of all applications. That fact should not be used for ignoring genetics in research. Either in formulating hypotheses or applying techniques, it is certain that any research program can be enhanced by implementing some sort of genetic analysis. Stress is certainly not a genetic condition; however, genetics plays a large role in stress acquisition, maintenance, and extinction. Human immunodeficiency virus (HIV) is not inherited genetically, but genetics plays a huge role in not just patient response but also in viral adaptation and subsequent drug development. In other words, applying genetics can only add to one's arsenal of understanding and discovery.

Breeding and Breeds

No researcher would ever recommend breeding a mammalian animal strain unless absolutely necessary. It is time-consuming, costly, difficult, and expensive, and the results are far from certain. It is a commitment with no guarantees. Rats and mice have long generational times and the amount of attention is immense. Luckily, companies sell breeds that have been selected for certain behaviors, anatomies, and disorders. Elsewhere in this book you will find animals bred based on alcohol consumption, for example.

Even with these "warnings," you may be interested in a behavior or disorder that does not exist in a certain breed. Breedings have been based on tone preference and the ability to associate tones with sucrose in fruit flies because stocks of these flies were not available, so we developed our own. It is noted that flies were chosen in part because they are invertebrates and the animal care of these organisms is much easier. In fact, a word of advice is that if behavior can be modified in an invertebrate, consider doing so. Insects are quicker (for the most part) in terms of generational times and the ethical guidelines much less strict. They eat less, require less space, and are often easier to test. However, mammals are often the 'go-to' animal model.

Breeding different mouse strains while measuring exposure to environmental stress can be an excellent measure for screening for genotypic hardiness (Turner & Burne, 2013). Environmental stress responses can be employed in the selection of mice strains for breeding. Let us take one example to walk through a typical process using easily purchased mouse strains. This model used selective breeding of both C57BL/6J and C57BL/6N mouse strains, as well as NMRI mice, which were investigated to see if different behavioral repertoires in response to the tail suspension test would emerge (Chmielarz, Kreiner, Kuśmierczyk, Kowalska, Roman, Tota, et al., 2016). The C57BL/6J and C57BL/6N strains of mice are separated by 220 generations, and they demonstrate many separate phenotypic features, with the genetic differences well mapped. The tail suspension, as it sounds, suspends a mouse from its tail and records behavioral responses. One might already see the relation to health psychology, as there may be genetic differences in response to an external stressor.

In the experiment, the responses of the strains were tested in some detail; key components will be provided, though readers should read the article in its entirety. Handling the different breeds of mice by the tail acts as a stress inducer that triggers a fighting response; however, due to the persistence of the stress, the mice despair and become immobile. Inbred mice species exhibit different levels of rigidity when subjected to the stressful stimulus as compared to cross-breed colonies. When subjected to the tail suspension test C57BL/6J and C57BL/6N breeds of mice were compared for different mobility levels (Chmielarz, et al., 2016).

It was discovered that regardless of breed, stressed mice exhibited a reduced body weight gain compared to the controls. Stress also increased the size of the adrenal cortex. In terms of breed differences, it was found that Naval Medical Research Institute mice spent less time immobile when compared to C57BL/6J mice (45% vs. 69%, respectively). This was an expected finding. Of certain note is that there was a difference between the immobility times of C57BL/6J and C57BL/6N mice (69% vs. 52%). There were further strain differences. For example, only the NMRI breed displayed increased immobility time after chronic stress.

While there are many results not detailed here, the sample presented here demonstrates that some characteristics vary regardless of breed and some are breed specific. The authors would acknowledge that that alone means little; however, when considered with the literature, these differences paint a picture. The first inclination is that certain characteristics are less dependent on inheritance. That is, if *all* breeds show the same reaction, then genetics may not play as large or any role. While this is possible, it is also possible that these breeds have the same genotypes in regard to *this* trait. Future studies, whether at the molecular or behavioral level, can determine this.

The fact that breed differences lead to behavioral differences is a strong case for genetic mechanisms at play, as it is difficult to argue the opposite. However, replication of this as well as a molecular factor (e.g., an allele) would make this a much stronger claim. If these breed differences bear out in terms of the tail suspension test, then one could use these differences for a wide variety of applications. If the differences are not there, as may be the case in weight changes when exposed to stress, one may think of establishing a breed that does show such differences.

Basic Sanger Sequencing

How does one actually find the DNA sequence? It is well known that G, C, A, T (guanine, cytosine, adenine, and thymine) are the "base pairs" or the nucleotides. Alterations of this genomic sequence lead to alterations in phenotype. That is, one's phenotype depends on the genotype. However, how does one figure out if a person is GGCCAC or CACCAC? What we are really asking is: How do we identify each nucleotide on a DNA strand? Knowing this changes everything, and the ability to identify the genome of any individual has changed science in ways we cannot even imagine.

In 1977, Frederick Sanger and colleagues published the nucleotide sequence of the bacteriophage phiX174 using a novel and effective technique for DNA sequencing. This lead to a Nobel Prize, as it made actual sequencing possible on a semi-grand scale. A phage is a virus that invades a bacteria, and by all means phiX174 is unremarkable in the virus world. It is, however, similar to the finch (a rather standard bird) that helped identify evolution.

First a simple explanation. The first step in identifying a genome using what is now called *Sanger sequencing* is isolating DNA (getting rid of all the other cell parts). Once the DNA is isolated, many copies are made of the DNA segment of interest. Four tubes are set up, each of which can identify one nucleotide only. Thus, in the guanine tube, only G is identified. The nature of the identification is such that once a G is encountered, the DNA stops growing; thus, a sequence is CAAATG. To know that a G is the sixth nucleotide (or that the strand is six letters, long with the last one having to be a G), electrophoresis is done. In electrophoresis one can tell how long a strand of DNA is, but not what the base pair is. Thus, combining the two can identify where all the Gs are. I use the three other tubes to identify the other letters.

Specifically, this technique, also called the ***dideoxy method***, capitalizes on the need for a 3'-OH group on a nucleotide for DNA to be present for sequence extension (Sanger, Donelson, Coulson, Kössel, & Fischer, 1973). Sanger synthesized all four nucleotides—dATP, dTTP, dCTP, and dGTP *without* the 3'-OH group (dideoxy nucleotides, ddNTPs). The absence of the 3'-OH group prevents DNA polymerase from recognizing the nucleotide and thereby stops further DNA chain extension. By mixing radiolabeled ddNTPs in the reaction mix along with DNA polymerase and normal deoxyribonucleotide triphosphates (dNTPs), DNA fragments of different lengths can be generated. Since these fragments may be separated based on molecular weight, running them on a gel could provide bands corresponding to the position of each ddNTP, which can help 'read' the sequence of the DNA strand.

Although a breakthrough, the *dideoxy method* came with several challenges. First, it utilized radiolabeled nucleotides, which carried significant challenges in handling and usage. In time, fluorescent ddNTPs replaced the radiolabeled ones, significantly improving the safety of the technique (Ansorge, Sproat, Stegemann, Schwager, & Zenke, 1987). Other chemical modifications (nanopore sequencing) have been introduced in recent years, especially with automated methods of DNA sequencing (Riedl, Ding, Fleming, & Burrows, 2015; Fuller, Kumar, Porel, Chien, Bibillo, Stranges, et al., 2016). Another drawback of the technique was that the sequence fragments generated by the prokaryotic Klenow fragment (DNA polymerase) were less than 1000 bps in size (Chen, 2014). To apply this technique to sequence larger DNA sequences (the human genome is 3 billion base pairs), a method called shotgun sequencing was developed. In this technique, overlapping DNA sequences are first sequenced and then put together to form a long contiguous sequence in silico (Heather & Chain, 2016). Yet another challenge with the Sanger method involved the use of a prokaryotic DNA polymerase. While the Klenow fragment could effectively use ddNTPs, it was also error-prone, especially when differently labeled ddNTPs were used. To overcome this problem, synthetically modified polymerases and species-specific polymerases have been utilized (Heather & Chain, 2016).

Over time, DNA sequencing has become automated and this has significantly reduced the time of the sequencing reaction, allowing scientists to sequence large DNA molecules and whole genomes with accuracy and efficiency. Some of these automated sequencers are capable of sequencing over 10-kb-long DNA sequences, allowing for large genome sequencing experiments (Heather & Chain, 2016).

With advances in DNA sequencing, specific information regarding sequence alterations in DNA (like mutations and polymorphisms) could be identified and associations between such alterations in DNA sequence and function could be made. Single-nucleotide polymorphism (SNP) refers to changes in single DNA bases (A, T, G, or C) within the genome or among members of a species or population. Also noted is that the different allelic variants found on the same chromosome are termed a haplotype. Genotyping, or the process by which such SNPs can be identified, and the presence or absence of specific SNPs have been associated with susceptibility to diseases, including cystic fibrosis (Mouradian, Gaurav, Pugliese, El Kasmi, Hartman, Hernandez-Lagunas, et al., 2017), Alzheimer's disease (Sleegers, Bettens, De Roeck, Van Cauwenberghe, Cuyvers, Verheijen, et al., 2015), sickle cell anemia (Upadhye, Jain, Trivedi, Nadkarni, Ghosh & Colah, 2016), and chronic obstructive pulmonary diseases (Wang, Li, Zhou, Zeng, Xu, Xu, et al., 2015).

Sequencing the FTO Gene

More recently, SNPs in the fat mass and obesity (FTO) gene have been identified and associated with an individual's susceptibility to obesity (increased body fat and lowered muscle content; Fawcett & Barroso, 2010; Saldaña-Alvarez, Salas-Martínez, García-Ortiz, Luckie-Duque, García-Cárdenas, Vicenteño-Ayala, et al., 2016). While the association is established, the underlying mechanism is as yet undetermined. In their latest study, Kalantari, Keshavarz Mohammadi, Izadi, Gholamalizadeh, Doaei, Eini-Zinab, et al. (2018) sought to determine the association between FTO gene polymorphisms and anthropometric indices (height, weight, body mass index [BMI], body fat percentage, and skeletal muscle percentage). Additionally, data on average daily calorie intake and physical activity per week were measured. The sample population was a voluntary group of adolescent male students (N = 233) between 12 and 16 years of age from two schools in a district in Tehran, Iran. This study was conducted over a period of a year and during this time, the subjects were assessed for all the aforementioned anthropometric indices. Genotyping of SNPs in the FTO gene was undertaken by extracting DNA from venous blood followed by polymerase chain reaction to amplify the specific gene followed by DNA sequencing for SNP identification. The authors searched for all SNPs from 300 bp upstream to 300 bp downstream of the FTO gene, especially focusing on the already identified SNP rs9930506, which had been associated with obesity (Qi, Kang, Zhang, van Dam, Kraft, Hunter, et al., 2008).

Genotype analysis determined that the haplotype block in the first region of the FTO gene consisted of three SNPs (rs993275 [allele G], rs9930506 [allele G], and rs9930501 [allele C]) (Kalantari, et al., 2018). Specifically, the rs9930506 GG genotype was positively associated with overweight and obese subjects compared to those that were of normal weight—after confounding factors such as age, dietary intake, and physical activity levels were controlled. The same genotype was negatively associated with skeletal muscle percentage, also after controlling for confounding factors.

Studies such as this are actually simple in concept. Identify differences in genotypes and determine if those differences result in any phenotypic differences. At this level, the why (i.e., protein mechanisms/identification) does not come into play. Thus the conclusion of the study is that there is a significant association between the rs9930506 GG genotype and body fat and skeletal muscle percentages. Obese and overweight subjects with lower skeletal muscle percentages had this genotype at a higher frequency compared to those that were of a more optimal body composition, irrespective of the quantity of food consumed or physical activity levels. With the gene pinpointed, future research will examine what else this SNP does, as well as potential mechanisms of action.

Employing ELISA for Ghrelin

Several techniques that can be used in the research method of health psychology have advanced over the years, making it easier for an individual to use the technique. ***Enzyme-linked immunosorbent assay (ELISA)*** is a test that can detect infectious agents or antibodies in a specific sample that are created through infections. *ELISA* is composed of a plate made out of polystyrene, proteins, and peptides. An *ELISA* test can be performed on blood or urine. The *ELISA* test works by relying on the interaction between parts of the immune system, which include antigens and antibodies. *ELISA* may be useful when detecting diseases. Under optimal conditions, *ELISA* gives either a positive or negative result when the test is conducted, which means that an antibody is either present or absent in an individual's body.

Genetic and environmental stimuli are two essential factors affecting food intake. With an emphasis on cognitive control or restrained eating, the study evaluated the effects of "restraining" on the secretion of appetite-regulating hormones. Additionally, the researchers employed *ELISA* to examine glucose and insulin interactions as influenced by the intake of meals to measure the concentration of ghrelin secretions in the stomach. Increased ghrelin production results from the cognitive and physiologic interactions of appetite-regulating hormones due to restraining as opposed to genetic factors.

ELISA is often used when attempting to detect the presence of a specific antigen in a person's blood. *ELISA* is performed by placing the patient's serum in the plate, where any proteins present in the patient will coat the plastic well and adhere to it. To avoid any reaction from occurring, a blocking agent is added to the *ELISA* plate. In this case, *ELISA* can be used to determine the level of insulin in human serum. After any type of food enters the body, the beta cells, located in the pancreas, release a signal to increase the levels of insulin. The insulin then works with the beta cells to lower the glucose levels within the cell.

Myhre, Kratz, Goldberg, Polivy, Melhorn, Buchwald and colleagues (2014) aimed at evaluating how restrained eating or attempted cognitive control of food intake affects the levels of appetite-regulating hormones. The research used a control setup that included restrained and unrestrained co-twins using ghrelin *ELISA* and radioimmunoassay (RIA) (Myhre, et al., 2014). The *ELISA* method detects and quantifies particular antigens and antibodies in a provided sample (Gan & Patel, 2013). The technique emanated from RIA, which detects and measures molecules such as hormones and peptides present in small quantities (Gan & Patel, 2013). In this study RIA was employed to detect ghrelin levels.

Therefore, the study aimed at evaluating ghrelin concentration in the blood using the *ELISA* and RIA in restrained and unrestrained groups. Ghrelin, a peptide hormone, regulates hunger sensations in the body (Barington, Brorson, Hofman-Bang, Rasmussen, Holst, & Feldt-Rasmussen, 2017). Ghrelin increases appetite, as evidenced through its rapid production before food intake and substantial depreciation after meals (Atalayer, Gibson, Konopacka, & Geliebter, 2013).

What makes this study particularly interesting is that it was a twin study, allowing one to examine the genetic influences determined by the assays. The study included 16 monozygotic twin pairs, in which one twin was restrained and the co-twin unrestrained (Myhre, et al., 2014). It is worth noting here that adding gender-matched dizygotic twins would have improved the study as that would control for environmental factors. Eating (restrained or unrestrained) was measured via survey.

The main finding was that restrained twins had higher ghrelin levels during the preload study. The preload study consisted of consuming a high-calorie/fat milkshake. This was followed by ice cream. The ghrelin difference was present despite the fact that restrained and unrestrained twins consumed identical meals prior to the preload study and almost identical amounts of milkshake and ice cream in the course of the preload study. In fact, the controls were held dramatically constant in this study, lending confidence to the study's results.

Because the authors examined monozygotic (MZ) twins, they suggest that these differences were independent of age, genetics, and family background. The differences found were largest in the context of the preload study; ghrelin levels in restrained twins were higher at all of the earlier sampling times and the differences disappeared at later points in the study. In terms of the overall genetic conclusion, "Although the initial predisposition to restrain eating **may** have a genetic component, our findings suggest that once restrained eating behavior is acquired, endogenous levels of ghrelin are increased independent of genetic influence (bold added; Myhre et al., 2014)". In other words, since genetics were controlled for by the use of MZ twins, it is unlikely that genotype had any influence on the differences observed.

CRISPR/Cas9

CRISPR/Cas9 was discovered in prokaryotic organisms that do not have a proper immune system. In this bacteria, the system is employed as a defense against viruses. It can identify, destroy, and "remember" viruses, creating a library for future defenses. The technique is simple, perhaps due to its prokaryotic origins, which has made it perfect for use across all organisms, including humans. Simply, the system identifies targeted sequences (e.g., CCGAT), and it takes those sequences and places them in its own DNA to later "know its enemy" and have it on record. While this is an oversimplification, one should be aware what CRISPR has the capability of doing. It can identify gene sequences, cut sequences, and insert sequences. That is, if we know that CCGAT causes congenital blindness, we can search for that sequence and destroy it, or destroy it and replace it. Like *Sanger sequencing*, CRISPR is a "science changer".

For example, CRISPR/Cas9 is easily imagined to be an effective technique that will detect and alter age-related brain diseases such as Alzheimer's, Parkinson's, and Huntington's disease (Raikwar, Thangavel, Dubova, Selvakumar, Ahmed, Kempuraj, et al., 2018; Yan, Tu, Li, & Li, 2018). Given its amazing flexibility, it is surprisingly inexpensive and relatively easy to build a lab using this technique. It is noted, as of this writing, that human trials are just underway.

CRISPR/Cas9 and Obesity

One of the leading causes of death and illness globally is obesity. Obesity is associated with several health issues involving heart disease, type 2 diabetes, and hypertension (Cummings, Weigle, Frayo, Breen, Ma, Dellinger, et al., 2002). It is clearly beneficial to understand the different mechanisms that control food intake, along with body weight, for clinical medication and public health (Altman, 2002). Ghrelin, as we have seen, is a hormone released from the stomach that is associated with several behaviors such as feeding, stress, reward, and addiction, which may persist upon binding to the growth hormone secretagogue receptor (GHSR; Guan, Yu, Palyha, McKee, Feighner, Sirinathsinghji, et al., 1997). GHSR regulates homeostasis, along with body weight, and plays a vital role when binding with ghrelin. When GHSR binds with ghrelin, metabolic activity, homeostasis, and energy metabolism are strongly influenced (Zallar, Tunstall, Richie, Zhang, You, Gardner, et al., 2018). Under negative conditions such as starvation and anorexia nervosa, ghrelin hormone becomes more active (Schanze, Reulbach, Scheuchenzuber, Groschl, Kornhuber, & Kraus, 2008).

Because CRISPR/Cas9 can be used to add, remove, and change sections of the DNA sequence (Belhaj, Chaparro-Garcia, Kamoun, Patron, & Nekrasov, 2015), it was thought that ghrelin levels could be controlled by the use of editing. In the current Zallar, et al. (2018) study, a GHSR Knockout (KO) Wistar rat was 'created' using CRISPR/Cas9. This was achieved by deleting the GHSR gene, which led to a novel GHSR KO Wistar rat. The data were confirmed a number of ways, but put simply, this new breed of rat lost GHSR messenger ribonucleic acid (mRNA) expression. These organisms, as one would do in a classic genetic study, were then comparted to wild-type (WT), genetically unaltered rats. Any emerged differences would be attributed to the loss of GHSR function.

How was this done? The ghrelin gene contains four exons and three introns, and it is located on chromosome 3 (exons code information associated with the gene, and introns do not code information associated with the gene) (Yang, Li, Zhao, Zhang, Song, Xiao, et al., 2012). A nickase is an enzyme that binds to specific regions in the DNA and breaks (nicks) a strand of DNA, causing it to unwind (Portin, 2014). Guide RNA (gRNA) are RNAs that can guide genomic deletion or insertion (Vidigal & Ventura, 2015). Here the researchers wanted the gRNA to identify the GHSR gene. This is done relatively simply, and in this case one can purchase a gRNA creator such as the Guide-IT synthesis kit (Zallar, et al., 2018).

The synthesized gRNAs are then injected into Wistar rat embryos along with the Cas9 nickase (Zallar, et al., 2018). Cas9 is a protein that is used to cut or bind targeted RNA sequences. This allows isolation of specific RNA sequences (O'Connell, Oakes, Sternberg, East-Seletsky, Kaplan, & Doudna, 2014). These injected embryos were then placed in pseudopregnant females until the pregnancy reached full term.

Upon birth, the genetic makeup of the newborn rats were determined by polymerase chain reaction (PCR) (Saiki, Scharf, Faloona, Mullis, Hoorn, & Arnheim et al., 1985). A tail biopsy, as we have seen in other portions of this book, was employed. In this study, 12 deletion alleles were identified among 57 rats, and the selected mutant GHSR was named W-Ghsr[em1Ottc] and is registered with the Rat Genome Database (#12879386). This was also inputted into the Rat Resource and Research Center (RRRC#827, University of Missouri, Columbia MO); thus, rats containing this mutant GHSR are now referred as GHSR KO rats (Zallar, et al., 2018). This is a standard way of registering new knockouts.

During the early development and experimental phases, the body weight of each rat was monitored weekly. There was a difference in body weight between the WT and GHSR KO groups, in which GHSR KO weighed significantly less and had a higher amount of brown adipose tissue. Meal consumption was higher among KO rats compared to WT rats. In the midbrain, hippocampus, and hypothalamus, a larger amount of GHSR mRNA expression was revealed among the WT rats, but not among the GHSR KO rats (Zallar, et al., 2018). Both WT and KO rats displayed almost identical levels of motor activity when tested in a locomotor chamber and in the open field. Importantly, moreover, the WT and GHSR KO rats did *not* differ in terms of gross body composition except for higher levels of brown adipose tissue observed in KO rats.

The authors speculate about the results by noting that the GHSR KO rats had increased brown adipose tissue as a percentage of total body weight compared to WT rats. They point out that brown adipose tissue is primarily responsible for energy expenditure via thermogenesis. Further, both obese humans and rodents have decreased brown adipose tissue activity. The lowered overall body weight of the GHSR KO rats compared with the WT rats may be not only due to reduction in food consumption but also to increased thermal energy output due to higher brown adipose tissue content.

It is noted that harmful and unintended edits with the CRISPR/Cas9 can be created since the technology is still imprecise (Sas & Martinlawrenz, 2017). Further, human trials are only starting now (as of 2020), and we really do not know what the consequences will be. Given the ease with which it is performed, CRIPR/Cas9 is going to fall into many hands and it is going to be difficult to regulate.

This being stated, one can immediately determine how promising this and related techniques are. As the authors point out, "The present GHSR KO rat model has the potential to facilitate our understanding of . . . a wide range of diseases, including medical disorders that represent leading causes of mortality and morbidity worldwide" (Zallar, et al., 2014, p. 350).

Conclusion

There is no shortage of ways to answer questions involving genetics. Even labs or researchers with few resources can address many questions within a small budget and limited skill sets. Given the yield of information, one is encouraged to ask about any health psychology topic, "What role are genes playing in that?"

From the simple (e.g., discovering if there is a genetic influence) to the most complex (e.g., knocking out genes and determining health impact), any researcher can perform what was once thought of as impossible studies. In terms of practical advice to leave one with, a few things have helped in terms of performing or starting out in genetics research. For the complete novice, start with a recent molecular biology text. This will give the basics of what is going on in the field and cover topics such as RNA, protein expression, and recent advances. Second, work with a genetics colleague who knows what kits to order, how to run PCR, and can find things like the electrophoresis equipment. Oftentimes, this person will be delighted to help. One can also follow advances in the popular press using resources such as *Scientific American* or *The Scientist*. Rather than start at a top-level genetics journal, one might be best off reading summaries. Finally, jump in! Some in our lab have used 23andMe and have found relatives (albeit third cousins) using DNA kits from commercial companies. Within a year, one will be able to actually perform techniques, even CRISP/Cas9. Given the wealth of information that one can achieve, it is a beneficial investment.

References

Altman, J. (2002). Weight in the balance. *Neuroendocrinology*, *76*(3), 131–136. https://doi.org/10.1159/000064528

Ansorge, W., Sproat, B., Stegemann, J., Schwager, C., & Zenke, M. (1987). Automated DNA sequencing: Ultrasensitive detection of fluorescent bands during electrophoresis. *Nucleic Acids Research*, *15*(11), 4593–4602. https://doi.org/10.1093/nar/15.11.4593

Atalayer, D., Gibson, C., Konopacka, A., & Geliebter, A. (2013). Ghrelin and eating disorders. *Progress in Neuro-Psychopharmacology & Biological Psychiatry*, *40*, 70–82. https://doi.org/10.1016/j.pnpbp.2012.08.011

Barington, M., Brorson, M. M., Hofman-Bang, J., Rasmussen, Å. K., Holst, B., & Feldt-Rasmussen, U. (2017). Ghrelin-mediated inhibition of the TSH-stimulated function of differentiated human thyrocytes ex vivo. *PLoS One*, *12*(9), e0184992. https://doi.org/10.1371/journal.pone.0184992

Belhaj, K., Chaparro-Garcia, A., Kamoun, S., Patron, N. J., & Nekrasov, V. (2015). Editing plant genomes with CRISPR/Cas9. *Current Opinion in Biotechnology*, *32*, 76–84. https://doi.org/10.1016/j.copbio.2014.11.007

Canli, T., & Lesch, K.-P. (2007). Long story short: The serotonin transporter in emotion regulation and social cognition. *Nature Neuroscience*, *10*(9), 1103–1109. https://doi.org/10.1038/nn1964

Chen, C.-Y. (2014). DNA polymerases drive DNA sequencing-by-synthesis technologies: Both past and present. *Frontiers in Microbiology*, *5*, 305. https://doi.org/10.3389/fmicb.2014.00305

Chmielarz, P., Kreiner, G., Kuśmierczyk, J., Kowalska, M., Roman, A., Tota, K., et al. (2016). Depressive-like immobility behavior and genotype × stress interactions in male mice of selected strains. *Stress*, *19*(2), 206–213. https://doi.org/10.3109/10253890.2016.1150995

Cummings, D. E., Weigle, D. S., Frayo, R. S., Breen, P. A., Ma, M. K., Dellinger, E. P., et al. (2002). Plasma ghrelin levels after diet-induced weight loss or gastric bypass surgery. *The New England Journal of Medicine*, *346*(21), 1623–1630. https://doi.org/10.1056/NEJMoa012908

Fawcett, K. A., & Barroso, I. (2010). The genetics of obesity: FTO leads the way. *Trends in Genetics: TIG*, *26*(6), 266–274. https://doi.org/10.1016/j.tig.2010.02.006

Fuller, C. W., Kumar, S., Porel, M., Chien, M., Bibillo, A., Stranges, P. B., et al. (2016). Real-time single-molecule electronic DNA sequencing by synthesis using polymer-tagged nucleotides on a nanopore array. *Proceedings of the National Academy of Sciences of the United States of America*, *113*(19), 5233–5238. https://doi.org/10.1073/pnas.1601782113

Gan, S. D., & Patel, K. R. (2013). Enzyme immunoassay and Enzyme-Linked Immunosorbent Assay. *The Journal of Investigative Dermatology*, *133*(9), e12. https://doi.org/10.1038/jid.2013.287

Guan, X. M., Yu, H., Palyha, O. C., McKee, K. K., Feighner, S. D., Sirinathsinghji, D. J., et al. (1997). Distribution of mRNA encoding the growth hormone secretagogue receptor in brain and peripheral tissues. *Brain Research. Molecular Brain Research*, *48*(1), 23–29. https://doi.org/10.1016/S0169-328X(97)00071-5

Heather, J. M., & Chain, B. (2016). The sequence of sequencers: The history of sequencing DNA. *Genomics*, *107*(1), 1–8. https://doi.org/10.1016/j.ygeno.2015.11.003

Kalantari, N., Keshavarz Mohammadi, N., Izadi, P., Gholamalizadeh, M., Doaei, S., Eini-Zinab, H., et al. (2018). A complete linkage disequilibrium in a haplotype of three SNPs in Fat Mass and Obesity associated (FTO) gene was strongly associated with anthropometric indices after controlling for calorie intake and physical activity. *BMC Medical Genetics*, *19*(1), 146. https://doi.org/10.1186/s12881-018-0664-z

Mouradian, G. C., Gaurav, R., Pugliese, S., El Kasmi, K., Hartman, B., Hernandez-Lagunas, L., et al. (2017). Superoxide dismutase 3 R213G single-nucleotide polymorphism blocks murine bleomycin-induced fibrosis and promotes resolution of inflammation. *American Journal of Respiratory Cell and Molecular Biology*, *56*(3), 362–371. https://doi.org/10.1165/rcmb.2016-0153OC

Myhre, R., Kratz, M., Goldberg, J., Polivy, J., Melhorn, S., Buchwald, D., et al. (2014). A twin study of differences in the response of plasma ghrelin to a milkshake preload in restrained eaters. *Physiology & Behavior*, *129*, 50–56. https://doi.org/10.1016/j.physbeh.2014.02.008

O'Connell, M. R., Oakes, B. L., Sternberg, S. H., East-Seletsky, A., Kaplan, M., & Doudna, J. A. (2014). Programmable RNA recognition and cleavage by CRISPR/Cas9. *Nature*, *516*(7530), 263–266. https://doi.org/10.1038/nature13769

Portin, P. (2014). The birth and development of the DNA theory of inheritance: Sixty years since the discovery of the structure of DNA. *Journal of Genetics*, *93*(1), 293–302. https://doi.org/10.1007/s12041-014-0337-4

Qi, L., Kang, K., Zhang, C., van Dam, R. M., Kraft, P., Hunter, D., et al. (2008). Fat mass-and obesity-associated (FTO) gene variant is associated with obesity: Longitudinal analyses in two cohort studies and functional test. *Diabetes, 57*(11), 3145–3151. https://doi.org/10.2337/db08-0006

Raikwar, S. P., Thangavel, R., Dubova, I., Selvakumar, G. P., Ahmed, M. E., Kempuraj, D., et al. (2018). Targeted gene editing of glia maturation factor in microglia: A novel Alzheimer's disease therapeutic target. *Molecular Neurobiology.* https://doi.org/10.1007/s12035-018-1068-y

Riedl, J., Ding, Y., Fleming, A. M., & Burrows, C. J. (2015). Identification of DNA lesions using a third base pair for amplification and nanopore sequencing. *Nature Communications, 6,* 8807. https://doi.org/10.1038/ncomms9807

Saiki, R. K., Scharf, S., Faloona, F., Mullis, K., Hoorn, G. T., & Arnheim, N. (1985). Polymerase chain reaction. *Science, 230,* 1350–1354. https://doi.org/10.1126/science.2999980

Saldaña-Alvarez, Y., Salas-Martínez, M. G., García-Ortiz, H., Luckie-Duque, A., García-Cárdenas, G., Vicenteño-Ayala, H., et al. (2016). Gender-dependent association of FTO polymorphisms with body mass index in Mexicans. *PLoS One, 11*(1), e0145984. https://doi.org/10.1371/journal.pone.0145984

Sanger, F., Donelson, J. E., Coulson, A. R., Kössel, H., & Fischer, D. (1973). Use of DNA polymerase I primed by a synthetic oligonucleotide to determine a nucleotide sequence in phage f1 DNA. *Proceedings of the National Academy of Sciences of the United States of America, 70*(4), 1209–1213. https://doi.org/10.1073/pnas.70.4.1209

Sas, D. F., & Martinlawrenz, H. (2017). Crispr-CAS9: The latest fashion in designer babies. *Ethics & Medicine: An International Journal of Bioethics, 33*(2).

Schanze, A., Reulbach, U., Scheuchenzuber, M., Groschl, M., Kornhuber, J., & Kraus, T. (2008). Ghrelin and eating disturbances in psychiatric disorders. *Neuropsychobiology, 57*(3), 126–130. https://doi.org/10.1159/000138915

Sleegers, K., Bettens, K., De Roeck, A., Van Cauwenberghe, C., Cuyvers, E., Verheijen, J., et al. (2015). A 22-single nucleotide polymorphism Alzheimer's disease risk score correlates with family history, onset age, and cerebrospinal fluid Aβ42. *Alzheimer's & Dementia: The Journal of the Alzheimer's Association, 11*(12), 1452–1460. https://doi.org/10.1016/j.jalz.2015.02.013

Turner, K. M., & Burne, T. H. J. (2013). Interaction of genotype and environment: Effect of strain and housing conditions on cognitive behavior in rodent models of schizophrenia. *Frontiers in Behavioral Neuroscience, 7,* 97. https://doi.org/10.3389/fnbeh.2013.00097

Upadhye, D., Jain, D., Trivedi, Y., Nadkarni, A., Ghosh, K., & Colah, R. (2016). Influence of single nucleotide polymorphisms in the BCL11A and HBS1L-MYB gene on the HbF levels and clinical severity of sickle cell anaemia patients. *Annals of Hematology, 95*(7), 1201–1203. https://doi.org/10.1007/s00277-016-2675-1

Vidigal, J. A., & Ventura, A. (2015). Rapid and efficient one-step generation of paired gRNA CRISPR-Cas9 libraries. *Nature Communications, 6,* 8083. https://doi.org/10.1038/ncomms9083

Wang, R., Li, M., Zhou, S., Zeng, D., Xu, X., Xu, R., et al. (2015). Effect of a single nucleotide polymorphism in miR-146a on COX-2 protein expression and lung function in smokers with chronic obstructive pulmonary disease. *International Journal of Chronic Obstructive Pulmonary Disease, 10,* 463–473. https://doi.org/10.2147/COPD.S74345

Yan, S., Tu, Z., Li, S., & Li, X.-J. (2018). Use of CRISPR/Cas9 to model brain diseases. *Progress in Neuro-Psychopharmacology & Biological Psychiatry, 81,* 488–492. https://doi.org/10.1016/j.pnpbp.2017.04.003

Yang, Y., Li, W., Zhao, J., Zhang, H., Song, X., Xiao, B., et al. (2012). Association between ghrelin gene (GHRL) polymorphisms and clinical response to atypical antipsychotic drugs in Han Chinese schizophrenia patients. *Behavioral and Brain Functions: BBF, 8,* 11. https://doi.org/10.1186/1744-9081-8-11

Zallar, L. J., Tunstall, B. J., Richie, C. T., Zhang, Y. J., You, Z. B., Gardner, E. L., et al. (2018). Development and initial characterization of a novel ghrelin receptor CRISPR/Cas9 knockout wistar rat model. *International Journal of Obesity.* https://doi.org/10.1038/s41366-018-0013-5

5
RESEARCH METHODS IN ALCOHOLISM

Maya Crawford, Liliia Savitska, Janet Brenya, Katherine Chavarria,
and Julian Paul Keenan

Overview

At a time when almost all humans are touched by alcoholism, research into the field could not be more welcome. The abuse of alcohol has been acknowledged for thousands of years and yet our understanding remains limited. That does not mean we do not know a lot about alcoholism—we do. It *does* mean that despite tens of thousands of researchers and billions of dollars invested, we have no definitive cause and no definitive treatment identified. Therefore, research in this area is highly encouraged.

Research in Practice

Using the Alcohol Self-Administration Experiment to Test Genetic Differences Between Adolescents, Men, and Women

The relationship between humans and the evolution of alcoholism can be traced far back in human evolutionary history. Humans have been exposed to ethanol, which is the most common type of naturally produced and consumed alcohol, through eating ripened fruit (Levey, 2004). Although alcoholism is a complex genetic disease, some genes have been identified, and current studies are making more discoveries and advancements (Edenberg & Foroud, 2013). Studying alcoholism is complex due to the various factors such as incomplete penetrance, phenocopies, different expression of genes, and environmental influences (Ducci & Goldman, 2012). This is an important topic to study because alcoholism is a serious disease that accounts for 3.3 million deaths per year worldwide when alcohol is misused (Sudhinaraset, Wigglesworth, & Takeuchi, 2016). Recent studies have shown that alcohol consumption has increased in adolescents. This change has led to more studies that focus on adolescent relationships with alcoholism (Keenan, Freeman, & Harrell, 1997). Therefore, this method section involves investigating whether there are genetic variations that contribute to the differences between alcohol consumption of adolescent men and women and the effects it has on them.

Since alcohol use disorder (AUD) is outlined by the *Diagnostic and Statistical Manual of Mental Disorders* (DSM-IV) as one of the most widespread and common disorders in the world, extensive research on the subject should be considered crucial in order to learn more about it (Gonzalez, Jia, Pinzón, Acevedo, Ojelade, Xu, et al., 2018). The benefits of using human participants include observing and relating the results directly to humans in society rather than observing results from fruit flies or rodents. The results obtained from research using humans provide meaningful data that can benefit the public as a whole (Resnik, 2008).

The article being used investigates how genetic influences such as sex and family history of alcohol play a role in alcohol consumption in young adults. Arterial blood alcohol concentration (aBAC) was used because it is a more accurate form of measuring blood alcohol concentrations than venous blood. The difference in accuracy is due to the different mechanisms of alcohol absorption between the veins and arteries (Martin, Moll, Schmid, & Dettli, 1984). This study concluded that women had significantly less real-life drinking (drinking in everyday life rather than intravenous [IV] administration in the lab) than men and also had lower mean arterial aBACs. In addition, the study used a self-administration experiment and concluded that adolescent women prefer having *lower* aBACs than men because of their relation to high sedation rates (Jünger, Gan, Mick, Seipt, Markovic, Sommer, et al., 2016).

Adolescents are used in this study because this developmental stage is critical for the development of AUD. Also, because the study wanted to investigate sex, it was necessary to use both male and female candidates. The participants were 18- to 19-year-olds who were recruited from the surrounding area. They were then required to provide information regarding family history of alcoholism. Because the researchers wanted to test genetic differences, they needed to make sure the participants had a history of alcoholism, and major genetically determined factors are known to affect the risk for AUDs, namely sex and family history of alcoholism. The researchers also sought out adolescents (18- to 19-year-olds) that experienced at least one episode of drunkenness and reported having two or more alcoholic drinks per week during the last two months. The study excluded participants for reasons such as having any previous alcohol-related treatments; a medical disorder that would place them at risk if consuming alcohol; current or past substance dependence (except nicotine dependence); elevated aspartate transaminase, alanine aminotransferase, or gamma-glutamyl transferase; any severe current or past axis I disorder according to DSM-IV; a urine drug screen positive for cocaine, amphetamines, cannabinoids, benzodiazepines, opiates, barbiturates, ecstasy, or antidepressants; pregnancy or breastfeeding; current desire to become pregnant; taking medication that might interact with alcohol; and drinking alcohol on the test day or the day before (Jünger, et al., 2016). Those that fit the criteria were invited for a laboratory screening for family history of alcoholism.

All materials associated with the study *Adolescent women induce lower blood alcohol levels than men in a laboratory alcohol self-administration experiment* (Jünger, et al., 2016) called for approval from the ethics committee. Once the study was approved, 3,580 invitation letters were sent out to 18- to 19-year-olds. This study obtained addresses from the recruitment office of Dresden, Germany; however, participants could also be recruited from college and community settings (Hendershot, Wardell, McPhee, & Ramchandani, 2017). A functional magnetic resonance image (fMRI) was needed to measure brain activity. Urine sample kits and pregnancy test kits were needed to make sure none of the women were pregnant. This study used medical pregnancy and urine drug screening tests. Any drug screening and pregnancy tests can be used. For the self-administration experiment, an 18G IV line was administered. A comfortable armchair was provided and an Alcotest 6810med breathalyzer was used to record aBAC levels. A television with sitcoms was needed to keep the participants engaged, and a full meal was provided.

The variables being investigated were genetic factors such as sex and family history of alcoholism. The results were measured in four ways, which were family history of alcoholism, real-life drinking, free-access IV alcohol self-administration, and subjective ratings Measuring in four ways allowed the researchers to accurately interpret the results. Also, a computer was used for subjective ratings. The participants were provided with ratings from 1 to 7 and told to click on how he or she was feeling. Rating number 1 was *stimulation*, and the participants clicked on a statement that suggested stimulating alcohol effects (e.g., cheerful, excited, full of energy). Rating number 2 was *sedation*, suggesting an experience of sedating alcohol effects (e.g., relaxed, tired). Rating number 3 was *negative effects*, suggesting negative alcohol effects (e.g., nausea, dizziness). The fourth rating was *alcohol desire*, suggesting a desire for alcohol at the moment. *Overall well-being* was the fifth rating assessing the participant's overall assessment at that point in time. The sixth rating was the *number of drinks* equating the participant's current feelings with past experiences after having *x* number of drinks. The last rating was *feeling drunk*, asking participants to assess whether they felt drunk at that moment. The statements were programmed with a presentation from Neurobehavioral Systems in Albany, California, to ensure that the participants received proper directions and to clarify how to answer the questions using the mouse and the monitor screen.

The participants that responded were called and pre-checked for a family history of alcoholism. The adolescents that reported having a family history of alcoholism were invited for laboratory screenings. Participants received written informed consent information. Liver enzymes were then obtained to check for inclusion and exclusion criteria. The adolescents were also interviewed using the Munich Composite International Diagnostic Interview, the Diagnostisches Interview Psychischer Störungen, and the Family History Assessment Module to further check on inclusion and exclusion in order to make sure the participants were fully qualified for the study. After going through the exclusion phase, the final sample size was 82 adolescents between 18 and 19 years of age. Out of the 82 participants, 35 were women and 38 were positive for family history of alcoholism.

The participants underwent two identical sessions separated by three days. The first day consisted of training sessions and two fMRIs. The study started at 1 p.m., and urine samples for pregnancy testing were obtained, along with drug screenings. At around 1:30 p.m. an 18G IV line was administered via the antecubital fossa vein of the participant's nondominant arm. After that, participants were given the Brief Alcohol Expectancy Questionnaire, Alcohol Use Disorders Identification Test, and the Beck Depression Inventory for about 45 minutes. To ensure comfort, the participants sat in a comfortable armchair facing a window. They were also allowed to watch television and use the restroom anytime. The alcohol self-administration (ASA) began at 2:15 p.m. and ended at 4:40 p.m. Subjective ratings were obtained after 10 minutes and every 20 minutes. Subjective ratings included the participants verbally expressing how they felt. The ratings were assessed in order, ranging from one to seven. Eight aBAC readings were obtained using an Alcotest 6810med breathalyzer and entered into the CAIS software. After the IV line was removed, participants were provided a full meal in order to provide them with nutrients and to help slow down the rate at which the alcohol was absorbed into the bloodstream. The participants were allowed to leave the lab as soon as their aBAC was below 45 mg%, if picked up by car, or below 20 mg% if they went home unaccompanied. (Jünger, et al., 2016).

The Washington University Twin Study of Alcoholism: A Study Method Analysis

Biological offspring of alcoholic parents are about three to five times more likely to develop alcoholism during their lifespan than the biological offspring of nonalcoholics (McGue, 1999). Using twins to study the genetics of AUDs will clarify the genetic contributions to the development of AUDs in individuals and its nuances in terms of traits, behaviors, and disease. Conclusions derived from this study rely on shared and unshared genetic and environmental factors between identical/monozygotic (MZ) and fraternal/dizygotic (DZ) twins (Iyer-Eimerbrink & Nurnberger, 2014). If MZ twins show more resemblance than DZ twins for a specific trait, this can be evidence that genetic factors influence the trait; however, if both MZ twins and DZ twins share a resemblance for a specific trait, this can be simply due to the environment around them. The study of gene–environment interactions (G×E) on alcohol use suggests that a person's genes interact with factors in their environment. This interaction may be better able to account for alcohol use patterns than either factor alone (Davis, Natta, & Slutske, 2017). Twin studies allow heritability estimates to be obtained. Not much is known about the role genetics plays in the development of AUDs; however, using twins to study alcoholism can not only prove genetic contributions but also give an insight into genetic variation during development. A study titled "The Washington University Twin Study of Alcoholism" used this method to study the role genetic influences play on alcoholism.

For Washington University's twin study of alcoholism, twins were recruited from alcohol rehab centers and psychiatric facilities. Twins experiencing alcohol abuse and dependence were verified through assessments, medical records, and interviews, and thus were conducted by professionals. Genetic similarity was taken into account to provide the most accurate results. Headshots and information on the physical attributes, through the use of a questionnaire, were obtained from each twin. For this particular study, 154 pairs of twins were analyzed, which included pairs of 28 monozygotic male (MZM), 17 monozygotic female (MZF), 26 dizygotic male (DZM), 24 dizygotic female (DZF), and 59 opposite-sex (OS) twins. In total, 167 males and 141 females participated in this study. The participants' ages varied between 15 and 76 years old, the mean being 34.7 years old, and 31.8% of the participants were African American.

Another study entitled "A National Swedish Longitudinal Twin-Sibling Study of Alcohol Use Disorders Among Males" used different registries such as the Swedish Twin Registry and the Swedish Inpatient Register to identify twins with AUDs. Zygosity was verified through mail-back questionnaires, which were compared to biological markers. Another study obtained their data through telephone interviews (Liu, Blacker, Xu, Fitzmaurice, Tsuang & Lyons, 2004).

After confirming the diagnosis of alcoholism of the participants, research assistants reviewed all demographics and documents, including the amount of alcohol consumed both before diagnosis and during diagnosis, medical records, and family history. A symptom score for each participant was calculated based on 23 items listed for the diagnosis of alcoholism, such as blackouts. Another study measured the level of alcohol dependence based on drinking quantity, drinking frequency, age at the individual's first alcoholic drink, and the number of alcoholic drinks in the last week. The responses to these questions were mailed via questionnaires. For drinking quantity, respondents were asked to indicate how many drinks specific people usually have in a typical week. For drinking frequency, respondents were asked to indicate how many drinks specific people had during the last 12 months, or in a typical year if the person is deceased. For the age of first drink, respondents were asked when they or their twin first drank alcohol. Lastly, for the number of drinks last week, respondents were asked to fill in the number of drinks for each type of alcoholic drink category for every day of the week. Another study only included the symptoms that lasted at least a month in their data. They determined this by asking two questions: when they first experienced the symptom and when they experienced the symptom.

Data collected in this study was used to determine twin pair similarity, the distinction between gender and ethnicity, any co-occurring conditions, and common signs and symptoms. Twin pair similarity was evaluated using two statistical analyses methods, probandwise concordance, and tetrachoric correlations. Twin pair correlation was calculated using Smith's method, based on Falconer's formula. Age- and sex-adjusted prevalence of alcohol consumption were obtained from the St. Louis site of the Epidemiological Catchment Area Study (ECA). Comorbidity prevalence estimates were also obtained from ECA. The Natural Language Processing (NLP) procedure in SAS version 8 was used to fit models to the data and to obtain the number of unaffected twin pairs. The findings from this procedure, presented in 2×2 tables for both unaffected and affected groups, were then put into Mx, a structural equation modeling software. Proportions of variance and 95% confidence intervals were obtained from models using maximum likelihood estimation. The differences in heritability for AUD between both sexes (female twins and male twins) were also evaluated in this study. Lifetime DSM-IV alcohol abuse, alcohol dependence, binge drinking frequency, and self-perceived lifetime alcohol consumption were used as indicators in this model, while AUD was the latent variable. The WLSMV-estimator in Mplus version 6.11 was utilized to approximate the confirmatory fit index and the root mean square error of approximation (Ystrom, Kendler, & Reichborn-Kjennerud, 2014).

An independent-sample t-test was used to test sex differences in the mean age of alcohol initiation (Ystrom, et al., 2014). Male/female risk ratios and $\chi 2$-based ratios were measured using "tables for epidemiologist" from Strata (Ystrom, et al., 2014). "Extended Twin Study of Alcohol Use in Virginia and Australia" not only studied the correlation between twins and alcoholic drinking behaviors for their study but also correlations between various familial relationships, such as parent and child and grandparent and child. This allows for AUD symptoms and drinking patterns to be detected within generations. This study used likelihood ratio tests (LRTs) to obtain model-fitting results for their data.

The Leu72Met Polymorphism of the Prepro-Ghrelin Gene Is Associated With Alcohol Consumption and Subjective Responses to Alcohol: Preliminary Findings: Study Method Analysis

For many years now, alcohol has been the drink of choice for many individuals when it comes to celebrations, recreation, and dealing with personal and stressful situations. However, this recreational drink that has the ability to hinder one's awareness and senses has also become more of a problematic issue in society. People react differently to alcohol. The effects of alcohol on an individual are influenced by the genetic composition of the particular person. Over time, alcoholism has been considered more of a medical condition as opposed to a mental or psychological condition. Thus, a study titled, *The Leu72Met Polymorphism of the Prepro-ghrelin Gene Is Associated with Alcohol Consumption and Subjective Responses to Alcohol: Preliminary Findings* aims to look into these claims by determining how the gene of an individual has a direct relation to alcohol and alcoholism (Suchankova, Yan, Schwandt, Stangl, Jerlhag, Engel, et al., 2017).

For this study to come to life, the methodology applied is known as association analysis, which was performed using the National Institution on Alcohol Abuse and Alcoholism (NIAAA) clinical sample. Association analysis has the ability to offer better understanding as well as identifying items that happen to have a close association for or affinity with each other (Wang, Feng, Ren, Huang, Zhou, Wen, et al., 2016). This methodology happens to look into the relation of a gene and a phenotype, which is usually derived and from the statistics of single nucleotide polymorphisms (SNPs) that are present within that particular gene. Thus, this study is not affected or influenced by data from outside of the given gene or environment (Yan, Du, Yao, & Shen, 2016). This methodology is strongly used and applied as a result of it having the following advantages:

1. A gene happens to be a functional unit of a given genome that is consistent throughout an individual.
2. When used in comparison to SNP-level association tests, this form of analysis results in a greater reduction on corrections.
3. Lastly, the findings that are made under this form of analysis (gene-based analysis association) can strongly and relevantly be used in other studies over time.

For this case, the participants were of a subset from a larger sample. The subset contained a total of 1,127 participants of a larger sample of 1,325. The participants were recruited at the NIH Clinical Centre in Bethesda, Maryland, USA. Eight hundred and sixteen of the participants had experienced past cases or were currently facing AUD, whereas the remaining portion of 311 participants had no past or present cases of AUD. The study mainly focused on major ancestries (i.e., Caucasian and African American). The age bracket of the participants ranged from 21 to 44 years of age for both male and female parties. The total nondependent social drinkers were 114 in total.

The participants had to hand in a written consent before taking part in the study. In addition, the participant's alcohol levels were measured in order to determine the levels of the participants before the examination/study. This was done to ensure that no external attributes would hinder or affect the final results that were collected at the end of the study. The study also had limits when it came to the AUD grouped in terms of average drinks per day and the number of heavy drinking days the participants were involved in, and the number was estimated at a 90-day state.

This simply means that the participants who would have had more than four or three drinks per day for men or women, respectively, were not to be included in the study. To attain the best results possible, the study first conducted a diagnostic on the AUD participants using the Structural Clinical Interview for DSM-IV-TR Axis I disorders (SCID; Spitzer, Gibbon, Gibbons, Janet, Gibbon Miriam, et al., 2002).

The main stimulus that was used in the study was alcohol, which participants administered to themselves after pressing a button. This was the IV-ASA procedure. The infusion of the IV alcohol infusion rate was determined by the individual's age, weight, height, and gender, all under a physiologically based pharmacokinetic model (Plawecki, Durrani, Boes, Wetherill, Kosobud, O'Connor, et al., 2019). The attributes were implemented through the use of computerized alcohol infusion systems to avoid external sources of error (Zimmermann, O'Connor, & Ramchandani, 2011).

Part of the research material that was used in the study was data from a human laboratory study of IV self-administration of alcohol by individuals, and the data was compared against subjective responses (Suchankova, et al., 2017). The study also made use of a handheld breathalyzer device. For the "open bar" phase, a linear regression was used to conduct the tests and results using the AUD participants, whereas the controlled phase used a logistic regression controlling to attain the scores in relation to the age and gender of participants.

This study applied a repeated measure experimental design where the participants were used in both phases of the study. This was done to determine the responsiveness of the patients between the two phases (a controlled phase and an "unregulated alcohol intake" phase). The unregulated phase was termed an "open bar" experiment phase. The dosages were also fixed and well regulated. Each button press consisted of a total of 7.5 mg% in increments in the breath alcohol concentrations (BrAC), which was at a fixed rate of 3 mg% for every minute, which was under a duration of 2.5 minutes. This was followed up with a 1 mg% decrease for every passing minute until the button was pressed next.

Data in the study was collected in a number of ways. The use of a handheld breathalyzer was also used in the study; this particular device is an Alcotest 7410. The device was used after every 15 minutes during the whole session of the study. A questionnaire was also used in the study; the participants were asked to fill up a rather modified version of the Drug Effects Questionnaire (DEQ). This questionnaire was designed to contain five items that were supposed to be selected by the participants using a 100-mm visual analog scale. The options included feel drug, like drug, like more drug, feel high, and feel intoxicated (Suchankova, et al., 2017).

The questionnaire was filled out after every 10 minutes during the primary phase of the study and after every 15 minutes during the self-administration study phase. In the self-administration phase, the participants had free will to press the button as many times as they wished. This was made so in order to attain the best results of overconsumption of alcohol. This would assist the study in understanding the effects of too much alcohol in short duration, since the phase only lasted for a total of 25 minutes (Cann, De Toma, Cazes, Legrand, Morel, Piouffre, et al., 2002).

On the other hand, genotyping was performed at the NIAAA Lab of Neurogenetics. Whole blood was used to attain the genomic deoxyribonucleic acid (DNA) needed for the study under standard protocols; the genotypes were classified using two applications:

1.   Illumina OmniExpress BeadChip
2.   Illumina HumanOmniExpressExome array

The Arf6 Activator Efa6/PSD3 Confers Regional Specificity and Modulates Ethanol Consumption in Drosophila and Humans: Methodology

Exploring the various ways in which the genetics of alcoholism can be studied may be done so via different organisms. The methods for this section involve using **Drosophila melanogaster**, or the fruit fly, to study the genetics of alcoholism. Ultimately, the question being investigated is whether the fruit fly is an ideal organism that can be used to study the genes involved in alcoholism and the ways in which the experiment will be conducted. AUD is outlined by the DSM-IV and is one of the most widespread and common disorders in the world (Grant, Goldstein, Saha, Chou, Jung, Zhang, et al., 2015). In addition to its complicated phenotype, AUD is influenced by environmental factors (Engel, Taber, Vinton, & Crocker, 2019). The use of *Drosophila* to study the characteristics of the genes in AUD is paramount for many reasons, especially discovering new treatment options (Engel, et al., 2019).

There are many studies that use flies to study the effects of alcohol. For example, Engel et al. used *Drosophila* to study AUD; Rodan and Rothenfluh studied the genetics of behavioral alcohol responses; additionally, Signor and Nuzhdin used *Drosophila* to study acute alcohol exposure using gene expression and alternative splicing. Specifically, this methodology will focus on investigating the specific mechanism behind alcohol consumption response. This study concluded that the Arf6 gene regulates ethanol-induced sedation within the nervous system of adult *Drosophila*, but it also showed that Efa6 is an activator of Arf6 and that both are required for ethanol-induced tolerance. Arf6 and Efa6 are involved in the growth and regulation of axons, thus playing a critical role in the nervous system of *Drosophila* (Qu, Hahn, Lees, Parkin, Voelzmann, Dorey, et al., 2019). In addition, Arf6 is part of the Rho family of small guanosine triphosphatase (GTPase) and is involved in the signaling and regulation action and neuronal processes (Gonzalez, et al., 2018). GTPases are a large family of enzymes that can bind and hydrolyze guanosine triphosphate (GTP). Because Arf6 plays a significant role in the nervous system, it is an ideal gene to use to study the behavioral effects of alcohol, since alcohol is a depressant that affects the nervous system. The effects observed on *Drosophila* are similar to mammals, and the genes that regulate ethanol response are orthologs to human genes, such as *PSD3* (Gonzalez, et al., 2018).

D. melanogaster is a model organism when it comes to genetic research. The use of *Drosophila* is efficient because it has a short life cycle, has low-maintenance breeding, is cost-effective, and has similar human genes (Lewis, 2004). Most importantly, *D. melanogaster* possess and display related behaviors and characteristics, such as disinhibition, locomotor hyperactivity, and sedation, which are related to those of mammals (Gonzalez, et al., 2018). Also, *Drosophila* has conserved genes such as the Rho family that is associated with human alcohol characteristics (Gonzalez, et al., 2018). To continue, flies have a 75% homology with the genomes of humans, making it a convenient organism for this study (Engel, et al., 2019). According to Signor and Nuzhdin, *Drosophila* is an ideal organism to study AUD because they acquire tolerance after long periods of exposure, which aligns with the criteria in the DSM-IV (2018). Overall, using *Drosophila* is a cost-effective, convenient, and efficient way of studying AUD. The study of interest, *The Arf6 Activator Efa6/PSD3 Confers Regional Specificity and Modulates Ethanol Consumption in Drosophila and Humans*, used *Drosophila* because of the similarity in genes that regulate alcohol behavior; thus, the flies were used to isolate conserved genes that were linked with human alcohol behaviors (Gonzalez, et al., 2018).

Design

Materials associated with the Gonzalez et al. study included obtaining flies from the Bloomington *Drosophila* Stock Center, specifically Efa6[PB], Stock #10314. Standard cornmeal and molasses will be needed to maintain the flies. The source of alcohol can be from fermented fruits, ethanol-containing foods, or ethanol (Rodan & Rothenfluh, 2010); however, Gonzalez et al. used a combination of ethanol and air. Also, chambers or tubes were used to house the flies and expose them to ethanol. A capillary feeder (CAFE) assay and an ethanol vapor assay are needed. A CAFE assay is a method in which the precise amount of food administered to the flies can be tracked (Ja, Carvalho, Mak, de la Rosa, Fang, Liong, et al., 2007). To analyze the data, Prism, specifically the GraphPad 6 Software, was used.

The flies were outcrossed for five generations to the *w− Berlin* before implementing the behavioral experiments. The data was collected by simply observing sedation and tolerance, which occurred when the flies had a loss of righting reflex, which is when the flies regained coordinated motor control to resume an upright position after stimulation, such as a gentle tap. Prism and Chi-square tests were used to analyze the data.

The flies were kept on a standard cornmeal/molasses food diet at 25 °C at 76% humidity and on a 12 hours light and 12 hours dark cycle (Gonzalez, et al., 2018). They were grown to a density of 200 to 400 F1 flies per tube. The flies were then outcrossed to the *w− Berlin* for about five generations. Along with having Efa6[PB], Stock #10314, Efa6KO, a knockout line generated by homologous recombination was obtained from Dr. Yang Hong. Adult males were used for the study one to five days after they emerged from the pupae stage. To observe the effects of sedation and tolerance, the flies were exposed to a combination of water-saturated airflow and ethanol. The flow rate of the mixture was kept at 150 units. The flies were visually observed every five minutes for loss of righting reflex. This was done by gently tapping the flies after exposure to the mixed airflow. To test for rapid tolerance, the flies were exposed to ethanol for 30 minutes and then exposed again after four hours. A sample size of 6 flies was used for sedation and tolerance, while 12 groups of flies were used for the CAFE assay. Genotypes were randomly assigned to different tubes and labeled.

The presence of Arf6 GTPase was determined by using GG3A-PBD, which is a specific protein-binding domain that only binds to activate Arf6. Next, Arf6 was pulled down or separated from the column, using affinity chromatography and glutathione agarose beads. Affinity chromatography is used to separate or pull down the protein of interest from other proteins, and glutathione agarose beads were used to bind the Arf6 and help pull it out of the column. Finally, Western blots were carried out using anti-Arf6 to test for the presence of the protein.

Transgenic Mice With Increased Astrocyte Expression of CCL2 Show Altered Behavioral Effects of Alcohol

Transgenic Mice with Increased Astrocyte Expression of CCL2 Show Altered Behavioral Effects of Alcohol might seem like an unlikely study (Bray, Roberts, & Gruol, 2017). However, mice have been employed for decades as a model organism for alcohol studies, with lines going back close to half a century.

Why mice? Clearly there are plenty of humans that qualify for any level of alcohol consumption. It seems the loss of extrapolation across species would be drastic. While this is true, the advantage, as one sees in this study, is that not only can invasive techniques be used but addiction can be examined through its stage-wise progress. We can examine organisms as they go from naive to dependent.

Why then examine brains? Simply put, different brains lead to different alcohol responses, be they acute or chronic responses. While this assumption is most certainly true, the notion that all behavioral responses are neuron based is absolutely false. Over the past three decades, and increasingly in the last few years, there has been a focus on white matter and glial cells as they relate to cognition, behavior, aberrant functioning, and addiction. This study examined such a relationship in the astrocyte, a glial cell. The astrocyte is the main source of CCL2, which is involved in the neuroimmune response in disorders such as Alzheimer's (Banisadr, Gosselin, Mechighel, Rostène, Kitabgi, & Mélik

Parsadaniantz, 2005); in relation to alcohol consumption, it has been presented that acute as well as chronic alcohol intake can increase the activation of the chemokine CCL2. In this study, the authors were interested in knowing if increased levels of CCL2 in the central nervous system (CNS) produce neuroadaptive changes that modify the actions of alcohol on the CNS.

Here mice present two distinct advantages. The first is that we have breeds that are dependent and those that are not. Second, we can model an individual's response to alcohol dependence. In this study, two methods of 'drinking' were used: one that results in dependence and one that does not (Blizard, Vandenbergh, Lionikas, & McClearn, 2008). Therefore, having breed data and the ability to cause addiction makes this model an extremely powerful one, and clearly its advantages outweigh the extrapolation dilemma.

Design

This study did follow all the animal procedures in relation to the National Institutes of Health Guidelines for the Care and Use of Laboratory Animals. This is perhaps the critical research point to make here. Unless one has a large university or a large grant, mice studies are not feasible. Properly caring for animals in an ethical manner is not easy, nor is it cheap. What then is a person to do from a smaller school or with no grant money? The answer is generally collaboration, and it has been our experience that if the idea is good, the collaboration will come to fruition.

The participants were split into two groups, where one sample of mice was not dependent on alcohol (and left as such) and the other set was made dependent on alcohol after being exposed to alcohol vapor fumes.

To ensure that this was consistent throughout all the mice, the enhanced expression of CCL2 in the CCL2-tg mice was targeted to astrocytes by insertion of the murine CCL2 gene under control of the human glial fibrillary acidic protein (huGFAP) promoter. As a result, the mice had to be genotyped from the weaning stage through the use of DNA samples obtained from their tails using the Mouse Tail Quick Extraction Kit. This is, as it sounds, extracting DNA from the tail of the mouse. Male and female CCL2-tg mice heterozygous for the transgene and their age-matched non-transgenic (non-tg) littermates were used for all experiments.

This study used a number of standard materials, such as alcohol that was diluted to different percentage levels. The study also used some specialized setups, such as the two-bottle choice–chronic ethanol intermittent vapor exposure (2BC/CIE) model, which involves the application of chronic intermittent vapor exposure (CIE) and 2BC limited-access drinking (Huang, Tani, Wang, Han, He, Weaver, et al., 2002). The idea here is to get some of the animals dependent and some of them not. Most of the materials here are standard to an animal lab, including timers to control daylight hours, feeders, bedding, and others.

A matched-pairs experimental design was used to ensure participant balance. In the first week, the mice were offered a 3% alcohol-to-water ratio. This value changed over time from 6%, 9%, and 12% and culminated at a 15% ratio for the fourth week. Typical controls were used here, demonstrating the advantages of animal designs: time of feeding, time of testing, temperature, etc., were all controlled. Again, the ability to detect subtle changes is what one looks for in any animal study.

Many measures were employed here, and the interested reader can seek out these from the original paper. However, we will note a few here. A Barnes maze was used, which is a fairly common tool. It tests the animal's spatial memory by placing holes on a large tabletop surface. Only one of the holes provides an escape, which gives the animal a feeling of comfort. At first, it is trial and error, but soon (within about five trials), a mouse or rat instantly goes to the safe zone. To collect data from the Barnes maze, a number of cameras were placed around the maze—always a good way of recording data. Again, attention to detail is important. For example, the maze was also well cleaned to ensure that any scent left by a previous mouse was not present in a manner that would guide the mice.

The study also used cued and contextual fear conditioning—this enabled the test to have an assessment of both hippocampus-dependent and amygdala-dependent learning processes (Rudy, Huff, & Matus-Amat, 2004). Another behavioral study portion of the study was utilizing a forced-swim test to determine the resilience and spatial abilities of the mice after exposure.

Results and Discussion

Not much was found in terms of breed. Using traditional statistics, it was found that breed did not exert much of an influence, though there were a few effects. As stated by the authors, "neither the non-dependent nor the alcohol dependent CCL2-tg mice showed increased alcohol drinking compared to their respective non-dependent or alcohol dependent non-tg control mice". CCL2 did have an influence, but again, not a dramatic one. The main finding was "CCL2/alcohol interactions produced neuroadaptive changes that impaired hippocampal mechanisms involved in spatial learning and memory in the CCL2-tg mice" (Bray, et al., p. 120). This could be taken to mean that CCL2 interacts with alcohol to impair the hippocampus.

It is noted that the statistics here are basic. There is no need to run structural models just because you are performing assays.

Conclusion

People, including the most qualified researchers, can be dismissive of a technique because it has been around for a long time. Recently our lab published a number of *Drosophila* papers, and a dean asked if people still *really* used fruit flies in behavioral genetics! Human twin studies do not have the innovative sound of theta-burst transcranial magnetic stimulation (TMS) or CRISPR-CAS9. However, it is difficult to find a more applicable technique for alcoholism than the human MZ/DZ or a more flexible one than that of the *Drosophila*.

Those in the know have realized that all techniques have a place. Alcoholism needs to be solved. We understand that solving the puzzle(s) will likely come via a breakthrough using these or other methods. As we chip away at the mountain that alcoholism appears to be, one tool will not suffice.

While no one knows the future, we can conservatively predict that mastering one (or all) or the techniques highlighted here will lead to fruitful results.

References

Banisadr, G., Gosselin, R. D., Mechighel, P., Rostène, W., Kitabgi, P., & Mélik Parsadaniantz, S. (2005). Constitutive neuronal expression of CCR2 chemokine receptor and its colocalization with neurotransmitters in normal rat brain: Functional effect of MCP-1/CCL2 on calcium mobilization in primary cultured neurons. *Journal of Comparative Neurology, 492*(2), 178–192. https://doi.org/10.1002/cne.20729

Bray, J. G., Roberts, A. J., & Gruol, D. L. (2017). Transgenic mice with increased astrocyte expression of CCL2 show altered behavioral effects of alcohol. *Neuroscience, 354*, 88–100. https://doi.org/10.1016/j.neuroscience.2017.04.009

Blizard, D. A., Vandenbergh, D. J., Lionikas, A., & McClearn, G. E. (2008). Learning in the 2-bottle alcohol preference test. *Alcoholism: Clinical and Experimental Research, 32*(12), 2041–2046. doi:10.1111/j.1530-0277.2008.00791.x

Cann, H. M., De Toma, C., Cazes, L., Legrand, M. F., Morel, V., Piouffre, L., et al. (2002). A human genome diversity cell line panel. *Science, 296*(5566), 261–262.

Davis, C. N., Natta, S. S., & Slutske, W. S. (2017). Moderation of genetic influences on alcohol involvement by rural residency among adolescents: Results from the 1962 national merit twin study. *Behavior Genetics, 47*(6), 587–595. doi:10.1007/s10519-017-9867-x

Ducci, F., & Goldman, D. (2012). The genetic bBasis of addictive disorders. *The Psychiatric Clinics of North America, 35*(2), 495–519. doi:10.1016/j.psc.2012.03.010

Edenberg, H. J., & Foroud, T. (2013). Genetics and alcoholism: Nature reviews. *Gastroenterology & Hepatology*, *10*(8), 487–494. doi:10.1038/nrgastro.2013.86

Engel, G. L., Taber, K., Vinton, E., & Crocker, A. J. (2019). Studying alcohol use disorder using Drosophila melanogaster in the era of "big data". *Behavioral and Brain Functions*, *15*(1), 7–7. doi:10.1186/s12993-019-0159-x

Gonzalez, D. A., Jia, T., Pinzón, J. H., Acevedo, S. F., Ojelade, S. A., Xu, B., et al. (2018). The Arf6 activator Efa6/PSD3 confers regional specificity and modulates ethanol consumption in Drosophila and humans. *Molecular Psychiatry*, *23*(3), 621–628. doi:10.1038/mp.2017.112

Grant, B. F., Goldstein, R. B., Saha, T. D., Chou, S. P., Jung, J., Zhang, H., et al. (2015). Epidemiology of DSM-5 alcohol use disorder: Results from the national epidemiologic survey on alcohol and related conditions III. *JAMA Psychiatry*, *72*(8), 757–766. doi:10.1001/jamapsychiatry.2015.0584

Hendershot, C. S., Wardell, J. D., McPhee, M. D., & Ramchandani, V. A. (2017). A prospective study of genetic factors, human laboratory phenotypes, and heavy drinking in late adolescence. *Addiction Biology*, *22*(5), 1343–1354. doi:10.1111/adb.12397.Levey

Huang, D., Tani, M., Wang, J., Han, Y., He, T. T., Weaver, J., et al. (2002). Pertussis toxin-induced reversible encephalopathy dependent on monocyte chemoattractant protein-1 overexpression in mice. *Journal of Neuroscience*, *22*(24), 10633–10642. doi:10.1523/JNEUROSCI.22-24-10633.2002

Iyer-Eimerbrink, P. A., & Nurnberger, J. I. (2014). Genetics of alcoholism. *Current Psychiatry Reports*, *16*(12), 518. doi:10.1007/s11920-014-0518-0

Ja, W. W., Carvalho, G. B., Mak, E. M., de la Rosa, N. N., Fang, A. Y., Liong, J. C., et al. (2007). Prandiology of drosophila and the CAFE assay. *Proceedings of the National Academy of Sciences of the United States of America*, *104*(20), 8253–8256. doi:10.1073/pnas.0702726104

Jünger, E., Gan, G., Mick, I., Seipt, C., Markovic, A., Sommer, C., et al. (2016). Adolescent women induce lower blood alcohol levels than men in a laboratory alcohol self-administration experiment. *Alcoholism, Clinical and Experimental Research*, *40*(8), 1769–1778. doi:10.1111/acer.13122.

Keenan, J. P., Freeman, P. R., & Harrell, R. (1997). The effects of family history, sobriety length, and drinking history in younger alcoholics on P300 auditory-evoked potentials. *Alcohol and Alcoholism (Oxford, Oxfordshire)*, *32*(3), 233–239. https://doi.org/10.1093/oxfordjournals.alcalc.a008262

Levey, D. J. (2004). The evolutionary ecology of ethanol production and alcoholism1. *Integrative and Comparative Biology*, *44*(4), 284–289. doi:10.1093/icb/44.4.284

Lewis, E. B. (2004). Developmental genetics of drosophila. *Annals of the New York Academy of Sciences*, *1038*(1), 94–97. doi:10.1196/annals.1315.016

Liu, I. C., Blacker, D. L., Xu, R., Fitzmaurice, G., Tsuang, M. T., & Lyons, M. J. (2004). Genetic and environmental contributions to age of onset of alcohol dependence symptoms in male twins. *Addiction*, *99*(11), 1403–1409. doi:10.1111/j.1360-0443.2004.00877.x

Martin, E., Moll, W., Schmid, P., & Dettli, L. (1984). The pharmacokinetics of alcohol in human breath, venous and arterial blood after oral ingestion. *European Journal of Clinical Pharmacology*, *26*(5), 619–626. doi:10.1007/BF00543496.

McGue, M. (1999). The behavioral genetics of alcoholism. *Current Directions in Psychological Science*, *8*(4), 109–115. doi:10.1111/1467-8721.00026

Plawecki, M. H., Durrani, A. M., Boes, J., Wetherill, L., Kosobud, A., O'Connor, S., et al. (2019). Comparison of subjective responses to oral and intravenous alcohol administration under similar systemic exposures. *Alcoholism: Clinical and Experimental Research*, *43*(4), 597–606. doi:10.1111/acer.13970

Qu, Y., Hahn, I., Lees, M., Parkin, J., Voelzmann, A., Dorey, K., et al. (2019). Efa6 protects axons and regulates their growth and branching by inhibiting microtubule polymerisation at the cortex. *eLife*, *8*, e50319. doi:10.7554/eLife.50319

Resnik, D. B. (2008). Social benefits of human subjects research. *Journal of Clinical Research Best Practices*, *4*(11), 1–7. doi:10.1126/science.296.5566.261b. https://pubmed.ncbi.nlm.nih.gov/24526930. Retrieved from www.ncbi.nlm.nih.gov/pmc/articles/PMC3920587/

Rodan, A. R., & Rothenfluh, A. (2010). The genetics of behavioral alcohol responses in Drosophila. *International Review of Neurobiology*, *91*, 25–51. doi:10.1016/S0074-7742(10)91002-7

Rudy, J. W., Huff, N. C., & Matus-Amat, P. (2004). Understanding contextual fear conditioning: Insights from a two-process model. *Neuroscience and Biobehavioral Reviews*, *28*, 675–685. doi:10.1016/j.neubiorev.2004.09.004

Signor, S., & Nuzhdin, S. (2018). Dynamic changes in gene expression and alternative splicing mediate the response to acute alcohol exposure in Drosophila melanogaster. *Heredity*, *121*(4), 342–360. doi:10.1038/s41437-018-0136-4

Spitzer, R. L., Robert, L., Gibbon, M., Gibbons, W., Janet, B. W., Gibbon Miriam, R. L., et al. (2002). Structured clinical interview for DSM-IV-TR axis I disorders, research version, non-patient edition. (SCID-I/NP). doi:10.1001/archpsyc.1992.01820080032005

Suchankova, P., Yan, J., Schwandt, M. L., Stangl, B. L., Jerlhag, E., Engel, J. A., et al. (2017). The Leu72Met polymorphism of the prepro-ghrelin gene is associated with alcohol consumption and subjective responses to alcohol: Preliminary findings. *Alcohol and Alcoholism*, *52*(4), 425–430. doi:10.1093/alcalc/agx021

Sudhinaraset, M., Wigglesworth, C., & Takeuchi, D. T. (2016). Social and cultural contexts of alcohol use: Influences in a social-ecological framework. *Alcohol Research: Current Reviews*, *38*(1), 35–45, PubMed, https://pubmed.ncbi.nlm.nih.gov/27159810. Retrieved from www.ncbi.nlm.nih.gov/pmc/articles/PMC4872611/

Wang, S. B., Feng, J. Y., Ren, W. L., Huang, B., Zhou, L., Wen, Y. J., et al. (2016). Improving power and accuracy of genome-wide association studies via a multi-locus mixed linear model methodology. *Scientific Reports*, *6*, 19444. doi:10.1038/srep19444

Yan, J., Du, L., Yao, X., & Shen, L. (2016). Machine learning in brain imaging genomics. In *Machine learning and medical imaging* (pp. 411–434). Academic Press. doi:10.1109/JPROC.2019.2947272

Ystrom, E., Kendler, K. S., & Reichborn-Kjennerud, T. (2014). Early age of alcohol initiation is not the cause of alcohol use disorders in adulthood, but is a major indicator of genetic risk: A population-based twin study. *Addiction*, *109*(11), 1824–1832. doi:10.1111/add.12620

Zimmermann, U. S., O'Connor, S., & Ramchandani, V. A. (2011). Modeling alcohol self-administration in the human laboratory. In *Behavioral neurobiology of alcohol addiction* (pp. 315–353). Berlin, Heidelberg: Springer. doi:10.1007/7854_2011_149

6

BEST PRACTICES FOR STUDYING ADDICTION

Heather E. Soder, Jessica L. Hoffman, Constanza de Dios, and Troy A. Webber

Overview

Drugs and alcohol are a large part of American culture and are often at the center of social gatherings and traditions. However, abuse of drugs and alcohol has serious financial, social, and health-related consequences. It is estimated that over $740 billion are spent yearly on substance use because of crime and healthcare costs (National Drug Intelligence Center, 2011). Socially, addiction can have a toll on the individual's mental health as well as introduce strain on relationships at home and in the workplace. Further, using drugs and alcohol can lead to serious physical health complications, such as heart and lung disease, cancer, HIV/AIDS, and numerous preventable deaths in the United States. Apart from health complications, overdose deaths have steadily risen since 1999, when there was a great rise in prescribing opioids, with over 67,000 Americans dying of overdose in 2018 (CDC Wonder, 2019). A second and third wave of overdose deaths occurred in 2010 and 2013, involving heroin and the synthetic opioid, fentanyl, respectively (Rudd, Paulozzi, Bauer, Burleson, Carlson, Dao, et al., 2014; Gladden, Martinez, & Seth, 2016). The Centers for Disease Control and Prevention (CDC) estimates that 128 people die of an opioid-related overdose each day in the United States. To address these striking statistics and the ongoing opioid epidemic, funding initiatives from the government and other agencies employ research methods aimed at better understanding addiction.

A common misunderstanding regarding addiction is that people who become addicted to drugs do not have enough willpower or lack morality. However, years of research efforts have shown that drug addiction is a complicated brain disease that involves changes in the way humans perceive the world (Volkow, Wang, Fowler, Tomasi, & Telang, 2011). For example, in nonaddicted persons, things that signify or evoke emotion (good or bad) are salient to us, meaning that they catch our attention. However, things that become salient change with drug use. For one, cues related to drug use (e.g., a crack pipe, a small plastic baggie, a lighter) become extremely salient to the user but would normally not draw the same attention in a person who is not using that drug. For example, animals will spend more time in an area that is associated with receiving a rewarding drug (Katz & Gormezano, 1979). Another change that occurs with repeated drug use is a decrease in the interest in naturally occurring rewards, such as feeling pleasure from eating your favorite food, hanging out with friends, or riding a thrilling rollercoaster. Such changes in attention contribute to maintaining an addiction, as exposure to cues can induce craving for the drug, and lack of pleasure from everyday activities may increase the need to seek out a "high." These changes are attributable to drug effects on the brain and help explain altered decision-making in those experiencing addiction.

73

While researchers have discovered a biological basis for drug addiction, even with all the time and money spent, there are still many incomplete answers. The research methods highlighted in this chapter are useful tools in answering some of our most pressing questions. Why are some substances addictive and others are not? How does an addiction develop, and why can it be so difficult to recover? Is it possible to treat addiction, and how can we improve abstinence rates? And perhaps most pressing, can we avoid addiction all together through active prevention strategies such as pharmacotherapies or even vaccination? The methods outlined here include behavioral and neuroimaging methods, animal and human models, correlational and experimental approaches, and cross-sectional and longitudinal designs that exemplify how researchers have begun to answer these questions.

Research in Practice

Classical Conditioning as a Tool to Understand Drug Abuse

The field of behavioral pharmacology emerged in the 1950s alongside the psychotherapeutic revolution as scientists began to link specific behavioral changes to various drugs, including drugs of abuse. With the development of this new field, the basic understanding of addiction as a sign of moral weakness slowly started to be reframed as a physiological reaction to the drugs (Schuster & Thompson, 1969). Animal models were established and fine-tuned in an effort to understand how these drugs were able to change the brain, body, and behavior.

Some of the very first studies investigating the effects of drugs on physiology and behavior utilized classical conditioning. Many people are familiar with the basic principles of classical conditioning established by Ivan Pavlov in the early 1900s. He was also the first to discover that drugs can be used in associative conditioning pairs, allowing previously unrelated stimuli to gain rewarding value by being paired with naturally rewarding stimuli (Pavlov, 1927). In later decades, the study of opioids through classical and operant conditioning would create the foundation for the experimental investigation of addiction using animal models (Siegel, 1983).

These models are versatile and thus have been adopted in the study of numerous drugs of abuse, but our focus for this chapter will remain with the opioid family, and specifically, the incredibly potent synthetic opioid, *fentanyl*. While *fentanyl* was developed in the 1960s for use in cardiac surgery (Stanley, 1992), it has gained a notorious reputation in the last decade, as it has increasingly contributed to opioid overdoses. In the study by Bryant, Roberts, Culbertson, Le, Evans, and Fanselow (2009), the researchers used *fentanyl*, a highly selective *mu* opioid receptor agonist, to investigate the conditioned effects of opioids and possible conditioned expectation effects. The methods employed in this study will be important to understand, as they are fundamental paradigms often used to behaviorally assess drugs of abuse in rodent models.

The subjects in these studies were adult male **C57BL/6J** mice naïve to all drugs. The studies were all approved and conducted in accordance with the Institutional Animal Care and Use Committee at University of California, Los Angeles (UCLA). The mice were group-housed and given unrestricted access to food and water in their home cages.

Fentanyl (0.2 mg/kg, i.p.) was the primary drug of interest in these experiments; however, **cocaine (15 mg/kg, i.p.)** has been used also in parallel studies as a drug comparison. In all studies, control groups received a placebo solution of the same volume.

Design

In this study, a series of experiments were designed to assess a variety of conditioned behaviors. Each experiment had enough subjects in the drug and control conditions to statistically compare the groups. The total number of mice in each experiment reflected the normally occurring individual variability that can be observed in that test using naïve mice. To avoid concerns about tolerance and experience, each experiment was conducted separately, and the mice were not reused for additional experiments.

In one experiment, an open field box lined with **photobeams** was used to test locomotion. As the mice explored the arena, the *photobeam* breaks were recorded for each 30-minute session. To assess conditional locomotion, mice were assigned to either a "conditioned" or "unconditioned" group. The goal was to condition the mice to *fentanyl* in the **open field** environment. On day one, mice in the "conditioned" group received *fentanyl* and were placed in the *open field* for 30 minutes. On day two, these mice received a placebo injection and were placed into their **home cage**. Days one and two were counterbalanced so that the order of injection did not interfere with the results. On day three, the test day, mice received a placebo and were placed into the *open field* again for 30 minutes. Mice in the "unconditioned" group received *fentanyl* in the *home cage* and a placebo in the *open field*. A group of control mice received placebo injections in both environments.

A second study explored the **Straub tail assay**, a paradigm that measures the height of a mouse's stiffened tail following the administration of an opioid. This reaction is a natural physiological response to opioids caused by a contraction of sacrococcygeal dorsalis muscles. Researchers placed a piece of white tape on the tip of the mouse's tail immediately prior to an injection of *fentanyl* or placebo. Then they measured the duration of this reaction. This test follows a similar conditioning schedule to the locomotion test. Due to an order effect in the data, "conditioned" mice were all injected with *fentanyl* on the first day, then placed on either an unheated hot plate or into their *home cage*. On day two, these mice were injected with a placebo and placed in the alternative location. On the test day, mice were injected with placebo and placed on the unheated hot plate for one minute to measure the *Straub tail*. "Unconditioned" mice received *fentanyl* in the *home cage* and a placebo on the unheated plate.

In the third experiment, **analgesia** (pain relief) was measured using the standard **hot plate assay**. During this *assay*, mice were confined to a hot plate heated to 52.5°C after receiving an injection, and the amount of time that lapsed before the animal began to lick its paws (a sign of discomfort) was measured. The animal was removed immediately and returned to its *home cage*. In this experiment, the temperature was warm enough to induce discomfort with prolonged exposure but did not cause injury to the mice. Mice were conditioned using the same paradigm as described earlier using an unheated hot plate during the training session and a heated hot plate on the test day.

The fourth experiment entailed a **conditioned place preference**, a paradigm that measures the reinforcing value of a drug. Most drugs of abuse create a conditioned preference, demonstrating the rewarding nature of the drug. This experiment used the **three-chambered place preference** test, so that one chamber was paired with *fentanyl*, a second assigned as a neutral chamber in the middle, and a third chamber was paired with a placebo. Doors that could be raised and lowered, distinguishable by both visual and olfactory cues, separated the chambers. Prior to training, the mice were allowed to explore all three chambers freely to determine an initial preference. The mice underwent a single training session per day for eight days (four *fentanyl*, four placebo). During each training session, a mouse was injected with either a placebo or *fentanyl* and then confined to the assigned chamber for 30 minutes. On the test day, the mouse received a placebo injection and then was allowed to explore all three chambers for 15 minutes to determine if there was a preference of either the drug or placebo chamber. The time spent in the drug-paired chamber was compared with the final preference to determine if a *place preference* had been established while also accounting for individual differences.

Finally, researchers also attempted to measure **drug expectation** using demonstrator and observer mice in the conditional locomotion and conditioned place preference paradigms. These studies deemed the experimental mice receiving *fentanyl* on the test day of these assays **demonstrator mice** and their cage mates that receive no treatment were deemed **observer mice**. Prior to the conditioned tests, *demonstrator mice* were placed into the *home cage* with the *observer mice* for 10 minutes before completing the assay. The *observer mice* were then tested in the assay after receiving a placebo injection. The goal was to determine if the *demonstrator mice* would act as a drug cue for the *observer mice* in the conditioned tests.

Results and Conclusions

The researchers demonstrated a simple associative conditioning effect of *fentanyl* in all of the standard paradigms, suggesting the mice were responding to the *fentanyl-paired* environment as if they received *fentanyl* even after a placebo was administered. This study represents a novel demonstration of the placebo effect in mice, extending the utility of rodent models when studying drugs of abuse. The authors acknowledge with a more substantial classical conditioning training schedule (more trials), the observed effects would likely change. This is especially likely with opioid drugs such as *fentanyl* because they are known to produce opposing responses such as **hyperalgesia** (increased pain) after repeated pairings in a classical conditioning paradigm. Finally, the researchers' findings did not support an effect of *demonstrator mice* on *observer mice*. This paradigm was innovative, but it is a more difficult experiment to conduct with mice. It requires the *observer mice* to recognize the drug state of the *demonstrator mice* and use that information as a cue. While this is a behavior that can be studied in humans, it has yet to be shown in mice; however, the authors described possible changes to the paradigm that may lead to future success. Although standardized animal models are instrumental to the field, it is also vital that researchers continue to develop clever assays to target additional behaviors in order to push the field forward.

Immunohistochemical Investigation of Long-Term Brain Damage After Drug Exposure in Nonhuman Primates

There are a number of advantages to using animal models to study addiction, including the ability to administer drugs that have unknown risk to human participants. In neuroscience addiction research, it is often also necessary to extract brain tissue for in-depth probing to understand drug-induced changes at a neurochemical and morphological level. Many of the animal models use smaller species such as mice and rats that also have much shorter life spans, allowing studies to examine effects on development and to be completed in a matter of weeks or months. However, rodents are not always similar enough to humans for the research to have translational value. This is where nonhuman primate models can be especially useful. Ethical committees regulate research on all mammals from rodents, to nonhuman primates, to humans in an effort to ensure that all of these studies answer important questions and are conducted responsibly. Nonhuman primate research is the most highly regulated of the animal models, so very few labs conduct them, but they have the greatest potential to inform human studies.

Previous studies in rodents and nonhuman primates strongly suggest acute use of the popular club drug, **(±)3,4-methylenedioxymethamphetamine (MDMA)** could lead to sustained damage to serotonin neurons. However, the studies differed regarding the extent of recovery and reported differing recovery periods after administration of *MDMA* (Insel, Battaglia, Johannessen, Marra, & De Souza, 1989; Lew, Sabol, Chou, Vosmer, Richards, & Seiden, 1996; Scanzello, Hatzidimitriou, Martello, Katz, & Ricaurte, 1993). Researchers sought to reconcile these discrepancies by conducting a study with an extended recovery period after administration of recreational levels of *MDMA* in a highly translational animal model (Hatzidimitriou, McCann, & Ricaurte, 1999).

The subjects were male and female adult squirrel monkeys (*Saimiri sciureus*), euthanized at two weeks (*n* = 3 *MDMA*-treated; *n* = 2 saline-treated), and six—seven years (*n* = 3 *MDMA*-treated; *n* = 2 saline-treated) after *MDMA* administration.

Racemic MDMA hydrochloride (5 mg/kg, twice daily) or saline was administered for four consecutive days. Following the drug administration, the monkeys were housed with free access to food, water, and enrichment according to the Animal Care and Use Committee of the Johns Hopkins Medical Institutions until they were euthanized. The brain vasculature was cleared of all blood prior to the brain removal and fixation in paraformaldehyde.

Design

The goal of this experiment was to execute an *immunohistochemical study* of the squirrel monkey brain tissue to assess the long-term neurotoxic effects of *MDMA* on serotonergic neurons. The fixed tissue was sliced and incubated with antibodies that would detect neurons containing serotonin, tyrosine hydroxylase, and tryptophan hydroxylase. The stained tissue sections were then enhanced and visualized to assess short- (two weeks) and long-term (six to seven years) serotonergic damage. Numerous brain regions were identified using a squirrel monkey brain atlas, and stained cell bodies were quantified. In addition to a simple cell body count, the axons of the neurons were observed for changes in the shape and quality. The axons were classified as either fine axons or beaded axons. Analyses were conducted to compare control brains with short- and long-term recovery periods.

Results and Conclusions

The results of this study precisely demonstrate the advantage of detailed histological studies of brain tissue using animal models. In this type of study, researchers are able to provide images that show serotonergic neurons in a high level of detail and compare the placebo-exposed brains to the *MDMA*-exposed brains (two week and seven years). The researchers examined the neurotoxic effects of *MDMA* on numerous brain regions and found that even after seven years, a few brain regions never recovered from the insult to the serotonergic neurons. In some regions, the natural complexity of the healthy neurons are in stark contrast with the two-week recovery group, with little improvement in the seven-year recovery condition. Other areas show patterns that suggests the neurons have returned to a normal state by the two-week or seven-year mark. These results show the complexity of the brain's reaction to drugs and emphasize a need to explore numerous brain regions over extended periods when studying drugs of abuse. While this type of study is both time- and labor-intensive, it can provide a level of detail that surpasses the current in vivo imaging technology available for use in human or animals, and therefore remains a fundamental technique in addiction research.

Using Event-Related Potentials to Assess Brain Reactivity to Cues and Other Rewards

One method to measure brain activity in humans is through an *electroencephalogram (EEG)*. Usually a net of small metal sensors detect electrical activity produced by the summed activity of large groups of neurons firing in unison over the scalp. *Event-related potentials (ERPs)* are fluctuations in the voltage of electrical activity in response to a specific event, such as viewing an image or making a button press. When particular groups of neurons fire in response to an event, the electrical activity is spread over the scalp, making it difficult to know where the activity is coming from. However, the activity being measured is almost instantaneous, allowing researchers to see what is occurring in the brain within milliseconds after an event occurs. This allows for excellent temporal resolution compared to other brain imaging methods such as *functional magnetic resonance imaging (fMRI)* or *positron emission tomography (PET)*, which are much slower but can provide information about where the activity is occurring. Measuring *ERPs* is also relatively inexpensive and comfortable compared to the other imaging methods and can be easily incorporated into a lab or even a clinical setting. Another major advantage of measuring *ERPs* is that there are several **ERP components** related to a wide range of cognitive, motor, and affective processes. *ERP components* are defined by several factors: 1) their polarity (whether the amplitude is positive or negative), 2) where they occur (the area of the scalp in which they appear), and 3) when they occur (how many milliseconds before or after an event).

One way to better understand changes in attention that occur with addiction is to measure how the brain responds to viewing images of cues and other emotional stimuli with *ERPs*. For example, there is a positive-going brain wave called the **late positive potential (LPP)** that is observed over the central-parietal area of the scalp. This positivity occurs within *400 ms* of viewing any type of image that is emotionally salient to the viewer (Figure 6.1). Pleasant images such as happy romantic couples, cute animals or babies, or even sweet foods elicit this positivity over the back of the head. Unpleasant images like violence or accidents also elicit this positivity, whereas neutral or boring images do not. Importantly, cigarette cues elicit an *LPP wave*, but only in smokers, indicating that these cues are only salient to those who are using cigarettes.

While scientists have investigated the *LPP* in drug users for decades, an important unanswered question is whether brain responses have anything to do with treatment. Does the *LPP* tell us how likely it is that someone will be able to quit while in treatment? We know that treating drug addiction

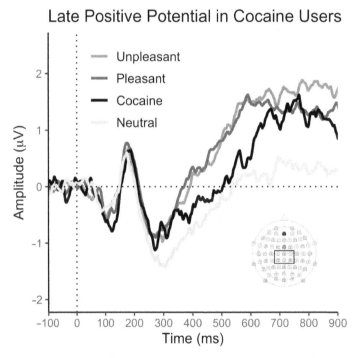

Figure 6.1   The late positive potential (LPP) component in a cocaine-using sample. In a typical ERP graph, the y-axis shows the amplitude of the brain waves in microvolts and the x-axis shows time in milliseconds following an important event. The zero point on the x-axis indicates when an image was shown on the screen. Within about 400 ms, the positivity begins to emerge, differentiating salient (i.e., pleasant and unpleasant) images from neutral images. As this sample was in cocaine users, it is expected that cocaine images will also produce a more positive LPP compared to neutral images, as shown here. The bottom-right corner displays an electrode map with the nose on top and highlights the electrodes where the LPP was measured (central-parietal area).

Source: **Citation:** Soder, H.E., Schmitz, J.M., Lane, S.D., & Versace, F. (2020). *The Late Positive Potential in Cocaine Use Disorder* [Unpublished data]. Faillace Department of Psychiatry, University of Texas Health Science Center at Houston, Texas, USA.

is difficult and that while good treatments exist, not everyone is able to quit. The study described here takes an innovative and interesting approach to study which individuals are more likely to quit and remain abstinent compared to others.

In their study, Versace, Lam, Engelmann, Robinson, Minnix, Brown, et al. (2012) investigated the *LPP* in a sample of 180 smokers. The participants had to smoke at least five cigarettes per day and also be willing to receive treatment to help them quit smoking. Because the treatment involved medications, it was important that the participants not be on any other medications or have any uncontrolled psychological disorders. It was also critical that the participants were not using any other substances—this allowed the researchers to maintain good control and rule out confounding factors

Baseline brain activity was collected with an *EEG* machine while the participants completed a picture viewing task on a computer. The task was a simple slideshow of images. Each image fit into one major category, with 24 images per category: pleasant, unpleasant, cigarette cue, or neutral. The images were presented on the screen for four seconds. In between each image, a small fixation cross was presented on the screen. The fixation was used to gather information about what the brain was doing during rest. This comparison of brain reactivity in response to the image, to a *baseline* (fixation) period, is important to ensure that the brain activity was not occurring prior to the image being presented on screen. The images presented were tested in hundreds of participants who rated them in terms of happy versus sad and excited versus calm to ensure that the images actually fit into the said categories.

One limitation of utilizing *ERPs* is that processing is complicated and should only be performed by researchers or students with training. Briefly, in Versace et al.'s experiment the process involved first filtering the data to reduce inference from electrical activity not due to the brain. The data were then inspected and corrected for artifacts (e.g., eye blinks or facial movements that showed up in the waveforms). Next, the data were segmented (cut) around the time the images came on the screen. Specifically, Versace, and colleagues (2012) looked at 100 milliseconds before the onset of the image to 800 milliseconds after the onset of the image. The segments were averaged together by category. Finally, the researchers identified the electrodes where the *LPP* occurred. In this case, the authors chose to calculate an average amplitude from 400 to 700 milliseconds for a group of electrodes over the central-parietal area. Notably, the researchers were able to identify where these *ERP components* occurred over the scalp but did not know what brain structure was responsible for generating them. Thus, *ERPs* are useful for telling the timing and strength of neurons firing, while other imaging methods are useful for telling us where the neurons are firing.

Design

First, participants were allowed to smoke before entering the lab to make sure they were not in a withdrawal state. Then they were fitted for an *EEG* cap with 129 electrodes and completed the picture viewing task. After completion of the task, the participants entered a 10-week treatment program where they attempted to quit.

The authors used a statistical analysis known as ***k-means cluster analysis***, which groups people by identifying similar patterns in their data (i.e., where individuals within-cluster have reduced variance, while variance between different clusters is maximized). This is a statistical method that can be performed by most statistical software packages, including ones that are commonly available to students, such as SPSS or Statistica. As the authors hypothesized that there would be two groups of individuals, they set the cluster number to two. Each participant's mean *LPP* amplitude for each category of images (i.e., pleasant, unpleasant, cigarette cue, and neutral) was entered into the analysis. The algorithm then classified each participant into one of two clusters, based on these values.

Results and Conclusions

The cluster analysis revealed two types of cigarette smokers. The people in Cluster One had an enhanced *LPP* to pleasant images compared to cigarette cues. The people in Cluster Two had an enhanced *LPP* to cigarette cues compared to pleasant images. Both clusters had similar *LPPs* to unpleasant and neutral images, indicating that the real difference between the groups has to do with how much the brain reacts to drug reward vs. everyday reward. Importantly, people in Cluster Two were less likely to be abstinent at 10, 12, and 24 weeks after the quit day, indicating that those who are more reactive to cues and less reactive to other rewards found it difficult to remain abstinent. This study highlights the utility of assessing *ERPs* during treatment programs. Future research could tailor treatments to help reduce attention to cues and increase attention to other everyday rewards. Future research could also test if *ERPs* can help match individuals to different treatments geared to their brain reactivity profile.

The Clinical Trial as a Test of Pharmacotherapy and Psychotherapy's Effects

Clinical trials represent attempts to test the safety, effectiveness, and efficacy of treatments prior to public use. Commonly, clinical trials seeking to establish effectiveness and efficacy compare two or more treatments (or "conditions") to assess the relative benefits of one condition versus the other. In clinical trials, random assignment of participants to conditions minimizes selection effects. The use of placebos minimizes participant expectancy effects on the efficacy of the experimental substance. Blinded studies circumvent demand characteristics, or features of the study that influence the participants' behavior implicitly or otherwise. Combining these three key elements produces a ***double-blind, placebo-controlled clinical trial***. It is double-blind as opposed to single-blind because in addition to the participants being "blind" to their assigned condition, the researchers administering the manipulation similarly are blind. Such a design has utility in testing the effects of pharmacotherapy and of psychotherapy on drug dependence in humans. While a medication (pharmacotherapy) targets one's biology, psychotherapy, as the name suggests, targets one's psychology. One kind of psychotherapy is cognitive-behavioral therapy (Beck, 2011), an approach that focuses on the client's thoughts (cognitions) and actions (behaviors). Medications and psychotherapy can act alone or in conjunction with each other to effect changes in drug dependence. Using a *double-blind, placebo-controlled trial* in which these two independent variables are "crossed" with each other allows us to parse out these effects.

Schmitz, Stotts, Rhoades, and Grabowski (2001) investigated the treatment of cocaine-dependent participants with ***naltrexone*** and relapse prevention (RP) therapy—a type of cognitive-behavioral therapy aimed at reducing the potential for relapse by helping the client develop coping skills in response to high-risk situations. *Naltrexone* is a *mu* opiate antagonist that has previously been shown to be effective at reducing alcohol use in persons dependent on both alcohol and cocaine. The imperative question, then, was: How effective would it be in persons solely dependent on cocaine?

Eighty-five participants between the ages of 18 and 50 were recruited through local flyers seeking persons who met the *Diagnostic and Statistical Manual of Mental Disorders* (DSM-IV) criteria for dependence on cocaine. During the first screening, researchers excluded individuals with co-occurring dependence on alcohol or other primary disorders and those on medication for other psychiatric symptoms. This critical exclusion ruled out effects of substances or conditions present prior to the manipulation.

Invited participants were to demonstrate initial abstinence, defined as producing at least five cocaine-negative urine toxicology tests in a row within ten days. If they did not achieve initial abstinence, they were referred to alternative studies or services. But if they achieved abstinence, they were included in the study and randomized into one of four conditions described next. All participants took part in the study for 12 weeks over 20 therapy sessions: twice weekly for the first eight weeks, then once weekly for each of the remaining four. Within a week of completion, participants underwent post-treatment assessment. Participants were paid for each scheduled visit they completed.

Design

The study employed a full factorial design with the independent variables (factors) being medication and therapy. Medication had two levels: 50 mg naltrexone or placebo. Similarly, therapy consisted of two levels: Drug Counseling (DC) or RP. Fully "crossing" these factors (i.e., taking all possible combinations of their respective levels) resulted in the four conditions to which participants were randomly assigned: naltrexone and RP, naltrexone and DC, placebo and RP, and placebo and DC.

The dependent variable was cocaine use, operationally defined as the presence of cocaine metabolite in the urine sample. The researchers hypothesized that the combination of naltrexone and RP would result in the greatest probability of abstinence from cocaine. Hence, they predicted that individuals in the naltrexone-RP group would have the fewest cocaine-positive urines over the course of the study, relative to the three other conditions.

Urine toxicology was conducted by detecting the concentration of **benzoylecgonine**, a cocaine metabolite, in urine specimens collected weekly. A specimen was considered cocaine-positive if the metabolite concentration exceeded 300 *ng/mL*, indicating recent cocaine use.

To manipulate pharmacotherapy, participants in the naltrexone condition received *50 mg* of the medication. Participants were administered their assigned medication in the clinic (in a double-blind fashion) and given take-home medication. Riboflavin was added to the medications to mark compliance; participants who showed subsequent urine samples where riboflavin was detected were considered compliant.

Psychotherapy was manipulated as follows. Standard DC served as the comparison therapy condition for RP. While RP focuses on developing coping skills, DC provides general support and praise for abstinence-oriented behaviors. Both therapy conditions were delivered by trained therapists, supervised on video and coded by raters blind to condition. These independent raters assessed the extent to which target behaviors in each therapy were present as a measure of construct validity. In addition, participants were given self-report tests to measure treatment integrity: one to rate their coping ability during high-risk situations (a hallmark of RP) and the other to measure their involvement in outside support groups (a target of DC).

The study also employed the following secondary measures: the self-reported measures of cocaine craving (Cocaine Craving Scale), side effects (Side Effects Checklist), and drug problem severity (Addiction Severity Index), collected weekly, and the clinician-rated assessment of their clients' overall well-being (Clinical Global Impression).

The primary outcome, percentage of cocaine-negative urines, was analyzed through a repeated-measures analysis of covariance (ANCOVA), which permits the testing of the impact of both categorical (medication, therapy) and continuous independent variables (time) on a continuous outcome.

Results and Conclusions

The main finding was a statistically significant three-way interaction between time, therapy, and medication on percentage of cocaine-negative urines. Specifically, there was less cocaine use over time, but this effect was strongest in the group receiving both naltrexone and RP compared to the other three groups, hence supporting the primary hypothesis. No effects were observed on self-reported cocaine craving. There was a main effect of time on drug problem severity, indicating less severity over time. Both the naltrexone and placebo groups exhibited no differences in medication compliance, hence ruling out adherence as a confounding variable. Clinicians rated RP participants as having significantly greater clinical global improvement than the DC group over time. RP showed larger improvements in self-efficacy relative to DC, while DC increased support group attendance relative to RP, thus showing that the therapy manipulation worked as intended.

This study demonstrates how the fully crossed factorial clinical trial design permits research on moment-to-moment changes of the interactive effects of pharmacotherapy and psychotherapy. Researchers found that naltrexone and RP worked together to produce the best abstinence results possible, potentially through complementary mechanisms. It could be that naltrexone reduced the reinforcing aspects of cocaine, so through RP, the individual sought new coping skills to compensate. Alternatively, a person in RP used more coping strategies, thus using cocaine less, making them more sensitive to the opiate-blocking effects of naltrexone. The research also serves as positive evidence for the case that the combination of psychological and biological interventions can be strengthened and built upon for further study.

Utility of Longitudinal Designs and the Classical Twin Study for Understanding Addiction

Correlational methods, broadly including cross-sectional and longitudinal designs, are commonly used to study addictions. Cross-sectional designs represent a convenient means of understanding addiction by studying individuals at a fixed point in time. Alternatively, longitudinal designs study individuals across multiple measurement occasions and afford the benefit of observing the temporal order of events. For instance, although well-established evidence from cross-sectional studies suggests substance use problems are associated with insecure attachment styles in relationships (Hayre, Goulter, & Moretti, 2019), the temporal precedence of this relationship is unclear (e.g., whether substance use or insecure attachments styles occur first). Longitudinal designs have been leveraged to answer this question and repeatedly suggest that insecure attachment styles more commonly precede substance use problems and may serve as a risk factor for later addiction (Fairbairn, Briley, Kang, Fraley, Hankin, & Ariss, 2018).

A specific and frequently utilized correlational method for studying addiction (both cross-sectional and longitudinal) is the *classical twin study (CTS),* which allows researchers to understand the etiology (i.e., underlying causes) of the addiction phenotype (i.e., observable characteristic). The *CTS* identifies the relative contribution of genetic and environmental influences on phenotypic expression in humans and is a popular tool because different types of twins conveniently vary in their genetic resemblance (Evans & Martin, 2000). Monozygotic (MZ), or identical, twins are genetically identical (100% genetic resemblance), while dizygotic (DZ), or fraternal, twins resemble each other approximately 50% genetically. Genetic similarity alone is thought to distinguish MZ and DZ twins, given that these two types of twins experience the same degree of environmental similarity; they share the same womb, are born at the same time, and (typically) share the same family. As such, the genetic differences across MZ and DZ twin pairs provide a natural experiment on genetic and environmental contributions to addiction. Indeed, extensive evidence based on the *CTS* design clearly indicates that genetic influences predominantly affect most (if not all) types of addiction (Agrawal & Lynskey, 2008), including alcohol (Huggett, Hatoum, Hewitt, & Stallings, 2018), nicotine (Huggett, et al. 2018), illicit drug (e.g., cocaine; Waaktaar, Kan, & Torgersen, 2018), and gambling addiction (King, Keyes, Winters, McGue, & Iacono, 2017).

To better understand the precursors and/or consequences of addiction and the corresponding impact of genes and environment on those precursors/consequences, several research groups (e.g., Virginia Commonwealth University, University of Colorado, University of Minnesota, the Swedish Twin Registry) have invested considerable time and large sums of money into developing twin registries with longitudinal addictions data (Corley, Reynolds, Wadsworth, Rhea, & Hewitt, 2019;

Lilley, Morris, & Silberg, 2019; Wilson, Haroian, Iacono, Krueger, Lee, Luciana, et al., 2019; Zagai, Lichtenstein, Pedersen, & Magnusson, 2019). Bornovalova, Verhulst, Webber, McGue, Iacono, and Hicks (2018) exemplify how the *CTS* can be intermixed with a longitudinal design in a study on the course of substance use disorders in adolescence and early adulthood, the interrelationships of drug use disorder (DUD) and alcohol use disorder (AUD) symptoms with other forms of psychopathology (i.e., major depressive disorder [MDD] symptoms and borderline personality disorder [BPD] traits), and how genetic and environmental influences differentially affect the relationships between development of these conditions.

To this end, the authors utilized a sample of 1,763 female twins from the Minnesota Twin Family Registry (Wilson, et al., 2019) with longitudinal data collected at ages 14, 17, 20, and 24. The number of AUD, DUD, and MDD symptoms were indexed by interviewing twins with structured diagnostic interviews. Interviews of twins assessed at the age of 14 and 17 were supplemented with parent interviews concerning of the twin's symptoms, with the symptom considered present if endorsed by either the twin or the parent. BPD features were measured via a self-report personality inventory.

Results

The authors utilized parallel process biometric latent growth modeling, which simultaneously models the initial amount of AUD, DUD, MDD, and BPD symptoms and growth in these constructs over the course of the study, while estimating the relative impact of genetic and environmental influences on the relationships among these symptoms. As demonstrated repeatedly in the literature (see citations earlier), genetic influences predominantly accounted for the level of AUD and DUD symptoms and increases in these symptoms throughout adolescence and early adulthood. Higher MDD symptoms were associated with greater increases in DUD and AUD symptoms, which was accounted for by genetic influences. Alternatively, higher DUD and AUD symptoms did not predict a change in MDD symptoms. Higher AUD and DUD symptoms predicted a slower rate of decline in BPD symptoms, while higher BPD traits predicted greater increases in AUD and DUD symptoms. Genetic influences similarly accounted for relationships among AUD, DUD, and BPD. These results suggest that genetic influences account for both the development of AUD and DUD and the development of comorbid psychopathology in addictions. The longitudinal design also affords the benefit of demonstrating that MDD symptoms tended to occur prior to the development of AUD and DUD symptoms in this sample, while AUD, DUD, and BPD appeared to develop simultaneously.

Limitations and Conclusions

While combining strengths of the *CTS* (e.g., relatively better replicability of genetic effects than candidate gene approaches) with those of longitudinal designs (e.g., establishing temporal precedence) affords notable benefits that other correlational methods cannot, a key limitation is that both the *CTS* and longitudinal designs require hundreds, if not thousands, of participants to maximize statistical power and corresponding confidence in the findings derived from these data (Kelley & Rausch, 2011; Verhulst, 2017). Combined with following participants across extended periods (up to years or decades), integrating twin studies with longitudinal data collection can be prohibitively costly and time consuming. Another key limitation is that although longitudinal designs help establish temporal precedence, the influence of confounding variables cannot be ruled out and causality cannot be inferred because there is no experimental control or random assignment. While the exorbitant cost of these methods and limits on causal inferences represent key drawbacks to these designs, these methods can facilitate some of the more meaningful inferences researchers can make when using correlational/observational data to study addictions.

Conclusion

While these methods have been useful tools in understanding addiction, they represent a very small sample of the larger body of research methods that can be employed to study several aspects of addiction. For example, paralleling the *MDMA* studies in primates, pharmacological studies on humans who have used *MDMA* have demonstrated the potential long-term effects of the drug on serotonin receptors (Reneman, Endert, de Bruin, Lavalaye, Feenstra, de Wolff, et al., 2002). Another example emerges in the *ERP* literature. In addition to the *LPP*, there are other *ERP* components related to addiction, including the feedback-related negativity, which is thought to reflect the ability to learn from positive and negative feedback. The feedback-related negativity is smaller in college students who drink alcohol, suggesting they are less sensitive to punishing outcomes, which could contribute to a difficulty in learning from the negative consequences of their choices (Soder, Suchting, & Potts, 2020). Finally, the behavior genetics literature has also demonstrated that the etiology of nonaggressive externalizing behaviors (to include addiction) may be strikingly altered by the degree of neighborhood disadvantage in childhood (Burt, 2016), necessitating replication of previously demonstrated effects in datasets designed to oversample participants with demographic or other characteristics relevant to addition.

Thus far, these methods and rigorous clinical trials have also led to the development of treatments that show at least low-to-moderate efficacy. For example, contingency management was developed to replace drug reward with monetary reward—patients are given money when they are able to demonstrate abstinence, such as passing a urine drug screen (Prendergast, Podus, Finney, Greenwell, & Roll, 2006). These types of treatments in conjunction with psychotherapy can work quite well. There are also several current Food and Drug Administration (FDA)–approved medications to treat opioid, alcohol, and nicotine use disorders that help either alleviate withdrawal symptoms or reduce the reward effects of the drug. Notably, there is no FDA-approved medication for the treatment of cocaine use disorder, so there is still important work to be done.

The research methods described here and others have contributed greatly to our understanding of the etiology, development, maintenance, and treatment of substance use problems. Thanks to cutting-edge research, we are now beginning to lift the stigma on addiction and understand the biological basis of the disease. While it may seem that there are many unanswered questions concerning addiction, these methods give us hope for the future.

References

Agrawal, A., & Lynskey, M. T. (2008). Are there genetic influences on addiction: Evidence from family, adoption and twin studies. *Addiction, 103*(7), 1069–1081. https://doi.org/10.1111/j.1360-0443.2008.02213.x

Beck, J. S. (2011). *Cognitive behavior therapy: Basics and beyond.* New York, NY: Guilford Press.

Bornovalova, M. A., Verhulst, B., Webber, T., McGue, M., Iacono, W. G., & Hicks, B. M. (2018). Genetic and environmental influences on the codevelopment among borderline personality disorder traits, major depression symptoms, and substance use disorder symptoms from adolescence to young adulthood. *Development and Psychopathology, 30*(1), 49–65. https://doi.org/10.1017/S0954579417000463

Bryant, C. D., Roberts, K. W., Culbertson, C. S., Le, A., Evans, C. J., & Fanselow, M. S. (2009). Pavlovian conditioning of multiple opioid-like responses in mice. *Drug and Alcohol Dependence, 103*(1–2), 74–83. https://doi.org/10.1016/j.drugalcdep.2009.03.016

Burt, S. A., Klump, K. L., Gorman-Smith, D., & Neiderhiser, J. M. (2016). Neighborhood disadvantage alters the origins of children's nonaggressive conduct problems. *Clinical Psychological Science, 4*(3), 511–526. https://doi.org/10.1177/2167702615618164

Centers for Disease Control and Prevention, National Center for Health Statistics. (2019, January). Multiple cause of death 1999–2018 on CDC wonder online database.

Corley, R. P., Reynolds, C. A., Wadsworth, S. J., Rhea, S. A., & Hewitt, J. K. (2019). The Colorado twin registry: 2019 update. *Twin Research and Human Genetics*, 1–9. https://doi.org/10.1017/thg.2019.50

Evans, D. M., & Martin, N. G. (2000). The validity of twin studies. *GeneScreen, 1*(2), 77–79. https://doi.org/10.1046/j.1466-9218.2000.00027.x

Fairbairn, C. E., Briley, D. A., Kang, D., Fraley, R. C., Hankin, B. L., & Ariss, T. (2018). A meta-analysis of longitudinal associations between substance use and interpersonal attachment security. *Psychological Bulletin*, *144*(5), 532. https://doi.org/10.1037/bul0000141

Gladden, R. M., Martinez, P., & Seth, P. (2016). Fentanyl law enforcement submissions and increases in synthetic opioid-involved overdose deaths: 27 states, 2013–2014. *MMWR Morbidity Mortality Weekly Report*, *65*, 837–843. Retrieved from www.jstor.org/stable/24858927

Hatzidimitriou, G., McCann, U. D., & Ricaurte, G. A. (1999). Altered serotonin innervation patterns in the forebrain of monkeys treated with (±) 3, 4-methylenedioxymethamphetamine seven years previously: Factors influencing abnormal recovery. *Journal of Neuroscience*, *19*(12), 5096–5107. https://doi.org/10.1523/JNEUROSCI.19-12-05096.1999

Hayre, R. S., Goulter, N., & Moretti, M. M. (2019). Maltreatment, attachment, and substance use in adolescence: Direct and indirect pathways. *Addictive Behaviors*, *90*, 196–203. https://doi.org/10.1016/j.addbeh.2018.10.049

Huggett, S. B., Hatoum, A. S., Hewitt, J. K., & Stallings, M. C. (2018). The speed of progression to tobacco and alcohol dependence: A twin study. *Behavior Genetics*, *48*(2), 109–124. https://doi.org/10.1007/s10519-018-9888-0

Insel, T. R., Battaglia, G., Johannessen, J. N., Marra, S., & De Souza, E. B. (1989). 3,4-methylenedioxymethamphetamine ("ecstasy") selectively destroys brain serotonin terminals in rhesus monkeys. *Journal of Pharmacology and Experimental Therapeutics*, *249*(3), 713LP–720LP.

Katz, R. J., & Gormezano, G. (1979). A rapid and inexpensive technique for assessing the reinforcing effects of opiate drugs. *Pharmacology Biochemistry and Behavior*, *11*(2), 231–233. https://doi.org/10.1016/0091-3057(79)90019-4

Kelley, K., & Rausch, J. R. (2011). Sample size planning for longitudinal models: Accuracy in parameter estimation for polynomial change parameters. *Psychological Methods*, *16*(4), 391. https://doi.org/10.1037/a0023352

King, S. M., Keyes, M., Winters, K. C., McGue, M., & Iacono, W. G. (2017). Genetic and environmental origins of gambling behaviors from ages 18 to 25: A longitudinal twin family study. *Psychology of Addictive Behaviors: Journal of the Society of Psychologists in Addictive Behaviors*, *31*(3), 367–374. https://doi.org/10.1037/adb0000266

Lew, R., Sabol, K. E., Chou, C., Vosmer, G. L., Richards, J., & Seiden, L. S. (1996). Methylenedioxymethamphetamine-induced serotonin deficits are followed by partial recovery over a 52-week period. Part II: Radioligand binding and autoradiography studies. *Journal of Pharmacology and Experimental Therapeutics*, *276*(2), 855LP–865.

Lilley, E. C., Morris, A. T., & Silberg, J. L. (2019). The mid-atlantic twin registry of Virginia Commonwealth University. *Twin Research and Human Genetics*, 1–4. https://doi.org/10.1017/thg.2019.87

National Drug Intelligence Center. (2011). *National drug threat assessment*. Washington, DC: United States Department of Justice.

Pavlov, I. (1927). *Conditioned reflexes*. New York, NY: Dover. doi:10.5214/ans.0972-7531.1017309

Prendergast, M., Podus, D., Finney, J., Greenwell, L., & Roll, J. (2006). Contingency management for treatment of substance use disorders: A meta-analysis. *Addiction*, *101*(11), 1546–1560. https://doi.org/10.1111/j.1360-0443.2006.01581.x

Reneman, L., Endert, E., de Bruin, K., Lavalaye, J., Feenstra, M. G., de Wolff, F. A., et al. (2002). The acute and chronic effects of MDMA ("ecstasy") on cortical 5-HT 2A receptors in rat and human brain. *Neuropsychopharmacology*, *26*(3), 387–396. https://doi.org/10.1016/S0893-133X(01)00366-9

Rudd, R. A., Paulozzi, L. J., Bauer, M. J., Burleson, R. W., Carlson, R. E., Dao, D., et al. (2014, October 3). Increases in heroin overdose deaths: 28 states, 2010 to 2012. *MMWR Morbidity Mortality Weekly Report*, *63*(39), 849. Retrieved from www.jstor.org/stable/24855364

Scanzello, C. R., Hatzidimitriou, G., Martello, A. L., Katz, J. L., & Ricaurte, G. A. (1993). Serotonergic recovery after (+/-)3,4-(methylenedioxy) methamphetamine injury: Observations in rats. *Journal of Pharmacology and Experimental Therapeutics*, *264*(3), 1484LP–1491.

Schmitz, J. M., Stotts, A. L., Rhoades, H. M., & Grabowski, J. (2001). Naltrexone and relapse prevention treatment for cocaine-dependent patients. *Addictive Behaviors*, *26*(2), 167–180. https://doi.org/10.1016/S0306-4603(00)00098-8

Schuster, C. R., & Thompson, T. (1969). Self-administration of and behavioral dependence on drugs. *Annual Review of Pharmacology*, *9*, 483–502. https://doi.org/10.1146/annurev.pa.09.040169.002411

Siegel, S. (1983). Classical conditioning, drug tolerance, and drug dependence. In R. G. Smart, F. B. Graser, Y. Israel, H. Kalant, R. E. Popham, & W. Schmidt (Eds.), *Research advances in alcohol and drug problems* (Vol. 7, pp. 207–246). New York, NY: Plenum Press. https://doi.org/10.1007/978-1-4613-3626-6_6

Soder, H. E., Suchting, R., & Potts, G. F. (2020). Electrophysiological responses to appetitive and aversive outcomes: A comparison of college drinkers and non-drinkers. *Neuroscience Letters*, *714*, 134549. https://doi.org/10.1016/j.neulet.2019.134549

Stanley, T. H. (1992). The history and development of the fentanyl series. *Journal of Pain and Symptom Management*, 7(3). doi:10.1016/0885-3924(92)90047-1

Verhulst, B. (2017). A power calculator for the classical twin design. *Behavior Genetics*, 47(2), 255–261. https://doi.org/10.1007/s10519-016-9828-9

Versace, F., Lam, C. Y., Engelmann, J. M., Robinson, J. D., Minnix, J. A., Brown, V. L., et al. (2012). Beyond cue reactivity: Blunted brain responses to pleasant stimuli predict long-term smoking abstinence. *Addiction Biology*, 17(6), 991–1000. https://doi.org/10.1111/j.1369-1600.2011.00372.x

Volkow, N. D., Wang, G. J., Fowler, J. S., Tomasi, D., & Telang, F. (2011). Addiction: Beyond dopamine reward circuitry. *Proceedings of the National Academy of Sciences*, 108(37), 15037–15042. https://doi.org/10.1073/pnas.1010654108

Waaktaar, T., Kan, K. J., & Torgersen, S. (2018). The genetic and environmental architecture of substance use development from early adolescence into young adulthood: A longitudinal twin study of comorbidity of alcohol, tobacco and illicit drug use. *Addiction (Abingdon, England)*, 113(4), 740–748. https://doi.org/10.1111/add.14076

Wilson, S., Haroian, K., Iacono, W. G., Krueger, R. F., Lee, J. J., Luciana, M., et al. (2019). Minnesota center for twin and family research. *Twin Research and Human Genetics*, 1–7. https://doi.org/10.1017/thg.2019.107

Zagai, U., Lichtenstein, P., Pedersen, N. L., & Magnusson, P. K. (2019). The Swedish twin registry: Content and management as a research infrastructure. *Twin Research and Human Genetics*, 1–9. https://doi.org/10.1017/thg.2019.99

7

APPLICATIONS OF NEXT-GENERATION SEQUENCING IN HEALTH PSYCHOLOGY

Matthew L. Aardema

Overview

Next-generation sequencing (NGS) technologies, in particular **Illumina sequencing**, have revolutionized genetic, genomic, and transcriptomic approaches to biology (Goodwin, McPherson, & McCombie, 2016). Compared to more traditional **Sanger** technology, *NGS* has substantially reduced the cost of sequencing and significantly increased the amount of data that can be generated (The ENCODE Project Consortium, 2012). *Sanger* and *NGS* technologies work in similar ways, with both technologies using deoxyribonucleic acid (DNA) polymerases (enzymes that synthesize DNA molecules from deoxyribonucleotides) to add fluorescent nucleotides one at a time to lengthening DNA templates. The added nucleotides are then recognized by a fluorescent tag. However, while the *Sanger* method allows the sequencing of only one DNA fragment at a time, *NGS* is massively parallel, allowing the sequencing of millions of fragments concurrently. Combined with an array of bioinformatics programs and utilities, *NGS* has facilitated an immense number of discoveries, broadly allowing for improved diagnoses and better treatment of psychologically associated diseases (Ashbrook, Mulligan, & Williams, 2018; Hitzemann, Darakjian, Walter, Iancu, Searles, & McWeeney, 2014).

Typically, *Illumina technology* is used to produce 'short' reads, which are sequences less than 500 nucleotides long. Advances in the generation of longer reads (>1 Kb), such as PacBio and Nanopore, are opening up many new and exciting avenues in biological research (Bleidorn, 2016). For example, longer reads are proving valuable for examining large structural variation in human genomes (e.g., Mizuguchi, Suzuki, Abe, Umemura, Tokunaga, Kawai, et al., 2019). While such variation may have relevance to human diseases (Feuk, 2010), long-read technology is predominately being applied to **nonmodel organisms** that lack high-quality reference genomes (species other than humans, mice, *Drosophila*, etc.). As the human reference genome is one of the highest-quality **eukaryotic genomes** (genomes from organisms whose DNA is in the form of chromosomes and is contained within a distinct nucleus) available, short reads are generally sufficient (and even preferable), given their lower error rates (Bleidorn, 2016). Furthermore, the generation of hundreds of millions of short reads gives researchers immense flexibility with regard to study design and analyses. Accordingly, the majority of studies utilizing *NGS* in health psychology exploit this form of data. For these reasons, for the remainder of the chapter I will focus predominately on the applications of short-read technologies, specifically *Illumina*.

The technology behind *Illumina sequencing* is relatively straightforward and as described earlier, similar to *Sanger sequencing*. After short fragments of double-stranded DNA have been prepared (a variety of methods will be discussed), specific adaptors are ligated (the joining of two DNA strands by an enzyme) to the fragments. The fragments are then annealed (heated and then cooled) to a slide. ***Polymerase chain reaction (PCR)*** amplifies each annealed fragment, generating a spot with many identical copies of the read. Next, the double-stranded DNA is separated into single strands. The strands are then sequenced by flooding the slide with nucleotides and DNA polymerase. These nucleotides are fluorescently labeled, with different colors corresponding to each of the four genetic bases. Each nucleotide also has a terminator so that only one base can be added at a time. An image is taken of the slide, revealing the fluorescent signal at each position and indicating which base has been added. The slide is then prepared for the next cycle by removing the terminators, thus allowing the next base to be added. To prevent the previous fluorescent signal from contaminating the current image, the signal is also removed. This entire process is repeated over and over, with one nucleotide added each round. The base at each site in each image is then determined computationally to construct the sequences. This process can result in hundreds of millions of unique sequence reads, all of which are the same length (typically between 50 and 250 nucleotides) depending on the specific sequence technology and chemistry used.

The origins of the starting material and the goals of the study determine whether these reads will next be aligned to a reference genome ('mapped') or assembled *de novo* (i.e., without additional information or outside guidance; Flicek & Birney, 2009). In most human studies, reads are mapped to a reference. This strategy of sequencing many millions of short sequence reads has made necessary the development of numerous bioinformatics tools to deal with the large amounts of data generated (Magi, Benelli, Gozzini, Girolami, Torricelli, & Brandi, 2010). These programs help to trim and filter low-quality reads, remove *PCR* duplicates, map the reads to a reference, identify genetic variation, and much more. Fortunately, much of this development has been driven by academic researchers, and open-source research options for analyzing data are available for nearly every application (Nagarajan & Pop, 2013; reviewed in Pabinger, Dander, Fischer, Snajder, Sperk, Efremova, et al., 2014).

Presently, the data generation component of studies utilizing *NGS* technology is relatively routine, with many companies and services established to provide sample preparation, sequencing library preparation kits, sequencing services, and bioinformatics assistance. The real challenge is devising biologically relevant studies with appropriate samples for exploratory discovery or hypothesis testing. It is important to plan the best strategies for generating useful data in cost-effective ways. The human genome is composed of over 3 billion nucleotides. Of this, 1.22% represents protein-coding exons. However, 80.4% of the human genome contributes to gene regulation and other biological process. Although whole-genome sequencing of samples is typically the most straightforward approach, when thousands of samples are being compared, this may not be cost-effective. Rather, some manner of reduced representation of the genome may be necessary.

There are many ways to focus a study on specific regions of interest. For example, if only variation in protein coding regions is important, then researchers may choose to begin their study by isolating messenger ribonucleic acid (RNA) from their samples (***RNA-seq***). It is also possible to develop specific probes that allow only regions of interest (such as exons) to be isolated and amplified in the sequencing library preparation (the methods used to prepare a nucleic acid–based sample for sequencing). Still other studies may want to focus on how specific genomic features aside from DNA information itself (i.e., methylation and/or other epigenetic factors) may influence gene regulation. In this case, a study could be designed that focuses on just ***epigenetic*** signatures in the ***genome***. *Epigenetics* is the study of heritable changes that do not involve alterations in the DNA sequence, but which do influence individual phenotype. For example, DNA methylation (the addition of a methyl group to a DNA molecule) can prevent a gene from being expressed. Still other studies may seek to examine nonhuman biological entities living within or on the human body (e.g., bacteria, protists) that correlate with particular phenotypes. Again, this would require specific library preparation methods.

In the remainder of this chapter, I will discuss each of these approaches in some detail, the kinds of questions they best address, and, briefly, how samples are prepared and analyzed. I will also present a case study for each method to illustrate their usage. I have selected mainly examples that explore Alzheimer's disease. This disease is the leading cause of dementia in elderly individuals and the sixth leading cause of death in the United States (Alzheimer's Association, 2020). It is highly heritable, yet genetically very complex. This means that there are a wealth of studies exploring its manifestation and identification in patients (Jiang, Li, Huang, Liu, & Zhao, 2017; reviewed in Naj, Schellenberg, & Alzheimer's Disease Genetics Consortium, 2017; Yokoyama, Rutledge, & Medici, 2017), a selection of which will be explored next.

Research in Practice

Genome-Wide Association Studies

Of all the uses of *NGS* for research in health psychology, perhaps none is more widely utilized than ***genome-wide association studies*** (***GWAS***; reviewed in Collins & Sullivan, 2013; Jensen, 2016). The ability to sequence large numbers of genomes relatively cheaply has facilitated hundreds of studies attempting to associate specific genetic variants with disease phenotypes. Such knowledge can prove invaluable for accurate diagnoses, preventative treatment, and the improvement of drug development.

Of all sample preparation methods, whole-genome sequencing for *GWAS* is perhaps the most straightforward. Typically, blood or tissue samples are collected from individuals displaying the phenotype of interest, here referred to as ***cases***, as well as a similar number of ***controls***, individuals who do not exhibit the phenotype. Sample sizes sufficient to obtain statistical power are largely dependent on the strength of associations, with larger samples needed to detect small-to-moderate associations (Visscher, Wray, Zhang, Sklar, McCarthy, Brown, et al., 2017). Once samples have been collected, the DNA within the sample is isolated, usually using a commercially available extraction kit. Next, the samples are prepared for sequencing, also generally using a commercial library preparation kit. Library preparation involves a series of steps. First, the DNA is sheared into small fragments (either chemically or mechanically), followed by DNA end repair, ligation of adapters (often with unique barcodes), and if necessary, fragment amplification (via PCR). Once these steps are completed, individual libraries may be pooled into a single multisample library for sequencing. The amount of sequencing to be done depends on the desired ***coverage***, defined here as the average number of sequencing reads that cover each nucleotide in a sample (e.g., '5x' means there is an average of five reads overlapping each location in the targeted region). Greater *coverage* may result in more confident assessments of genetic variation, especially when a site is heterozygous. However, targeting lower coverage often means more samples can be analyzed. Balancing these two competing factors is one of the biggest challenges for designing a successful *GWAS* study. Fortunately, humans are among the best-studied species and genetic variation found within the human population is well characterized, with variants segregating at frequencies as low as 1% worldwide having been classified (1000 Genomes Project Consortium, 2012). This means relatively low *coverage*, sometimes less than 1x, is possible for a successful *GWAS* study (Pasaniuc, Rohland, McLaren, Garimella, Zaitlen, Li, et al., 2012).

After sequencing the samples, the resulting data (referred to as ***sequence reads***) are generally filtered to remove low-quality reads and sequence adaptors. In some studies, *PCR* duplicates are also removed. Next, the reads are mapped to a human reference *genome*. The specific *genome* used may depend on the particular study, but generally it is preferable to select the highest-quality *genome* available with regard to number of gaps (fewer is better) and limited sequencing error. This may be preferable to genetically similar references in part because humans exhibit such low genetic variation.

As of this writing, the **Genome Reference Consortium Human genome, build 38** (**GRCh38**) is considered the highest-quality human *genome* available (Schneider, Graves-Lindsay, Howe, Bouk, Chen, Kitts, et al., 2017).

After the reads have been mapped to a reference *genome*, many tools are available for characterizing genetic variation (reviewed in Pabinger, et al., 2014). **Variant calling** involves comparing the mapped reads to the reference and classifying deviations from the reference. The tools to do this use different computational strategies and algorithms, and the one selected depends on the inferred nature of the variants, as well as the goals of the study. Much effort has been given to benchmarking various *variant calling* programs (e.g., Hwang, Kim, Lee, & Marcotte, 2015; Li, Wang, & Wang, 2018; Warden, Adamson, Neuhausen, & Wu, 2014), and researchers should review this literature to determine which program is best suited to their needs.

Finally, the last step in a *GWAS* study is to use computational methods to perform association tests between *case* and *control* samples. While easy to implement, it is important to choose thresholds carefully to avoid both false-negatives (rejecting variants associated with phenotypes) and false-positives (accepting variants that are not associated with phenotypes). Marees, de Kluiver, Stringer, Vorspan, Curis, Marie-Claire and colleagues (2018) have written an excellent reference for analyzing human *GWAS* data and discuss several programs available for this process.

A *GWAS* approach was used to identify segregating genetic variants associated with Alzheimer's disease in the Chinese population (Zhou, Chen, Mok, Zhao, Chen, Chen, et al., 2018). The authors of this study utilized samples from 972 individuals, which included 489 subjects with Alzheimer's disease, 260 subjects with mild cognitive impairment, and 223 control subjects who did not display a disease phenotype. These controls were age- and gender-matched to the case samples. Each sample was sequenced on an *Illumina Hiseq X Ten* to an average genome depth of 5x coverage. The resulting data were trimmed to remove adapters and low-quality nucleotides, then mapped to the **GRCh37 reference genome** using the program BWA-MEM (Li, 2013). BWA is a popular software package for mapping short reads with minimal divergence against a large reference genome (such as human data to a human reference genome). The programs Samtools (Li & Durban, 2009) and glfFlex were used to identify and classify variants, and then PLINK (Purcell, Neale, Todd-Brown, Thomas, Ferreira, Bender, et al., 2007) was used to test for associations between genetic variants and the Alzheimer's phenotype. PLINK is another popular analysis toolset that can perform a range of basic, large-scale genetic analyses (such as genetic associations) in a manner that is computationally efficient. In the study, multiple variants were identified in and around the well-known **apolipoprotein E (APOE)** locus, as well as other variants known to be associated with Alzheimer's disease. In particular, the authors revalidated associations with two identified risk loci: GCH1 and KCNJ15. In genetics, a locus is a specific location in the genome where a gene or other feature can be found. For example, **APOE** is mapped to chromosome 19 in the human genome, between nucleotides 44,905,791 and 44,909,393. This gene encodes a protein that is involved in the metabolism of fats in the body, and genetic polymorphism in this gene correlates strongly with late-onset Alzheimer's disease (reviewed in Yamazaki, Zhao, Caulfield, Liu, & Bu, 2019).

Differential Expression

The goal of a *GWAS* study is typically to identify genetic differences between *case* and *control* phenotypes, often focusing on nonsynonymous changes in protein coding sequence or loss-of-function mutations. However, it is well established that differences in the expression of particular genes can also have a substantial effect on how a phenotype (such as disease state) manifests itself (Emilsson, Thorleifsson, Zhang, Leonardson, Zink, Zhu, et al., 2008). While *GWAS* studies may locate genetic variations that contribute to differences in gene expression, a distinct and often complementary approach to investigating this issue is to look at differences in gene expression directly using **transcriptome** *sequencing*. When an organism requires a specific protein, the gene that encodes for this protein is transcribed into **messenger RNA (mRNA)** from the DNA code for this protein found in the genome. This *mRNA* is then translated into an amino acid sequence, which most often then folds into a protein. In the laboratory, *mRNA* molecules in a sample can be isolated and then sequenced. Some proteins are constructed more frequently than others depending on a wide variety of factors such as tissue type, the age of the individual from which the sample was taken, environmental factors, or disease state. The complete set of genes that are transcribed for a specific set of conditions is known as the *transcriptome*. The process of determining the proportions that the genes within a *transcriptome* are expressed (either relative to other genes or other samples) can be an important aspect of *transcriptome sequencing*. Gene expression is the aforementioned process through which the information encoded in a gene is converted into a functional gene product, typically a protein.

Examinations of **gene expression** differences, generally between phenotypes of interest and controls, is a common usage of *NGS* technology. For example, differences in *gene expression* could be examined between the brain tissue of individuals that suffered from Alzheimer's disease and healthy individuals who died of other causes. Many of the initial preparation methods for examining differential expression are similar to those used in *whole-genome sequencing* for *GWAS*. The primary difference is that the starting material for examining differential expression is generally RNA, rather than DNA. This means that for such studies, only expressed genes in the tissue at the time of isolation will be sequenced.

Once RNA has been isolated, the first step is to reverse-transcribe fragments back into double-stranded molecules. After this, steps proceed in a similar fashion to *WGS* preparation, noted previously. For an expression study, the number of samples that can be pooled is typically far less than in a *GWAS* study. This is because differences in expression level between genes within a sample exhibit high levels of variation. Effectively, this means that some RNA molecules may have thousands of copies represented in a sequencing library, whereas other RNA molecules may have only a few dozen or even less. A good rule of thumb is to target at least 30 million reads per sample (Williams, Thomas, Wyman, & Holloway, 2014). This will give sufficient data to look at differences in expression patterns between even moderately expressed genes. Therefore, the number of reads to expect on the chosen sequencer will dictate the level of **multiplexing**, or library pooling, possible. This also means that differential expression studies tend to have more restricted sampling because they are limited to dozens of samples compared to hundreds or thousands as in *GWAS* studies.

After sequencing, the *transcriptome sequencing* data are processed computationally. Unlike with *whole-genome sequencing* and many other next-generation applications, it may not be advisable to trim the reads for quality. This is because the trimming process may alter inferences about expression patterns (Williams, Baccarella, Parrish, & Kim, 2016). Sequencing adapters should still be removed, however.

For human studies, after initial read processing, the reads are generally mapped to a genome reference so that differences in gene expression patterns can be examined. There are many programs for doing this, and they each have distinct statistical methods for assessing whether genes are differentially expressed. Often it is prudent within a study to use more than one program and compare the results. There are excellent reviews discussing these various tools (e.g., Costa-Silva, Domingues, & Lopes, 2017; McDermaid, Monier, Zhao, Liu, & Ma, 2019). Additionally, there are many excellent guides for designing *RNA-seq* experiments to examine *gene expression* differences (Finotello & Di Camillo, 2015; Wolf, 2013).

In one differential study examining individuals with late-onset Alzheimer's, researchers compared the expression profiles of patients with Alzheimer's to cognitively normal controls (Annese, Manzari, Lionetti, Picardi, Horner, Chiara, et al., 2018). For this study, the authors extracted RNA from brain tissue samples, then prepared libraries for sequencing using a standard *RNA-seq* preparation kit. An *Illumina* 'NextSeq 500' system was used to then sequence the libraries. After quality filtering the data, reads were aligned to the human genome (hg19) using the program GSNAP (Wu & Nacu, 2010). The program CuffDiff2 (Trapnell, Hendrickson, Sauvageau, Goff, Rinn, & Pachter, et al., 2013) was used to quantify expression levels and identify differentially expressed genes. From this analysis, the authors discovered 2,064 genes that were regulated differently between the control samples and the samples that came from individuals with Alzheimer's disease. This means that these genes were either expressed statistically more or less often in one group compared to the other. Many of the discovered genes in this study are involved in neurodegenerative and inflammatory pathways, response to unfolded proteins (proteins that have failed to form their proper 3D structure), positive regulation of immune response, and toll-like receptor signaling.

One final note: Similar methods to those described here are also applicable to examinations of splicing difference between *case* and *control* phenotypes (Wang, Gerstein, & Snyder, 2009). Such gene-splicing variation is known to be a contributing factor for many diseases (Kim, Pham, Ko, Rhee, & Han, 2018; reviewed in Tazi, Bakkour, & Stamm, 2009).

Exome Sequencing

Most genetic variations that have large effects on phenotypes, including disease phenotypes, have been found in protein coding sequences despite the fact that such sequences only make up approximately 1.2% of the entire genome (The ENCODE Project Consortium, 2012). This is because variations in protein-coding sequence are more easily analyzed and understood due to our clear knowledge of how amino acid changes, insertions/deletions (INDELs), and missense mutations influence the structure of proteins. Despite this focus on protein coding regions, in *whole-genome sequencing (WGS) efforts*, the vast majority of the data produced comes from intergenic regions of the genome (stretches of DNA that occur between protein coding sequences). Therefore, it will be substantially more challenging to determine potential functional relevance for a phenotype of interest. For this reason, many sequencing efforts to examine variation between control and disease phenotypes explicitly focus on **exons** (regions of DNA that encode for a protein).

Exome sequencing, although seemingly similar to **transcriptome sequencing**, has an important difference. Specifically, the starting material for *exome* sequencing is genomic DNA compared to RNA as in the *transcriptome sequencing* described earlier. Rather than sequencing all mRNA molecules present in the sample at the time of its isolation, *exome* capture utilizes known *exon* sequences to isolate the regions of interest. This is both cost-effective and allows researchers to focus on well-characterized regions of the human genome (Bamshad, Ng, Bigham, Tabor, Emond, Nickerson, et al., 2011). Post-sequencing data processing and analyses are very similar to those used in *WGS* and *GWAS*.

One example of this approach used *exome* capture to identify novel genes associated with Alzheimer's disease in extended families (Cukier, Kunkle, Hamilton, Rolati, Kohli, Whitehead, et al., 2017). DNA from 99 individuals with Alzheimer's disease within 23 extended families were obtained, as well as from four family members with mild cognitive impairment and 18 unaffected family members. This DNA was prepared using the SureSelect Human All Exon Mb Kit from Agilent Technologies. The resulting libraries were sequenced on an *Illumina* HiSeq 2000 for paired-end reads, 100 nucleotides in length. After sequencing, the resulting data were mapped to the human reference genome (hg19) using the program BWA (Li & Durbin, 2009). Genetic variants within the *exons* were called using the Genome Analysis Toolkit (GATK; McKenna, Hanna, Banks, Sivachenko, Cibulskis, Kernytsky, et al., 2010), while small insertions or deletions were assessed using Bowtie2 (Langmead & Salzberg, 2012) and Pindel (Ye, Schulz, Long, Apweiler, & Ning, 2009). This study identified 14 variants associated with the Alzheimer's disease phenotype, including 10 in known Alzheimer's disease genes. Thirteen of these were single-nucleotide changes, and one was a four–base pair deletion, meaning that four DNA nucleotides were absent from the gene. Such a deletion may cause a protein to form incorrectly, in which case it may not be able to perform its normal function.

Targeted Gene Sequencing

An even more directed approach to examine specific genetic variation is **targeted gene sequencing.** Such studies are used to investigate the presence or prevalence of known functional variants in specific populations. This approach can also be used to examine the genes of specific chemical pathways or to follow up on studies from *GWAS* and/or *WGS* (Mertes, Elsharawy, Sauer, van Helvoort, van der Zaag, Franke, et al., 2011). *Targeted gene sequencing* necessarily requires knowledge of the gene or regions of interest to be examined.

First in a *targeted gene sequencing* study, specific probes that will capture the desired regions are designed. Predesigned commercially available probes are available for humans, although many studies require custom-designed probes for the regions of interest. One benefit of a *targeted sequencing* approach is that in addition to coding sequences, introns and intergenic regions around genes of interest may also be examined. Much of the cost of *targeted gene sequencing* depends on the amount of data per sample that is desired.

In one study, a *targeted sequencing* approach was used to investigate Alzheimer's disease in African Americans (Logue, Lancour, Farrell, Simkina, Fallin, Lunetta, et al., 2018). In this study, 107 genes were sequenced from 643 case individuals and 623 control individuals. The genes sequenced included many previously associated with Alzheimer's disease in African Americans, including *ABCA7, AKAP9, COBL, MS4A6A, PTK2B, SLC10A2,* and *ZCWPW1.* In addition, the researchers selected additional genes that were identified as potentially associated with Alzheimer's disease. The probes that were generated for this study included the *exons* for the genes as well as introns and regions both 5,000 bp upstream and 1,000 bp downstream of the gene boundaries. Overall, there were 10,906 capture targets in the study, covering 122 targeted regions. Sequencing was done on an *Illumina* HiSeq 2500, with the resulting data mapped to the *GRCh37* human reference genome using BWA-MEM (Li, 2013). After mapping, variants were called using GATK (McKenna, et al., 2010), and variants were annotated with SnpEff (Cingolani, Platts, Wang, Coon, Nguyen, Wang, et al., 2012) and SnpSift (Cingolani, et al., 2012). Variants of potential functional significance, such as loss-of-function mutations or missense variants, were tested for association with Alzheimer's using PLINK (Purcell, et al., 2007). One of the most substantial observations from this study was an association between Alzheimer's and an 11-nucleotide loss-of-function mutation that caused a frameshift in the *ABCA7* gene. A second important observation was an association with a nine-nucleotide deletion close to the transcription start site of *AKAP9.* These types of genetic changes, where a small number of nucleotides are missing from a gene region, can have very significant effects on how a protein forms and its ability to function correctly.

Epigenetics

Increasingly, it is being recognized that information stored within genomes but that is not a genetic variation itself can have substantial influence on disease phenotypes (Zoghbi & Beaudet, 2016). This **epigenetic** variation can be transmitted between generations (inheritance) but can also change much more quickly due to environmental influences. *Epigenetics* is the study of such heritable changes, and *epigenetic* studies encompass multiple related areas of focus, including DNA methylation, histone modification, and noncoding RNA variation. **DNA methylation** occurs when methyl groups are added to a DNA molecule, which can change the activity of a DNA segment without changing the sequence (Robertson, 2005). In particular, *DNA methylation* can act to suppress gene transcription.

Post-translational modifications made to histones can affect gene expression by altering chromatin structure or recruiting histone modifiers (Ye, Feng, Gao, Mu, Zhu, & Yang, 2017). Noncoding RNA functions to regulate gene expression at the transcriptional and post-transcriptional level by inducing cleavage, degrading the molecule, or blocking translation (Esteller, 2011).

There are several methods to examine *epigenetic* signatures within a sample, each of which requires its own preparation approach. To examine *DNA methylation*, researchers employ a **bisulfite treatment** to their samples, which converts unmethylated cytosine residues into uracil, while methylated residues are left unmodified. These samples can then be sequenced using *NGS* technology and the resulting data bioinformatically assessed to determine which locations are methylated versus unmethylated. To examine histone modifications, researchers can use a targeted antibody selection to enrich DNA fragments of interest bound to particular proteins. Finally, an assay for transposase-accessible chromatin sequencing may determine regions of chromatin accessibility and map DNA-binding proteins. This makes it possible to identify active promoters, enhancers, and other cis-regulatory elements. The methods selected will generally depend on the nature of the study and type of *epigenetic* changes being analyzed.

One study examining *epigenetic methylation* in relation to Alzheimer's disease used tissue samples from 34 deceased case patients and 34 deceased nondemented control patients (Watson, Roussos, Garg, Ho, Azam, Katsel, et al., 2016). DNA from these samples was extracted and then treated with sodium bisulfate. The samples were then processed on an *Illumina* HumanMethylation450 array platform. Data processing and calculation of methylation values were done using the GenomeStudio Methylation Module Package (Illumina). For the 461,272 potentially methylated autosomal sites available for analysis after quality controls, the authors first used linear regression to examine differences between *cases* and *controls*. Sites that were significantly different were then clustered into regions, and these regions were examined for the presence of genes and promotor regions. Many regions associated with Alzheimer's disease were found to be hypermethylated. Furthermore, many of these regions correlated with genes previously reported in Alzheimer's genome-wide association studies. This is strong evidence that these genes are important for proper brain functioning and that any disruption to them, whether through mutation or changes in their ability to be expressed, results in a detrimental phenotype.

The Microbiome

One final area in which *NGS* has facilitated a wealth of new and important studies for human health is in the analysis of the microbiome (Mohajeri, Brummer, Rastall, Weersma, Harmsen, Faas, et al., 2018). The **microbiome** can be defined as the bacteria, protists, and other nonhuman living organisms that reside on or within a human, or even within a specific tissue, organ, etc. Many recent studies have shown how strongly correlated the community that makes up the *microbiome* is with specific disease phenotypes (reviewed in Liang, Leung, Guan, & Au, 2018; Mohajeri, et al., 2018). *NGS* technology allows for this community to be studied in greater detail.

Most commonly, primers specific to regions of the *16S* ribosomal RNA gene are used to amplify this genomic region from samples taken from individuals with both the control and the disease phenotype (Kuczynski, Lauber, Walters, Parfrey, Clemente, Gevers, et al., 2011). These regions are then sequenced, resulting in millions of genetic reads. The reads are bioinformatically analyzed in a metagenomic context to determine the presence or absence of specific species or taxa, as well as their relative abundance. Many computational tools are available to perform metagenomic analyses (reviewed in Ladoukakis, Kolisis, & Chatziioannou, 2014; Oulas, Pavloudi, Polymenakou, Pavlopoulos, Papanikolaou, Kotoulas, et al., 2015).

In a recent study, the gut *microbiome* of 25 patients with Alzheimer's disease was compared to 94 patients without dementia (Vogt, Kerby, Dill-McFarland, Harding, Merluzzi, Johnson, et al., 2017). The researchers collected stool samples from both patient groups. From these samples, microbial

DNA was extracted and the *V4* region of the *16S* gene was amplified using *PCR*. After amplification and purification, the amplicons were sequenced on an *Illumina* MiSeq. The data that resulted were quality filtered and chimeric sequences (sequences formed from two or more separate molecules joined together) were removed. Finally, the sequences were clustered into operational taxonomic units (OTUs) using the OptiClust algorithm (Westcott & Schloss, 2017). This study showed that microbial diversity tended to be lower within patients with Alzheimer's disease. It also showed that their microbial composition (i.e., species present/absent) differed between the case and control samples. Future work will be needed to determine the causal mechanisms for these observed differences.

Conclusion

The advent of *NGS* technology has both greatly increased the amount of data that is possible to collect and lowered the costs of collecting it. Furthermore, as studies are published, the data generated typically become available, making possible many additional secondary studies (van Dijk, Auger, Jaszczyszyn, & Thermes, 2014). Together, this work is allowing for major breakthroughs that have important implications for diagnosing and treating many challenges in health psychology. Importantly, it must be remembered that the majority of these methods allow researchers to identify potentially contributing factors to specific phenotypes. Often, it is necessary to follow up such studies with additional tests or experiments to determine how specific variation relates to a particular disease or other trait of interest. Methods for such studies are covered in other chapters of this book.

References

1000 Genomes Project Consortium, Abecasis, G. R., Auton, A., Brooks, L. D., DePristo, M. A., Durbin, R. M., et al. (2012). An integrated map of genetic variation from 1,092 human genomes. *Nature*, *491*(7422), 56–65. https://doi.org/10.1038/nature11632

2020 Alzheimer's disease facts and figures. (2020). Alzheimer's & dementia: The journal of the Alzheimer's Association, 10.1002/alz.12068. Advance online publication. https://doi.org/10.1002/alz.12068

Annese, A., Manzari, C., Lionetti, C., Picardi, E., Horner, D. S., Chiara, M., et al. (2018). Whole transcriptome profiling of Late-Onset Alzheimer's Disease patients provides insights into the molecular changes involved in the disease. *Scientific Reports*, *8*(1), 4282. https://doi.org/10.1038/s41598-018-22701-2

Ashbrook, D. G., Mulligan, M. K., & Williams, R. W. (2018). Post-genomic behavioral genetics: From revolution to routine. *Genes, Brain, and Behavior*, *17*(3), e12441. https://doi.org/10.1111/gbb.12441

Bamshad, M. J., Ng, S. B., Bigham, A. W., Tabor, H. K., Emond, M. J., Nickerson, D. A., et al. (2011). Exome sequencing as a tool for Mendelian disease gene discovery. *Nature Reviews: Genetics*, *12*(11), 745–755. https://doi.org/10.1038/nrg3031

Bleidorn, C. (2016). Third generation sequencing: Technology and its potential impact on evolutionary biodiversity research. *Systematics and Biodiversity*, *14*(1), 1–8. doi:10.1080/14772000.2015.1099575

Cingolani, P., Patel, V. M., Coon, M., Nguyen, T., Land, S. J., Ruden, D. M., et al. (2012). Using Drosophila melanogaster as a model for genotoxic chemical mutational studies with a new program, SnpSift. *Frontiers in Genetics*, *3*, 35. https://doi.org/10.3389/fgene.2012.00035

Cingolani, P., Platts, A., Wang, L., Coon, M., Nguyen, T., Wang, L., et al. (2012). A program for annotating and predicting the effects of single nucleotide polymorphisms, SnpEff: SNPs in the genome of Drosophila melanogaster strain w1118; iso-2; iso-3. *Fly*, *6*(2), 80–92. https://doi.org/10.4161/fly.19695

Collins, A. L., & Sullivan, P. F. (2013). Genome-wide association studies in psychiatry: What have we learned? *The British Journal of Psychiatry: The Journal of Mental Science*, *202*(1), 1–4. https://doi.org/10.1192/bjp.bp.112.117002

Costa-Silva, J., Domingues, D., & Lopes, F. M. (2017). RNA-seq differential expression analysis: An extended review and a software tool. *PLoS One*, *12*, 12, e0190152. doi:10.1371/journal.pone.0190152

Cukier, H. N., Kunkle, B. K., Hamilton, K. L., Rolati, S., Kohli, M. A., Whitehead, P. L., et al. (2017). Exome sequencing of extended families with Alzheimer's disease identifies novel genes implicated in cell immunity and neuronal function. *Journal of Alzheimer's Disease & Parkinsonism*, *7*(4), 355. https://doi.org/10.4172/2161-0460.1000355

Emilsson, V., Thorleifsson, G., Zhang, B., Leonardson, A. S., Zink, F., Zhu, J., et al. (2008). Genetics of gene expression and its effect on disease. *Nature*, *452*(7186), 423–428. https://doi.org/10.1038/nature06758

ENCODE Project Consortium. (2012). An integrated encyclopedia of DNA elements in the human genome. *Nature, 489*(7414), 57–74. https://doi.org/10.1038/nature11247

Esteller, M. (2011). Non-coding RNAs in human disease. *Nature Reviews: Genetics, 12*(12), 861–874. https://doi.org/10.1038/nrg3074

Feuk, L. (2010). Inversion variants in the human genome: Role in disease and genome architecture. *Genome Medicine, 2*(2), 11. https://doi.org/10.1186/gm132

Finotello, F., & Di Camillo, B. (2015). Measuring differential gene expression with RNA-seq: Challenges and strategies for data analysis. *Briefings in Functional Genomics, 14*(2), 130–142. https://doi.org/10.1093/bfgp/elu035

Flicek, P., & Birney, E. (2009). Sense from sequence reads: Methods for alignment and assembly. *Nature Methods, 6*(Suppl. 11), S6–S12. https://doi.org/10.1038/nmeth.1376

Goodwin, S., McPherson, J. D., & McCombie, W. R. (2016). Coming of age: Ten years of next-generation sequencing technologies. *Nature Reviews: Genetics, 17*(6), 333–351. https://doi.org/10.1038/nrg.2016.49

Hitzemann, R., Darakjian, P., Walter, N., Iancu, O. D., Searles, R., & McWeeney, S. (2014). Introduction to sequencing the brain transcriptome. *International Review of Neurobiology, 116*, 1–19. https://doi.org/10.1016/B978-0-12-801105-8.00001-1

Hwang, S., Kim, E., Lee, I., & Marcotte, E. M. (2015). Systematic comparison of variant calling pipelines using gold standard personal exome variants. *Scientific Reports, 5*, 17875. https://doi.org/10.1038/srep17875

Jensen, K. P. (2016). A review of genome-wide association studies of stimulant and opioid use disorders. *Molecular Neuropsychiatry, 2*(1), 37–45. https://doi.org/10.1159/000444755

Jiang, C., Li, G., Huang, P., Liu, Z., & Zhao, B. (2017). The gut microbiota and Alzheimer's disease. *Journal of Alzheimer's Disease: JAD, 58*(1), 1–15. https://doi.org/10.3233/JAD-161141

Kim, H. K., Pham, M., Ko, K. S., Rhee, B. D., & Han, J. (2018). Alternative splicing isoforms in health and disease. *Pflugers Archiv: European Journal of Physiology, 470*(7), 995–1016. https://doi.org/10.1007/s00424-018-2136-x

Kuczynski, J., Lauber, C. L., Walters, W. A., Parfrey, L. W., Clemente, J. C., Gevers, D., et al. (2011). Experimental and analytical tools for studying the human microbiome. *Nature Reviews: Genetics, 13*(1), 47–58. https://doi.org/10.1038/nrg3129

Ladoukakis, E., Kolisis, F. N., & Chatziioannou, A. A. (2014). Integrative workflows for metagenomic analysis. *Frontiers in Cell and Developmental Biology, 2*, 70. https://doi.org/10.3389/fcell.2014.00070

Langmead, B., & Salzberg, S. L. (2012). Fast gapped-read alignment with Bowtie 2. *Nature Methods, 9*(4), 357–359. https://doi.org/10.1038/nmeth.1923

Li, H. (2013). Aligning sequence reads, clone sequences and assembly contigs with BWA-MEM. arXiv 2013;1303.3997v2

Li, H., & Durbin, R. (2009). Fast and accurate short read alignment with Burrows-Wheeler transform. *Bioinformatics (Oxford, England), 25*(14), 1754–1760. https://doi.org/10.1093/bioinformatics/btp324

Li, Z., Wang, Y., & Wang, F. (2018). A study on fast calling variants from next-generation sequencing data using decision tree. *BMC Bioinformatics, 19*(1), 145. https://doi.org/10.1186/s12859-018-2147-9

Liang, D., Leung, R. K., Guan, W., & Au, W. W. (2018). Involvement of gut microbiome in human health and disease: Brief overview, knowledge gaps and research opportunities. *Gut Pathogens, 10*, 3. https://doi.org/10.1186/s13099-018-0230-4

Logue, M. W., Lancour, D., Farrell, J., Simkina, I., Fallin, M. D., Lunetta, K. L., et al. (2018). Targeted sequencing of Alzheimer disease genes in African Americans implicates novel risk variants. *Frontiers in Neuroscience, 12*, 592. https://doi.org/10.3389/fnins.2018.00592

Magi, A., Benelli, M., Gozzini, A., Girolami, F., Torricelli, F., & Brandi, M. L. (2010). Bioinformatics for next generation sequencing data. *Genes, 1*(2), 294–307. https://doi.org/10.3390/genes1020294

Marees, A. T., de Kluiver, H., Stringer, S., Vorspan, F., Curis, E., Marie-Claire, C., et al. (2018). A tutorial on conducting genome-wide association studies: Quality control and statistical analysis. *International Journal of Methods in Psychiatric Research, 27*(2), e1608. https://doi.org/10.1002/mpr.1608

McDermaid, A., Monier, B., Zhao, J., Liu, B., & Ma, Q. (2019). Interpretation of differential gene expression results of RNA-seq data: Review and integration. *Briefings in Bioinformatics, 20*(6), 2044–2054. https://doi.org/10.1093/bib/bby067

McKenna, A., Hanna, M., Banks, E., Sivachenko, A., Cibulskis, K., Kernytsky, A., et al. (2010). The genome analysis toolkit: A map reduce framework for analyzing next-generation DNA sequencing data. *Genome Research, 20*(9), 1297–1303. https://doi.org/10.1101/gr.107524.110

Mertes, F., Elsharawy, A., Sauer, S., van Helvoort, J. M., van der Zaag, P. J., Franke, A., et al. (2011). Targeted enrichment of genomic DNA regions for next-generation sequencing. *Briefings in Functional Genomics, 10*(6), 374–386. https://doi.org/10.1093/bfgp/elr033

Mizuguchi, T., Suzuki, T., Abe, C., Umemura, A., Tokunaga, K., Kawai, Y., et al. (2019). A 12-kb structural variation in progressive myoclonic epilepsy was newly identified by long-read whole-genome sequencing. *Journal of Human Genetics, 64*(5), 359–368. https://doi.org/10.1038/s10038-019-0569-5

Mohajeri, M. H., Brummer, R., Rastall, R. A., Weersma, R. K., Harmsen, H., Faas, M., et al. (2018). The role of the microbiome for human health: From basic science to clinical applications. *European Journal of Nutrition, 57*(Suppl. 1), 1–14. https://doi.org/10.1007/s00394-018-1703-4

Nagarajan, N., & Pop, M. (2013). Sequence assembly demystified. *Nature Reviews: Genetics, 14*(3), 157–167. https://doi.org/10.1038/nrg3367

Naj, A. C., Schellenberg, G. D., & Alzheimer's Disease Genetics Consortium (ADGC). (2017). Genomic variants, genes, and pathways of Alzheimer's disease: An overview. *American Journal of Medical Genetics. Part B: Neuropsychiatric Genetics: The Official Publication of the International Society of Psychiatric Genetics, 174*(1), 5–26. https://doi.org/10.1002/ajmg.b.32499

Oulas, A., Pavloudi, C., Polymenakou, P., Pavlopoulos, G. A., Papanikolaou, N., Kotoulas, G., et al. (2015). Metagenomics: Tools and insights for analyzing next-generation sequencing data derived from biodiversity studies. *Bioinformatics and Biology Insights, 9*, 75–88. https://doi.org/10.4137/BBI.S12462

Pabinger, S., Dander, A., Fischer, M., Snajder, R., Sperk, M., Efremova, M., et al. (2014). A survey of tools for variant analysis of next-generation genome sequencing data. *Briefings in Bioinformatics, 15*(2), 256–278. https://doi.org/10.1093/bib/bbs086

Pasaniuc, B., Rohland, N., McLaren, P. J., Garimella, K., Zaitlen, N., Li, H., et al. (2012). Extremely low-coverage sequencing and imputation increases power for genome-wide association studies. *Nature Genetics, 44*(6), 631–635. https://doi.org/10.1038/ng.2283

Purcell, S., Neale, B., Todd-Brown, K., Thomas, L., Ferreira, M. A., Bender, D., et al. (2007). PLINK: A tool set for whole-genome association and population-based linkage analyses. *American Journal of Human Genetics, 81*(3), 559–575. https://doi.org/10.1086/519795

Robertson, K. D. (2005). DNA methylation and human disease. *Nature Reviews: Genetics, 6*(8), 597–610. https://doi.org/10.1038/nrg1655

Schneider, V. A., Graves-Lindsay, T., Howe, K., Bouk, N., Chen, H. C., Kitts, P. A., et al. (2017). Evaluation of GRCh38 and de novo haploid genome assemblies demonstrates the enduring quality of the reference assembly. *Genome Research, 27*(5), 849–864. https://doi.org/10.1101/gr.213611.116

Tazi, J., Bakkour, N., & Stamm, S. (2009). Alternative splicing and disease. *Biochimica et Biophysica Acta, 1792*(1), 14–26. https://doi.org/10.1016/j.bbadis.2008.09.017

Trapnell, C., Hendrickson, D. G., Sauvageau, M., Goff, L., Rinn, J. L., & Pachter, L. (2013). Differential analysis of gene regulation at transcript resolution with RNA-seq. *Nature Biotechnology, 31*(1), 46–53. https://doi.org/10.1038/nbt.2450

van Dijk, E. L., Auger, H., Jaszczyszyn, Y., & Thermes, C. (2014). Ten years of next-generation sequencing technology. *Trends in Genetics: TIG, 30*(9), 418–426. https://doi.org/10.1016/j.tig.2014.07.001

Visscher, P. M., Wray, N. R., Zhang, Q., Sklar, P., McCarthy, M. I., Brown, M. A., et al. (2017). 10 years of GWAS discovery: Biology, function, and translation. *American Journal of Human Genetics, 101*(1), 5–22. https://doi.org/10.1016/j.ajhg.2017.06.005

Vogt, N. M., Kerby, R. L., Dill-McFarland, K. A., Harding, S. J., Merluzzi, A. P., Johnson, S. C., et al. (2017). Gut microbiome alterations in Alzheimer's disease. *Scientific Reports, 7*(1), 13537. https://doi.org/10.1038/s41598-017-13601-y

Wang, Z., Gerstein, M., & Snyder, M. (2009). RNA-seq: A revolutionary tool for transcriptomics. *Nature Reviews: Genetics, 10*(1), 57–63. https://doi.org/10.1038/nrg2484

Warden, C. D., Adamson, A. W., Neuhausen, S. L., & Wu, X. (2014). Detailed comparison of two popular variant calling packages for exome and targeted exon studies. *PeerJ, 2*, e600. https://doi.org/10.7717/peerj.600

Watson, C. T., Roussos, P., Garg, P., Ho, D. J., Azam, N., Katsel, P. L., et al. (2016). Genome-wide DNA methylation profiling in the superior temporal gyrus reveals epigenetic signatures associated with Alzheimer's disease. *Genome Medicine, 8*(1), 5. https://doi.org/10.1186/s13073-015-0258-8

Westcott, S. L., & Schloss, P. D. (2017). OptiClust, an improved method for assigning amplicon-based sequence data to operational taxonomic units. *mSphere, 2*(2), e00073–17. https://doi.org/10.1128/mSphereDirect.00073-17

Williams, A. G., Thomas, S., Wyman, S. K., & Holloway, A. K. (2014). RNA-seq data: Challenges in and recommendations for experimental design and analysis. *Current Protocols in Human Genetics, 83*, 11.13.1–11.13.20. https://doi.org/10.1002/0471142905.hg1113s83

Williams, C. R., Baccarella, A., Parrish, J. Z., & Kim, C. C. (2016). Trimming of sequence reads alters RNA-seq gene expression estimates. *BMC Bioinformatics, 17*, 103. https://doi.org/10.1186/s12859-016-0956-2

Wolf, J. B. (2013). Principles of transcriptome analysis and gene expression quantification: An RNA-seq tutorial. *Molecular Ecology Resources, 13*(4), 559–572. https://doi.org/10.1111/1755-0998.12109

Wu, T. D., & Nacu, S. (2010). Fast and SNP-tolerant detection of complex variants and splicing in short reads. *Bioinformatics (Oxford, England), 26*(7), 873–881. https://doi.org/10.1093/bioinformatics/btq057

Yamazaki, Y., Zhao, N., Caulfield, T. R., Liu, C. C., & Bu, G. (2019). Apolipoprotein E and Alzheimer disease: Pathobiology and targeting strategies. *Nature Reviews: Neurology, 15*(9), 501–518. https://doi.org/10.1038/s41582-019-0228-7

Ye, K., Schulz, M. H., Long, Q., Apweiler, R., & Ning, Z. (2009). Pindel: A pattern growth approach to detect break points of large deletions and medium sized insertions from paired-end short reads. *Bioinformatics (Oxford, England), 25*(21), 2865–2871. https://doi.org/10.1093/bioinformatics/btp394

Ye, X., Feng, C., Gao, T., Mu, G., Zhu, W., & Yang, Y. (2017). Linker histone in diseases. *International Journal of Biological Sciences, 13*(8), 1008–1018. https://doi.org/10.7150/ijbs.19891

Yokoyama, A. S., Rutledge, J. C., & Medici, V. (2017). DNA methylation alterations in Alzheimer's disease. *Environmental Epigenetics, 3*(2), dvx008. https://doi.org/10.1093/eep/dvx008

Zhou, X., Chen, Y., Mok, K. Y., Zhao, Q., Chen, K., Chen, Y., et al. (2018). Identification of genetic risk factors in the Chinese population implicates a role of immune system in Alzheimer's disease pathogenesis. *Proceedings of the National Academy of Sciences of the United States of America, 115*(8), 1697–1706. https://doi.org/10.1073/pnas.1715554115

Zoghbi, H. Y. & Beaudet, A. L. (2016). Epidenesis and human disease. Cold Spring Harbor Perspectives in Biology, 8(2), a019497.

8

THE ETHICS OF GENETICS RESEARCH

Curtis R. Coughlin II

Overview

The field of human genetics is often associated with an ominous past. Over a century ago, Francis Galton coined the term **eugenics** referring to the systematic study of inherited traits. The initial eugenic studies were voluntary and emphasized genetic education (Galton, 1884). Surprisingly, these studies emphasized important tenets of ethical research performed today. Yet most people associate the idea of *eugenics* with the atrocities of Hitler's death camps or the involuntary sterilization policies of the 20th century. In fact, the very horrific and villainous actions of World War II emphasized the need for voluntariness and informed consent that are central to all human subject research today (Shuster, 1997). Similarly, it may seem as though the popular media is dominated by stories consisting of DNA-based crime investigations or misuse of genome editing. These unfortunate missteps have guided ethical standards surrounding genetic research. By understanding potential ethical dilemmas, the health psychology researcher can feel more confident applying exciting genetic tools to research.

Historically, ethical issues associated with genetic testing were theoretical or at least limited to the infrequent instances of misattributed paternity (i.e., "nonpaternity"). In the last decade, technological advancements have made **genome sequencing** cost-effective and relatively easy for the non-geneticist. Commercially available high-throughput platforms can sequence millions of small segments of DNA in parallel (Bick & Dimmock, 2011). Although many variants are identified through such sequencing approaches, bioinformatic platforms allow variants to be filtered based upon evolutionary conservation, population data, inheritance patterns, and phenotypic presentation (Richards, Aziz, Bale, Bick, Das, Gastier-Foster, et al., 2015; Tabor, Auer, Jamal, Chong, Yu, Gordon, et al., 2014). As a result of low-cost sequencing platforms and automated bioinformatics pipelines, *genomic sequencing* has become a ubiquitous tool. The vast amount of information obtained from *genomic sequencing* allows researchers to identify new genes associated with **Mendelian disease**, complex human traits, and pathways associated with pharmacologic response. It may also uncover unexpected genetic results ranging from misattributed paternity to increased risk of treatable cancers. These unexpected genetic results are most commonly referred to as secondary findings, and the debate surrounding the return of secondary findings has been referred to as "arguably the most pressing issue in genetics today" (Couzin-Frankel, 2011, p. 662).

The field of human genetics has attempted to distance itself from the *eugenics* movement even as patients, subjects, and popular news articles (or book chapters, such as this one) remind us of the past. Until now, such criticism has been limited. The prospective selection of embryos and fetuses based on genetic status has focused on severe, often life-threatening, disease. And although selecting embryos based on qualitative traits such as hair color are compelling news stories, there are relatively few documented cases of genetic selection for nondisease traits. Yet the world of genetics has changed dramatically in the last few years. Once only found in science fiction, genetic modification techniques now allow researchers to edit the genome of living organisms almost at will.

Recently, a scientist infamously announced the use of genetic modification techniques to knockdown the *CCR5* gene in twin girls (Cyranoski & Ledford, 2018; Normile, 2018). It is fair to say that most scientists, researchers, and even geneticists were not familiar with the *CCR5* gene prior to this story. The **CCR5** mutations were intended to reduce the twins' risk of HIV infections, although it may have had unintended effects. The *CCR5* gene may have a protective role against West Nile virus, and individuals with *CCR5* mutations have had severe reactions to some vaccines (Lim & Murphy, 2011; Pulendran, Miller, Querec, Akondy, Moseley, Laur, et al., 2008). At least in mice, mutations in *CCR5* are also associated with improvement in cognition (Zhou, Greenhill, Huang, Silva, Sano, Wu, et al., 2016). It is important to emphasize that the genetic manipulation of human embryos was not supported by any oversight organization or the scientist's university. In fact, the scientist was removed from the university's faculty and is currently facing criminal charges. It is unfortunate that this is the first case of genetic modification leading to the live birth of a child. Despite the many ethical questions about the use of this technology in general, and specifically in this case, the era of genetic modification has begun. It is reasonable to assume that the advances in genome sequencing and genome editing will result in increasing adaption of genetic research. This chapter is intended to guide the reader through ethical principles that apply to current and future genetic research. Careful planning about possible ethical concerns will aid both the scientist and subjects during this exciting era of genomic research.

Ethical Framework

The four principles of biomedical ethics, colloquially referred to as **principlism**, are most likely familiar to the psychological researcher (Beauchamp & Childress, 2013). **Principlism** is a common framework for conceptualizing ethics in biomedical research and is often taught in postgraduate education programs and emphasized on medical or board exams. The four principles provide a general ethical framework and are not intended to replace all ethical thought or moral theory. Similarly, the following discussion is intended to provide a framework for the author to discuss ethical issues related to genetic research and not intended to answer all possible ethical dilemmas the psychological researcher may face.

The Four Principles

It is also important to note that while Tom Beauchamp (2005) was working on *Principles of Biomedical Ethics*, he was also recruited by the National Commission for the Protection of Human Subjects of Biomedical and Behavioral Research. The commission was charged with establishing the ethical principles for biomedical and behavioral research involving human subjects. The commission's final recommendations were detailed in *The Belmont Report*, and the two texts, published less than one year apart, heavily influenced the other (Beauchamp, 2005). In this chapter, we will treat both works as a single ethical framework, which can be applied equally to clinical, medical, and research ethics.

Beauchamp and Childress (2013) identified fundamental moral considerations or obligations that underlie clinical ethics and human subject research. These obligations can be described by the following concepts. **Autonomy** is an obligation to respect a person's choice. **Beneficence** involves maximizing to benefits others. **Nonmaleficence** means not to harm others. **Justice** distributes benefits and harms fairly. It is likely that the reader will be familiar with these core principles and providing details on each would be pedantic. Instead, we will apply these principles to genetic research throughout the chapter.

Limitations of the Four Principles

Although *principlism* is arguably the most widely recognized ethical framework, it is not without limitations. Indeed, many have questioned whether the principlist paradigm limits the number of moral obligations recognized by the clinician or researcher (Fiester, 2007). Virtue-based bioethics has gained popularity as a reaction to the perceived oversimplification of principle-based bioethics. Moral obligations are often attributed to virtue ethics. **Virtue ethics** focuses on the professional character and conduct of clinicians and researchers (Holland, 2011; Oakley, 2010), including obligations such as truthfulness, honesty, and the protection of privacy (Childress, 2010). Although we will refer to them individually, *virtue-based ethics* and principle-based ethics are complementary approaches to most ethical or moral issues.

Veracity and Fidelity

The principles of veracity and fidelity are integral to ethical research in the current era of genomic research. As these principles may be less familiar to the reader, the following is provided as a brief overview. **Veracity** refers to the obligation for the researcher to be truthful or honest. The principle of *veracity* is especially critical in the current landscape of genome sequencing. As researchers are faced with whether to return secondary findings, it is imperative that they be truthful about whether secondary findings could be identified, will be identified, and will be returned to subjects. Although the obligation to return secondary findings may be debated, the obligation for the researcher to be honest about the possibly of secondary findings is clear.

The principle of **fidelity** refers to the researcher's obligation to protect a subject's confidentiality. The arrest of Joseph DeAngelo, the alleged Golden State Killer, highlighted the power of DNA-based technology to identify potential criminals. It also emphasized how easy it is to identify an individual when genetic information is made publicly available. Currently there is tension between funding agencies requiring genetic data be publicly available and the researcher's obligation to protect confidentiality. The principle of *fidelity* also refers to the trusted relationship between researcher and subject. It is not an oversimplification to state that honesty (i.e., *veracity*) is integral to building a trusting relationship. It is paramount that the psychology researcher be honest about how genetic information will be used and with whom it will be shared.

The ethical framework described herein is meant as a general guide for the psychological researcher. Discussion of all ethical dilemmas that arise from genetic-based research is beyond the scope of any single book chapter. Therefore, the ethical framework will be applied to three common ethical issues: genetic testing and secondary findings, genetic testing and privacy, and genetic modification.

Research in Practice

Genetic Testing and Secondary Findings

In this chapter, **secondary findings** refer to a genetic result that is not related to the primary research question. This is the broadest possible definition of *secondary finding*, as it does not include interpretation of the medical or social implication of the result. *Secondary findings* have historically been referred to as incidental findings (Cohen, 1971; Geelhoed & Druy, 1982), although many have suggested that the term "incidental" may minimize a result that could have life-altering implications (Christenhusz, Devriendt, & Dierickx, 2013). Terminology is not as important as ensuring that each researcher and subject have a clear understanding of the plan to identify and disclose *secondary findings* identified during the research study.

The following is provided as an example to clarify the concept of secondary findings for the reader: *Genome sequencing* is performed in a cohort of subjects with major depressive disorder to identify genes associated with a positive response to a pharmacologic intervention. During the genetic analysis, a missense mutation in the *BRCA1* gene (associated with breast cancer) is identified in a single subject. This variant is not associated with the onset of major depressive disorder or metabolism of pharmacologic agents and is therefore a secondary finding.

It may not be immediately clear to the reader why the decision to disclose a genetic result is considered an ethical dilemma. It can reasonably be assumed a subject is both aware of and consented to the use of genetic testing. In our example, the subject consented to genetic testing related to major depressive disorder. It cannot be assumed that the subject also consented to receive personal genetic results about breast cancer. Receiving such a genetic result has been associated with short-term depression and anxiety (Mella, Muzzatti, Dolcetti, & Annunziata, 2017), can have medical implications for other family members, and can affect life insurance policies. It is also reasonable that the researcher does not have formal training or experience providing genetic counseling to subjects. This is one reason why many researchers have avoided returning secondary findings.

In this example, the researcher was using *genome sequencing* in a study that may have previously used a genotyping array. *Genome sequencing* is often used as a general term, although two sequencing approaches are often used. **Whole-exome** sequencing targets the part of the genome that encodes proteins (Bamshad, Ng, Bigham, Tabor, Emond, Nickerson, et al., 2011). Most of the disease-causing variants are in these genes (Monroe, Frederix, Savelberg, de Vries, Duran, van der Smagt, et al., 2016), and *whole-exome* sequencing is an ideal approach for identifying rare Mendelian disorders. *Whole-genome* sequencing includes all of the human genome, which has both the added benefit and disadvantage of more information requiring robust bioinformatic pipelines. *Whole-genome* sequencing can be performed quicker than *whole-exome* sequencing, as the latter requires the amplification of selected genes. As a result, *whole-genome* sequencing has been preferred in time-sensitive situations such as the diagnosis of critically ill patients (Saunders, Miller, Soden, Dinwiddie, Noll, Alnadi, et al., 2012; Willig, Petrikin, Smith, Saunders, Thiffault, Miller, et al., 2015).

In general, genome sequencing provides a lot more genetic information than single-**nucleotide polymorphism (SNP)–based genotyping** arrays. *SNP-based genotyping* arrays detect common polymorphisms or single-nucleotide changes. Using *SNP* genotypes, a researcher can gauge the dosage of gene and genomic fragments to identify known genetic syndromes, as well as the degree of relation between a patient's biological parents (i.e., consanguinity; Coughlin, Scharer, & Shaikh, 2012). *Genome sequencing* is becoming popular, as the data is more flexible for both current and future studies. Although genotyping arrays also identify medically actionable results (Coughlin, et al. 2012), *genome sequencing* platforms are much more likely to identify a secondary result. It has been estimated that approximately 1% to 5% of subjects will have a medically actionable result (Kim, Luo, Wang, Wegman-Ostrosky, Frone, Johnston, et al., 2018; Olfson, Cottrell, Davidson, Gurnett, Heusel, Stitziel, et al., 2015). This number is only expected to grow as more is learned about the role of genetics in disease and as genetic-based treatments improve.

As we just discussed, the disclosure of genetic results can be difficult. It is not possible for the psychological researcher, or any individual, to be an expert on all genetic disorders identified through genomic sequencing. Some researchers have partnered with genetic-trained colleagues, although this may not always be practical. It is estimated that there is only one genetic counselor or medical geneticist for every 132,000 and 650,000 persons in the United States, respectively (Cooksey, Forte, Flanagan, Benkendorf, & Blitzer, 2006; Summar & Watson, 2015). As a result, it is important to determine who is going to return any secondary findings (or at least how).

For a moment, let us assume that a researcher is considering returning secondary findings. This immediately raises the question: What secondary findings should be disclosed? Recently, the American College of Medical Genetics and Genomics (ACMGG) published a statement supporting disclosure of secondary results with high medical value for the patient (Green, Berg, Grody, Kalia, Korf, Martin, et al., 2013). The high medical value is colloquially referred to as "medical actionable" results and has been interpreted as a result that has medical treatment implications for the individual subject. The ACMGG further recommended that pathogenic findings in 59 genes be disclosed to all patients regardless of the reason for genetic testing (Kalia, Adelman, Bale, Chung, Eng, Evans, et al., 2017). It is easy to criticize the specific list of genes, and many clinicians, researchers, bioethicists, and organizations have made custom lists of medically actionable genes. Any list is certain to be changed often as our understanding of genetics continues to improve. It is also easy to overlook this significant paradigm change in the field of genetics. The ACMGG statement said that clinicians have an obligation to return medically actionable results, *even if patients have not consented to such results.*

Historically, many researchers chose to ignore secondary findings and debate whether researchers have the same obligation to report secondary findings as clinical colleagues (Fernandez, Strahlendorf, Avard, Knoppers, O'Connell, Bouffet, et al., 2013). Although it may feel like a recent phenomenon, the National Bioethics Advisory Commission (in 1999), the Centers for Disease Control and Prevention (in 2001), and the National Institutes of Health (in 2007) recommended returning secondary findings to research participants over a decade ago. It is important for each researcher to follow the recommendations of their funding agency, although regulatory requirements are not necessarily the same as ethical obligations.

Ethical Framework

Respect for persons (or *autonomy*) is central to all research. It is reasonable to assume that all psychological researchers support this tenet of research demonstrated by the care taken to write assent and consent forms and the time spent to consent research subjects. *Autonomy* emphasizes that subjects be fully informed to make the best possible decisions for themselves. This includes the information about what genetic testing results will be analyzed and reported.

In fact, having misinformation about the genetic testing has the potential for harm. In the author's experience, individuals have declined *clinical* genetic testing when indicated because they already had genetic testing in a research study. Often these subjects incorrectly assumed that the research genetic testing was comprehensive. Most of these subjects did not even receive a note or discussion about a negative genetic result from the researcher, assuming that "no news is good news." The research team also did a disservice to the subject and should have attempted to mitigate such a misunderstanding.

I have also spent significant time calling research participants about secondary findings who had no idea such results could be identified. I cannot emphasize enough that the researcher has a duty to clearly communicate *if* secondary findings will be analyzed and *if* secondary results will be returned (Coughlin, 2015). This is supported by the principle of *veracity* or truthfulness. It may be ethically justified for a researcher to not disclose secondary findings, but it is hard to justify a researcher not being honest with a subject about how the genetic information will be analyzed or used.

Admittedly, most researchers have elected to return a limited set of medically actionable results. This is due to a combination of regulatory changes by funding agencies and the increasing recognition of the obligation to return such results. For a moment, let us assume that most researchers will disclose medically actionable results. In fact, many researchers have even provided a list of such genes in information packets or consent forms. Although it is clearly outlined what will happen if a secondary finding is identified, it is hardly ever clear whether each genome will be systematically evaluated for these results. It is paramount that researchers have honest discussions about the genetic results, the methods (or lack thereof) for returning results, and the limitations of research testing in general.

It has also been suggested that medically actionable results should always be returned to subjects. Some question whether results will be forced upon unwilling recipients (Dimmock, 2012). It may be immediately obvious to the reader that not all subjects will want to receive genetic results. In fact, there was no consensus about receiving genetic results in a recent survey of current research participants (Viberg Johansson, Langenskiöld, Segerdahl, Hansson, Hösterey, Gummesson, et al., 2019). *Autonomy* emphasizes that subjects be fully informed to make the best possible decisions for themselves. This includes the decision to decline genetic results—even results that have high medical actionability.

Many researchers have elected to disclose any results identified in one of the genes recommended by the ACMGG. This approach is practical, as these genes have been curated by experts, sequencing platforms are designed to capture these sequences, and most analytical pipelines have been optimized to interpret these results. In a minority of studies, there appears to be a recruitment initiative (or simply a point of pride) to state that "our study returns more genes than other studies." The principles of *beneficence* and *nonmaleficence* should guide the researcher when deciding which results to return to participants.

There is a strong argument for disclosing secondary results when there is a high clinical utility (i.e., medically actionable) associated with the result. This is supported by the principle of *beneficence* (discussed extensively earlier). It is just as important to note that there is a strong argument against disclosing a secondary result where there is unclear significance. Results with unclear significance may also be referred to as **variants of unknown significance (VOUS**; Richards, Aziz, Bale, Bick, Das, Gastier-Foster, et al., 2015). These results are neither pathogenic nor benign. Returning such results can result in harm to subjects and for this reason should be avoided (i.e., violating the principle of *nonmaleficence*). Patients have reported anxiety, worry, and general uncertainty when receiving a *VOUS* (Makhnoon, Shirts, & Bowen, 2019). Although it may be justified to return such results in a clinical setting, it is hard to justify returning a VOUS to a research subject.

There will be nuanced situations that may affect the researcher's decision to disclose a secondary result. One such situation is when an adult-onset condition, such as breast cancer risk or Alzheimer's disease risk, is identified in a minor. In general, it is recommended that genetic testing for adult-onset conditions in a minor be delayed until that individual can consent to the testing. This supports the future autonomy of that individual, who may not want to know his or her risk for a genetic condition (Botkin, Belmont, Berg, Berkman, Bombard, Holm, et al., 2015; Ross, Ross, Saal, David, Anderson, American Academy of Pediatrics, et al., 2013). In the case of an unexpected finding, it is justified to report the result even in the case of a minor. Disclosure in these cases is often complex. Results will need to be disclosed to a family member or legal guardian, although the researcher should discuss a formal plan to disseminate the result to the subject at an appropriate age. In such situations, it may be important to involve a genetics-trained health care provider due to both the complications of disclosure and the need for long-term genetic counseling.

Recommendations and Future Research

There is increased recognition of the obligation to disclose medically actionable genetic results to research participants. Many researchers focus on practical concerns such as who should return the genetic results and whether every subject should receive genetic counseling. There are no easy (or right) answers to these questions, as it is easy to see how many different permutations would be ethically justified. It is important to focus on an ethical approach to results disclosure. Researchers should be transparent with subjects about genetic testing. Emphasis should be placed on what genes or diseases will be identified, whether every subject will have those genes analyzed, how results will be returned, and whom the subjects could talk to about the results. Through these honest conversations, researchers will support a subject's decision to participate in genetic research and the subject's decision to receive a secondary result.

By now, it may be clear to the reader that genetic testing itself has become rather accessible to the non-geneticist. As a result, it is tempting to collect and store DNA on all subjects. Yet disclosure of genetic results has become increasingly complex. This section was meant to guide the researcher who may simply store DNA for future studies without thought about disclosure of results. Future studies are also needed to determine how to disclose research results to subjects, as many different methods have been used, including letters from research staff, forwarding results to primary care providers, or having each subject receive an individual genetic counseling appointment. It is likely that each psychological researcher will find a reasonable solution to returning genetic results. What is paramount is that each subject has a reasonable understanding of the genetic testing performed as part of the research study.

Genetic Testing and Privacy

A tension exists between the desire to both openly share genetic data and protect subjects' privacy. As our understanding of genetic traits and disease grew, there were many concerns about the possible misuse of genetic testing. For example, individuals were concerned that law enforcement, governmental agencies, or private companies would use an individual's genetic results for nonmedical reasons. Although these fears seldom materialized, there were examples of misuse. In the 1990s, the Burlington Northern and Santa Fe Railway Company forced all employees who claimed a work-related carpal tunnel syndrome injury to provide a DNA sample to the company. The workers eventually sued the company, stating the company was using genetic information to avoid paying compensation to workers or to screen potential employees for a susceptibility to carpal tunnel syndrome (Lewin, 2001). There are now numerous legislative and regulatory rules to protect individuals from possible misuses of genetic information (Friedrich, 2002).

Currently, the biggest threat to breach of privacy is the voluntary sharing of genetic information through consumer genetic platforms such as Ancestry or genealogy platforms. *Direct-to-consumer (DTC)* genetic companies do not require a prescription from a medical provider, advertise widely to consumers, and offer social media–style sharing of results. *DTC* platforms use genotyping arrays to evaluate common *SNPs* associated with health risks, common traits, and ancestry. Many third-party services also offer to further interpret genotype data and to identify genetic relatives.

In 2012, investigators evaluated the *Y-chromosome haplotypes* of research subjects and compared them to publicly available genealogy databases (Gymrek, McGuire, Golan, Halperin, & Erlich, 2013). *Haplotypes*, a combination of normal variations or polymorphisms that are inherited together, can be used to identify genetic family members. At that time, many genealogy companies were offering to reunite relatives by genotyping *polymorphic short tandem repeats* on the Y chromosome (*Y-STR*; Calafell & Larmuseau, 2017). Researchers were able to correctly identify the surname of research participants, as well as identify many members of their entire family, using the limited amount of genetic information. Authors warned that a few genetic markers from one individual could "lead to the identification of another person who might have no acquaintance with the person who released his genetic data" (Gymrek, et al., 2013, p. 324). This remarkable study received little press, and there is little evidence it slowed down the use of public genealogy websites.

In 2018, law enforcement agencies used a DNA sample from a crime scene attributed to the Golden State Killer and cross-referenced it on a genealogy website. The authorities were able to identify a third-degree cousin of the suspect, which ultimately led to the arrest of Joseph DeAngelo. This very public use of a consumer genetic website raised many questions about whether anyone can expect to have true genetic privacy. Researchers recently evaluated 1.28 million individuals who participated in *DTC* testing and identified a third cousin in 60% of cases and a second cousin in 15% of individuals (Erlich, Shor, Pe'er, & Carmi, 2018). It is likely that these numbers will only increase as ancestry algorithms improve and as more individuals participate in consumer and ancestry genetic platforms.

Ethical Framework

Protecting genetic privacy is difficult. It is not uncommon for some individuals to have grave concerns over genetic privacy and may avoid enrolling in studies that use genetic testing. That same individual may have a distant relative who already shared DNA results with multiple entities. Such concerns about sharing results are justified. Yet when any one family member elects to share DNA results, it affects all other family members. It goes without saying that Joseph DeAngelo never elected to share his DNA results. Despite the nature of shared genetic information, researchers have a duty to protect his or her subject's privacy.

Fidelity is an often-overlooked ethical principle, which refers to an obligation to duties such as being trustworthy. Researchers trust that subjects will do what is requested, such as take a study medication or honestly fill out a questionnaire. In turn, subjects must also trust that researchers will fulfill their duties, including informing them of all risks and potential benefits of the research study. It may already be evident to the reader that one core component of trust is maintaining subject confidentiality.

True genetic privacy is difficult, especially as genetic data is increasingly incorporated into our health care (Collins & Varmus, 2015), consumer products, and even aid in our decisions about wine selection (viome.com). There are ways to increase genetic privacy by encrypting of DNA results and only sharing aggregate genetic data. What is paramount is that the psychological researcher attempts to fulfill his or her duty to protect subject privacy *and* that each researcher be transparent with subjects about the limitations of genetic privacy.

Genetic Selection and Genetic Modification

Genetic Selection

There is a seminal moment in the popular film *Gattaca* where the geneticist convinces a couple to select an embryo for positive genetic traits. He states, "We want to give your child the best possible start. Believe me, we have enough imperfection built in already. Your child doesn't need any additional burdens" (DeVito, Shamberg, & Sher, 1997). The movie received critical acclaim but heightened the concern about genetic selection for nondisease traits. Shortly after the release of *Gattaca*, commercial laboratories started advertising **pre-implementation genetic diagnostic (PGD)** or **screening (PGS) services** aimed at selection of sex, hair color, and eye color (see www.fertility-docs.com).

PGD/S was first reported in 1990 to select female embryos in couples who were at risk of having male children with an X-linked disease (Handyside, Kontogianni, Hardy, & Winston, 1990). Over the past three decades, improvements in *in vitro* fertilization (IVF) techniques in genetic testing have greatly expanded the number of disorders that can be screened by *PGD/S*. Embryos can now be screened for single-gene disorders, multiple single-gene disorders, and chromosomal anomalies. Despite a few laboratories offering services to select qualitative traits such as eye color, the vast majority of individuals who use *PGD/S* services are at an increased risk of having a child with a severe genetic disorder. The majority of individuals have used *PGD/S* services in order to avoid severe, often life-limiting, genetic diseases.

The 2004 novel *My Sister's Keeper* popularized a story of a couple that screened embryos based on human leukocyte antigen (**HLA)** status. Although many may remember both the novel and subsequent movie, a number of similar cases were reported in the literature (Grewal, Kahn, MacMillan, Ramsay, & Wagner, 2004; Verlinsky, Rechitsky, Schoolcraft, Strom, & Kuliev, 2001). These cases represented a significant philosophical change to previous uses of **PGD/S**. In the past, embryos were selected to limit the risk of disease in the future child. Selection of embryos based on *HLA* status was intended to increase the likelihood a future child would be a compatible donor for a **haemopoietic stem cell**(HSCS)—the stem cells that develop into white blood cells, red blood cells, and platelets—transplant for an older sibling. The *HLA* status benefited an individual other than the embryo and future child. It also represented the first case where an embryo was selected for a nondisease trait. *HLA* status itself is not associated with a disease or even a risk of disease in the future child. Many bioethicists were concerned about the intention to have a "savior child" and what would happen to that child if he or she was not able to be, or refused to be, a stem cell donor (Devolder, 2005; Pennings, Schots, & Liebaers, 2002).

While many philosophers were concerned about the possibility of selecting embryos based on the nondisease trait of *HLA* status, one philosopher famously argued that all couples should select the best-possible embryos. In 2001, Julian Savulescu published his seminal paper on *Procreative Beneficence* and argued that couples should "select embryos or fetuses which are mostly likely to have the best life, based on available genetic information, including information about non-disease genes" (Savulescu, 2001, p. 413).

Procreative Beneficence attempts to reframe the debate from whether it is permissible to select embryos based on nondisease traits to question whether it is permissible to select an embryo without considering every disease and nondisease trait. This also raised significant questions about what constitutes a disease. For example, many readers may think of hearing impairment or deafness as a disability. Yet many view deafness as a culture that should be celebrated and conserved, which includes positive selection for embryos or fetus that have an inherited form of deafness (Dennis, 2004; Munoz-Baell & Ruiz, 2000). In a survey of *PGD/S* clinics in the United States, 3% of clinics reported providing services to couples who selected an embryo based on the presence of a disability such as deafness (Karpin, 2007).

The psychological researcher sits at the edge of the scientific and philosophical debate. Traits such as anxiety, depression, substance abuse, alcoholism, and Alzheimer's disease have a clear hereditary component, although the inheritance is far from Mendelian. Yet questions remain about whether individuals select embryos with lower risk for such traits. Even now, experts are wary of genetic selection of embryos for nondisease traits. Yet the definition of disease is complex. It is reasonable to assume that not all individuals would classify common disorders such as Down syndrome, deafness, and anxiety in the same manner.

Genetic selection is still quite limited. First, an individual must either know they are at risk for a genetic disease or be interested in choosing an embryo based on a genetic trait. Second, *PGD/S* requires the use of *IVF* procedures. In the United States, access to *IVF* is limited, and few insurance plans cover the services even in the cases of documented infertility (let alone for the purpose of genetic selection). Finally, such a decision must be made before an individual is pregnant. Studies have suggested that 45% to 51% of all pregnancies in the United States are unintended (Finer & Zolna, 2016). Although genetic selection may have been limited, the precedent has been set, including selection for and against disability traits and selection based on nondisease traits.

Genetic Modification

Recently there has been a renewed concern over possible genetic manipulation, or "genome editing." In this chapter, **genome editing** refers to various techniques used to modify DNA sequences in the genomes of organisms. The most widely reported technique is based on a **CRISPR/Cas9 mechanism**, which is used by organisms to fend off viral infections (Gupta & Musunuru, 2014; Hsu, Lander, & Zhang, 2014).

Scientists and philosophers have been discussing the possibility of genome editing since the 1970s, although these arguments were limited to theoretical situations or the distant future (Fletcher, 1974; Ramsey, 1970). Current genome editing techniques allow scientists to precisely pinpoint areas of the genome to edit, delete, or alter the expression of specific areas of the genome (Salsman & Dellaire, 2017). Certainly, there are potential therapeutic uses of this technology, as a number of diseases are genetic in nature. It is reasonable to assume that genome modification will be intended to "fix" errors in the genetic code associated with disease.

Correcting the genome of an embryo with a genetic disease is like the previously discussed paradigm of genetic selection. For a moment let's assume a couple is known to be carriers of *cystic fibrosis (CF)*, an autosomal recessive disorder characterized by lung and digestive defects caused by biallelic (in both copies of the gene) mutations in the *CFTR* gene. The couple could undergo pre-natal genetic testing or *PGD/S* in order to ensure a future child does not have *CF*. Alternatively, an embryo affected with *CF* could undergo genome editing so that it no longer has the mutations in the *CFTR* gene. The intention of both techniques is similar—a future child who is free from disease. In both cases, the couple could also limit the risk of *CF* in future generations of their family.

The use of such modification techniques is not limited to the embryonic DNA. For example, if a two-year-old child were diagnosed with *CF*, it would be impossible to use genetic selection or embryo genome modification to avoid that disease. Genetic modification of the *CFTR* gene in affected organs, such as the lungs and pancreas, could still be an important treatment option for this individual. It is important to note that even if successful, this individual may still be at risk of having a child with *CF*. As we already discussed, few families know they are at risk of having a child with a genetic disease, and not all pregnancies are planned. As a result, genetic modification is an exciting possible therapeutic approach to many genetic diseases.

Genetic modification also raises some concerns that are unique. In general, the number of embryos and the combination of genetic traits from any given couple are limited. As a result, the focus of genetic selection is often on the absence of disease. Genome modification is theoretically unlimited. Therefore, scientists could edit the genomes in ways never identified in nature. For example, if the amount of a protein were associated with cognitive ability, one could use genome editing techniques to increase the expression of the protein to supraphysiological levels. As a result, many are concerned that there will be a shift from genetic-based therapies towards genetic enhancement (Resnik, 2000).

Ethical Framework

Often referred to as a risk–benefit ratio, the ethical principles of *beneficence* and *nonmaleficence* guide many of our ethical decisions. Initially, these decisions may seem easy, as genetic selection and modi-fication hold the promise to treat and even eliminate genetic disease. Let us examine one more example that will highlight that such decisions are not always so straightforward.

A researcher intends to add genomic sequencing to an existing study of subjects with early-onset Alzheimer's disease. The researcher's intent is to identify genes enriched in his patient population. This study design appears to be low risk for subjects. After all, they are in the study because they have Alzheimer's disease. The researcher has educated each subject about the potential for identifying sec-ondary findings and supported his or her decision for a return of results. The study is successful, and the researcher reports a novel *SNP* associated with early Alzheimer's disease. The underlying biology is not yet understood, but the results are shared at a family meeting. One of the participant's daugh-ters is considering her first pregnancy. At the end of the lecture, she approaches the microphone and asks whether she should test her embryos for this genetic result.

This may seem unlikely, although I have experienced many individuals requesting *PGD/S* for genetic variants scribbled on paper or based on emails from researchers. These are often very motivated patients who are only interested in genetic testing for this one disease without regard for more common disorders. Many readers may question whether this is even a difficult question—what could the harm be of selecting an embryo with a lower risk of Alzheimer's disease? As a reminder, there is a cost associated with *IVF* and *PGD/S*. This cost is both financial and emotional. Second, it is important to understand the patient's goal. It is not unusual for couples to endure the difficulty of *IVF* in order to ensure their child is "healthy" only to later find out that it is impossible to ensure a child will not have a disease. This is especially true when considering non-Mendelian disorders such as Alzheimer's disease when the absence of one risk allele will not guarantee that an individual will not have the disease.

The solution to this appears practical, if not simple. As we previously discussed, there is a duty for researchers to be truthful to subjects. Although simple, this is often difficult. Speaking as a researcher, it is often difficult to admit how little we understand about genetics. This is especially true when talking with subjects who have participated in and advocated for our own research.

We then must consider the benefit and harm of pursuing genetic selection for the Alzheimer's risk allele. Such a decision is often nuanced. The benefit of genetic selection based on a well-studied genetic risk such as *apolipoprotein E*, which is a well-defined genetic risk for developing late-onset Alzheimer disease (Liu, Liu, Kanekiyo, Xu, & Bu, 2013), may be different from a newly identified and poorly studied allele. The risk of genetic selection may also be different for the individual who has no known infertility compared to the individual who is already pursing *IVF* due to a personal history of infertility. These decisions are complex and often benefit from multiple points of view, including the psychological researcher, reproductive medicine colleagues, and, occasionally, genetic experts.

Genetic modification is still in its infancy. Unfortunately, we have yet to understand all of the potential concerns associated with genetic modification. Recently a joint statement on human germline genome editing was released with representation from a large number of international medical societies (Ormond, Mortlock, Scholes, Bombard, Brody, Faucett, et al., 2017). The working group stated that there were several scientific, ethical, and policy questions about the use of germline genome editing and did not support the use of genetic modification that would result in a pregnancy. The group also stated that before germline genome editing should proceed, there needed to be "a) a compelling medical rational, b) an evidence base that supports its clinical use, c) an ethical justification, and d) a transparent public process to solicit and incorporate stakeholder input" (Ormond, et al., 2017, p. 167).

To date, there has been only one instance where genome editing resulted in the birth of a child (Normile, 2018). This single case did not meet any of the ethical justifications agreed upon in the initial guideline. First, it is not clear that the *CCR5* variants in these two twins will significantly lower the risk of *HIV* infection. At the very least, there are alternative treatment options to decrease the risk of *HIV* infection that do not raise the same "off-target" genetic effects associated with *CRISPR-Cas9* methods. There has been limited stakeholder involvement, let alone scientific peer or ethics review. There have been limited details provided about the case and no peer-reviewed publication. This has led to speculation about the details of the case.

As previously noted, this single case of germline genome modification was not supported by local ethics committees, the university (Southern University of Science and Technology in Shenzhen, China), or even close scientific colleagues. Yet the misuse of this genetic technology may result in significant regulation around this promising tool (Daley Lovell-Badge & Steffann, 2019). Genetic selection, genetic modification, and even the historical *eugenic* studies are not unethical in themselves. Rather, ethics become relative to the researchers' processes. Therefore, it is paramount that the researcher applies these tools and study designs in an ethical manner.

Conclusion

For the uninitiated, there may be an element of scientific fantasy to genetic research. At the very least, it is easy to dismiss genomic medicine and genome editing as the distant future. After all, President Bill Clinton and British Prime Minister Tony Blair may have prematurely ushered in the era of genetic medicine in the year 2000. After all, the human genome was not even completed until 2003, which took over 13 years of work at the cost of over $3 billion (International Human Genome Sequencing Consortium, 2004). Today, genetics is ubiquitous throughout science and society. Once the domain of the geneticist, genome sequencing is now used as a tool in most scientific disciplines. Genotyping arrays are often mentioned on best-gift lists and purchased for friends on Christmas and Mother's Day. Commercial genetic testing companies such as 23andMe are so well known that it does not even require an explanation to friends or family. And we have already heard of the birth of the children born after germline genome editing.

Unfortunately, numerous stories about potential misuse or harm from genetics have also been well reported. Anecdotally, marriages have ended after commercial genetic testing companies revealed children who were conceived from marital affairs (Zhang, 2018). And in a survey of DTC companies, 34 companies advertised surreptitious infidelity testing (Phillips, 2016). Public databases that share DNA results to aid in finding long-distant relatives have also been used to identify crime suspects, raising questions about privacy. And the scientific community's misuse of genetic editing technology has been widely reported in the popular media. It is important to remember how both science fiction and popular media affect the views of our subjects on genetic research.

It is likely that genetic technology will continue to change, as will the way that we use both genetic results and genetic modification. More than ever, it is important to protect the trusted research relationship. It is paramount that health psychology researchers continue to be honest and transparent about the use of genetics. After all, the era of genomic research has only just begun. Genetic technology will change faster than books can be published, but ethical approaches to research that support subject autonomy and fulfill our ethical duties to subjects will always be important.

References

Bamshad, M. J., Ng, S. B., Bigham, A. W., Tabor, H. K., Emond, M. J., Nickerson, D. A., et al. (2011). Exome sequencing as a tool for Mendelian disease gene discovery. *Nature Reviews: Genetics, 12*(11), 745–755. https://doi.org/10.1038/nrg3031

Beauchamp, T. L. (2005). *The origins and evolution of the Belmont report.* Retrieved from https://repository.library.georgetown.edu/handle/10822/985464

Beauchamp, T. L., & Childress, J. F. (2013). *Principles of biomedical ethics.* Oxford, UK: Oxford University Press.

Bick, D., & Dimmock, D. (2011). Whole exome and whole genome sequencing. *Current Opinion in Pediatrics, 23*(6), 594–600. https://doi.org/10.1097/MOP.0b013e32834b20ec

Botkin, J. R., Belmont, J. W., Berg, J. S., Berkman, B. E., Bombard, Y., Holm, I. A., et al. (2015). Points to consider: Ethical, legal, and psychosocial implications of genetic testing in children and adolescents. *American Journal of Human Genetics, 97*(1), 6–21. https://doi.org/10.1016/j.ajhg.2015.05.022

Calafell, F., & Larmuseau, M. H. D. (2017). The Y chromosome as the most popular marker in genetic genealogy benefits interdisciplinary research. *Human Genetics, 136*(5), 559–573. https://doi.org/10.1007/s00439-016-1740-0

Childress, J. F. (2010). A principle-based approach. In *A companion to bioethics* (pp. 65–76). John Wiley & Sons, Ltd. https://doi.org/10.1002/9781444307818.ch7

Christenhusz, G. M., Devriendt, K., & Dierickx, K. (2013). Secondary variants: In defense of a more fitting term in the incidental findings debate. *European Journal of Human Genetics: EJHG.* https://doi.org/10.1038/ejhg.2013.89

Cohen, M. M., Jr. (1971). Variability versus "incidental findings" in the first and second branchial arch syndrome: Unilateral variants with anophthalmia. *Birth Defects Original Article Series,* 7(7), 103–108.

Collins, F. S., & Varmus, H. (2015). A new initiative on precision medicine. *The New England Journal of Medicine, 372*(9), 793–795. https://doi.org/10.1056/NEJMp1500523

Cooksey, J. A., Forte, G., Flanagan, P. A., Benkendorf, J., & Blitzer, M. G. (2006). The medical genetics workforce: An analysis of clinical geneticist subgroups. *Genetics in Medicine*, *8*(10), 603–614. https://doi.org/10.1097/01.gim.0000242307.83900.77

Coughlin, C. R. (2015). These are not the genes you are looking for: Incidental findings identified as a result of genetic testing. In *Ethical dilemmas in genetics and genetic counseling* (p. 226). Oxford, UK: Oxford University Press.

Coughlin, C. R., 2nd, Scharer, G. H., & Shaikh, T. H. (2012). Clinical impact of copy number variation analysis using high-resolution microarray technologies: Advantages, limitations and concerns. *Genome Medicine*, *4*(10), 80. https://doi.org/10.1186/gm381

Couzin-Frankel, J. (2011). Human genome 10th anniversary: What would you do? *Science (New York, N.Y.)*, *331*(6018), 662–665. https://doi.org/10.1126/science.331.6018.662

Cyranoski, D., & Ledford, H. (2018). Genome-edited baby claim provokes international outcry. *Nature*, *563*(7733), 607–608. https://doi.org/10.1038/d41586-018-07545-0

Daley, G. Q., Lovell-Badge, R., & Steffann, J. (2019). After the storm: A responsible path for genome editing. *The New England Journal of Medicine*, *380*(10), 897–899. https://doi.org/10.1056/NEJMp1900504

Dennis, C. (2004). Genetics: Deaf by design. *Nature*, *431*(7011), 894–896. https://doi.org/10.1038/431894a

DeVito, D., Shamberg, M., Sher, S. (Producers), & Niccol, A. (Director). (1997). *Gattaca* [Motion Picture]. United States: Columbia Pictures.

Devolder, K. (2005). Preimplantation HLA typing: Having children to save our loved ones. *Journal of Medical Ethics*, *31*(10), 582–586. https://doi.org/10.1136/jme.2004.010348

Dimmock, D. (2012). A personal perspective on returning secondary results of clinical genome sequencing. *Genome Medicine*, *4*(6), 54. https://doi.org/10.1186/gm353

Erlich, Y., Shor, T., Pe'er, I., & Carmi, S. (2018). Identity inference of genomic data using long-range familial searches. *Science (New York, N.Y.)*, *362*(6415), 690–694. https://doi.org/10.1126/science.aau4832

Fernandez, C. V., Strahlendorf, C., Avard, D., Knoppers, B. M., O'Connell, C., Bouffet, E., et al. (2013). Attitudes of Canadian researchers toward the return to participants of incidental and targeted genomic findings obtained in a pediatric research setting. *Genetics in Medicine: Official Journal of the American College of Medical Genetics*. https://doi.org/10.1038/gim.2012.183

Fiester, A. (2007). Viewpoint: Why the clinical ethics we teach fails patients. *Academic Medicine: Journal of the Association of American Medical Colleges*, *82*(7), 684–689. https://doi.org/10.1097/ACM.0b013e318067456d

Finer, L. B., & Zolna, M. R. (2016). Declines in unintended pregnancy in the United States, 2008–2011. *The New England Journal of Medicine*, *374*(9), 843–852. https://doi.org/10.1056/NEJMsa1506575

Fletcher, J. F. (1974). *The ethics of genetic control: Ending reproductive roulette: Artificial insemination, surrogate pregnancy, nonsexual reproduction, genetic control*. Buffalo, NY: Prometheus Books.

Friedrich, M. J. (2002). Preserving privacy, preventing discrimination becomes the province of genetics experts. *JAMA*, *288*(7), 815–816, 819.

Galton, F. (1884). Mr. Francis Galton's proposed "family registers". *Science (New York, N.Y.)*, *3*(48), 3. https://doi.org/10.1126/science.ns-3.48.3

Geelhoed, G. W., & Druy, E. M. (1982). Management of the adrenal "incidentaloma". *Surgery*, *92*(5), 866–874.

Green, R. C., Berg, J. S., Grody, W. W., Kalia, S. S., Korf, B. R., Martin, C. L., et al. (2013). ACMG recommendations for reporting of incidental findings in clinical exome and genome sequencing. *Genetics in Medicine: Official Journal of the American College of Medical Genetics*. https://doi.org/10.1038/gim.2013.73

Grewal, S. S., Kahn, J. P., MacMillan, M. L., Ramsay, N. K. C., & Wagner, J. E. (2004). Successful hematopoietic stem cell transplantation for Fanconi anemia from an unaffected HLA-genotype-identical sibling selected using preimplantation genetic diagnosis. *Blood*, *103*(3), 1147–1151. https://doi.org/10.1182/blood-2003-02-0587

Gupta, R. M., & Musunuru, K. (2014). Expanding the genetic editing tool kit: ZFNs, TALENs, and CRISPR-Cas9. *The Journal of Clinical Investigation*, *124*(10), 4154–4161. https://doi.org/10.1172/JCI72992

Gymrek, M., McGuire, A. L., Golan, D., Halperin, E., & Erlich, Y. (2013). Identifying personal genomes by surname inference. *Science (New York, N.Y.)*, *339*(6117), 321–324. https://doi.org/10.1126/science.1229566

Handyside, A. H., Kontogianni, E. H., Hardy, K., & Winston, R. M. (1990). Pregnancies from biopsied human preimplantation embryos sexed by Y-specific DNA amplification. *Nature*, *344*(6268), 768–770. https://doi.org/10.1038/344768a0

Holland, S. (2011). The virtue ethics approach to bioethics. *Bioethics*, *25*(4), 192–201. https://doi.org/10.1111/j.1467-8519.2009.01758.x

Hsu, P. D., Lander, E. S., & Zhang, F. (2014). Development and applications of CRISPR-Cas9 for genome engineering. *Cell*, *157*(6), 1262–1278. https://doi.org/10.1016/j.cell.2014.05.010

International Human Genome Sequencing Consortium. (2004). Finishing the euchromatic sequence of the human genome. *Nature*, *431*(7011), 931–945. https://doi.org/10.1038/nature03001

Kalia, S. S., Adelman, K., Bale, S. J., Chung, W. K., Eng, C., Evans, J. P., et al. (2017). Recommendations for reporting of secondary findings in clinical exome and genome sequencing, 2016 update (ACMG SF v2.0):

A policy statement of the American college of medical genetics and genomics. *Genetics in Medicine: Official Journal of the American College of Medical Genetics*, *19*(2), 249–255. https://doi.org/10.1038/gim.2016.190

Karpin, I. (2007). Choosing disability: Preimplantation genetic diagnosis and negative enhancement. *Journal of Law and Medicine*, *15*(1), 89–102.

Kim, J., Luo, W., Wang, M., Wegman-Ostrosky, T., Frone, M. N., Johnston, J. J., et al. (2018). Prevalence of pathogenic/likely pathogenic variants in the 24 cancer genes of the ACMG secondary findings v2.0 list in a large cancer cohort and ethnicity-matched controls. *Genome Medicine*, *10*(1), 99. https://doi.org/10.1186/s13073-018-0607-5

Lewin, T. (2001, February 10). Commission sues railroad to end genetic testing in work injury cases. *The New York Times*. Retrieved from www.nytimes.com/2001/02/10/us/commission-sues-railroad-to-end-genetic-testing-in-work-injury-cases.html

Lim, J. K., & Murphy, P. M. (2011). Chemokine control of West Nile virus infection. *Experimental Cell Research*, *317*(5), 569–574. https://doi.org/10.1016/j.yexcr.2011.01.009

Liu, C.-C., Liu, C.-C., Kanekiyo, T., Xu, H., & Bu, G. (2013). Apolipoprotein E and Alzheimer disease: Risk, mechanisms and therapy. *Nature Reviews: Neurology*, *9*(2), 106–118. https://doi.org/10.1038/nrneurol.2012.263

Makhnoon, S., Shirts, B. H., & Bowen, D. J. (2019). Patients' perspectives of variants of uncertain significance and strategies for uncertainty management. *Journal of Genetic Counseling*. https://doi.org/10.1002/jgc4.1075

Mella, S., Muzzatti, B., Dolcetti, R., & Annunziata, M. A. (2017). Emotional impact on the results of BRCA1 and BRCA2 genetic test: An observational retrospective study. *Hereditary Cancer in Clinical Practice*, *15*, 16. https://doi.org/10.1186/s13053-017-0077-6

Monroe, G. R., Frederix, G. W., Savelberg, S. M. C., de Vries, T. I., Duran, K. J., van der Smagt, J. J., et al. (2016). Effectiveness of whole-exome sequencing and costs of the traditional diagnostic trajectory in children with intellectual disability. *Genetics in Medicine: Official Journal of the American College of Medical Genetics*, *18*(9), 949–956. https://doi.org/10.1038/gim.2015.200

Munoz-Baell, I. M., & Ruiz, M. T. (2000). Empowering the deaf: Let the deaf be deaf. *Journal of Epidemiology and Community Health*, *54*(1), 40–44. https://doi.org/10.1136/jech.54.1.40

Normile, D. (2018). Shock greets claim of CRISPR-edited babies. *Science (New York, N.Y.)*, *362*(6418), 978–979. https://doi.org/10.1126/science.362.6418.978

Oakley, J. (2010). A virtue ethics approach. In *A companion to bioethics* (pp. 91–104). John Wiley & Sons, Ltd. https://doi.org/10.1002/9781444307818.ch10

Olfson, E., Cottrell, C. E., Davidson, N. O., Gurnett, C. A., Heusel, J. W., Stitziel, N. O., et al. (2015). Identification of medically actionable secondary findings in the 1000 genomes. *PLoS One*, *10*(9), e0135193. https://doi.org/10.1371/journal.pone.0135193

Ormond, K. E., Mortlock, D. P., Scholes, D. T., Bombard, Y., Brody, L. C., Faucett, W. A., et al. (2017). Human germline genome editing. *American Journal of Human Genetics*, *101*(2), 167–176. https://doi.org/10.1016/j.ajhg.2017.06.012

Pennings, G., Schots, R., & Liebaers, I. (2002). Ethical considerations on preimplantation genetic diagnosis for HLA typing to match a future child as a donor of haematopoietic stem cells to a sibling. *Human Reproduction (Oxford, England)*, *17*(3), 534–538. https://doi.org/10.1093/humrep/17.3.534

Phillips, A. M. (2016). Only a click away: DTC genetics for ancestry, health, love . . . and more: A view of the business and regulatory landscape. *Applied & Translational Genomics*, *8*, 16–22. https://doi.org/10.1016/j.atg.2016.01.001

Pulendran, B., Miller, J., Querec, T. D., Akondy, R., Moseley, N., Laur, O., et al. (2008). Case of yellow fever vaccine: Associated viscerotropic disease with prolonged viremia, robust adaptive immune responses, and polymorphisms in CCR5 and RANTES genes. *The Journal of Infectious Diseases*, *198*(4), 500–507. https://doi.org/10.1086/590187

Ramsey, P. (1970). *Fabricated man: The ethics of genetic control*. New Haven, CT: Yale University Press.

Resnik, D. B. (2000). The moral significance of the therapy-enhancement distinction in human genetics. *Cambridge Quarterly of Healthcare Ethics: CQ: The International Journal of Healthcare Ethics Committees*, *9*(3), 365–377.

Richards, S., Aziz, N., Bale, S., Bick, D., Das, S., Gastier-Foster, J., et al. (2015). Standards and guidelines for the interpretation of sequence variants: A joint consensus recommendation of the American college of medical genetics and genomics and the association for molecular pathology. *Genetics in Medicine: Official Journal of the American College of Medical Genetics*. https://doi.org/10.1038/gim.2015.30

Ross, L. F., Ross, L. F., Saal, H. M., David, K. L., Anderson, R. R., American Academy of Pediatrics, et al. (2013). Technical report: Ethical and policy issues in genetic testing and screening of children. *Genetics in Medicine: Official Journal of the American College of Medical Genetics*, *15*(3), 234–245. https://doi.org/10.1038/gim.2012.176

Salsman, J., & Dellaire, G. (2017). Precision genome editing in the CRISPR era. *Biochemistry and Cell Biology = Biochimie Et Biologie Cellulaire*, *95*(2), 187–201. https://doi.org/10.1139/bcb-2016-0137

Saunders, C. J., Miller, N. A., Soden, S. E., Dinwiddie, D. L., Noll, A., Alnadi, N. A., et al. (2012). Rapid whole-genome sequencing for genetic disease diagnosis in neonatal intensive care units. *Science Translational Medicine*, *4*(154), 154ra135. https://doi.org/10.1126/scitranslmed.3004041

Savulescu, J. (2001). Procreative beneficence: Why we should select the best children. *Bioethics*, *15*(5–6), 413–426.

Shuster, E. (1997). Fifty years later: The significance of the Nuremberg code. *The New England Journal of Medicine*, *337*(20), 1436–1440. https://doi.org/10.1056/NEJM199711133372006

Summar, M. L., & Watson, M. S. (2015). LDTs, incidental findings, and the need for more geneticists. *Medscape*. Retrieved from www.medscape.com/viewarticle/853979

Tabor, H. K., Auer, P. L., Jamal, S. M., Chong, J. X., Yu, J.-H., Gordon, A. S., et al. (2014). Pathogenic variants for Mendelian and complex traits in exomes of 6,517 European and African Americans: Implications for the return of incidental results. *American Journal of Human Genetics*, *95*(2), 183–193. https://doi.org/10.1016/j.ajhg.2014.07.006

Verlinsky, Y., Rechitsky, S., Schoolcraft, W., Strom, C., & Kuliev, A. (2001). Preimplantation diagnosis for Fanconi anemia combined with HLA matching. *JAMA*, *285*(24), 3130–3133.

Viberg Johansson, J., Langenskiöld, S., Segerdahl, P., Hansson, M. G., Hösterey, U. U., Gummesson, A., et al. (2019). Research participants' preferences for receiving genetic risk information: A discrete choice experiment. *Genetics in Medicine: Official Journal of the American College of Medical Genetics*. https://doi.org/10.1038/s41436-019-0511-4

Willig, L. K., Petrikin, J. E., Smith, L. D., Saunders, C. J., Thiffault, I., Miller, N. A., et al. (2015). Whole-genome sequencing for identification of Mendelian disorders in critically ill infants: A retrospective analysis of diagnostic and clinical findings. *The Lancet: Respiratory Medicine*, *3*(5), 377–387. https://doi.org/10.1016/S2213-2600 (15)00139-3

Zhang, S. (2018, October 12). *When a DNA test leads to divorce*. Retrieved from www.theatlantic.com/science/archive/2018/10/dna-test-divorce/571684/

Zhou, M., Greenhill, S., Huang, S., Silva, T. K., Sano, Y., Wu, S., et al. (2016). CCR5 is a suppressor for cortical plasticity and hippocampal learning and memory. *ELife*, *5*. https://doi.org/10.7554/eLife.20985

PART III

Physiological Studies and Health

9

PHYSIOLOGICAL RESEARCH

Matthew J. Criscione, Jordanne Nelson, and Julian Paul Keenan

Overview

Physiology research has changed and so has access to physiological data for studies. Previous barriers such as expense or invasiveness are now outdated. Armed with a catalog or a smartphone, assays are simple. Furthermore, expertise is not needed, nor is a lab full of equipment. A study involving cortisol data takes only an hour or two of training and practice and costs a few hundred dollars (depending on sample size), rather than thousands, requiring no dedicated space. In this chapter we review some of the classic physiological techniques but with a twist. We focus on the techniques that take advantage of the new technologies.

But first, a word on safety. If the COVID-19 crisis taught us anything, it is to wash our hands and to protect ourselves from pathogens. At all phases of physiological research, safety should come first and be in the forefront of everyone's mind.

Research in Practice

Accuracy of Smartphone Apps

The ubiquitous use of mobile smartphones and other technology could change the way health is accessed and monitored because of the new elements of connectivity (Coppetti, Brauchlin, Müggler, Attinger-Toller, Templin, Schönrath, et al., 2017). Many electronic devices, such as the iPhone, are gaining popularity throughout the world. The number of smartphone subscriptions is expected to equal about 70% of the world's population, or approximately 7.6 billion (Budde, 2013). As the population increases, new methods of health monitoring will be needed to meet population needs. An ability to communicate across multiple spectrums would allow scientists to connect through these electronic applications using something currently called mobile health technologies, or *mHealth*. Essentially, *mHealth* is the practice of medicine with the aid of portable diagnostic devices (Bhavnani, Narula, & Sengupta, 2016). Technological strategies, such as *mHealth*, have demonstrated their importance for research by allowing easy and accurate diagnoses of health and disease (Bhavnani, et al., 2016). For example, heart rate monitoring is an essential assessment for almost all health conditions (Coppetti, et al., 2017). Smartphone-connected cardiac monitoring devices and health apps are now available for the diagnosis of cardiovascular disease (Nguyen & Silva, 2016). With improved accuracy of such smartphone applications, future healthcare practitioners and researchers will have a wide array of new diagnostic capabilities through technology.

Coppetti, et al. (2017) conducted a case study demonstrating the application of this new camera technology by examining the accuracy of smartphone apps for heart rate measurement. Coppetti et al. used a method called ***photoplethysmography (PPG)***, a procedure based on the principle that blood absorbs more light than the surrounding tissue (Coppetti, et al., 2017). In addition, systole and diastole were used in variations of blood volumes to study the transmission or reflection of light (Verkruysse, Svaasand, & Nelson, 2008). Together, these two methods measured blood flow. Their experiment used both the ***contact PPG*** method, which involves a subject placing a finger on the built-in camera of the smartphone, and the ***noncontact PPG*** method, which involves using the classic way (i.e., by holding the camera in front of the patient's face, up to 1.5 m away), without the need for direct skin contact (Coppetti, et al., 2017). *PPG* is feasible using only visible light and the smartphone's own flash camera (Verkruysse, et al., 2008). Nearly all smartphones have a built-in flash, which provides sufficient light for reflection by blood cells (Coppetti, et al., 2017).

In this study, four different apps were downloaded from the iTunes Store for the study, using the iPhone 4 and iPhone 5. Similar apps are available on other online stores, such as Google Play for Android devices. For *contact PPG*, "Instant Heart Rate" (IHR) and "Heart Fitness" (HF) were used. For *noncontact PPG*, "What's My Heart Rate" (WMH) and "Cardiio" (CAR) were tested.

Coppetti, et al. (2017) studied a random selection of willing adult patients (n = 108) who required heart rate monitoring in the chest pain unit or the emergency department of the University Hospital Zurich, Switzerland. Patients with critical medical conditions were excluded from the study. Initial heart rates and rhythms were collected for the control group using ***electrocardiography (ECG)*** and simultaneous ***pulse oximetry***. Both are monitoring devices not typically found in the average biology lab. Initial heart rates were also collected by the iPhone applications.

The mean absolute error was computed to assess the level of agreement between methods. Analyses such as linear and multiple regression models were performed to define factors influencing the mean absolute error of the four different apps. A chi-squared test was used to analyze categorical data. A variety of different factors were also recorded (e.g., body weight, temperature, systolic and diastolic blood pressures, age, and arterial and oxygen saturation).

ECG measurements using the app-based technology showed promising results when using *contact PPG*. The ECG-derived heart rate correlated well with both IHR (r = .83) and HF (r = .96), but less with WMH (r =.62) and CAR (r = .60). Analyses found that *noncontact PPG* measurements performed significantly worse compared to fingertip-based (contact) measurements, having the tendency to "underestimate higher heart rates." It can be concluded that the reason for *noncontact PPG* resulting in significantly worse measurement may be due to camera technology and/or performance capabilities. Many influences could affect light sensing from 1.5 meters away such as the light environment and the iPhone version.

The potential to increase patient engagement, to reduce healthcare costs, and to improve technological healthcare is exciting. However, obtaining reliable and meaningful digital health data is troublesome; in the present study, the performance of different apps for heart rate measurements by a smartphone was very mixed. It was concluded that careful analysis of app accuracy is warranted before using these apps in clinical practice. Most reasonably, the cameras for iPhones 4 and 5 do not deliver reliable results for medical practitioners in clinical settings. Also, there are many unregulated healthcare applications, which can be confusing for consumers. If such applications were to be used, careful consideration of these applications would be necessary to ensure accurate assessment of a patient's health.

The future for research has many unique opportunities. With the wide array of technological advances currently available, possibilities will soon be infinite. Many methods of noninvasive research now can be easily conducted just by using a smartphone. However, any human involvement in physiological and health research becomes slightly troublesome. Typically, for most invasive procedures that can potentially affect or interfere with normal human functioning, nonhuman animals are used.

Does Exposure to Chronic Stress Affect Blood Pressure?

Human participants for any type of research must take into account the participant's safety, must obtain informed consent, and ensure confidentiality. Human subjects research also requires adherence to ethical principles such as dignity, bodily integrity, autonomy, and privacy (Kapp, 2006). Research for biological science and data is primarily used for the purpose of analyzing and collecting data to generalize conclusions to benefit and improve future science (Code of Federal Regulations, Part 46.102(d)). Much of the biomedical research is conducted on nonhuman animals with the goal of improving human welfare and to gain basic knowledge that can benefit humans and animals in the future (National Research Council Institute of Medicine, Institute for Laboratory Animal Research, Commission on Life Science, and Committee on the Use of Laboratory Animals in Biomedical and Behavioral Research, 1988). There is a considerable variation in how some animals are used in research settings, as well as what type of animals are used in these experiments (National Research Council, et al., 1988).

An interesting case study using nonhuman animals by Bobrovskaya, Beard, Bondarenko, Beig, Jobling, and Walker (2013) included adult male Wistar rats, or *Rattus norvegicus*, the brown rat. Wistar rats are highly popular for scientific research in psychology or biomedical science. Bobrovskaya et al. wanted to determine whether chronic stress could ultimately affect sustained changes in blood pressure by administering a series of foot shocks to rats. There have been many studies to show that stress-linked hypertension can persist after the discontinuance of stress events (Schnall, Schwartz, Landsbergis, Warren, & Pickering, 1992), as recorded by variations in an elevated **arterial pressure (AP)**. Having any control, or even *perceived* control, over a stressful environment or situation can significantly reduce any negative psychological consequences (Bobrovskaya, et al, 2013). Bobrovskaya et al. sent various uncontrolled and random foot shocks to the subjects to understand whether the elevated *AP* could last for an extended period of time (six weeks). By also examining the **sympathoadrenal system**, a physiological system that responds to outside stimuli, Bobrovskaya et al. measured catecholamine release from nerve terminals and adrenal glands. Increased release of catecholamine can lead to cardiovascular diseases such as hypertension (Grassi, Seravalle, & Quarti-Trevano, 2010; Lee, Borkowski, Leenen, Tsoporis, & Coughlin, 1991; Parati & Esler, 2012).

Wistar rats can be obtained easily, and they are housed in quite a few biological and medical facilities. In Bobrovskaya, et al.'s (2013) setup, all animals were housed individually in an animal holding facility, with rat chow and water available ad libitum. The room temperature was maintained at 21 °C ± 1 °C and animals were kept on a reversed 12 h:12 h light/dark cycle. These are typical conditions for housed rats.

The foot shock (*FS*) protocol in this procedure was performed by placing the test subjects in a Perspex FS cylinder within another cage. An electric current was delivered for 1 second at 1.5 mA. Six shocks were delivered randomly within a 40-minute period. The condition of the animals' feet was monitored regularly to ensure that there were no adverse effects of the FS procedure. This experiment lasted seven weeks. Shocks were delivered four times a day (weeks one to four) or seven times a day (weeks five to seven).

Prior to week one, subjects were implanted with telemetry probes. The **radiotelemetry system** employed in this study allowed recording of *AP*, heart rate, and locomotor activity. It is always the goal to record while minimizing natural movement; because of this, many researchers now employ wireless/Bluetooth transmission. Raw data were compressed into daily and weekly averages to observe differences in blood pressure. Blood pressure is the force of blood pushing against the walls of the arteries as the heart pumps blood and can be measured in two ways: systolic and diastolic pressures (National Heart, Lung, and Blood Institute, 2005). Systolic refers to blood pressure when the heart beats while pumping blood. Diastolic refers to blood pressure when the heart is at rest between beats (Chhajer, 2014). It is a general rule of thumb that blood pressure increases when one is excited, nervous, or active (Chhajer, 2014). For this particular experiment, the average change in systolic blood pressure was significantly higher in FS+ rats in comparison to FS− rats during a stress period ($p <$ .05). The increase was sustained during post-stress week seven but did not reach statistical significance ($p =$ .053). In the adrenal gland, there was a significant increase in pSer40TH (3.3-fold, $p <$ .05) and AT1R proteins (1.8-fold, $p <$ .05) in the FS+ group relative to the FS− group. These were measured by homogenizing tissue samples. Membranes were immunoblotted with total TH, phospho-Ser40-specific TH, or AT1R antibodies overnight at 4 °C. These lab samples were sent to Santa Cruz Biotechnology for processing. As a note, we have discovered that oftentimes it is much cheaper and the data much more accurate when specialized labs analyze samples. The casual saying in our lab is, "There is no shame in sending it out." However, understanding what the other labs are doing is critical.

It was found that chronic stress caused pronounced behavioral and neurochemical changes. These changes were associated with neurochemical alterations in the sympathoadrenal system, with increases in AT1R expression and pSer40TH within the adrenal gland. Chronic stress significantly reduced body weight gain, locomotor activity, and social interaction of the FS+ rats relative to FS− rats. Social activity was measured by pairing rats with naive and size-matched target rats. Social activity was manually scored offline by an observer blind to treatment. Chronic stress did not influence *AP*, but it did increase systolic and pulse blood pressure. It was found that there was an increase of TH activity and, as a result, increased capacity to synthesize catecholamines. This suggests that chronic stress leads to the activation of the sympathoadrenal system (Bobrovskaya, et al., 2013).

This study exemplifies a typical examination in the stress/animal field. Alterations of this are typical, for example, the introduction of social variables or pheromones.

Cortisol in a Hair Biomarker in Youth

Karlén, Ludvigsson, Frostell, Theodorsson, and Faresjö (2011) report an interesting method for measuring stress via biomarkers. **Biological markers**, or **biomarkers**, are entities within the body capable of providing objective information on the current physiological state of a living organism (Yoshizawa, Schafer, Schafer, Farrell, Paster, & Wong, 2013). Within the field of public health, the social environment plays a crucial role in understanding psychosocial factors such as anxiety, social isolation, and major life events that ultimately affect mental health and stability. It is worth reiterating that health is affected by stress; therefore, researchers in health psychology often explore the physiological mechanisms that regulate stress within the body.

The human hair follicle (HF) acts as a mini organ (Schneider, Schmidt-Ullrich, & Paus, 2009). The HF contains numerous amounts of neurohormones (Costa-e-Sousa & Hollenberg, 2012) and neuromodulators (Zmijewski & Slominski, 2011) that aid in the regulation of HF growth, pigmentation (Gáspár, Nguyen-Thi, Hardenbicker, Tiede, Plate, Bodó, et al., 2011), stem cells (Stenn & Paus, 2001), and energy metabolism (Paus, Langan, Vidali, Ramot, & Andersen, 2014). The HF continuously engages in the processing of important signals from the internal and external environment, leading to major adaptive modifications of the integument (Paus, et al., 2014). This is the reason why hormones are secreted to HF and why it acts as such a potential identifier for hormones. For years, HF have been used to detect agents of drugs, toxins, and environmental agents (Boumba, Ziavrou, & Vougiouklakis, 2006).

An interesting case study conducted by Karlén et al. measured the cortisol levels in hair within young adults to examine how it can be a biomarker for major life stressors. ***Cortisol*** is a type of steroid from the glucocorticoid class of hormones that is routinely analyzed by endocrinologists to reiterate the importance of glucocorticoids as a mediator of negative stress response (Haussmann, Vleck, & Farrar, 2007). Karlén et al. decided to examine a physiological pathway that governs many of our stress responses: the neuroendocrine ***hypothalamic-pituitary-adrenocortical* (HPA) axis**. Each section of this axis regulates particular hormones within the body that aid the regulation of the immune and inflammatory processes (Costa-e-Sousa & Hollenberg, 2012; Slominski, Zbytek, Pisarchik, Slominski, Zmijewski, & Wortsman, 2006). High levels of cortisol within the body can have deleterious effects on sleep/wake patterns, digestion, blood pressure, and physical activity (Karlén, et al., 2011) *Cortisol* is regulated by the *HPA* that is released from the adrenal cortex when we experience stress (Cohen, Doyle, & Skoner, 1999; Hostinar, Sullivan, & Gunnar, 2014). Karlén et. al. chose to observe the levels of cortisol within HFs and determine the correlation between cortisol and major life stressors in youth.

There are many ways of measuring cortisol in the body such as urine, saliva, and blood. However, methods such as these only cover a specific time interval and cannot detect stress longitudinally or retrospectively. Furthermore, these methods are either invasive or seen as invasive and often create an excess of biohazard. The aim in this particular study was to determine if cortisol in hair can serve as a longitudinal biomarker of chronic stress. Medical and nursing students ($n = 99$) in their second semester at the Faculty of Health Sciences at Linköping University voluntarily cut their hair and filled out questionnaires regarding *serious* life events within the last three months (e.g., death of a close relative, serious illness, or divorce). Hair samples were then obtained. The lowest coefficient of variation in hair samples was cut and analyzed from the posterior vertex of the head at least 3 centimeters closest to the root (Sauvé, Koren, Walsh, Tokmahjian, van Uum., 2007).

As indicated previously, one option after performing the hair extraction would be to send the samples out to an independent lab for measurement of cortisol levels. However, one can also perform cortisol sampling in-house. Here we detail some of what in-house analysis looks like. Karlén et al. took the hair samples in their lab and weighed them between 5 mg and 17 mg to ensure a usable/practical amount of cortisol would be able to be extracted. Once the sample was weighed and pressed, the hair was placed into liquid nitrogen for two minutes and quickly minced into a fine powder. Hair was then placed in methanol (due to its powerful properties as a solvent for polar and nonpolar molecules, methanol is used to extract bioactive compounds). The hair was pressed again. Afterward, all the supernatant was put into a centrifuge. The separated supernatant was moved to another sample tube for lyophilization, which is the process of water being removed from the sample after it is frozen using a vacuum. The vacuum used in this sample was an Edwards XDS 5 vacuum pump. The samples were dissolved in 150 μL 0.1 mol/L phosphate buffer, pH 7.4 containing 0.02% bovine serum albumin (BSA) and 0.01% triton X-100 to allow levels of cortisol to precipitate. There were four recorded outliers who had considerably higher than the average cortisol concentrations and were consequently omitted from further statistical analyses. Two of the subjects who produced the outliers reported a serious life event within the last three months, and they were dealing with major psychological issues. As per almost every experimental design, the manner in which one deals with outliers has no definitive answer.

After collecting the hair and isolating the cortisol, the authors wished to compare these data to major life stressors. As expected, increased cortisol levels in hair were found among participants reporting that they had experienced serious life events compared to the levels of those who did not have any recent serious life experiences. There were other minor correlations, but this served as the main finding. In short, this study suggests that hair could serve as a biomarker for any life stressors. Extracting hair is a safe, noninvasive technique that does not increase participant's stress (compared to drawing blood, for instance).

If hair grows about 1 cm/month, an adaption of this could be 'splitting hairs'. Taking 36 cm of hair is in some sense a record of three years of data, and thus one could obtain pre/post data following a stressor. This method is still in need of perfection, but the results are positive to this point (Kalliokoski, Jellestad, & Murison, 2019).

Salivary Cortisol and ELISA

Saliva is widely recognized as an important resource for evaluating physiological and pathological conditions in humans. Considering its simple, noninvasive method of collection and its easy storage, saliva usage has many advantages. Due to the implementation of modern techniques and chemical instrumentation equipment, there has been an increase in its use for laboratory investigations, basic research, clinical analyses, and medicine. The importance of these methods for the diagnosis of oral and systemic diseases has been sought with goals to implement its use for a variety of exams. (Lima, Garcia Diniz, Moimaz, Sumida, & Okamoto, 2010).

Enzyme-linked immunosorbent assay (*ELISA*) is a commonly used tool for analytical biochemistry, and its use is scattered throughout this volume. In a modern laboratory, the technique is used to find the amount of endogenous antigens within the blood plasma or saliva (Lima, et al., 2010). With commercial kits based on ELISA's techniques, physiologists and endocrinologists are now easily and quickly able to detect and measure substances such as peptides, proteins, antibodies, and hormones (Pokhrel, 2015). While there are many types of ELISA, some of the most popular are competitive ELISA, sandwich ELISA, and indirect ELISA (Haussmann, et al., 2007). The goal of competitive ELISA is to measure the concentration of a specific antigen within a sample (Pokhrel, 2015). The other two ELISA techniques aim to detect antibodies or antigens.

There are many experiments designed to illustrate how psychological and physiological stressors affect the release of cortisol by the *HPA* axis in an interactive laboratory setting using current research diagnostic tools. Both real and perceived stress activates the *HPA* axis, resulting in the release of glucocorticoids into the systemic circulation. **Glucocorticoids** are responsible for elevating blood glucose, while providing the required energy for the organism to cope with the added stress (Haussmann, et al., 2007).

In order to assess the effects of stress on salivary cortisol, an ethical manipulation inducing stress may be used. Haussman, and colleagues (2007) recruited 12 biology and genetics students (eight women and four men) aged 20 to 22 years. Over the course of one semester, three lab experiments were conducted: Experiment 1 was designed to combine two potential stressors, in this case, public speaking and exams. Saliva was taken before the presentation, and it was compared to those watching in the audience. Experiment 2 was designed to explore whether fasting, a known stressor, would affect salivary cortisol levels. Experiment 3 was designed to explore how competitive games, a known psychosocial stressor, affected a student's salivary cortisol levels. Saliva was taken after each game and compared with basal levels that were taken beforehand.

In short, an ELISA works based on the principles of a competitive binding *assay*: a tool used to provide quantitative or qualitative data regarding an analyte. To begin, the wells of the ELISA plate were coated with an antigen. In this study, the ELISA microplate was coated with monoclonal antibodies with respect to cortisol (Haussmann, et al., 2007). After that, each well was filled with an antigen–antibody mixture. The cortisol in saliva samples was added to wells of the microplate followed by cortisol linked to horseradish peroxidase, a commonly used enzyme labeler (Overview of ELISA: US, n.d.). The sample and labeled cortisol then competed for a limited number of antibody-binding sites, and all the unbound components were washed away (Pokhrel, 2015). The amount of labeled cortisol was measured by the reaction of its peroxidase enzyme on the substrate. As is typical in these studies, the reaction between the two produces a color that can be measured on a plate reader. The intensity of the color indicates the amount of peroxidase or enzyme label found in the sample, and this finding is inversely proportional to the amount of cortisol present. A weak chromogenic or fluorescent signal suggests a stronger concentration of the sample antigen.

It is suggested that ELISA tests are also more accurate than their predecessor, radioimmunoassay, due to their high sensitivity and strong specificity (competitive ELISA). In addition to its ability to measure analytes from a crude sample, ELISA's popularity stemmed from its relatively simple lab procedure. ELISA's low cost and efficiency make it well suited for point-of-care diagnosis, especially in resource-poor settings (Thiha & Ibrahim, 2015). All of these factors deem ELISA kits an optimal tool for clinical diagnostics but also research investigations.

sAA and Stress

Stress has become a major causative factor in the precipitation of a multitude of medical problems in today's society. Through basic physiological methods, researchers have been able to assess the role of stress in disease and the risk factors associated with stress. The biological tradition of stress analysis focuses on specific physiological systems repeatedly shown to be induced by both psychologically and physically demanding conditions. Since chronic psychological stress is known to negatively affect physical, mental, and social well-being, health psychologists have explored various biomarkers that indicate stress within the human body (Vineetha, Pai, Vengal, Gopalakrishna, & Narayanakurup, 2014). In order to have a better understanding of stress's responsibility for disease, valid and reliable measurements are extremely important.

While we introduced saliva in the last section, it is worth remembering that saliva is a significant source of indicators for local, systemic, and infectious disorders. Saliva's main purpose is to begin breaking down lipids and starches because of the enzymes found within it. Biomarkers exist in several different forms, including proteins, which is why enzymes found in saliva often make great biomarkers. Saliva-based biomarkers offer unique opportunities to bypass invasive measures by utilizing oral fluids to evaluate the condition of both healthy and diseased individuals (Yoshizawa, et al., 2013).

Stress can be considered a multifaceted dilemma and therefore should require a holistic measurable approach (Vineetha, et al., 2014). While a wide variety of anxiety questionnaires are available to assess the psychological factors of human stress, these methods rely heavily on the mood and attitude of the patient, both of which are subject to fluctuations, and oftentimes the results are inaccurate, thus suggesting the addition of salivary measures (Centre D'études Sur Le Stress Humain).

A pilot study by Vineetha, and colleagues (2014) examined whether participants diagnosed with chronic psychosocial stress had higher levels of salivary alpha amylase (*sAA*). These complaints included dry mouth, burning sensation, lichen planus, or ulcerations (Vineetha, et al., 2014). *sAA* is one of the major enzymes in the oral cavity. In addition to its primary function of hydrolyzing starch and glycogen, it is involved in defense against bacteria; low sAA activity has been related to a higher risk of oral infection (Petrakova, Doering, Vits, Engler, Rief, Schedlowski, et al., 2015).

In order to measure sAA's correlation to stress, subjects "diagnosed to be suffering from chronic psychosocial stress after a detailed subjective and objective evaluation by the experts" were recruited. Additionally, a control group consisting of 50 subjects . . . age and sex matched" with the study group were selected from a pool of people visiting a dental outpatient department for a routine checkup (Vineetha, et al., 2014, p. 133). Individual evaluation of the anxiety levels was performed using a questionnaire that assesses psychological stress for additional screening; in this case, the one used in this study was a State-Trait Anxiety Inventory (STAI) questionnaire. After identifying the two groups, "a detailed case history and oral examination was carried out by [a] trained oral diagnostician to see whether the participants suffered from stress related oral mucosal complaints" (Vineetha, et al.,

2014, p. 133). This step was to ensure that the subjects did not have any differential diagnoses and to detect any other conditions known to be associated with psychological stress.

After the subjects were classified into groups based on the absence or presence of oral mucosal complaints, saliva was collected. The authors reminded the participants not to eat in order to avoid contradiction of the naturally occurring circadian pattern and chewing activity that would affect enzyme levels. For example, each subject had to wash his or her mouths to remove any extra food debris that may be present (which is typical of any salivary study). Once approximately one ml of saliva was collected by asking the patient to expectorate a few times into a sterile disposable container, evaluation began.

Salivary amylase levels may be estimated with a kinetic enzyme kit or any other analyzer that uses synthetic substrates. A Hitachi 912 Automatic analyzer was used for analysis in this pilot study. Again, like other studies, a kit to send out is available if one does not have access to their own Hitachi. After examining sAA levels and their relation to oral complaints, Vineetha et al. investigated the correlation between the two.

For the oral mucosal complaints, the results suggest that there was no correlation or significant difference ($p = .204$ in the study group and $p = .757$ within the control group). However, increased alpha amylase levels in saliva were found among participants diagnosed with psychosocial stress and not in those in the control group ($p = .002$). This study suggests that sAA could serve as a possible biomarker for stress. However, the results of comparison of alpha amylase levels between the two groups (those with and those without oral mucosal changes) suggested that sAA levels *do not* have a relationship with oral mucosal changes. As the researchers put it, it was concluded that the correlation between sAA does not increase oral mucosal changes in relation to stress.

sAA has recently become a recognized indicator for sympathetic activity. "Measuring sAA may be more practical in an undergraduate laboratory setting than measuring cortisol, since sAA seems to be influenced less by sex, menstrual cycle, and oral contraceptives" (Bañuelos, Musleh, & Olson, 2017). Therefore, sAA should be considered in one's future research.

Conclusion

As physiological techniques improve in accuracy, become more cost-effective, and become simple to employ, one expects the breadth of our understanding of health psychology to grow. No longer are major research grants (R01) needed to obtain replicable and important data. What once was conceived of as a survey study can now, with very little effort, become a full-blown physiological examination.

In our laboratory, we just finished running a study in which oxytocin was being assayed. For less than $500, we were able to sample 90 people and have the results tabulated for us using the methods described here. We needed a freezer, gloves and masks, and some test tubes and that was about it in terms of additional equipment. Given that our institution is not attached to a medical school, nor is it a major research institution, the ease with which physiological data can now be obtained cannot be overstated. Similar to women entering science, or minorities given equal opportunities, the ability for small labs to contribute can only make science better. While we only examined a few techniques here, we implore anyone reading this to pick up a catalog or browse the Web to see how adding physiological measures can improve their future health psychology research.

References

Bañuelos, M. S., Musleh, A., & Olson, L. (2017). Measuring salivary alpha-amylase in the undergraduate neuroscience laboratory. *Journal of Undergraduate Neuroscience Education: June: A Publication of FUN, Faculty or Undergraduate Neuroscience, 16*(1), A23–A27.

Bhavnani, S. P., Narula, J., & Sengupta, P. P. (2016). Mobile technology and the digitization of healthcare. *European Heart Journal, 37*(18), 1428–1438. https://doi.org/10.1093/eurheartj/ehv770

Bobrovskaya, L., Beard, D., Bondarenko, E., Beig, M. I., Jobling, P., & Walker, F. R. (2013). Does exposure to chronic stress influence blood pressure in rats? *Autonomic Neuroscience: Basic & Clinical, 177*(2), 217–223. https://doi.org/10.1016/j.autneu.2013.05.001

Boumba, V. A., Ziavrou, K. S., & Vougiouklakis, T. (2006). Hair as a biological indicator of drug use, drug abuse or chronic exposure to environmental toxicants. *International Journal of Toxicology, 25*(3), 143–163. https://doi.org/10.1080/10915810600683028

Budde, P. (2013). The UN broadband commission for digital development. *Telecommunications Journal of Australia, 63*(1). https://doi.org/10.7790/tja.v63i1.392

Centre D'études Sur Le Stress Humain (CESH). (n.d.). Retrieved October 27, 2018, May 20, 2020, from www.stresshumain.ca.

Chhajer, B. (2014). *High blood pressure.* Diamond Pocket Books Pvt Ltd.

Cohen, S., Doyle, W. J., & Skoner, D. P. (1999). Psychological stress, cytokine production, and severity of upper respiratory illness. *Psychosomatic Medicine, 61*(2), 175–180. https://doi.org/10.1097/00006842-199903000-00009

Competitive ELISA. (n.d.). Retrieved October 27, 2018, from www.elisa-antibody.com/ELISA-Introduction/ELISA-types/competitive-elisa

Coppetti, T., Brauchlin, A., Müggler, S., Attinger-Toller, A., Templin, C., Schönrath, F., et al. (2017). Accuracy of smartphone apps for heart rate measurement. *European Journal of Preventive Cardiology, 24*(12), 1287–1293. https://doi.org/10.1177/2047487317702044

Costa-e-Sousa, R. H., & Hollenberg, A. (2012). Minireview: The neural regulation of the hypothalamic-pituitary-thyroid axis. *Endocrinology, 153*(9), 4128–4135. https://doi.org/10.1210/en.2012-1467

Gáspár, E., Nguyen-Thi, K., Hardenbicker, C., Tiede, S., Plate, C., Bodó, E., et al. (2011). Thyrotropin-releasing hormone selectively stimulates human hair follicle pigmentation. *The Journal of Investigative Dermatology, 131*(12), 2368–2377. https://doi.org/10.1038/jid.2011.221

Grassi, G., Seravalle, G., & Quarti-Trevano, F. (2010). The "neuroadrenergic hypothesis" in hypertension: Current evidence. *Experimental Physiology, 95*(5), 581–586. https://doi.org/10.1113/expphysiol.2009.047381

Haussmann, M. F., Vleck, C. M., & Farrar, E. (2007). A laboratory exercise to illustrate increased salivary cortisol in response to three stressful conditions using competitive ELISA. *Advances in Physiology Education, 31*(1), 110–115. https://doi.org/10.1152/advan.00058.2006

Hostinar, C. E., Sullivan, R. M., & Gunnar, M. R. (2014). Psychobiological mechanisms underlying the social buffering of the hypothalamic-pituitary-adrenocortical axis: A review of animal models and human studies across development. *Psychological Bulletin, 140*(1), 256–282. https://doi.org/10.1037/a0032671

Kalliokoski, O., Jellestad, F. K., & Murison, R. (2019). A systematic review of studies utilizing hair glucocorticoids as a measure of stress suggests the marker is more appropriate for quantifying short-term stressors. *Sci Rep, 9*, 11997. https://doi.org/10.1038/s41598-019-48517-2

Kapp, M. B. (2006). Ethical and legal issues in research involving human subjects: Do you want a piece of me? *Journal of Clinical Pathology, 59*(4), 335–339. https://doi.org/10.1136/jcp.2005.030957

Karlén, J., Ludvigsson, J., Frostell, A., Theodorsson, E., & Faresjö, T. (2011, October). Cortisol in hair measured in young adults: A biomarker of major life stressors? *BMC Clinical Pathology, 11*, 12. https://doi.org/10.1186/1472-6890-11-12

Lee, R. M., Borkowski, K., Leenen, F., Tsoporis, L., & Coughlin, M. (1991). Interaction between sympathetic nervous system and adrenal medulla in the control of cardiovascular changes in hypertension. *Journal of Cardiovascular Pharmacology, 17*(Suppl. 2), S114–116. https://doi.org/10.1097/00005344-199117002-00025

Lima, D., Garcia Diniz, D., Moimaz, S. A. S., Sumida, D. H., & Okamoto, A. C. (2010). Saliva: Reflection of the body. *International Journal of Infectious Diseases: IJID: Official Publication of the International Society for Infectious Diseases, 14*(3), e184–188. https://doi.org/10.1016/j.ijid.2009.04.022

National Heart, Lung, and Blood Institute. (2005). *Your guide to a healthy heart.* National Heart, Lung, & Blood Institute.

National Research Council, Institute of Medicine, Institute for Laboratory Animal Research, Commission on Life Sciences, and Committee on the Use of Laboratory Animals in Biomedical and Behavioral Research. (1988). *Use of laboratory animals in biomedical and behavioral research.* National Academies Press.

Nguyen, H. H., & Silva, J. N. A. (2016). Use of smartphone technology in cardiology. *Trends in Cardiovascular Medicine, 26*(4), 376–386. https://doi.org/10.1016/j.tcm.2015.11.002

Overview of ELISA: US. (n.d.). Retrieved October 27, 2018, from www.thermofisher.com/us/en/home/life-science/protein-biology/protein-biology-learning-center/protein-biology-resource-library/pierce-protein-methods/overview-elisa.html

Parati, G., & Esler, M. (2012). The human sympathetic nervous system: Its relevance in hypertension and heart failure. *European Heart Journal, 33*(9), 1058–1066. https://doi.org/10.1093/eurheartj/ehs041

Paus, R., Langan, E. A., Vidali, S., Ramot, Y., & Andersen, B. (2014). Neuroendocrinology of the hair follicle: Principles and clinical perspectives. *Trends in Molecular Medicine*, *20*(10), 559–570. https://doi.org/10.1016/j.molmed.2014.06.002

Petrakova, L., Doering, B. K., Vits, S., Engler, H., Rief, W., Schedlowski, M., et al. (2015). Psychosocial stress increases salivary alpha-amylase activity independently from plasma noradrenaline levels. *PLoS One*, *10*(8), e0134561. https://doi.org/10.1371/journal.pone.0134561

Pokhrel, P. (2015, June 9). ELISA-principle, types and applications. *Microbiology Notes*. Retrieved October 27, 2018, from www.microbiologynotes.com/elisa-principle-types-and-applications/

Schnall, P. L., Schwartz, J. E., Landsbergis, P. A., Warren, K., & Pickering, T. G. (1992). Relation between job strain, alcohol, and ambulatory blood pressure. *Hypertension*, *19*(5), 488–494. https://doi.org/10.1161/01.HYP.19.5.488

Schneider, M. R., Schmidt-Ullrich, R., & Paus, R. (2009). The hair follicle as a dynamic miniorgan. *Current Biology*, *19*(3), R132–R142. https://doi.org/10.1016/j.cub.2008.12.005

Slominski, A., Zbytek, B., Pisarchik, A., Slominski, R. M., Zmijewski, A., & Wortsman, J. (2006). CRH functions as a growth factor/cytokine in the skin. *Journal of Cellular Physiology*, *206*(3), 780–791. https://doi.org/10.1002/jcp.20530

Stenn, K. S. Y., & Paus, R. (2001). Controls of hair follicle cycling. *Physiological Reviews*, *81*(1), 449–494. https://doi.org/10.1152/physrev.2001.81.1.449

Sauvé, B., Koren, G., Walsh, G., Tokmahjian, S., van Uum, S. H. M. (2007). Measurement of cortisol in hi=uman hair as a biomarker of systemic exposure. Clinical Investigation Medicine, 30(5), E113-E119.

Thiha, A., & Ibrahim, F. (2015). A colorimetric Enzyme-Linked Immunosorbent Assay (ELISA) detection platform for a point-of-care dengue detection system on a lab-on-compact-disc. *Sensors*, *15*(5), 11431–11441. https://doi.org/10.3390/s150511431

Verkruysse, W., Svaasand, L. O., & Nelson, J. S. (2008). Remote plethysmographic imaging using ambient light. *Optics Express*, *16*(26), 21434–21445. https://doi.org/10.1364/OE.16.021434

Vineetha, R., Pai, K.-M., Vengal, M., Gopalakrishna, K., & Narayanakurup, D. (2014). Usefulness of salivary alpha amylase as a biomarker of chronic stress and stress related oral mucosal changes: A pilot study. *Journal of Clinical and Experimental Dentistry*, *6*(2), e132–137. https://doi.org/10.4317/jced.51355

Yoshizawa, J. M., Schafer, C. A., Schafer, J. J., Farrell, J. J., Paster, B. J., & Wong, D. T. W. (2013). Salivary biomarkers: Toward future clinical and diagnostic utilities. *Clinical Microbiology Reviews*, *26*(4), 781–791. https://doi.org/10.1128/CMR.00021-13

Zmijewski, M. A., & Slominski, A. T. (2011). Neuroendocrinology of the skin: An overview and selective analysis. *Dermato-Endocrinology*, *3*(1), 3–10. https://doi.org/10.4161/derm.3.1.14617

10

STRESS PHYSIOLOGY AND PHYSIOMETRICS

Elana M. Gloger, Gregory T. Smith, and Suzanne C. Segerstrom

Overview

Psychological stressors, including acute stressors such as public speaking, short-term stressors such as exam periods, and long-term stressors such as caregiving have all been associated with changes in physiological systems. Some systems such as the cardiovascular system (heart rate, blood pressure) and the immune system (cell counts, cell function, cytokine levels) have established relationships with stressors, whereas knowledge of how molecular and cellular measures such as telomere length and mitochondrial function relate to stressors is emerging.

Much of the literature relating psychological stress and physiology has ignored how ***physiometrics***—the reliability and validity of physiological parameters and biomarkers—might affect the estimation of relationships between these parameters and measures of stress. Rather than attempt to sample the substantial and substantive literature on stressors and physiology, we hope to advance methodology in the area of stress physiology by reviewing the much smaller number of studies on *physiometrics*. By doing so, we not only draw attention to potential methodological problems in the literature but also hope to improve design of future studies.

Consideration of the generalizability of physiological measures to other time points—the surrounding days, weeks, or months—reveals that many biomarkers are relatively unstable and therefore generalize poorly, whereas others are quite stable (Reed, Al-Attar, Presnell, Lutz, & Segerstrom, 2019; Segerstrom, Boggero, Smith, & Sephton, 2014; see also Segerstrom & Smith, 2012; Strube, 2000). In many cross-sectional designs, a longer-term stressor or longer-term perceived stress is correlated with a single measurement of a biomarker. The low generalizability associated with unstable biomarkers (i.e., the level of that biomarker does not generalize to the surrounding weeks or, in some cases, days) can hinder investigations that want to know about longer-range relationships, for example, with the long-term demands of caregiving. On the other hand, stable biomarkers that do not vary over time can hinder investigations that wish to study change from day to day (Adam, Hawkley, Kudielka, & Cacioppo, 2006) or individual differences in variability (Almeida, Piazza, & Stawski, 2009).

In addition, poor reliability along with small sample size creates a misestimation of effects and can result in both Type I and Type II errors (Gelman & Carlin, 2014; Segerstrom, 2019). This is contrary to the popular opinion that a small sample with an unreliable measure can only result in a Type II error and the subsequent conclusion that a statistically significant effect must be accurate. Simulation of 100,000 datasets with $n = 130$ and reliability of $\gamma = 0.41$ found that after regressing y on x, only 42% of b weights were within .10 of the known relationship and b weights ranged from less than $b = -0.50$ to greater than $b = 0.80$ (Segerstrom & Boggero, 2020). This design scenario is not outlandish: the person-level variance (i.e., reliability with regard to person) is similar for *interleukin-6* (*IL-6*), a commonly studied proinflammatory cytokine. Likewise, over 6 months, the amount of stable variance in the 3-day average of the *diurnal cortisol slope* (the daily change from normally high morning cortisol to normally low evening cortisol) was also around 40% (Segerstrom, et al., 2014). Reliable measurement is especially important for smaller sample sizes; very large sample sizes ($n > 500$) are less likely to misestimate relationships even if there is lower reliability (Kraemer, 1991; Perkins, Wyatt, & Bartko, 2000; Segerstrom, 2019).

In this chapter, we consider studies of physiometrics across several different biomarkers—of neuroendocrine, immune, cardiovascular, and cellular function—which one might want to correlate with stress. For each kind of biomarker, we consider one method's estimate of reliability and generalizability in depth and then compare that study with others in the literature. Doing so highlights best practices for estimating physiometrics but also suggests best practices for biomarker measurement in substantive studies.

Research in Practice

Cortisol

Cortisol is a glucocorticoid hormone generated by the *hypothalamic–pituitary–adrenocortical (HPA) axis*, a negative-feedback regulatory system involved in metabolism and important for the body's adaptation to, and recovery from, environmental and physiological stressors. Importantly, chronically high *cortisol* levels can lead to system dysregulation and long-term health consequences such as cardiovascular disease, pain conditions, and psychiatric disorders. *Cortisol* therefore depicts a physiological response to stress that is established as a predictor for long-term health outcomes (Nicolson, 2008).

Cortisol dynamics are typically operationalized as a *diurnal slope*, a calculated estimate of the slope of (log) *Cortisol* from waking to evening; *diurnal area–under–the–curve (AUC)*, a calculated summary of collective *Cortisol* exposure throughout the day; and the *cortisol awakening response (CAR)*, a sharp increase in *Cortisol* levels that occurs, on average, 30 minutes after waking up and that precedes the daily diurnal cycle (see Adam & Kumari, 2009; Pruessner, Kirschbaum, Meinlschmid, & Hellhammer, 2003, for reviews). The *CAR* has different health outcomes and correlates compared with diurnal measures (Clow, Hucklebridge, Stalder, Evans, & Thorn, 2010). In most cases, *cortisol* samples are collected via saliva, as salivary cortisol contains the biologically active form. Alternatively, *Cortisol* can be found in blood or urine; however, these fluids also contain biologically inactive cortisol (Nicolson, 2008).

Cortisol has very high day-specific variance relative to longer-term or trait variance. That is, it can be especially difficult to generalize from one day's *cortisol* parameter to the next day, week, or month. Thus, estimates of the minimum number of days of cortisol sampling to yield generalizable measurements are useful in examining relationships with longer-term measures of stress and other psychosocial factors.

In a sample of younger and a sample of older adults, a generalizability study (Shavelson & Webb, 1991; Brennan, 2001) estimated the percentage of variance in *Cortisol diurnal slope*, mean *cortisol*, and *diurnal AUC* due to stable individual differences, measurement occasion, sampling day, or interactions among them. Subsequently, a decision study provided estimates of the number of days of cortisol sampling needed to achieve satisfactory measurement reliability and generalizability with regard to stable individual differences and within-person changes (Segerstrom, et al., 2014).

The first sample had 124 first-year law students ($M_{age} = 23.9$, 55% female, 90% Caucasian) who provided saliva samples over 3 consecutive weekdays on five different occasions throughout their first semester. The second sample had 148 older adults ($M_{age} = 74$, 58% female, 96% Caucasian) who provided saliva samples over 3 consecutive weekdays every 6 months on four different occasions. For law students, 10% of the variance in *diurnal slope*, 24% of the variance in ***diurnal mean***, and 19% of the variance in *AUC* was due to stable individual differences. Specific occasions (e.g., the first occasion vs. the third), specific days (e.g., the first day vs. the third), or *person x day* or *occasion x day* interactions accounted for negligible variance for any of the parameters. For older adults, 11% of the variance in *diurnal slope*, 28% of the variance in *diurnal mean*, and 11% of the variance in *AUC* were due to stable individual differences. Otherwise, main effects and *person x day* or *occasion x day* interactions accounted for negligible variance.

In addition, people varying across different occasions in different ways (*person x occasion* interaction) accounted for a moderate amount of variance in both samples: 14% to 20% of the variance in *diurnal slope*, 29% to 32% of the variance in *diurnal mean*, and 26% to 28% of the variance in *diurnal AUC*. This interaction indicates individual differences in how *cortisol* changed across occasions of measurement. For example, some law students in the first study might have felt more stressed than others at the onset of their first semester but more confident by the onset of their second, whereas some might have felt more confident at the onset of their first semester but more stressed as the semester progressed, with corresponding changes in *cortisol*.

The largest amount of variance in both samples was due to different people having different *Cortisol* parameters on different days and occasions (the three-way interaction). This variance is an "error" for studies wishing to generalize *cortisol* measurement beyond one specific day. Further, Study 1 and Study 2 had similar substantive results, suggesting that variability in *cortisol* might not increase or decrease across the lifespan. Therefore, to generalize to the occasion or trait level, multiple days of measurement are required. Table 10.1 shows the results of the decision study for cross-sectional (between-person) and longitudinal (within-person) designs to achieve reliability at .60 (minimal) to .80 (adequate). These recommendations resemble those suggested by the MacArthur Research Network on SES and Health (2000) for between-person designs: three days for *AUC* and seven days for *diurnal slope*.

Limitations of this particular study included lack of ethnic diversity in the samples and self-reported, rather than automatically recorded, *cortisol* collection times. However, several other studies with other samples and methods have obtained similar variance estimates, suggesting that the estimates are not specific to a particular demographic and method. Some studies also reported estimates for the *CAR*.

Other studies used the ***intraclass correlation (ICC)***, a ratio of between-person variance to all variance, to assess the reliability of *cortisol* measures (or reported variance partitions that could be used to calculate the *ICC*). Although methods for obtaining the *ICC* varied slightly among studies, at the person level, *ICCs* for *diurnal slope* were ~0.00 to 0.20 with six to 12 days of sampling; for *diurnal AUC*, 0.00 to 0.30; and for the *CAR*, 0.02 to 0.20 (Almeida, et al., 2009; Doane, Chen, Sladek, Van Lenten, & Granger, 2015; Ross, Murphy, Adam, Chen, & Miller, 2014; Wang,

Table 10.1 Days of sampling for diurnal cortisol parameters to reach reliability criteria .60 (minimal) and .80 (high) from decision studies of younger (Y) and older (O) adults

Reliability:		Days for Mean		Days for AUC		Days for Slope	
		.60	*.80*	*.60*	*.80*	*.60*	*.80*
Differences between people measured	Y	3	7	4	11	11	> 21
on a single occasion	O	3	6	8	21	10	> 21
Differences within a person measured	Y	2	5	3	8	8	21
on several occasions	O	3	6	3	9	5	14

Source: Segerstrom, Boggero, Smith, and Sephton (2014)

Sánchez, Golden, Shrager, Kirschbaum, Karlamangla, et al., 2014). These estimates were obtained from samples with participants ranging in age from eight to 87 and diverse with regard to gender and ethnicity. Some of the studies also used electronic verification of saliva sampling times but with little effect on estimates. Among older adults who had electronic verification at one occasion of data collection but not another, the *ICC* within occasions was virtually identical (Wang, et al., 2014). Among college-age adults, those who were time compliant (i.e., they collected samples at or near the target time) did not yield substantively different variance estimates than the total sample (Doane, et al., 2015).

One study of children reported higher *ICCs* than other studies (slope, 0.71; *CAR*, 0.46; Kuhlman, Robles, Dickenson, Reynolds, & Repetti, 2019), as did one study of younger (aged 25 to 40) and older (aged >60) adults (*CAR*, 0.71; Hellhammer, Fries, Schweisthal, Schlotz, Stone, & Hagemann, 2007). Methods for these studies were not substantially different from the others, but one sample did include prepubescent children and reported that pubertal onset and female gender were associated with lower *ICCs* (Kuhlman, et al., 2019). Increasing age across ages 33 to 84 was also associated with lower *ICCs* for the *CAR*, particularly among men (Almeida, et al., 2009).

In addition, these studies were all longitudinal. The *ICC* for occasions of data collection can be interpreted as the average correlation between any two occasions in the study after removing day variance (i.e., assuming reliable measurement within occasions). Intervals ranged from two months to six years. These estimates were around 0.20 to 0.45 for *diurnal slope*, 0.50 to 0.75 for *diurnal AUC*, and 0.10 to 0.20 for the *CAR*. Estimates for *diurnal slope* and *CAR* were higher when intervals between occasions were shorter, but this trend did not hold for *diurnal AUC*. Peri-adolescent children again had substantially higher estimates (Kuhlman, et al., 2019). One study sampled *cortisol* only on one day at each of three occasions (one year apart). For this study, the same variance estimate contained both occasion and day variance. As one might expect, these estimates were generally higher than day-only estimates and lower than occasion-only estimates (slope, .13; *AUC*, .36; *CAR*, .20; Skoluda, La Marca, Gollwitzer, Müller, Limm, Marten-Mittag, et al., 2017).

A comparison of occasion *ICC* using single days vs. the average of the days within occasions (two to three days) illustrates the benefits of more reliable measurements. The *ICC* for *diurnal slope* increased from .14 to .46 over an interval of six years (Wang, et al., 2014) and from .18 to .95 over an interval of four months (Doane, et al., 2015). The *ICC* for *diurnal AUC* increased from .07 to .09 over six years, and the *ICC* for the *CAR* increased from .02 to .09 over six years and from .15 to .83 over four months (Doane, et al., 2015; Wang, et al., 2014). Note that parameters with the most "error" or day variance, will benefit the most from adding more sampling days. Characterizing *cortisol* at the occasion level or the person level requires numerous days of data collection, with the number of days necessary to achieve good generalizability and reliability somewhat dependent on the measure of choice. With any measure, generalizing from one day to a longer time period is ill advised, with the vast majority of variance in all *diurnal cortisol* parameters due to idiosyncratic effects of that particular day.

Salivary α-Amylase (sAA)

α-amylase is a digestive enzyme produced by the salivary glands that reflects the activity of the **sympathetic nervous system (SNS)** and correlates with **plasma epinephrine** and **norepinephrine**. Whereas *plasma epinephrine* and *norepinephrine* only reliably reflect *SNS* activity when measured in blood, *sAA* is a noninvasive method for measuring real-time *SNS* activity, making it a feasible biomarker for tracking *SNS* activity in response to stress (Ditzen, Ehlert, & Nater, 2014; Granger, Kivlighan,

El-Sheikh, Gordis, & Stroud, 2007a, 2007b). Elevated levels of *sAA* have been related to illness vulnerability as well as poorer cognitive and psychological outcomes (for reviews, see Ali & Nater, 2020; Bauduin, van Noorden, van der Werff, de Leeuw, van Hemert, van der Wee, et al., 2018; Granger, et al., 2007a, 2007b).

sAA levels increase in response to physical and psychological stressors (Weiss, Venezia, & Smith, 2019). However, *sAA* levels and profiles are not the same as those of salivary cortisol. In response to acute stress, *sAA* increases at a steeper rate than *cortisol*, reflecting the more sensitive *SNS* response compared to the more gradual *HPA axis* response. It is not yet clear how the *HPA* and the *SNS* responses work together to respond to stressors (Engert, Kok, Puhlmann, Stalder, Kirschbaum, Apostolakou, et al., 2018; Granger, et al., 2007a, 2007b; for review, see Strahler, Skoluda, Kappert, & Nater, 2017).

sAA generalizability and reliability were estimated using the law student sample described earlier (Segerstrom, et al., 2014) and likewise applied generalizability theory to estimate the percentage of *sAA* awakening response, *diurnal slope*, *diurnal mean*, and *AUC* with respect to ground due to person, occasion, day, or the interactions among them (Out, Granger, Sephton, & Segerstrom, 2013). First-year law students (n = 122, M_{age} = 23.9, 55% female, 90% Caucasian) collected saliva on 3 consecutive days, with five occasions of measurement over their first semester in law school.

Compared with salivary cortisol, *sAA* showed more evidence of stable individual differences, but person variance varied substantially by measure. The awakening response (26% person variance) and *diurnal slope* (15%) were similar to *cortisol* parameters, but the *diurnal mean* (65%) and *diurnal AUC* (61%) had higher person variance; that is, they showed more evidence of stable individual differences. In addition, people varying across different occasions in different ways (*person x occasion* interaction) accounted for a moderate amount of variance: 6% of the variance in the awakening response, 17% of the variance in *diurnal slope*, 16% of the variance in *diurnal mean*, and 17% of the variance in *diurnal AUC*. These estimates indicate that the *diurnal slope* of *sAA* may be equally sensitive to changing conditions as the *diurnal slope* of *cortisol*, but the *diurnal mean* and *AUC* may be less sensitive.

Limitations of this sample, as noted earlier, include low diversity, self-reported sampling times, and in this single sample, a small age range. Due to conventions at the time of data collection, saliva production and oral health, which can confound *sAA* values, were not measured (Beltzer Fortunato, Guaderrama, Peckins, Garramone, & Granger, 2010; Strahler, et al., 2017).

Although *sAA* is a relatively novel biomarker of stress, one other longitudinal study found substantial person variance in *sAA AUC* (*ICC* = .75; compare .61 in Out, et al., 2013) and awakening response (*ICC* = .43; compare .26; in Out, et al., 2013; Skoluda, et al., 2017). An estimate for *diurnal slope* was not reported because the Hessian matrix used to compute the standard errors of the covariances was not positive definite, which is a multilevel modeling error that can occur with scaling (variable values are too close to 0) or overparameterization (linear dependencies; Kiernan, Tao, & Gibbs, 2012). Participants in this study had ages across middle adulthood (24 to 60 years old), but 99% were male, and their race or ethnicity was not reported. A large proportion (36.8%) were smokers, which was adjusted in analyses. This study also did not control for oral hygiene or saliva production. Despite the substantial demographic differences in the two studies, the estimates were similar and indicated that more variance in *sAA* is attributable to stable individual differences than is true for *cortisol*, with some parameters appearing highly stable (e.g., *diurnal AUC*). However, there was also enough change over time that individual differences in responses to occasions accounted for variance in *sAA*, including 17% of the variance in *diurnal AUC* (Out, et al., 2013). As research with *sAA* continues, we expect to see more studies examining the dynamics and reliability of various daily measures (e.g., output, slope, and awakening response).

Systemic Inflammation

Inflammation, an immune response to infection or injury, is the driving force of localized reactions, such as swelling, redness, heat, and fever, and is mediated by **cytokines** (molecules that act as communicators; Zimmerman, Bowden, & Vogel, 2014). Evolutionarily, the inflammatory response acted as protection from physical harm (e.g., foreign cells, pathogens), and evidence suggests that this system is similarly activated in times of acute, repeated, and chronic stress, despite the lack of cellular threat or injury (Maier & Watkins, 1998; for review, see Segerstrom & Miller, 2004)

Inflammation can also be chronic, low-grade, or systemic. **Systemic inflammation**, whether due to stress or other psychological and physical conditions, increases the risk for multiple psychological and physical morbidities as well as premature mortality (Franceschi & Campisi, 2014; Gregor & Hotamisligil, 2011; Marchand, Perretti, & McMahon, 2005; Milaniak & Jaffee, 2019; Pace & Heim, 2011; Rohleder, 2014; Slavich, 2014; Stolp & Dziegielewska, 2009). Inflammatory biomarkers most often include those involved in the cascade that progresses from **IL-1** to **tumor necrosis factor alpha (TNFα)** to **IL-6** to **C-reactive protein (CRP)**, which is not itself a *cytokine* but a product of the liver that activates antibody-mediated immunity (Du Clos, 2000; for a review, see Maier & Watkins, 1998).

These standard inflammatory biomarkers as well as soluble *TNFα* receptors (**sTNFR I and II**) and **IL-8** were assessed in a sample of 62 participants (M_{age} = 30.1, 50% female, 60% Caucasian, 31% Asian) at four time points over six months (Navarro, Brasky, Schwarz, Song, Wang, Kristal, et al., 2012). Biomarkers ranged in their stability (*ICC*) from very high among the *TNFα* markers (*TNFα*, 0.92; *sTNFR I*, 0.92; *sTNFR II*, 0.90) to high (*IL-8*, 0.73; *CRP*, 0.62). *IL-6*, although it had the lowest *ICC* (0.48), was nonetheless more stable than *cortisol* or *sAA*. Therefore, over a period of months, inflammatory biomarkers are sufficiently stable to suggest that one measurement will generalize to weeks or months. However, *IL-6* was more changeable and therefore more unreliable with regard to stable individual differences than other inflammatory biomarkers. Measurement of stable individual differences in *IL-6* requires either more measurements across the time period of interest or generalization to a shorter time period. Three averaged *IL-6* measurements would be necessary to achieve a reliability of 0.75.

Strengths of this study include the careful selection of participants and variety of biomarkers measured. However, limitations include a sample low in racial and ethnic diversity and a small age range (20 to 40 years old).

Other studies of inflammatory biomarker variability over periods of two weeks to five years have used diverse samples with regard to gender, ethnicity, and age, with generally similar results. However, the range of results varied: *TNFα ICCs* ranged from 0.39 to 0.89; *IL-6*, 0.36 to 0.87; *CRP*, 0.55 to 0.70; and *IL-8*, 0.55 to 0.73 (Agalliu, Xue, Cushman, Cornell, Hsing, Kaplan, et al., 2013; Cava, González, Pascual, Navajo, & González-Buitrago, 2000; Hardikar, Song, Kratz, Anderson, Blount, Reid, et al., 2014; Ho, Xue, Burk, Kaplan, Cornell, & Cushman, 2005; Hofmann, Yu, Bagni, Lan, Rothman, & Purdue, 2011; Kaplan, Ho, Xue, Rajpathak, Cushman, Rohan, et al., 2007; Picotte, Campbell, & Thorland, 2009; Rao, Pieper, Currie, & Cohen, 1994; Todd, Simpson, Estis, Torres, & Wub, 2013). Most studies used small samples (e.g., *n* < 50), which created large confidence intervals. For example, in 36 participants measured three times over two years, the *ICC* for *TNFα* was 0.73, but the 95% confidence interval was 0.49 to 0.79. Likewise, the *ICC* for *IL-6* was 0.48, but the 95% confidence interval was 0.25 to 0.58 (Ho, et al., 2005). By contrast, in 360 participants measured twice over two years, the *ICC* for *IL-6* was 0.55, with a 95% confidence interval of 0.50 to 0.64 (Hardikar, et al., 2014). Therefore, some of the large range of estimates may be due to sampling variation; other high estimates, particularly for *IL-6*, arose from studies with shorter elapsed time between measurements (Picotte, et al., 2009; Rao, et al., 1994).

The degree to which one can generalize from a single time point to the surrounding weeks, months, or years varies by the inflammatory biomarker one selects. The *ICC* point estimate for *IL-6* reported by the study reviewed earlier (0.48) (Navarro, et al., 2012) was representative of other estimates, and so the recommendation that more than one *IL-6* measurement be taken to accurately generalize to an occasion or to stable individual differences is supported by other findings. For other *cytokines*, that *ICC* point estimate agreed with some other studies but by no means all, and those other studies did not all agree with each other. In addition, for the most part, there was only one measurement of a biomarker at each time point, so the short-term variability (e.g., days) could not be separated from the long-term variability (e.g., months). Larger-scale studies that can estimate both short- and long-term variability could give important information about the generalizability and measurement requirements for inflammatory biomarkers.

Finally, individual and group differences in variability may be important. In one of the earliest reports, Black participants had significantly higher intraindividual variability than White participants (Rao, et al., 1994). More studies that specifically compare stability across gender, ethnicity, and age are needed to make measurement recommendations for different kinds of samples.

Stress Reactivity

Acute physiological reactivity to experimental stress can serve as a meaningful predictor of future health outcomes and disease risk (Chida & Steptoe, 2010; Manuck, Cohen, Rabin, Muldoon, & Bachen, 1991; Marsland, Bachen, Cohen, Rabin, & Manuck, 2002; Matthews, Katholi, McCreath, Whooley, Williams, Zhu, et al., 2004). Laboratory tasks that induce acute stress include mental arithmetic, cold pressor, and the Trier Social Stress Task (Marsland, Walsh, Lockwood, & John-Henderson, 2017). *Cardiovascular reactivity* is typically operationalized as a change in blood pressure, heart rate (HR), and heart rate variability (HRV) from baseline to stressor. *HPA axis* reactivity is typically operationalized as a change in salivary cortisol. *Immunological reactivity* has been operationalized as acute redistribution of immune cells into circulation or a change in the inflammatory biomarkers *IL-6* or *TNFα*, which significantly and reliably increase in response to acute laboratory stressors; less commonly studied inflammatory biomarkers, such as **interferon-γ** and *CRP*, typically do not (Marsland, et al., 2017).

The stability of cardiovascular reactivity was estimated from 134 participants (M_{age} = 42.5, 59% female, 90% Caucasian) who attended two experimental sessions three years apart (Dragomir, Gentile, Nolan, & D'Antono, 2014). Stability of the cardiovascular response was calculated as the test-retest **Spearman rank correlation** (ρ) of reactivity (stress value to baseline value) and recovery (post-stress value to baseline value) for **systolic blood pressure (SBP)**, **diastolic blood pressure (DBP)**, HR, **high-frequency heart rate variability (HF-HRV)**, **low-frequency heart rate variability (LF-HRV)**, **very low-frequency HRV (VLF-HRV)**, and *HF-HRV* and *LF-HRV* in normalized units. Individual differences in *SBP* and HR reactivity were most stable over three years (ρ = 0.48 and ρ = 0.68, respectively), whereas all others were moderately stable (ρ's = 0.23 to 0.38). Individual differences in recovery were less stable over three years; however, *SBP* and HR had the highest stability (ρ = 0.37 and ρ = 0.38, respectively), individual differences in *DBP* recovery were almost completely unrelated (ρ = 0.07), and all others fell in between (ρ = 0.17 to 0.26). There were no significant effects of age or gender in reactivity or recovery change.

The strengths of this study included a large sample size, a long interval between laboratory tasks, and a large age range (18 to 65 years). Limitations included low diversity in race and ethnicity and differences in the laboratory tasks at Time 1 and Time 2, which may have introduced instability.

High stability in *SBP* and HR reactivity and low stability in *DBP* reactivity were also observed over intervals of 2.5 to 10 years (Allen, Sherwood, Obrist, Crowell, & Grange, 1987; Sherwood,

Girdler, Bragdon, West, Brownley, Hinderliter, et al., 1997). However, higher estimates of stability in *DBP* reactivity over intervals of one to 18 years have also been reported (Burleson, Poehlmann, Hawkley, Ernst, Berntson, Malarkey, et al., 2003; Hassellund, Flaa, Sandvik, Kjeldsen, & Rostrup, 2010). Over shorter periods of time (two weeks), stable individual differences in cardiovascular reactivity are more evident (*SBP* and HR $r \approx .80$) (Cohen, Hamrick, Rodriguez, Feldman, Rabin, & Manuck, 2000; Marsland, Manuck, Fazzari, Stewart, & Rabin, 1995). Diversity in race and ethnicity does not appear to affect stability in cardiovascular reactivity, but stability may increase with age (Burleson, et al., 2003; Kamarck, Jennings, Stewart, & Eddy, 1993; Swain & Suls, 1996).

Compared with cardiovascular reactivity, individual differences in reactivity in immune cell redistribution, $r = 0.25$ to 0.53, may not be as stable (Marsland, 1995). One possibility has to do with the time scale of cardiovascular changes versus immunological changes. Direct innervation of the heart and blood vessels creates the possibility for an almost immediate response in the cardiovascular system, and the system can be assessed continuously through a stressor. By contrast, some immunological changes may be slower, or the peak change may be different in different people, such that a single blood draw may not capture the peak for all individuals. This is particularly true for inflammatory biomarkers, which peak many minutes after the stressor. Although we are not aware of studies of the stability of *HPA reactivity*, cortisol also peaks approximately 20 minutes after the stressor, and therefore few measurements across that time course may miss individual peaks and contribute to lower stability estimates for cortisol reactivity.

Across all studies, individual differences in cardiovascular reactivity, especially *SBP* and HR, appear highly stable across both the short and long term. *Cardiovascular reactivity* can therefore be measured once with sufficient reliability and used for important clinical risk and treatment evaluations (e.g., for behavioral interventions) (Boulware, Daumit, Frick, Minkovitz, Lawrence, & Powe, 2001). However, multiple measurements of DBP reactivity and immunological reactivity may be necessary to achieve sufficient reliability to generalize over the long term.

Telomere Length

Telomeres are caps on the ends of chromosomes that give DNA polymerase a platform on which to begin the process of DNA replication. *Telomeres* become shorter with each replication (the first *telomere*, acting as a platform, does not replicate, and thus the *telomere* length in the new cell is shorter). Very short *telomeres* indicate that the DNA "environment" is not safe for accurate replication. When *telomeres* become sufficiently short, cells become senescent and do not divide further (Montpetit, Alhareeri, Montpetit, Starkweather, Elmore, Filler, et al., 2014).

A seminal paper reported that life stress was associated with accelerated *telomere* shortening among adult women (Epel, Blackburn, Lin, Dhabhar, Adler, Morrow, et al., 2004). Attempts to link psychological and behavioral factors to **telomere length (TL)** and rate of shortening have since proliferated (see Epel & Prather, 2018, for a review). *Telomeres* are presumed to change with aging (as replications accumulate) and with stress, but there has been little examination of the natural dynamics of individual differences in *TL*.

One notable exception used data on over 1,000 adults from Israel, the United States, France, and Denmark with ages across the adult lifespan ($M_{age} = 38$, SD = 15; 44% women) who had blood drawn twice with an interval of more than 10 years (Benetos, Kark, Susser, Kimura, Sinnreich, Chen, et al., 2013). The correlation between **leukocyte TL** at baseline and follow-up was $r \geq .91$ in each of the samples, and 56% of participants remained in the same decile at baseline and follow-up. In all samples, after adjusting for age, sex, smoking, and body mass index (BMI), decile at baseline correlated .96 with decile at follow-up.

This is a remarkably high correlation. Although correlations do not speak to mean changes, they do indicate that *TL*-relative rank was more or less unchanging across more than a decade of adulthood. This stability is consistent with indications that the effect of stress on *TL* largely occurs prenatally or in early life (Epel & Prather, 2018). *Leukocyte TL* is about 5,000 ***base pairs (bp)*** at birth. By age 20, *leukocyte TL* is shorter by 60% and shortens from that point by approximately 1% per year (Benetos, et al., 2013). This shortening from prenatal or natal maximum *TL* to adult *TL* may be a sensitive period for the effects of stress.

A methodological strength of this longitudinal study was that the assays were done in the same lab, using ***Southern blot*** assays and examining each sample for DNA integrity. *Southern blot* is the most reliable method for measuring *TL* (Montpetit, et al., 2014). Less reliable methods not only affect the precision of measurement but also introduce a statistical artifact. When baseline values are related to change, which is true of *TL* as well as other biomarkers, unreliability in the baseline value carries over into the change score. This can artificially create a negative slope where none exists. This effect was demonstrated using duplicate *TL* measurements (i.e., two assays done on the same sample), for which there should be no relationship between TL_1 and the difference between TL_1 and TL_2. Nonetheless, there was a negative correlation on the order of $r = -.15$. This correlation was found using the highly reliable *Southern blot*; the less reliable the assay, the larger this negative correlation will be (Verhulst, Aviv, Benetos, Berenson, & Kark, 2013).

One weakness of this study was the use of *leukocyte TL*. ***Leukocytes***, or white blood cells, have different rates of division and therefore will be expected to have different *TLs*, different variation in *TL* from cell to cell, or both (Montpetit, et al., 2014). The proportions of different cell types are sensitive to both acute and longer-term stress (Segerstrom & Miller, 2004). Therefore, apparent change in *TL* can be a function of changes in cell proportion or turnover. One alternative is to use ***buccal cells*** from the inside of the mouth, which are more homogeneous (Epel & Prather, 2018).

Although adult *leukocyte TL* was extremely stable in a rank-order sense, correlations between stress and *TL* in adulthood still make sense. Stressors tend to cluster with other stressors within people, and maternal and early life conditions (e.g., socioeconomic status) may lay a foundation for the experience of further stressors in adulthood (Hobfoll, 1989; Johnson & Schoeni, 2011). The most compelling evidence for *TL* change in adulthood would come from intervention studies, which are beginning to appear (Epel & Prather, 2018). The natural stability of *TL* does not preclude such change, just as personality rank-order stability is high, but interventions can introduce change (Roberts, Wood, & Caspi, 2008; Roberts, Luo, Briley, Chow, Su, & Hill, 2017).

Strengths and Limitations

Biomarkers used in studies of stress and other psychosocial variables have a wide range of variability. *Cortisol*, for example, does not generalize well from one day to the next, but if multiple days are collected at each time point, stability over weeks to months is low to moderate. Levels of the *proinflammatory cytokine IL-6* have moderate stability. HR reactivity can be quite stable over longer periods of time. The stability of these biomarkers can be confidently characterized because there have been multiple studies of each of them. However, this is not true of all biomarkers being used in stress research. There are only two studies (to our knowledge) of *sAA* and only one of *TL*. Good study design for substantive questions about stress and biomarkers requires knowing the temporal dynamics of the latter, and more studies are needed for many biomarkers. Furthermore, most studies only characterize variability and stability at one level, typically the medium-to-long range. The exceptions are studies of ***salivary analytes*** (*cortisol* and *α-amylase*), which have been characterized at both the short (daily) and medium range. More such studies for biomarkers with potential short-term variation are needed. Furthermore, studies with multiple levels of measurement can detect person-by-situation interactions and provide study design recommendations for longitudinal studies (e.g., Out, et al., 2013; Segerstrom, et al., 2014).

The literature on the variability of inflammatory biomarkers illustrates the importance of large samples in studies estimating biomarker variability. Most of these studies had very small n's, and the large range of estimates for stability (e.g., $TNF\alpha \approx 0.40$ to 0.90) is very likely to be due in part to sampling error. One solution for biomarkers with sufficient numbers of studies would be meta-analysis of these estimates. A better solution would be new studies powered to provide more accurate point estimates with smaller confidence intervals.

Finally, there may be differences in biomarker variability across different ages, genders, and racial or ethnic groups. For *cortisol*, estimates seem to agree regardless of sample characteristics. However, for other biomarkers, agreement across different sample characteristics cannot be assumed, and there is some evidence that different groups have different levels of variability (e.g., for cardiovascular reactivity, age but not gender or ethnicity, appears to affect variability; for *IL-6*, Black samples may have higher variability than White). Studies of samples with different characteristics are important, as are studies with sufficiently large samples to compare subsamples with different characteristics.

Recommendations for Future Research

Every study of stress physiology should use sufficiently reliable and generalizable measurement to avoid misestimation and both Type I and Type II errors. However, all studies do not require the same kind of reliability or generalizability. A cross-sectional study of cumulative life stress should measure physiology in such a way as to achieve high reliability at the person level, that is, individual differences that are stable over a long period of time. However, a study of examination stress may only need to generalize to a week. A daily stress study only needs to generalize to the same day; in fact, measures that generalize to the person level with only a single measurement (e.g., *TNF\alpha*) would not be well suited for this kind of study. Careful consideration of what biomarker is relevant for a particular population (e.g., *systemic inflammation* is more relevant for older adults) and its physiometrics should be a part of every study of stress and physiology.

Furthermore, systems associated with stress are not interchangeable. In a network analysis of systems associated with the stress response ($n = 328$ psychologically and physically healthy adults, age range = 20 to 55, 59% women), clusters emerged for salivary cortisol, hair cortisol, inflammation, and subjective stress, but the clusters were themselves very modestly related (Engert, et al., 2018). Network analysis includes adjustment for all other relationships in the network, so a general stress relationship across all variables might have been missed, but zero-order correlations supported the independence of the clusters. Therefore, "stress" research should consider not only the physiometrics of different biomarkers but also potential substantive relationships. One interesting connection that did emerge linked depression, sleep, awakening time, and salivary cortisol. Another interesting connection that emphasizes the importance of generalizability linked stressors reported on saliva sampling days to cortisol in those saliva samples (zero-order $r = 0.14$); longer-term perceived stress was only linked to cortisol via its relationship with stressors on saliva sampling days. In this example, *cortisol* measures were only required to generalize to the days on which they were collected, an appropriate use of an unstable measure.

Conclusion

Too often, physiological measurement in stress studies is designed based on ease (e.g., saliva vs. blood) or cost (e.g., one day's sampling vs. multiple days'). We hope that this chapter illustrates the importance of considering both substantive and *physiometric* issues when selecting an appropriate biomarker and method. When methods are not appropriate and *physiometrics* are poor, misestimation occurs and leads both theory and future studies astray, at a cost to us all (Segerstrom & Boggero, 2020).

References

Adam, E. K., Hawkley, L. C., Kudielka, B. M., & Cacioppo, J. T. (2006). Day-to-day dynamics of experience: Cortisol associations in a population-based sample of older adults. *Proceedings of the National Academy of Sciences*, *103*, 17058–17063. https://doi.org/10.1073/pnas.0605053103

Adam, E. K., & Kumari, M. (2009). Assessing salivary cortisol in large-scale, epidemiological research. *Psychoneuroendocrinology*, *34*, 1423–1436. https://doi.org/10.1016/j.psyneuen.2009.06.011

Agalliu, I., Xue, X., Cushman, M., Cornell, E., Hsing, A. W., Kaplan, R. C., et al. (2013). Detectability and reproducibility of plasma levels of chemokines and soluble receptors. *Results in Immunology*, *3*, 79–84. https://doi.org/10.1016/j.rinim.2013.07.001

Ali, N., & Nater, U. M. (2020). Salivary alpha-amylase as a biomarker of stress in behavioral medicine. *International Journal of Behavioral Medicine*, 1–6. https://doi.org/10.1007/s12529-019-09843-x

Allen, M. T., Sherwood, A., Obrist, P. A., Crowell, M. D., & Grange, L. A. (1987). Stability of cardiovascular reactivity to laboratory stressors: A 2 1/2 yr follow-up. *Journal of Psychosomatic Research*, *31*, 639–645. https://doi.org/10.1016/0022-3999(87)90043-2

Almeida, D. M., Piazza, J. R., & Stawski, R. S. (2009). Interindividual differences and intraindividual variability in the cortisol awakening response: An examination of age and gender. *Psychology and Aging*, *24*, 819–827. https://doi.org/10.1037/a0017910

Bauduin, S. E., van Noorden, M. S., van der Werff, S. J. A., de Leeuw, M., van Hemert, A. M., van der Wee, N. J. A., et al. (2018). Elevated salivary alpha-amylase levels at awakening in patients with depression. *Psychoneuroendocrinology*, *97*, 69–77. https://doi.org/10.1016/j.psyneuen.2018.07.001

Beltzer, E. K., Fortunato, C. K., Guaderrama, M. M., Peckins, M. K., Garramone, B. M., & Granger, D. A. (2010). Salivary flow and alpha-amylase: Collection technique, duration, and oral fluid type. *Physiology & Behavior*, *101*, 289–296. https://doi.org/10.1016/j.physbeh.2010.05.016

Benetos, A., Kark, J. D., Susser, E., Kimura, M., Sinnreich, R., Chen, W., et al. (2013). Tracking and fixed ranking of leukocyte telomere length across the adult life course. *Aging Cell*, *12*, 615–621. https://doi.org/10.1111/acel.12086

Boulware, L. E., Daumit, G. L., Frick, K. D., Minkovitz, C. S., Lawrence, R. S., & Powe, N. R. (2001). An evidence-based review of patient-centered behavioral interventions for hypertension. *American Journal of Preventive Medicine*, *21*, 221–232. https://doi.org/10.1016/s0749-3797(01)00356-7

Brennan, R. L. (2001). *Generalizability theory*. New York, NY: Springer.

Burleson, M. H., Poehlmann, K. M., Hawkley, L. C., Ernst, J. M., Berntson, G. G., Malarkey, W. B., et al. (2003). Neuroendocrine and cardiovascular reactivity to stress in mid-aged and older women: Long-term temporal consistency of individual differences. *Psychophysiology*, *40*, 358–369. https://doi.org/10.1111/1469-8986.00039

Cava, F., González, C., Pascual, M. J., Navajo, J. A., & González-Buitrago, J. M. (2000). Biological variation of interleukin 6 (IL-6) and soluble interleukin 2 receptor (sIL2R) in serum of healthy individuals. *Cytokine*, *12*, 1423–1425. https://doi.org/10.1006/cyto.2000.0714

Chida, Y., & Steptoe, A. (2010). Greater cardiovascular responses to laboratory mental stress are associated with poor subsequent cardiovascular risk status: A meta-analysis of prospective evidence. *Hypertension*, *55*, 1026–1032. https://doi.org/10.1161/hypertensionaha.109.146621

Clow, A., Hucklebridge, F., Stalder, T., Evans, P., & Thorn, L. (2010). The cortisol awakening response: More than a measure of HPA axis function. *Neuroscience & Biobehavioral Reviews*, *35*, 97–103. https://doi.org/10.1016/j.neubiorev.2009.12.011

Cohen, S., Hamrick, N. M., Rodriguez, M. S., Feldman, P. J., Rabin, B. S., & Manuck, S. B. (2000). The stability of and intercorrelations among cardiovascular, immune, endocrine, and psychological reactivity. *Annals of Behavioral Medicine*, *22*, 171–179. https://doi.org/10.1007/BF02895111

Ditzen, B., Ehlert, U., & Nater, U. M. (2014). Associations between salivary alpha-amylase and catecholamines: A multilevel modeling approach. *Biological Psychology*, *103*, 15–18. https://doi.org/10.1016/j.biopsycho.2014.08.001

Doane, L. D., Chen, F. R., Sladek, M. R., Van Lenten, S. A., & Granger, D. A. (2015). Latent trait cortisol (LTC) levels: Reliability, validity, and stability. *Psychoneuroendocrinology*, *55*, 21–35. https://doi.org/10.1016/j.psyneuen.2015.01.017

Dragomir, A. I., Gentile, C., Nolan, R. P., & D'Antono, B. (2014). Three-year stability of cardiovascular and autonomic nervous system responses to psychological stress. *Psychophysiology*, *51*, 921–931. https://doi.org/10.1111/psyp.12231

Du Clos, T. W. (2000). Function of C-reactive protein. *Annals of Medicine*, *32*, 274–278. https://doi.org/10.3109/07853890009011772

Engert, V., Kok, B. E., Puhlmann, L. M., Stalder, T., Kirschbaum, C., Apostolakou, F., et al. (2018). Exploring the multidimensional complex systems structure of the stress response and its relation to health and sleep outcomes. *Brain, Behavior, and Immunity*, *73*, 390–402. https://doi.org/10.1016/j.bbi.2018.05.023

Epel, E. S., Blackburn, E. H., Lin, J., Dhabhar, F. S., Adler, N. E., Morrow, J. D., et al. (2004). Accelerated telomere shortening in response to life stress. *Proceedings of the National Academy of Sciences*, *101*, 17312–17315. https://doi.org/10.1073/pnas.0407162101

Epel, E. S., & Prather, A. A. (2018). Stress, telomeres, and psychopathology: Toward a deeper understanding of a triad of early aging. *Annual Review of Clinical Psychology*, *14*, 371–397. https://doi.org/10.1146/annurev-clinpsy-032816-045054

Franceschi, C., & Campisi, J. (2014). Chronic inflammation (inflammaging) and its potential contribution to age-associated diseases. *Journals of Gerontology Series A: Biomedical Sciences and Medical Sciences*, *69*, S4–S9. https://doi.org/10.1093/gerona/glu057

Gelman, A., & Carlin, J. (2014). Beyond power calculations: Assessing type S (sign) and type M (magnitude) errors. *Perspectives on Psychological Science*, *9*, 641–651. https://doi.org/10.1177/1745691614551642

Granger, D. A., Kivlighan, K. T., El-Sheikh, M., Gordis, E. B., & Stroud, L. R. (2007a). Assessment of salivary alpha-amylase in biobehavioral research. In L. J. Luecken & L. Gallo (Eds.), *Handbook of physiological research methods in health psychology* (pp. 95–114). New York: Sage Publications.

Granger, D. A., Kivlighan, K. T., El-Sheikh, M., Gordis, E. B., & Stroud, L. R. (2007b). Salivary α-amylase in biobehavioral research: Recent developments and applications. *Annals of the New York Academy of Sciences*, *1098*, 122–144. https://doi.org/10.1196/annals.1384.008

Gregor, M. F., & Hotamisligil, G. S. (2011). Inflammatory mechanisms in obesity. *Annual Review of Immunology*, *29*, 415–445. https://doi.org/10.1146/annurev-immunol-031210-101322

Hardikar, S., Song, X., Kratz, M., Anderson, G. L., Blount, P. L., Reid, B. J., et al. (2014). Intraindividual variability over time in plasma biomarkers of inflammation and effects of long-term storage. *Cancer Causes & Control*, *25*, 969–976. https://doi.org/10.1007/s10552-014-0396-0

Hassellund, S. S., Flaa, A., Sandvik, L., Kjeldsen, S. E., & Rostrup, M. (2010). Long-term stability of cardiovascular and catecholamine responses to stress tests: An 18-year follow-up study. *Hypertension*, *55*, 131–136. https://doi.org/10.1161/hypertensionaha.109.143164

Hellhammer, J., Fries, E., Schweisthal, O. W., Schlotz, W., Stone, A. A., & Hagemann, D. (2007). Several daily measurements are necessary to reliably assess the cortisol rise after awakening: State-and trait components. *Psychoneuroendocrinology*, *32*, 80–86. https://doi.org/10.1016/j.psyneuen.2006.10.005

Ho, G. Y., Xue, X. N., Burk, R. D., Kaplan, R. C., Cornell, E., & Cushman, M. (2005). Variability of serum levels of tumor necrosis factor-alpha, interleukin 6, and soluble interleukin 6 receptor over 2 years in young women. *Cytokine*, *30*, 1–6. https://doi.org/10.1016/j.cyto.2004.08.008

Hobfoll, S. E. (1989). Conservation of resources: A new attempt at conceptualizing stress. *American Psychologist*, *44*, 513–524. https://doi.org/10.1037/0003-066X.44.3.513

Hofmann, J. N., Yu, K., Bagni, R. K., Lan, Q., Rothman, N., & Purdue, M. P. (2011). Intra-individual variability over time in serum cytokine levels among participants in the prostate, lung, colorectal, and ovarian cancer screening trial. *Cytokine*, *56*, 145–148. https://doi.org/10.1016/j.cyto.2011.06.012

Johnson, R. C., & Schoeni, R. F. (2011). The influence of early-life events on human capital, health status, and labor market outcomes over the life course. *The BE Journal of Economic Analysis & Policy*, *11*, 2521. https://doi.org/10.2202/1935-1682.2521

Kamarck, T. W., Jennings, J. R., Stewart, C. J., & Eddy, M. J. (1993). Reliable responses to a cardiovascular reactivity protocol: A replication study in a biracial female sample. *Psychophysiology*, *30*, 627–634. https://doi.org/10.1111/j.1469-8986.1993.tb02088.x

Kaplan, R. C., Ho, G. Y., Xue, X., Rajpathak, S., Cushman, M., Rohan, T. E., et al. (2007). Within-individual stability of obesity-related biomarkers among women. *Cancer Epidemiology and Prevention Biomarkers*, *16*, 1291–1293. https://doi.org/10.1158/1055-9965.EPI-06-1089

Kiernan, K., Tao, J., & Gibbs, P. (2012). *Tips and strategies for mixed modeling with SAS/STAT® procedures* [PDF file]. Retrieved from https://support.sas.com/resources/papers/proceedings12/332-2012.pdf

Kraemer, H. C. (1991). To increase power in randomized clinical trials without increasing sample size. *Psychopharmacology Bulletin*, *27*, 217–224.

Kuhlman, K. R., Robles, T. F., Dickenson, L., Reynolds, B., & Repetti, R. L. (2019). Stability of diurnal cortisol measures across days, weeks, and years across middle childhood and early adolescence: Exploring the role of age, pubertal development, and sex. *Psychoneuroendocrinology*, *100*, 67–74. https://doi.org/10.1016/j.psyneuen.2018.09.033

MacArthur Research Network on SES and Health. (2000). Retrieved from https://macses.ucsf.edu/research/allostatic/salivarycort.php

Maier, S. F., & Watkins, L. R. (1998). Cytokines for psychologists: Implications of bidirectional immune-to-brain communication for understanding behavior, mood, and cognition. *Psychological Review, 105*, 83–107. https://doi.org/10.1037/0033-295x.105.1.83

Manuck, S. B., Cohen, S., Rabin, B. S., Muldoon, M. F., & Bachen, E. A. (1991). Individual differences in cellular immune response to stress. *Psychological Science, 2*, 111–115. https://doi.org/10.1111/j.1467-9280.1991.tb00110.x

Marchand, F., Perretti, M., & McMahon, S. B. (2005). Role of the immune system in chronic pain. *Nature Reviews Neuroscience, 6*, 521–532. https://doi.org/10.1038/nrn1700

Marsland, A. L., Bachen, E. A., Cohen, S., Rabin, B., & Manuck, S. B. (2002). Stress, immune reactivity and susceptibility to infectious disease. *Physiology & Behavior, 77*, 711–716. https://doi.org/10.1016/S0031-9384(02)00923-X

Marsland, A. L., Manuck, S. B., Fazzari, T. V., Stewart, C. J., & Rabin, B. S. (1995). Stability of individual differences in cellular immune responses to acute psychological stress. *Psychosomatic Medicine, 57*, 295–298. https://doi.org/10.1097/00006842-199505000-00012

Marsland, A. L., Walsh, C., Lockwood, K., & John-Henderson, N. A. (2017). The effects of acute psychological stress on circulating and stimulated inflammatory markers: A systematic review and meta-analysis. *Brain, Behavior, and Immunity, 64*, 208–219. https://doi.org/10.1016/j.bbi.2017.01.011

Matthews, K. A., Katholi, C. R., McCreath, H., Whooley, M. A., Williams, D. R., Zhu, S., et al. (2004). Blood pressure reactivity to psychological stress predicts hypertension in the CARDIA study. *Circulation, 110*, 74–78. https://doi.org/10.1161/01.cir.0000133415.37578.e4

Milaniak, I., & Jaffee, S. R. (2019). Childhood socioeconomic status and inflammation: A systematic review and meta-analysis. *Brain, Behavior, and Immunity, 78*, 161–176. https://doi.org/10.1016/j.bbi.2019.01.018

Montpetit, A. J., Alhareeri, A. A., Montpetit, M., Starkweather, A. R., Elmore, L. W., Filler, K., et al. (2014). Telomere length: A review of methods for measurement. *Nursing Research, 63*, 289–299. https://doi.org/10.1097/nrr.0000000000000037

Navarro, S. L., Brasky, T. M., Schwarz, Y., Song, X., Wang, C. Y., Kristal, A. R., et al. (2012). Reliability of serum biomarkers of inflammation from repeated measures in healthy individuals. *Cancer Epidemiology, Biomarkers, and Prevention, 21*, 1167–1170. https://doi.org/10.1158/1055-9965.epi-12-0110

Nicolson, N. A. (2008). Measurement of cortisol. In L. J. Luecken & L. Gallo (Eds.), *Handbook of physiological research methods in health psychology* (pp. 37–74). New York: Sage Publications.

Out, D., Granger, D. A., Sephton, S. E., & Segerstrom, S. C. (2013). Disentangling sources of individual differences in diurnal salivary α-amylase: Reliability, stability and sensitivity to context. *Psychoneuroendocrinology, 38*, 367–375. https://doi.org/10.1016/j.psyneuen.2012.06.013

Pace, T. W., & Heim, C. M. (2011). A short review on the psychoneuroimmunology of posttraumatic stress disorder: From risk factors to medical comorbidities. *Brain, Behavior, and Immunity, 25*, 6–13. https://doi.org/10.1016/j.bbi.2010.10.003

Perkins, D. O., Wyatt, R. J., & Bartko, J. J. (2000). Penny-wise and pound-foolish: The impact of measurement error on sample size requirements in clinical trials. *Biological Psychiatry, 47*, 762–766. https://doi.org/10.1016/s0006-3223(00)00837-4

Picotte, M., Campbell, C. G., & Thorland, W. G. (2009). Day-to-day variation in plasma interleukin-6 concentrations in older adults. *Cytokine, 47*, 162–165. https://doi.org/10.1016/j.cyto.2009.05.007

Pruessner, J. C., Kirschbaum, C., Meinlschmid, G., & Hellhammer, D. H. (2003). Two formulas for computation of the area under the curve represent measures of total hormone concentration versus time-dependent change. *Psychoneuroendocrinology, 28*, 916–931. https://doi.org/10.1016/s0306-4530(02)00108-7

Rao, K. M., Pieper, C. S., Currie, M. S., & Cohen, H. J. (1994). Variability of plasma IL-6 and crosslinked fibrin dimers over time in community dwelling elderly subjects. *American Journal of Clinical Pathology, 102*, 802–805. https://doi.org/10.1093/ajcp/102.6.802

Reed, R. G., Al-Attar, A., Presnell, S. R., Lutz, C. T., & Segerstrom, S. C. (2019). A longitudinal study of the stability, variability, and interdependencies among late-differentiated T and NK cell subsets in older adults. *Experimental Gerontology, 121*, 46–54. https://doi.org/10.1016/j.exger.2019.03.006

Roberts, B. W., Luo, J., Briley, D. A., Chow, P. I., Su, R., & Hill, P. L. (2017). A systematic review of personality trait change through intervention. *Psychological Bulletin, 143*, 117–141. https://doi.org/10.1037/bul0000088

Roberts, B. W., Wood, D., & Caspi, A. (2008). The development of personality traits in adulthood. In O. P. John, R. W. Robins, & L. A. Pervin (Eds.), *Handbook of personality: Theory and research* (3rd ed., pp. 375–398). New York: Guillford.

Rohleder, N. (2014). Stimulation of systemic low-grade inflammation by psychosocial stress. *Psychosomatic Medicine, 76*, 181–189. https://doi.org/10.1097/psy.0000000000000049

Ross, K. M., Murphy, M. L., Adam, E. K., Chen, E., & Miller, G. E. (2014). How stable are diurnal cortisol activity indices in healthy individuals? Evidence from three multi-wave studies. *Psychoneuroendocrinology, 39*, 184–193. https://doi.org/10.1016/j.psyneuen.2013.09.016

Segerstrom, S. C. (2019). Between the error bars: How modern theory, design, and methodology enrich the personality-health tradition. *Psychosomatic Medicine, 81*, 408–414. https://doi.org/10.1097/psy.00000 00000000701

Segerstrom, S. C., & Boggero, I. A. (2020). Expected estimation errors in studies of the cortisol awakening response: A simulation. Psychosomatic Medicine. Volume published ahead of print issue.

Segerstrom, S. C., Boggero, I. A., Smith, G. T., & Sephton, S. E. (2014). Variability and reliability of diurnal cortisol in younger and older adults: Implications for design decisions. *Psychoneuroendocrinology, 49*, 299–309. https://doi.org/10.1016/j.psyneuen.2014.07.022

Segerstrom, S. C., & Miller, G. E. (2004). Psychological stress and the human immune system: A meta-analytic study of 30 years of inquiry. *Psychological Bulletin, 130*, 601–630. https://doi.org/10.1037/0033-2909. 130.4.601

Segerstrom, S. C., & Smith, G. T. (2012). Methods, variance, and error in psychoneuroimmunology research: The good, the bad, and the ugly. In S. C. Segerstrom (Ed.), *Oxford handbook of psychoneuroimmunology* (pp. 421–432). New York: Oxford.

Shavelson, R. J., & Webb, N. M. (1991). *Generalizability theory: A primer* (Vol. 1). Thousand Oaks, CA: Sage Publications.

Sherwood, A., Girdler, S. S., Bragdon, E. E., West, S. G., Brownley, K. A., Hinderliter, A. L., et al. (1997). Ten-year stability of cardiovascular responses to laboratory stressors. *Psychophysiology, 34*, 185–191. https://doi.org/10.1111/j.1469-8986.1997.tb02130.x

Skoluda, N., La Marca, R., Gollwitzer, M., Müller, A., Limm, H., Marten-Mittag, B., et al. (2017). Long-term stability of diurnal salivary cortisol and alpha-amylase secretion patterns. *Physiology & Behavior, 175*, 1–8. https://doi.org/10.1016/j.physbeh.2017.03.021

Slavich, G. M. (2014). From stress to inflammation and major depressive disorder: A social signal transduction theory of depression. *Psychological Bulletin, 140*, 774–815. https://doi.org/10.1037/a0035302

Stolp, H. B., & Dziegielewska, K. M. (2009). Review: Role of developmental inflammation and blood: Brain barrier dysfunction in neurodevelopmental and neurodegenerative diseases. *Neuropathology and Applied Neurobiology, 35*, 132–146. https://doi.org/10.1111/j.1365-2990.2008.01005.x

Strahler, J., Skoluda, N., Kappert, M. B., & Nater, U. M. (2017). Simultaneous measurement of salivary cortisol and alpha-amylase: Application and recommendations. *Neuroscience & Biobehavioral Reviews, 83*, 657–677. https://doi.org/10.1016/j.neubiorev.2017.08.015

Strube, M. J. (2000). Psychometrics. In J. T. Cacioppo, L. G. Tassinary, & G. G. Berntson (Eds.), *Handbook of Psychophysiology* (2nd ed., pp. 849–869). Cambridge, MA: Cambridge University Press.

Swain, A., & Suls, J. (1996). Reproducibility of blood pressure and heart rate reactivity: A meta-analysis. *Psychophysiology, 33*, 162–174. https://doi.org/10.1111/j.1469-8986.1996.tb02120.x

Todd, J., Simpson, P., Estis, J., Torres, V., & Wub, A. H. B. (2013). Reference range and short-and long-term biological variation of interleukin (IL)-6, IL-17A and tissue necrosis factor-alpha using high sensitivity assays. *Cytokine, 64*, 660–665. https://doi.org/10.1016/j.cyto.2013.09.018

Verhulst, S., Aviv, A., Benetos, A., Berenson, G. S., & Kark, J. D. (2013). Do leukocyte telomere length dynamics depend on baseline telomere length? An analysis that corrects for "regression to the mean". *European Journal of Epidemiology, 28*, 859–866. https://doi.org/10.1007/s10654-013-9845-4

Wang, X., Sánchez, B. N., Golden, S. H., Shrager, S., Kirschbaum, C., Karlamangla, A. S., et al. (2014). Stability and predictors of change in salivary cortisol measures over six years: MESA. *Psychoneuroendocrinology, 49*, 310–320. https://doi.org/10.1016/j.psyneuen.2014.07.024

Weiss, L. R., Venezia, A. C., & Smith, J. C. (2019). A single bout of hard RPE-based cycling exercise increases salivary alpha-amylase. *Physiology & Behavior, 208*, 112555. https://doi.org/10.1016/j.physbeh.2019.05.016

Zimmerman, L. M., Bowden, R. M., & Vogel, L. A. (2014). A vertebrate cytokine primer for eco immunologists. *Functional Ecology, 28*, 1061–1073. https://doi.org/10.1111/1365-2435.12273

11
CARDIOVASCULAR REACTIVITY AND STRESS

Chun-Jung Huang, Andy V. Khamoui, Aaron L. Slusher, and Brandon G. Fico

Overview

Chronic psychological stress has been associated with the increased risk of cardiovascular disease (CVD), such as atherosclerosis (Olinski, Gackowski, Foksinski, Rozalski, Roszkowski, & Jaruga, 2002; Wirtz & von Kanel, 2017). An early indicator of subclinical stages of atherosclerotic development is endothelial dysfunction (Singhai, 2005). Approximately 20% of adults in the United States report inadequacies in managing psychological stress (APA, 2018). Chronic psychological stress has been shown to impair endothelial function, such as reduced ability of cells on the blood vessel to maintain vascular homeostasis (i.e., vasoconstriction/vasodilation (Williams, Kaplan, & Manuc, 1993), and deplete the number of circulating endothelial progenitor cells (Chen, Zhang, Zhang, Song, Zhang, Liu, et al., 2013). Furthermore, research has observed a negative association between *flow-mediated dilation* (**FMD**, an index of endothelium-dependent vasodilation) and the Framingham Risk Score (an index of 10-year CVD risk) (Maruhashi, Soga, Fujimura, Idei, Mikami, Iwamoto, et al., 2013).

Importantly, a brief period of laboratory-induced psychological stress has been demonstrated to elicit impaired *FMD* as a predictor of CVD (Ghiadoni, Donald, Cropley, Mullen, Oakley, Taylor, et al., 2000). Specifically, the physiological response to an acute mental stressor is detailed by the robust and coordinated activation of the *sympathoadrenal medullary* (**SAM**), which rapidly releases the *catecholamines epinephrine* (**EPI**) and norepinephrine (NOR) from the adrenal medulla and nerve endings, respectively (Flatmark, 2000). Shortly thereafter, the *hypothalamic-pituitary-adrenal* (**HPA**) axis releases the *glucocorticoid cortisol* (**CORT**) from the adrenal cortex as a negative-feedback mechanism to prevent overactivation of the *SAM*-associated stress response (Herman & Cullinan, 1997; Sapolsky, Romero, & Munck, 2000). In individuals who experience chronically elevated levels of psychological stress, the normal physiological operating range becomes altered and causes vital organ systems to adapt to new baseline level functions (e.g., progressive increases in resting heart rate [HR] and *blood pressure* [**BP**]). These adverse physiological adaptations are directly linked to the increased risk of early mortality from CVD (Carroll, Ginty, Der, Hunt, Benzeval, & Phillips, 2012; Chida & Steptoe, 2010). This chapter discusses how chronic elevation in these mediators (e.g., *EPI, NOR, and CORT*) modulate various biological mechanisms, such as elevated inflammation, as a major cause of CVD (Côco & de Oliveira, 2015). To further explore the link between CVD and other cellular mechanism(s) of mental health and psychological stress-related disorders (e.g., anxiety and depression), this chapter also addresses the role of mitochondria from an energetic perspective to sustain the energy demand of the resultant "fight or flight response".

Research in Practice

Psychoneuroimmunological Response to Psychological Stress

Overview of the Immunological Response to Psychological Stress

The neurological response to psychological stress exhibits profound effects on immune function, resulting in the emergence of psychoneuroimmunology as a field of scientific study (Elenkov, Wilder, Chrousos, & Vizi, 2000; Sapolsky, et al. 2000). The immune system is functionally characterized into two primary categories—innate and adaptive immunity—which are regulated by white blood cells termed **leukocytes**. Innate immune responses are primarily mediated by natural killer (NK) cells, **monocytes**, and **neutrophils** that provide a nonspecific and immediate defense against infectious pathogens. In addition, innate immune cells help facilitate debris clearance and the initiation of the healing process following injury. Adaptive, or acquired, immunity is mediated by **helper (CD4$^+$)** and **cytotoxic (CD8$^+$) T-cell lymphocytes**, and **B-cell lymphocytes** that communicate with innate immune cells and are responsible for the highly specific recognition of antigens upon secondary exposure to foreign pathogens.

In response to acute psychological stress, circulating concentrations of the psychological stress-related hormones *EPI* and *NOR* from *SAM* system activation, and *CORT* from *HPA* axis activation, are transiently elevated and interact with their respective cell-signaling receptors to increase the number of immune cells observed in circulation, referred to as **leukocytosis** (Benschop, Rodriguez-Feuerhahn, & Schedlowsk, 1996). In addition, these hormones help coordinate the activation and subsequent inactivation of the inflammatory signaling pathways within innate immune cells. Of particular importance are monocytes, the primary contributor to the cellular production of pro- and anti-inflammatory cytokines in response to acute psychological stress (Bierhaus, Wolf, Andrassy, Rohleder, Humpert, Petrov, et al., 2003; Brydon, Edwards, Jia, Mohamed-Ali, Zachary, Martin, et al., 2005). As a result of being exposed to an acute psychological stressor, an increased number of monocytes capable of producing and secreting the hallmark pro-inflammatory cytokines **interleukin 6** (*IL-6*) and **tumor necrosis factor alpha** (**TNF-α**) can be observed in circulation, thereby temporarily shifting the systemic and cellular microenvironment towards a pro-inflammatory milieu (Marsland, Walsh, Lockwood, & John-Henderson, 2017).

Chronic psychological stress alters *EPI, NOR, and CORT* concentrations in circulation observed under resting conditions. In addition, the density of their respective receptors and the sensitivity of their receptor's response on (*EPI* and *NOR* adrenergic receptors) or within (*CORT* glucocorticoid receptors) immune cells is altered (Huang, Acevedo, Mari, Randazzo, & Shibata, 2014; Miller, Murphy, Cashman, Ma, Ma, Arevalo, et al., 2014; Rouppe van der Voort, Kavelaars, van de Pol, & Heijnen, 2000). These adaptive changes contribute to dynamic shifts in the distributions of immune cell populations, their respective subsets (categorized subpopulations within each immune cell population), and the inflammatory phenotype/characteristics of circulating monocytes. These alterations further contribute to progressive low-grade elevations of systemic pro-inflammatory cytokine (e.g., *IL-6 and TNF-α*) concentrations and serve as a feed-forward mechanism to further increase the pro-inflammatory phenotype of monocytes in circulation. More worrisome may be that when monocytes migrate into inflamed tissues, they differentiate into resident macrophages. Under elevated pro-inflammatory conditions, monocytes appear to be predisposed to differentiate into a pro-inflammatory macrophage (Bories, Caiazzo, Derudas, Copin, Raverdy, Pigeyre, et al., 2012). As a result, the enhanced pro-inflammatory milieu adversely alters the cellular function of vital organ systems, including cardiac muscle and the vascular endothelium, which is considered to play a key role in the advanced development and early mortality from CVD (Elenkov, 2004; Gu, Tang, & Yang, 2012).

Academic Examinations to Study Psychological Stress Adaptations

Maydych, Claus, Dychus, Ebel, Damaschke, Diestel, colleagues (2017) recently examined the effects of academic stress as a temporally confined, naturalistic stressor to study the negative consequences of acute and chronic psychological stress on immune function in 20 healthy university students (85% female, aged 19 to 25 years old) over an eight-week continuum (Maydych, et al., 2017). Specifically, the timing of outcome measures in this study is as follows: 1) a baseline assessment 4.5 weeks prior to an examination period, 2) a follow-up assessment 1.5 weeks prior to the examination period, 3) an assessment the first day of and immediately following the two-week examination period, and 4) a final assessment occurring one week upon completion of the examination period (Maydych, et al., 2017). This methodological approach strengthened the researcher's ability to accurately assess adaptive changes in immune function during various phases of academic stress, including the anticipatory stress response (i.e., period leading up to the examination period) and their capacity to recover following the completion of the examination period. Furthermore, documentation of various physiological variables described later provides additional insight into an individual's perceived level of psychological stress prior to, during, and 1 week following the examination period. As a result, researchers provided a potential explanation for the level of dysregulation to immune function observed within each individual.

Compared to baseline, Maydych, et al. (2017) utilized flow cytometry to identify changes in immune cell profiles over the course of the examination period. Flow cytometry is a simple laboratory technique that enables researchers to quickly and accurately determine the proportion of cell populations using a small amount of blood sample (~100 µL of whole blood). More specifically, the flow cytometer takes up a small sample of suspended immune cells and uses fluidics to align cells into a single-file stream that passes through a laser to determine the distribution of immune cells based on their size and the structure of a cell. Using this technique, Maydych, et al. (2017) observed significant decreases in the absolute number of circulating NK cells and monocytes following completion of the academic period, whereas no differences in the number of *T-* and *B-cell lymphocytes* were observed at any time point throughout the study. These findings demonstrate that a prolonged period of psychological stress reduces the number of innate immune cells, whereas lymphocytes specific to the adaptive arm of the immune system may remain relatively unaltered.

Researchers also collected whole blood samples and cultured a small volume in an artificial environment (37°C at 5% CO_2) for 3 hours in the presence of a well-characterized inflammatory stimulant, **lipopolysaccharide** (**LPS**). This *ex vivo* (an experiment performed on human-derived cells in an externally controlled environment) approach enables researchers to measure changes in the production of various inflammatory cytokines produced predominately from monocytes. Interestingly, although the number of monocytes observed in circulation during and throughout recovery from the examination period were reduced, the production of *IL-6* and *TNF-α* increased at the end of the examination period compared to baseline. These findings demonstrate that an 8-week academic examination period designed to elicit a chronic psychological stress phenotype either 1) increases the number of monocytes specifically capable of producing and secreting pro-inflammatory cytokines following *LPS* stimulation or 2) individual monocytes are more sensitive to *LPS* stimulation and secrete greater pro-inflammatory cytokine concentrations in response.

As previously suggested, immune cells (e.g., monocytes) exposed to elevated concentrations of the psychological stress-related hormones *EPI* and *NOR* exhibit a progressively more pro-inflammatory phenotype under normal physiological conditions. Maydych, and colleagues (2017) did not investigate changes in *EPI* or *NOR* concentrations. However, salivary *CORT* concentrations were measured upon awakening and 30 minutes later as a biological measure of psychological stress. Significant increases in salivary *CORT* were observed during and following completion of the examination period. *CORT* is primarily responsible for the *deactivation* of the immune cell's inflammatory response during recovery from the stressful situation (McEwen, 2000), and the capacity of *CORT* to down-regulate or inhibit the pro-inflammatory signaling pathway becomes impaired in response to chronic psychological stress (Miller, Chen, Fok, Walker, Lim, Nicholls, et al., 2009; Sauer, Polack, Wikinski, Holsboer, Stalla, & Arzt, 1995). Maydych, et al. (2017) did not observe an association between changes in monocyte cell counts and their inflammatory response to *LPS* with increases in salivary *CORT* or other indices of chronic psychological stress (i.e., emotional exhaustion, depressive symptoms, ego depletion, and negative affect). Nonetheless, the decreased capacity of monocytes to respond to *CORT* signaling represents another important psychological stress-related characteristic. Whether or not sensitivity changes are observed in response to acute and chronic psychological stress are warranted to assess future CVD risk and progression (Miller, et al., 2009; van den Akker, Koper, van Rossum, Dekker, Russcher, de Jong, et al., 2008; Walker, 2007).

In summary, the psychoneuroimmunological field has provided a framework to understand how psychological stress-related alterations of immune profiles, which in part result from chronic dysregulation of the *SAM* system and *HPA* axis, directly contribute to four outcomes. First, an increase in the total number and proportion (relative to the entire population) of immune cells with a pro-inflammatory phenotype. Second, sensitivity of monocytes to respond to pro-inflammatory stimulants (e.g., *LPS*, and *NOR*). Third, production of pro-inflammatory proteins following the activation of their pro-inflammatory signaling pathways. Finally, the decreased ability of *CORT* to inactivate the pro-inflammatory response of immune cells during recovery from the stressor. The utilization of acute and prolonged academic stress therefore provides a valid model to examine various alterations in monocyte and global immune function associated with endothelial dysfunction and subsequent CVD risk.

Chronic Stress and Endothelial Dysfunction

A recent study investigated the association between chronic stress and biomarkers of endothelial dysfunction as an index of subclinical atherosclerosis (Kershaw, Lane-Cordova, Carnethon, Tindle, & Liu, 2016). In order to investigate this association, the authors used data from the Multi-Ethnic Study of Atherosclerosis, which is an observational cohort study intended to examine causes of subclinical CVD in 6457 adults aged 45 to 84 years. To evaluate chronic stress, each participant completed the Chronic Burden scale, ranging from 1 (not very stressful) to 3 (very stressful), that probes for ongoing financial-, job-, relationship-, and health-related difficulties. As a result, a chronic burden score (ranged from 0 to 5) was calculated by summing the domains containing reports of moderate-to-severe stress, which were then modeled categorically as high, medium, and low.

To measure endothelial dysfunction, brachial artery *FMD* was measured using a linear-array multifrequency transducer operating at 9 MHz (GE Logiq 700 Device) to acquire images of the brachial artery. Brachial artery baseline images taken 5 to 9 cm above the antecubital fossa were captured for 30 seconds. Subsequently, a BP cuff placed 2 inches below the antecubital fossa was inflated to 50 mmHg above ***systolic blood pressure*** (***SBP***) for 5 minutes to occlude blood flow to the forearm and hand. Upon deflation of the BP cuff, the brachial artery's responsiveness to reactive hyperemia was measured for 2 minutes, and images were analyzed using validated semi-automated software to measure baseline and maximum diameters of the brachial artery according to the following formulas: 1) absolute *FMD* = maximum diameter (mm) − baseline diameter (mm), and 2) *FMD* % = ([maximum diameter − baseline diameter] / baseline diameter) × 100 (lower *FMD* is indicative of endothelial dysfunction). Additionally, blood samples were collected to measure ***intercellular adhesion molecule-1*** (***ICAM-1***) and E-selectin by enzyme-linked immunosorbent assay methods to evaluate endothelial dysfunction. These cellular adhesion molecules are proportionately upregulated during the inflammatory response resulting from endothelial damage.

This study demonstrated that chronic stress was associated with lower *FMD* and with greater concentrations of *ICAM-1*, but not E-selectin. The authors concluded that psychological stress and repeated activation of the sympathetic nervous system are significant contributors to increased CVD risk. Although a major strength of this study was the large sample size ($n = 6489$), each dependent variable was evaluated across separate groups of subjects. Furthermore, another weakness of the cross-section study was an inability to establish a clear causation between chronic stress and endothelial dysfunction. Nonetheless, this study supports the growing body of literature regarding the association between chronic stress and endothelial dysfunction.

Another recent study aimed to determine if self-reported indices of psychological stress and depressive-like symptoms were associated with endothelial dysfunction in 203 adolescents from second grade into adolescents of tenth grade under the Lifestyle of our Kids project (Olive, Abhayaratna, Byrne, Richardson, & Telford, 2018). Psychological stress was assessed using the Children's Stress Questionnaire (CSQ), a 50-item questionnaire based on the Adolescent Stress Questionnaire, which utilized a 5-point Likert scale (1 = low stress; 5 = high stress) that probes the impact of stressor experiences within the last year. Furthermore, depression was assessed from a modified Children's Depression Inventory (CDI) questionnaire containing 19 items designed to determine whether or not depressive-like symptoms are present. Final values of the CDI range from 19 to 38, with a score ≥26 necessary to determine the presence of depression.

Endothelial function was assessed using the EndoPat 2000 (Itamar), a technique that is less technically demanding than FMD (Kuvin, Patel, Sliney, Pandian, Sheffy, Schnall, et al., 2003), requires little training, and has been validated in adolescent populations (Tierney, Newburger, Gauvreau, Geva, Coogan, Colan, et al., 2009). More specifically, the EndoPat 2000 records beat-to-beat arterial pressure waves in the finger using an inflatable cuff. The peripheral arterial tonometry is placed on the index finger of each hand (one serving as a control) and a baseline measurement is recorded for five minutes. Afterwards, a BP cuff placed around the testing upper arm is inflated above the *SBP* for five minutes to occlude blood flow. Following the occlusion period, the BP cuff on the testing arm is deflated, reactive hyperemia is recorded for five minutes, and the pulse amplitude response is measured simultaneously to indicate the degree of the endothelial function. Finally, a reactive hyperemia index is calculated, with a score ≤1.67 indicating endothelial dysfunction.

Interestingly, this study did not demonstrate early symptoms of psychological stress or depressive-like symptoms being associated with endothelial dysfunction in adolescents. A major limitation is likely that indices of psychological stress and depressive-like symptoms were self-reported. Self-reports are susceptible to biases and other limitations, which may have challenged the validity of the measures, especially among a sample of pediatric and adolescent participants. Furthermore, data on endothelial function using the Endo-Pat 2000 was among the first to measure endothelial function in adolescents and was only collected when the participants reached tenth grade. However, this was a longitudinal assessment with a relatively large sample size ($n = 203$) and potentially serves as a guide to help future studies in this area refine assessment techniques and methodologies.

Real-Life Stress and Cardiovascular Reactivity

To examine the impact of work stress on cardiovascular reactivity, Lumley, Shi, Wiholm, Slatcher, Sandmark, Wang, et al., (2014) investigated the relationships of chronic and momentary stress to heart rate (HR) reactivity in real-life work settings using a sample of 40 women in management positions. Participants were equipped with an HR monitor (Zephyr HxM BT), which was connected to a smartphone device (Nokia 553) via Bluetooth. Data was stored using the Java RecordStore application programming interface (API) on the smartphone device, and when the participant's HR increased by 20%, stress rating questionnaires were prompted on the smartphone device.

Chronic work stress was assessed by four questions regarding the participant's typical workday. On a 100-point scale, questioning included 1) "Overall, how stressful is your work?"; 2) "How intense is your work?"; 3) "Do you have regular opportunities to recover during work?"; and 4) "How often do you receive breaks during your work?" Participant responses were used to develop a single index of chronic work stress. For momentary work stress, the HR monitor triggered the smartphone device to prompt the question "How stressed are you?" and participants answered using a 6-point scale, with 6 being extremely stressed.

This study demonstrated that momentary work stress was associated with greater HR reactivity during work. Additionally, chronic stress predicted HR reactivity alone. When combined with momentary work stress, increased indices of chronic stress augment the physiological reactions observed during momentary stress. Despite limitations of this study, such as relying on HR alone (rather than collecting additional psychological stress-related cardiovascular measures, such as BP) and a relatively small sample size, Lumley and colleagues demonstrated an existing association between chronic stress and acute cardiac reactivity to momentary work stress.

More recently, Gnam, Loeffler, Haertel, Engel, Hey Boes, et al. (2019) aimed to determine whether or not higher physical activity/fitness would attenuate physiological and cognitive stress responses to real-life stressors among professional firefighters. More specifically, firefighters were administered an examination at the conclusion of a commander training course. Physical activity was assessed using the International Physical Activity Questionnaire, which subjectively quantifies physical activities of different intensities and provides a summed score of metabolic equivalent (estimated energy expenditure) of task minutes per week based on individual recall. Physical fitness was also measured quantitatively using a graded exercise test to determine *maximal oxygen uptake* (VO_{2max}). The protocol started at a speed of 6 km/hr and increased by 2 km/hr every three minutes until exhaustion, with oxygen uptake and carbon dioxide exhalation measured using a spirometer Meta-Max 3B (Cortex Biophysik GmbH, Leipzig, Germany).

To assess physiological stress, saliva *CORT* was measured using the DELFIA (time-resolved fluorescence immunoassay) method, and HR and HR variability (HRV) were measured using the Polar RS800 system (Polar Electro Oy, Kempele, Finland). To assess cognitive stress, a two-item scale was used. The first question asked participants how challenging the situation was using a Likert scale, with 1 representing no challenge and 5 representing high challenge. Similarly, the second question asked how manageable the situation was, with 1 (no manageability) and 5 (high manageability), and was inversely coded. The responses were then used to calculate an index ranging from 2 to 10, with lower scores indicating less cognitive stress.

This study did not observe any difference between the CORT, *HR*, or HRV stress responses between the lower and higher physical activity groups. As such, no attenuating effect was associated with increased physical activity or fitness on physiological stress responses to real-life stress reactivity. Although this study did not find any differences, it should be noted that the participants were all male firefighters who are typically more occupationally active than most other professions. Indeed, the less active subjects would be categorized as moderately active.

Acute Exercise Effect on Cardiovascular Reactivity With Stress

Aerobic Exercise

Research by Chandrakumar, Dyck, Boutcher, and Boutcher (2018) aimed to determine how 30 minutes of acute aerobic exercise on a cycle ergometer would influence cardiovascular reactivity to mental stress in overweight males. The cardiovascular response of the overweight males (*body mass index [BMI] ≥25 kg/m²*) was compared to age-matched individuals of normal weight (*BMI* between 18.5 and 24.9 kg/m²). Mental stress was applied using the Stroop Color and Word Test (SCWT) task before and after exercise. The SCWT is a color–word conflict test, in which participants are asked to name the color of a word rather than reading the word. The number of mistakes were summed to assess performance across time (before and after exercise) and between groups (overweight vs. normal weight).

Arterial stiffness was assessed using an ***augmentation index*** (***AIx***), which is an indirect measure of arterial stiffness. *AIx* was measured by placing a pressure sensor on the radial artery to record pressure waveforms. The *AIx* was derived from the ratio of augmented pressure (the degree of which reflected waveforms increase *SBP*) and pulse pressure (the difference between *SBP* and diastolic BP). ***Forearm blood flow*** (*FBF*) was measured using a strain gauge plethysmography with venous occlusion. Mercury strain gauges that measure changes in volume were placed on the right forearm five cm distal to the cubital fossa, while BP cuffs were placed on the wrist and upper arm. The wrist cuff was then inflated above *SBP* to occlude blood flow to the hand. Subsequently, *FBF* was assessed by inflating the upper arm cuff to 50 mmHg to occlude venous return for five seconds, every 15 seconds. The increase in volume of the arm (measured via strain gauges) is used to measure the arterial inflow, whereas BP was assessed using a beat-by-beat recording of the radial pulse waveform (Jentow, Colin Electronics, Komaki, Japan). Finally, electrodes were connected to the participant's chest to monitor HR via respiratory rate (RR) intervals (time elapsed between two successive R-waves determined by electrocardiogram).

This study demonstrated that the overweight participants had greater arterial stiffness throughout the mental challenge before and after acute aerobic exercise. Additionally, the overweight group had lower *FBF* during the SWCT before and after exercise. Although the overweight group had more mistakes during the SWCT, acute aerobic exercise elicited improvements (higher scores) in both groups, and HR and BP responses were similar throughout testing. As such, a short bout of aerobic exercise enhanced cardiovascular and *FBF* reactivity in both groups, with the overweight participants having greater atrial stiffness but less *FBF* responsiveness. Interestingly, although this study used indirect measures for both arterial stiffness and *FBF*, these techniques are still sensitive enough to pick up changes between groups and across time. A more direct measure of *FBF* would involve recording the diameter of the brachial via B-mode, and the blood velocity being measured using Doppler ultrasound. However, this technique requires more technical expertise and has been shown to provide similar results as strain gauge plethysmography (Brothers, Wingo, Hubing, & Crandall, 2010). Similarly, arterial stiffness is more directly measured using ***pulse wave velocity*** (***PVW***), yet many researchers measure carotid-femoral *PWV*, brachial-ankle *PWV*, or use the ***cardio–ankle vascular index*** (***CAVI***) (Fukuda Denshi; (Tanaka, 2018).

Resistance Exercise

The next study investigated the acute effects of traditional and circuit resistance exercise on BP and autonomic control (HRV) on mental stress (Gauche, Lima, Myers, Gadelha, Neri, Forjaz, et al., 2017). The participants included in the study were older hypertensive women. Mental stress was induced similarly to the previous study by using a computerized version of the SWCT. The computer program presented each slide for about one second with the names of colors being displayed in different colors. The participants were instructed to report the color of the word (not the written word) as fast as possible, with BP measured by a mercury-column sphygmomanometer and HRV examined by a chest strap cardiac monitor (RS800CX model; Polar Electro Oy, Kempele, Finland) to assess autonomic control.

This study demonstrated that both traditional and circuit resistance exercise attenuates BP reactivity to mental stress. Additionally, a reduction was observed in HRV. Moreover, circuit training takes less time to complete than traditional resistance exercise while providing similar benefits in cardiovascular reactivity with mental stress. A limitation in the methodology of this study may be the lack of sensitivity to reflect changes in autonomic function by using HRV. Baroreflex sensitivity testing may provide a more sensitive analysis for autonomic function, as baroreflex sensitivity is calculated as the slope of the linear regression between beat-to-beat *SBP* and the values of the RR interval (Zygmunt & Stanczyk, 2010). It is also suggested to measure BP with an automated device, although manually measuring BP did not negatively affect the results of this study. Other devices, such as the Finapres and Portapres, allow researchers to measure beat-to-beat BP, which can provide insight into momentary changes of the cardiovascular system (Langewouters, Settels, Roelandt, & Wesseling, 1998).

Mitochondrial Function and Responses to Psychological Stress

Overview of Mitochondrial Function

As the site of multiple nutrient oxidation pathways, mitochondria have a central role in cellular energy metabolism. Indeed, mitochondria have long been recognized as the powerhouse or powerplant of the cell due to their major role in the provision of cellular *adenosine triphosphate* (**ATP**), an important chemical responsible for providing cells with energy. Although once viewed as an end organelle with the singular role of generating *ATP* and serving the bioenergetic needs of the cell, the multifaceted and complex roles of mitochondria are now well-recognized and continue to emerge in exciting, ongoing areas of research (Picard, Wallace, & Burelle, 2016). Mitochondria partake in diverse signaling pathways and cell fate decisions and are dynamic rather than static organelles, undergoing constant remodeling and turnover in response to environmental stressors and cellular cues (Mishra & Chan, 2016). Given their central role in cellular metabolism, it is not very surprising that impairment of mitochondrial function has been linked to many chronic diseases. Mitochondria and their metabolic functions are, in fact, often cited as significant contributors to health and disease given their roles in aging, cancer, metabolic disease and CVD, and neurodegeneration (Mishra & Chan, 2016).

The electron transport chain, or respiratory chain, is synonymous with cellular *ATP* provision. The respiratory chain consists of a series of protein complexes embedded in the inner membrane of the mitochondria that includes complex I (CI), complex II (CII), complex III (CIII), and complex IV (CIV), along with *ATP* synthase (complex V [CV]). Electron input and transfer through the respiratory chain generate a proton motive force that enables phosphorylation—the chemical addition of a phosphoryl group to an organic molecule—of *adenosine diphosphate* (*ADP*) to *ATP* at CV. Oxygen is consumed during this process at CIV, whereby electron transfer to oxygen produces metabolic water. The coupling of the *electron transfer system* (**ETS**) to *ADP* phosphorylation (to yield *ATP*) is referred to as *mitochondrial oxidative phosphorylation* (**OXPHOS**). Disturbances to this aspect of mitochondrial function (i.e., respiration/oxygen consumption) are important because *OXPHOS* can affect redox status (a balance between oxidants and antioxidants), mitochondrial dynamics (i.e., fission and fusion), quality control (i.e., clearance of damaged mitochondria), and therefore the overall health of the mitochondrial network (Mishra & Chan, 2016).

In terms of human health and wellness, high mitochondrial oxidative capacity in energetically demanding tissues such as skeletal muscle is associated with trained athletes as well as systemic metabolic fitness, whereas impaired mitochondrial respiration correlates with disease (Dube, Coen, DiStefano, Chacon, Helbling, Desimone, et al., 2014). Recent work also suggests that mitochondrial function can reflect both acute and chronic psychological stress (Picard, McManus, Gray, Nasca, Moffat, Kopinski, et al., 2015; Picard, Prather, Puterman, Cuillerier, Coccia, Aschbacher, et al., 2018). Therefore, measurement of *OXPHOS* provides important information on mitochondrial and cellular health, could serve as a diagnostic indicator of disease state, or reveal some of the underlying energetic mechanisms that are either the cause or consequence of disease and stressors.

Assessment of Mitochondrial Respiratory Function

Measurements of mitochondrial respiratory function can be made in several types of sample preparations, including intact cells, chemically permeabilized cells, permeabilized tissues, tissue homogenates, or isolated mitochondria. A number of commercially available devices are used to evaluate mito-chondrial respiratory function in one or more of these mitochondrial preparations. The Seahorse Extracellular Flux analyzer (Agilent Technologies) is a plate reader–based assay of mitochondrial respiration. Because this device assays samples in either a 24- or 96-well format, it allows for high-throughput analysis of mitochondrial respiration. Another commonly used device is the Oxygraph-2k (O2k, Oroboros Instruments) for high-resolution respirometry, which will be the focus of this section.

The protocol consists of sequential injections of substrates, uncouplers, and inhibitors. Each num-ber in the table indicates the constituents injected into the respirometer chambers for that stage, as well as the corresponding respiratory state that is being measured. Syringe wash denotes the medium used to rinse and clean the Hamilton syringe before use. Also indicated are the required volumes injected per respirometer chamber in order to achieve the final concentration listed. After the appro-priate constituents are injected, the real-time recording of oxygen consumption is monitored until a steady state is reached (i.e., stable signal) before proceeding to the next step in the protocol.

The LEAK state refers to non-phosphorylating respiration without adenylates. Residual oxygen (O_2) consumption refers to the measurement of non-mitochondrial measurement that is obtained by using the CI and CIII inhibitors rotenone and antimycin A. The residual O_2 consumption is sub-tracted from all other respiratory states to correct for non-mitochondrial respiration.

This workstation contains two Oxygraph-2k respirometers that simultaneously measure oxygen concentration and oxygen consumption in a real-time read-out provided on a computer connected to the devices. The Hamilton syringes on the rack (left of the laptop computer) are used to inject various substrates, uncouplers, and inhibitors to evaluate mitochondrial respiration.

The O2k respirometer contains two chambers with oxygen sensors that simultaneously measure both oxygen concentration and oxygen consumption in real time (Pesta & Gnaiger, 2012). When performing *in situ* respiration experiments with permeabilized tissues (e.g., cardiac muscle, liver), the oxygen consumption recording is normalized to the mass of the tissue placed into each chamber as *pmol $O_2 \cdot s_{-1} \cdot mg_{-1}$*. Since each O2k device contains only two chambers, several devices are often used in tandem to allow for high-throughput capabilities. Any number of substrates, uncouplers, and inhibitors can be injected into the respirometer chambers using Hamilton syringes in order to mea-sure respiration supported by individual complexes of the respiratory chain, or by several respiratory complexes at the same time. For instance, after placing saponin-permeabilized muscle tissue into the respirometer chambers, injection of the CI-linked substrates malate, pyruvate, and glutamate would yield CI-supported LEAK respiration. The **LEAK** state refers to non-phosphorylating respiration, whereby *ADP* has not yet been added into the chambers, or where an *ATP* synthase inhibitor is injected into the chambers in order to arrest phosphorylating respiration. Subsequent titration of *ADP* would then yield CI-supported *OXPHOS*—in other words, phosphorylating/coupled respira-tion supported by electron supply into CI. To subsequently measure CII-supported respiration in the same experimental run, rotenone titration (to inhibit CI) would be followed by injection of suc-cinate (a CII-linked substrate) to supply electrons into CII, yielding a measurement of CII-supported *OXPHOS*.

Alternatively, the subsequent addition of succinate without being preceded by rotenone would yield coupled phosphorylating respiration with electron input into both *CI* and *CII* (i.e., CI + II *OXPHOS*). Doing so allows for convergent electron flux into CIII, and this is often referred to as maximal *OXPHOS* capacity, a state that can be considered a physiological maximal cellular oxy-gen consumption rate. At this point we could also titrate small volumes of the chemical uncoupler FCCP or CCCP. Injection of uncouplers at this stage would provide a measurement of the maximal capacity of the *ETS*, supported by CI- and CII-linked substrates. In other words, this would be a measurement of CI + II *ETS* because all of the previous CI- and CII-linked substrates are still in the chambers, but we are now measuring only the capacity of the *ETS* and not *OXPHOS*, which includes the phosphorylation system (e.g., CV). The uncouplers used in these protocols are titrated in small volumes in a graded, stepwise manner to slowly increase respiration up to a maximal level. Once the technician makes the judgment that additional titrations will not increase respiration, no additional uncoupler is added because further injections will impart inhibitory effects on respiration.

A sample protocol listing the full sequence of titrations that we typically use in our experiments with permeabilized tissues and the corresponding respiratory state being assessed are shown in Table 11.1. It should be mentioned that it is standard to integrate a quality control check into

Table 11.1 Sample mitochondrial respiration protocol used with the oxygraph-2k respirometer

Protocol constituents	Syringe wash	Volume per chamber	Final concentration	Respiratory state
1. Malate +	H_2O	5 ul	1 mM	CI LEAK
Pyruvate+	H_2O	5 ul	5 mM	
Glutamate	H_2O	10 ul	10 mM	
2. ADP	H_2O	20 ul	5 mM	CI OXPHOS
3. Succinate	H_2O	20 ul	10 mM	CI+II OXPHOS
4. Cyt c	H_2O	5 ul	10 μM	—
5. CCCP	EtOH	1 ul steps	0.5 μM	CI+II ETS
6. Rotenone	EtOH	1 ul	0.5 μM	CII ETS
7. Antimycin A	EtOH	1 ul	2.5 μM	Residual O_2

CI, complex I. CII, complex II. CI+II, complex I and II. Cyt c, cytochrome c. CCCP, carbonylcyanide m-cholorophenyl hydrazone. OXPHOS, oxidative phosphorylation. ETS, electron transfer system. EtOH, ethanol.

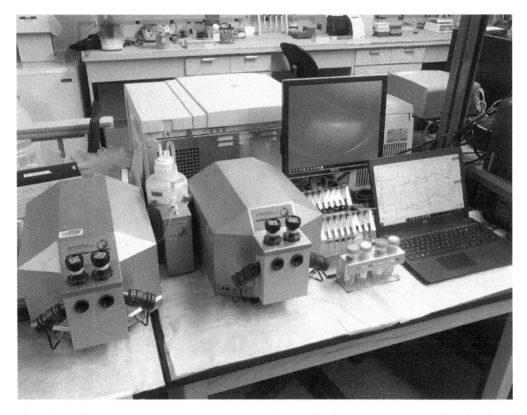

Figure 11.1 High-resolution respirometry workstation, Exercise Biochemistry Laboratory at Florida Atlantic University

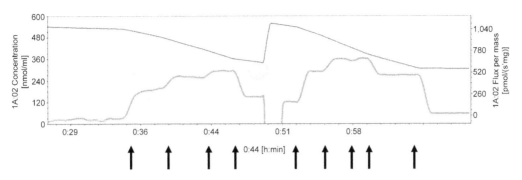

Figure 11.2   Sample Oxygraph recording from a full experimental run with the Oxygraph-2k device

the protocol by titration of **cytochrome c** into the chambers (when in the *OXPHOS* state; Pesta & Gnaiger, 2012). *Cytochrome c*, a protein attached to the inner membrane of the mitochondria, is responsible for electron transfer from CIII to CIV. If mitochondrial integrity is compromised during the course of sample preparation, such as during mechanical separation of whole muscle tissue into smaller fiber bundles, we would observe a very large increase in oxygen consumption upon addition of *exogenous cytochrome c*. This occurs because the *exogenous cytochrome c* would facilitate electron transfer and respiration, whereas we would not observe this exaggerated increase in respiration if *cytochrome c* remained in its normal position, as would be the case with samples where mitochondrial integrity was not compromised. At the end of each experimental run, we inject the CIII inhibitor antimycin *A* in order to terminate mitochondrial respiration. Any oxygen consumption recording made following antimycin *A* titration reflects non-mitochondrial sources of oxygen consumption, which we would then subtract from all other respiratory states examined. A sample Oxygraph trace from a full experimental run using the O2k device is shown in Figure 11.2.

The blue trace represents oxygen concentration, and the red trace indicates oxygen consumption, which is derived from the slope of the oxygen concentration curve. The vertical arrows indicate when substrates are injected into the respirometer chambers and a steady state is allowed to be achieved. When the oxygen consumption signal is stable, the next injection(s) can be performed. The oxygen concentration decreases over time as oxygen is being consumed. Periodic injections of 100% oxygen are performed to ensure that oxygen availability is not limiting to the experiment. The rise of the blue trace in the middle of the image reflects oxygen injection into the respirometer chambers.

Mitochondrial Function and Response to Psychological Stress

Evidence from basic science research supports a key role of mitochondria in mediating responses of different organ systems, including the cardiovascular system, to psychological stress. Picard, et al. (2015) used a genetic approach in which they studied mice with global (whole-body) mutations or deletions in mitochondrial genes encoded by both nuclear DNA (*ANT1; NNT*) and mitochondria DNA (respiratory chain subunits NADH dehydrogenase 6 [*ND6*] and *cytochrome c oxidase subunit I [COI]*). These genetic manipulations caused mitochondrial dysfunction as evidenced by impaired respiration. These mice were then subjected to a restraint procedure (30 minutes in a ventilated tube) to induce acute psychological stress. Afterwards, their physiological reactivity was assessed. The authors found that activation of the *HPA* axis depended on genotype. As expected, wild-type mice with normal mitochondria showed a rise in plasma *CORT* levels. Mice with a mutation in the CI subunit *ND6*, but not the CIV subunit COI, showed an even greater *CORT* increase compared to wild-type mice. In similar fashion, deletion of

ANT1 also caused an exaggerated *CORT* increase relative to wild-type mice, whereas the *CORT* response was blunted in mice with *NNT* deletion. These findings offer evidence to support the idea that mitochondria modulate the systemic response to acute psychological stress and this response is specific to a given mitochondrial gene. More broadly speaking, given that the cardiovascular consequences of excessive *CORT* are well established (Whitworth, Williamson, Mangos, & Kelly, 2005), repeated exposures to psychological stressors and continued activation of mitochondrial-mediated stress responses may have important implications for the development of CVD in humans.

Since the cardiovascular system is a principal organ system affected by stress, it would be of interest to better understand the mechanisms by which stress exposure causes cardiac injury. To that end, Liu, Qian, Gong, Shen, Zhang, & Qian (2004) conducted a proteomic analysis (a study of a set of proteins) of mitochondrial proteins in **cardiomyocytes**, a type of cell found in cardiac muscle, as well as an assessment of mitochondrial function, in rodents subjected to chronic restraint stress. The number of Terminal deoxynuckeotidyl transferase dUTP nick and labeling, referred to as TUNEL-positive cells, was greater in rats that experienced chronic restraint stress compared to controls, reflecting stress-induced cardiomyocyte **apoptosis**, or cell death. This is consistent with a previous report documenting significant mitochondrial structural alterations in the atrium of rodents after six hours of noise exposure, with damage extending to the ventricle after 12 hours of exposure (Gesi, Fornai, Lenzi, Ferrucci, Soldani, Ruffoli, et al., 2002). Liu et al. also found that proteins involved in the tricarboxylic acid cycle, or Krebs cycle, and lipid metabolism were decreased in the ventricle as a result of the chronic restraint stress. In addition, mitochondrial respiratory function was lower in the rodents exposed to chronic psychological stress compared to controls. Consistent with the impaired respiration, chronically stressed rats also had lower *ATP* content. Collectively, these findings suggest that chronic stress disrupts oxidative energy metabolism in cardiomyocytes, with specific impairment of fat metabolism that could contribute to injury and diseases of the heart.

In addition to basic research, work in clinical populations supports a role of mitochondria in mediating stress adaptation. For instance, the respiratory function of mitochondria in blood has been shown to reflect the severity of depression experienced by patients (Karabatsiakis, Bock, Salinas-Manrique, Kolassa, Calzia, Dietrich, et al., 2014). Major depression is a disease characterized by sleep disturbances, lack of energy and fatigue, and impaired concentration. It has been proposed that some of these features may be attributed to disrupted energy metabolism arising from dysfunctional mitochondrial *OXPHOS*. To explore this hypothesis, Karabatsiakis and colleagues collected blood from patients with major depression and a control group (Karabatsiakis, et al., 2014). **Peripheral blood mononuclear cells (PBMCs)** were isolated from the blood samples and mitochondrial respiration assayed using the O2k device.

In comparison to controls, *PBMCs* from patients with major depression exhibited dysregulation of mitochondrial respiration, as evidenced by significantly lower **routine respiration**, a measurement specific to cells supported by endogenous substrates because this oxygen consumption measurement is made before any substrates are injected into the respirometer chambers. Further, there was a tendency toward higher *LEAK* respiration, and substantially decreased *ETS* capacity. Aside from the lower maximal capacity of the *ETS* in patients with major depression, the greater *LEAK* respiration is suggestive of "looser" coupling of respiration to *ADP* phosphorylation. In agreement, the authors reported significantly lower coupling efficiency calculated from the *routine* and *LEAK* respiration measurements.

Therefore, the mitochondria in *PBMCs* from patients with major depression have looser coupling that may reflect inefficient *ATP* synthesis. Perhaps more importantly, mitochondrial respiration reportedly showed significant negative relationships with severity of depressive symptoms That is to say, lower mitochondrial respiration was associated with greater severity of depression. Collectively, these findings suggest that blood cell mitochondrial respiration can serve as an objective indicator of depression severity. Given that blood is routinely collected from clinical populations, an assay of mitochondrial respiration would have significant diagnostic value. It also indicates that targeted improvement of mitochondrial function could contain therapeutic value for patients with depression.

Extending the clinical and human health relevance of blood cell mitochondrial function, it has been proposed that a ***mitochondrial health index*** (***MHI***) derived from such measurements can reflect mood and stress associated with caregiving (Picard, et al., 2018). The *MHI* was determined from *PBMC* enzyme activity of CII, CIV, and citrate synthase, as well as mitochondrial DNA copy number. CII and CIV are encoded by the mitochondrial genome, while the latter two were assayed as proxies of mitochondrial content and represent the nuclear genome. To calculate the *MHI*, the enzyme activities for CII and CIV were added together and divided by the sum of citrate synthase activity and mitochondrial DNA copy number. Hence, the mitochondrial genome and nuclear genome occur in the numerator and denominator of this calculation, respectively, and represent equal contributions from both nuclear and mitochondrial DNA. More specifically, *MHI* represents respiratory chain function per unit of mitochondrial content. When the *MHI* was determined in healthy mothers of a child with autism spectrum disorder (high-stress caregivers), they showed a lower *MHI* compared to mothers of a neurologically typical child (controls). Further, across the entire sample, it was found that a higher *MHI* was associated with elevated positive mood at night. Overall, this data suggests that blood cell mitochondrial function can serve as an objective indicator of the degree of stress exhibited by individuals, and perhaps has broad use in clinical settings, given the routine nature of blood collection.

Conclusion

The literature evidently supports the adverse physiological effects from chronic psychological stress to enhance the risk of CVD incidence. Researchers should be aware of some limitations associated with varying methodology. For example, noninvasive endothelial function measurements can be made using *FMD* and Endo-PAT 2000, as previously described. *FMD* is validated as an endothelium-dependent measurement of vasodilation; however, the measurement is highly operator dependent and can be influenced by diet and environmental conditions (e.g., room temperature, lighting). As such, participants must be evaluated in a fasting condition and testing conditions must remain consistent. Regarding the Endo-PAT 2000, although the measurement is nonoperator dependent, the physiology remains partially unclear, as it measures microvessel dilation and is only partly dependent on nitric oxide availability (Premer, Kanelidis, Hare, & Schulman, 2019). Additionally, further investigations regarding the potential adaptive changes of inflammatory monocytes would provide novel insight into the mechanistic consequences responsible for the advanced development and increased mortality from CVD in individuals who experience chronic levels of psychological stress. Although the exact mechanisms of mitochondrial regulation by psychological stress-related hormones such as *CORT* remains to be elucidated, a low level of *CORT* provides a cardioprotective effect (Enc, Karaca, Ayoglu, Camur, Kurc, & Cicek, 2006), whereas chronic elevation enhances intrinsic mitochondrial-dependent apoptosis (Du, Wang, Hunter, Wei, Blumenthal, Falke, et al., 2009). A further understanding of this multifaceted interaction between mitochondria and these stress mediators would facilitate the knowledge of the mitochondrial biogenetic role in the pathophysiology of psychological stress-mediated CVD.

To conclude, research in the area of cardiovascular reactivity and psychological stress varies regarding study design (longitudinal, observational, cross-sectional), selection of populations, and assessments of various measures of dependent variables (endothelial function, biomarkers, arterial stiffness, FBF, HR, HRV, BP, mitochondrial function). This flexibility allows researchers across multiple disciplines (e.g., psychology, physiology, etc.) to study the degree to which stress modulates cardiovascular function and how interventions may attenuate potential negative effects.

Table of Abbreviations

Abbreviation	Meaning
ADP	Adenosine Diphosphate
ATP	Adenosine Triphosphate
Aix	Augmentation Index
ATP	Adenosine Triphosphate
BMI	Body Mass Index
BP	Blood Pressure
CI-IV	Complex I-IV
CAVI	Cardio-Ankle Vascular Index
CDI	Children's Depression Inventory
COI	Cytochrome c Oxidase subunit I
CORT	Cortisol
CSQ	Children's Stress Questionnaire
CVD	Cardiovascular Disease
DNA	Deoxyribonucleic Acid
EPI	Epinephrine
ETS	Electron Transfer System
FBF	Forearm Blood Flow
FMD	Flow-Mediated Dilation
HPA	Hypothalamic-Pituitary Adrenal Axis
HR	Heart Rate
HRV	Heart Rate Variability
ICAM-1	Intercellular Adhesion Molecule-1
IL	Interleukin
LPS	Lipopolysaccharides
MHI	Mitochondrial Health Index
NK	Natural Killer Cells
NOR	Norepinephrine
OXPHOS	Mitochondrial Oxidative Phosphorylation
PBMCs	Peripheral Blood Mononuclear Cells
PWV	Pulse Wave Velocity
SAM	Sympatho-Adrenal Medullary
SBP	Systolic Blood Pressure
SCWT	Stroop Color and Word Test
TNF-α	Tumor Necrosis Factor alpha
VO_{2max}	Maximal Oxygen Uptake

References

American Psychological Association. (2018). *Stress in America: Stress and generation Z*. Retrieved April 3, 2020, from www.apa.org/news/press/releases/stress/

Benschop, R. J., Rodriguez-Feuerhahn, M., & Schedlowski, M. (1996). Catecholamine-induced leukocytosis: Early observations, current research, and future directions. *Brain, Behavior, and Immunity, 10*(2), 77–91.

Bierhaus, A., Wolf, J., Andrassy, M., Rohleder, N., Humpert, P. M., Petrov, et al. (2003). A mechanism converting psychosocial stress into mononuclear cell activation. *Proceedings of the National Academy of Sciences, 100*(4), 1920–1925.

Bories, G., Caiazzo, R., Derudas, B., Copin, C., Raverdy, V., Pigeyre, M., et al. (2012). Impaired alternative macrophage differentiation of peripheral blood mononuclear cells from obese subjects. *Diabetes & Vascular Disease Research, 9*(3), 189–195.

Brothers, R. M., Wingo, J. E., Hubing, K. A., & Crandall, C. G. (2010, September). Methodological assessment of skin and limb blood flows in the human forearm during thermal and baroreceptor provocations. *Journal of Applied Physiology (1985), 109*(3), 895–900.

Brydon, L., Edwards, S., Jia, H., Mohamed-Ali, V., Zachary, I., Martin, J. F., et al. (2005). Psychological stress activates interleukin-1β gene expression in human mononuclear cells. *Brain, Behavior, and Immunity, 19*(6), 540–546.

Carroll, D., Ginty, A. T., Der, G., Hunt, K., Benzeval, M., & Phillips, A. C. (2012). Increased blood pressure reactions to acute mental stress are associated with 16-year cardiovascular disease mortality. *Psychophysiology, 49*(10), 1444–1448.

Chandrakumar, D., Dyck, D., Boutcher, S. H., & Boutcher, Y. N. (2018). Acute effect of aerobic exercise on cardiovascular reactivity of overweight males. *International Journal of Human Movement and Sports Sciences, 6*(3), 47–54.

Chen, H., Zhang, L., Zhang, M., Song, X., Zhang, H., Liu, Y., et al. (2013). Relationship of depression, stress and endothelial function in stable angina patients. *Physiology & Behavior, 118*, 152–158.

Chida, Y., & Steptoe, A. (2010). Greater cardiovascular responses to laboratory mental stress are associated with poor subsequent cardiovascular risk status: A meta-analysis of prospective evidence. *Hypertension, 55*(4), 1026–1032.

Côco, H., & de Oliveira, A. M. (2015). Endothelial dysfunction induced by chronic psychological stress: A risk factor for atherosclerosis. *Cardiovascular Pharmacology, 4*(5), 168–173.

Du, J., Wang, Y., Hunter, R., Wei, Y., Blumenthal, R., Falke, C., et al. (2009). Dynamic regulation of mitochondrial function by glucocorticoids. *Proceedings of the National Academy of Sciences, 106*(9), 3543–3548.

Dube, J. J., Coen, P. M., DiStefano, G., Chacon, A. C., Helbling, N. L., Desimone, M. E., et al. (2014, December 15). Effects of acute lipid overload on skeletal muscle insulin resistance, metabolic flexibility, and mitochondrial performance. *American Journal of Physiology-Endocrinology & Metabolism, 307*(12), E1117–E1124.

Elenkov, I. J. (2004). Glucocorticoids and the Th1/Th2 balance. *Annals of the New York Academy of Sciences, 1024*(1), 138–146.

Elenkov, I. J., Wilder, R. L., Chrousos, G. P., & Vizi, E. S. (2000). The sympathetic nerve: An integrative interface between two supersystems: The brain and the immune system. *Pharmacological Reviews, 52*(4), 595–638.

Enc, Y., Karaca, P., Ayoglu, U., Camur, G., Kurc, E., & Cicek, S. (2006). The acute cardioprotective effect of glucocorticoid in myocardial ischemia-reperfusion injury occurring during cardiopulmonary bypass. *Heart and Vessels, 21*(3), 152–156.

Flatmark, T. (2000). Catecholamine biosynthesis and physiological regulation in neuroendocrine cells. *Acta Physiologica Scandaniva, 168*(1), 1–17.

Gauche, R., Lima, R. M., Myers, J., Gadelha, A. B., Neri, S. G., Forjaz, C. L. M., et al. (2017). Blood pressure reactivity to mental stress is attenuated following resistance exercise in older hypertensive women. *Clinical Interventions in Aging, 12*, 793–803.

Gesi, M., Fornai, F., Lenzi, P., Ferrucci, M., Soldani, P., Ruffoli, R., et al. (2002). Morphological alterations induced by loud noise in the myocardium: The role of benzodiazepine receptors [Review]. *Microscopy Research and Technique, 59*(2), 136–146.

Ghiadoni, L., Donald, A. E., Cropley, M., Mullen, M. J., Oakley, G., Taylor, M., et al. (2000). Mental stress induces transient endothelial dysfunction in humans. *Circulation, 102*(20), 2473–2478.

Gnam, J.-P., Loeffler, S.-N., Haertel, S., Engel, F., Hey, S., Boes, K., et al. (2019). On the relationship between physical activity, physical fitness, and stress reactivity to a real-life mental stressor. *International Journal of Stress Management, 26*(4), 344–355.

Gu, H.-F., Tang, C.-K., & Yang, Y.-Z. (2012). Psychological stress, immune response, and atherosclerosis. *Atherosclerosis, 223*(1), 69–77.

Herman, J. P., & Cullinan, W. E. (1997). Neurocircuitry of stress: Central control of the hypothalamo-pituitary-adrenocortical axis. *Trends in Neuroscience, 20*(2), 78–84.

Huang, C. J., Acevedo, E. O., Mari, D. C., Randazzo, C., & Shibata, Y. (2014). Glucocorticoid inhibition of leptin- and lipopolysaccharide-induced interleukin-6 production in obesity. *Brain Behavior & Immunity, 35*, 163–168.

Karabatsiakis, A., Bock, C., Salinas-Manrique, J., Kolassa, S., Calzia, E., Dietrich, D. E., et al. (2014). Mitochondrial respiration in peripheral blood mononuclear cells correlates with depressive subsymptoms and severity of major depression. *Translational Psychiatry, 4*, e397.

Kershaw, K. N., Lane-Cordova, A. D., Carnethon, M. R., Tindle, H. A., & Liu, K. (2016). Chronic stress and endothelial dysfunction: The Multi-Ethnic Study of Atherosclerosis (MESA). *American Journal of Hypertension, 30*(1), 75–80.

Kuvin, J. T., Patel, A. R., Sliney, K. A., Pandian, N. G., Sheffy, J., Schnall, et al. (2003). Assessment of peripheral vascular endothelial function with finger arterial pulse wave amplitude. *American Heart Journal, 146*(1), 168–174.

Langewouters, G., Settels, J., Roelandt, R., & Wesseling, K. (1998). Why use Finapres or Portapres rather than intraarterial or intermittent non-invasive techniques of blood pressure measurement? *Journal of Medical Engineering & Technology, 22*(1), 37–43.

Liu, X. H., Qian, L. J., Gong, J. B., Shen, J., Zhang, X. M., & Qian, X. H. (2004). Proteomic analysis of mitochondrial proteins in cardiomyocytes from chronic stressed rat. *Proteomics, 4*(10), 3167–3176.

Lumley, M. A., Shi, W., Wiholm, C., Slatcher, R. B., Sandmark, H., Wang, S., et al. (2014). The Relationship of chronic and momentary work stress to cardiac reactivity in female managers: Feasibility of a smart phone-assisted assessment system. *Psychosomatic Medicine, 76*(7), 512–518.

Marsland, A. L., Walsh, C., Lockwood, K., & John-Henderson, N. A. (2017). The effects of acute psychological stress on circulating and stimulated inflammatory markers: A systematic review and meta-analysis. *Brain Behavior & Immunity, 64*, 208–219.

Maruhashi, T., Soga, J., Fujimura, N., Idei, N., Mikami, S., Iwamoto, Y., et al. (2013). Relationship between flow-mediated vasodilation and cardiovascular risk factors in a large community-based study. *Heart*, heartjnl-2013-304739.

Maydych, V., Claus, M., Dychus, N., Ebel, M., Damaschke, J., Diestel, S., et al. (2017). Impact of chronic and acute academic stress on lymphocyte subsets and monocyte function. *PLoS One, 12*(11), e0188108.

McEwen, B. S. (2000). Allostasis and allostatic load: Implications for neuropsychopharmacology. *Neuropsychopharmacology, 22*(2), 108–124.

Miller, G. E., Chen, E., Fok, A. K., Walker, H., Lim, A., Nicholls, E. F., et al. (2009). Low early-life social class leaves a biological residue manifested by decreased glucocorticoid and increased proinflammatory signaling. *Proceedings of the National Academy of Science of the United States of America, 106*(34), 14716–14721.

Miller, G. E., Murphy, M. L., Cashman, R., Ma, R., Ma, J., Arevalo, A., et al. (2014). Greater inflammatory activity and blunted glucocorticoid signaling in monocytes of chronically stressed caregivers. *Brain Behavior & Immunity, 41*, 191–199.

Mishra, P., & Chan, D. C. (2016). Metabolic regulation of mitochondrial dynamics [Research Support, N.I.H., Extramural Research Support, Non-U.S. Gov't Review]. *The Journal of Cell Biology, 212*(4), 379–387.

Olinski, R., Gackowski, D., Foksinski, M., Rozalski, R., Roszkowski, K., & Jaruga, P. (2002). Oxidative DNA damage: Assessment of the role in carcinogenesis, atherosclerosis, and acquired immunodeficiency syndrome1. *Free Radical Biology and Medicine, 33*(2), 192–200.

Olive, L. S., Abhayaratna, W. P., Byrne, D., Richardson, A., & Telford, R. D. (2018). Do self-reported stress and depressive symptoms effect endothelial function in healthy youth? The LOOK longitudinal study. *PloS One, 13*(4), e0196137.

Pesta, D., & Gnaiger, E. (2012). High-resolution respirometry: OXPHOS protocols for human cells and permeabilized fibers from small biopsies of human muscle [Research Support, Non-U.S. Gov't]. *Methods in Molecular Biology, 810*, 25–58.

Picard, M., McManus, M. J., Gray, J. D., Nasca, C., Moffat, C., Kopinski, et al. (2015). Mitochondrial functions modulate neuroendocrine, metabolic, inflammatory, and transcriptional responses to acute psychological stress [Research Support, N.I.H., Extramural Research Support, Non-U.S. Gov't]. *Proceedings of the National Academy of Sciences of the United States of America, 112*(48), E6614–6623.

Picard, M., Prather, A. A., Puterman, E., Cuillerier, A., Coccia, M., Aschbacher, K., et al. (2018). A mitochondrial health index sensitive to mood and caregiving stress. *Biological Psychiatry, 84*(1), 9–17.

Picard, M., Wallace, D. C., & Burelle, Y. (2016). The rise of mitochondria in medicine. *Mitochondrion, 30*, 105–116.

Premer, C., Kanelidis, A. J., Hare, J. M., & Schulman, I. H. (2019). Rethinking endothelial dysfunction as a crucial target in fighting heart failure. *Mayo Clinic Proceedings: Innovations, Quality & Outcomes, 3*(1), 1–13.

Rouppe van der Voort, C., Kavelaars, A., van de Pol, M., & Heijnen, C. J. (2000). Noradrenaline induces phosphorylation of ERK-2 in human peripheral blood mononuclear cells after induction of alpha(1)-adrenergic receptors. *Journal of Neuroimmunology, 108*(1–2), 82–91.

Sapolsky, R. M., Romero, L. M., & Munck, A. U. (2000). How do glucocorticoids influence stress responses? Integrating permissive, suppressive, stimulatory, and preparative actions. *Endocrine Reviews, 21*(1), 55–89.

Sauer, J., Polack, E., Wikinski, S., Holsboer, F., Stalla, G. K., & Arzt, E. (1995). The glucocorticoid sensitivity of lymphocytes changes according to the activity of the hypothalamic-pituitary-adrenocortical system. *Psychoneuroendocrinology, 20*(3), 269–280.

Singhai, A. (2005). Endothelial dysfunction: Role in obesity-related disorders and the early original of CVD. *Proceedings of the Nutrition Society, 64*, 15–22.

Tanaka, H. (2018). Various indices of arterial stiffness: Are they closely related or distinctly different? *Pulse (Basel), 5*(1–4), 1–6.

Tierney, E. S. S., Newburger, J. W., Gauvreau, K., Geva, J., Coogan, E., Colan, S. D., et al. (2009). Endothelial pulse amplitude testing: Feasibility and reproducibility in adolescents. *The Journal of Pediatrics, 154*(6), 901–905.

van den Akker, E. L. T., Koper, J. W., van Rossum, E. F. C., Dekker, M. J. H., Russcher, H., de Jong, F. H., et al. (2008). Glucocorticoid receptor gene and risk of cardiovascular disease. *Archives of Internal Medicine*, *168*(1), 33–39.

Walker, B. R. (2007). Glucocorticoids and cardiovascular disease. *European Journal of Endocrinology*, *157*(5), 545–559.

Whitworth, J. A., Williamson, P. M., Mangos, G., & Kelly, J. J. (2005). Cardiovascular consequences of cortisol excess [Review]. *Vascular Health and Risk Management*, *1*(4), 291–299.

Williams, J. K., Kaplan, J. R., & Manuck, S. B. (1993). Effects of psychosocial stress on endothelium-mediated dilation of atherosclerotic arteries in cynomolgus monkeys. *The Journal of Clinical Investigation*, *92*(4), 1819–1823.

Wirtz, P. H., & von Kanel, R. (2017). Psychological stress, inflammation, and coronary heart disease. *Current Cardiology Reports*, *19*(11), 111.

Zygmunt, A., & Stanczyk, J. (2010). Methods of evaluation of autonomic nervous system function. *Archives of Medical Science*, *6*(1), 11–18.

12

OBESITY AND NUTRITION
Physiological Studies

Diana M. Thomas and J. Kenneth Wickiser

Overview

Obesity and nutrition interventions often provide patients with a focused lifestyle change strategy such as altering energy consumed or physical activity (The Diabetes Prevention Program. Design and methods for a clinical trial in the prevention of type 2 diabetes, 1999; Kelley, 2002; Ross, Hudson, Day, & Lam, 2013). To effectively deliver the intervention, an investigator or clinician needs objective and accurate knowledge of how much energy is being consumed and/or expended during the intervention to monitor patient compliance. Despite this critical need, interventionists have struggled for nearly a century to find feasible, quantitative, noninvasive, and trustworthy methods to measure energy intake and physical activity–driven energy expenditure (Dhurandhar, Schoeller, Brown, Heymsfield, Thomas, Sorensen, et al., 2015).

Research in Practice

In 1915, Francis G. Benedict published a 31-day fasting-in-residence experiment using carefully collected psychological, metabolic, anthropometric (for example, weight, height, waist circumference), and biometric data from a single participant (Benedict, Goodall, Ash, Langfeld, Kendall, & Higgins, 1915). This landmark study provided stunning new insights into the changes in body weight regulation during weight loss. The results of the study are still being used for first principles–based models of human body weight regulation today (Song & Thomas, 2007). Benedict knew at the time that the only available method to collect objective data on a human participant undergoing fasting was by directly monitoring the participant in-residence in a metabolic ward. While full objective knowledge of energy intake and physical activity were known, the high cost of housing and monitoring subjects restricted Benedict to a sample size of one. In fact, until approximately the early 1970s, nutrition studies were performed largely in-residence and hence were limited to small participant samples (Grande, 1968; Passmore, 1963; University of Minnesota, Laboratory of Physiological Hygiene & Keys, 1950).

As obesity prevalence rates jumped in the early 1970s, funding agencies were less inclined to support small sample size experiments, and the obesity and nutrition research community moved away from direct monitoring of energy intake and energy expenditure. To estimate energy intake and expenditure in larger-sized populations, investigators began to rely on food intake and physical activity questionnaires. However, in 1982, Dale Schoeller was the first to employ a quantitative approach based on an analytical chemistry technique using an isotopically labeled molecule to directly measure energy expenditure in free-living humans (Schoeller & van Santen, 1982). From this **doubly labeled water method (DLW)**, it was revealed that individuals tended to underreport energy intake and overreport energy expenditure on questionnaires (Lichtman, Pisarska, Berman, Pestone, Dowling, Offenbacher, et al., 1992). Unfortunately, the *DLW* method is expensive and unfeasible to use in large-scale epidemiological studies. Thus, while *DLW* demonstrated the unreliability of questionnaires to measure energy intake and expenditure, the method is rarely used as a routine analytic tool for obesity and nutrition interventions. Despite the expense of *DLW* and the need for laboratory analysis of samples, *DLW* remains the gold standard for measuring energy intake in free-living humans. In addition, a wealth of new and existing biochemical methods are being developed to evaluate macronutrient-level (carbohydrate, protein, and fat) intake in free-living humans (Schoeller, 2013).

Recently, wearable technologies and digital imaging have revolutionized the field of nutrition and obesity research, allowing clinicians and researchers, for the first time, to quantitatively assess energy intake and expenditure in free-living individuals using these relatively inexpensive and noninvasive devices. Treatment plans guided by feedback from these technologies and customized for individuals are referred to as **just-in-time adaptive interventions** (**JITAI**; J. G. Thomas & Bond, 2015). *JITAI*, delivered to a patient's natural, free-living environment, leverages information from wearable sensors, mobile phones, and user-interface software. The technologies capture real-time patient behavior and biometric data, which are then used to continuously adapt and convey personalized treatment recommendations back to the patient.

Whereas clinical trials suffer from high patient dropout due to burdens of frequent in-person measurements (Little, D'Agostino, Cohen, Dickersin, Emerson, Farrar, et al., 2012), *JITAI* offer an opportunity to reduce this burden and provide instantaneous and adaptive feedback best suited for the individual patient. While the wearable technologies powering *JITAI* strategies have only recently emerged, the first sets of experimental data demonstrate highly promising results. We describe five recent obesity-related successful *JITAIs* with different primary outcomes based on a variety of wearable technologies.

A Just-in-Time Adaptive Intervention to Reduce Sedentary Behavior

Sedentary behavior and obesity-related comorbidities (Chaput, Barnes, Tremblay, Fogelholm, Hu, Lambert, et al., 2018; Shields & Tremblay, 2008) are highly correlated with mortality (Klenk, Dallmeier, Denkinger, Rapp, Koenig, Rothenbacher, et al., 2016; Nunez, Nair-Shalliker, Egger, Sitas, & Bauman, 2018; Patterson, McNamara, Tainio, de Sa, Smith, Sharp, et al., 2018). Increases in physical activity, on the other hand, have positive health effects (Burn, Norton, Drummond, & Ian Norton, 2017). Therefore, behavioral interventions that improve physical activity in sedentary populations are valuable and effective. With the affordability and accessibility of accelerometers, either through smartphones or as a stand-alone device, the opportunity for directly measuring movement to facilitate personalized physical activity behavior modification is now possible. Accelerometers are devices that can measure acceleration and are used to track movement in devices like Fitbits.

To interrupt sedentary time, a recent study encouraged 30 participants to take walking breaks, prompted by smartphone pings from a wearable fitness sensor, after sensing a period of sedentary time (Bond, Thomas, Raynor, Moon, Sieling, Trautvetter, et al., 2014; J. G. Thomas & Bond, 2015). To investigate the optimal time to break up inactive periods, three different strategies were delivered: The first was a prompt for a three-minute walking break after sensing a 30-minute continuous block of sedentary time. The second was a prompt for a six-minute walking break after a 60-minute block of inactivity. Finally, a 12-minute walking break prompt was delivered after sensing a 120-minute block of sedentary time. The three conditions were delivered to participants in a randomized, counterbalanced order through smartphones. Each condition was presented for a seven-day period after an initial seven-day baseline period with no prompts. The wearable sensor was used to measure total sedentary time, light physical activity time, and moderate-to-vigorous physical activity time in minutes.

All three prompts generated a decrease in sedentary time from baseline measurements. Inactivity was reduced by 5.9%, 5.6%, and 3.3% for three-, six-, and 12-minute prompts, respectively. The three-minute prompt led to the optimal decrease in sedentary time and an increase in light physical activity

Strengths and Weaknesses

One major strength of this study was the use of wearable technology to discover best practices quickly and effectively during the course of the experiment when the optimal strategy was unknown *a priori*. The authors determined that delivering prompts more frequently with smaller walking iterations proved most effective. They also found that all prompt conditions led to decreases in sedentary time.

The limitation of this preliminary study was its short duration. Future work should focus on conducting a longer study with a larger, more diverse cohort.

A Just-in-Time Adaptive Intervention to Reduce Energy Intake

As noted in the introduction, a major challenge in obesity and nutrition research is determining how much, when, and what individuals are consuming. Over the past decade, several novel portable eating sensors have been developed. A partial list of examples include a wrist-worn watch that detects movements from hand to mouth (Jasper, James, Hoover, & Muth, 2016), an ear-worn sensor that detects chewing and swallowing (Sazonov, Schuckers, Lopez-Meyer, Makeyev, Sazonova, Melanson, et al., 2008), and a fork sensor that detects biting and provides the subject physical feedback through fork vibrations if bites are taken too quickly (Hermsen, Frost, Robinson, Higgs, Mars, & Hermans, 2016). In the study outlined here (Farooq, McCrory, & Sazonov, 2017), a sensor was designed to capture movement of the temporalis muscles on both sides of the head that are used for chewing. Sensor feedback was provided to the participant to modify eating behavior in real time.

Eighteen adult participants were equipped in a laboratory with the sensor for three meals over three visits. Participants were provided a baseline meal to capture baseline chew counts. Enough food and water were provided so that the participants could consume as much as they desired until they felt full. During the second and third visits, a goal was set to either match 100% of the participant's baseline chew count or reduce their chew count by 25%. Participants were placed in one of two conditions using a randomized, counterbalanced order. During the meal, chew counts were monitored by the sensor and the participants were guided by audio as they approached their target number of chews. Participants heard messages indicating what percentage of the desired goal was reached. When they reached the limit, they were directed to stop. The participants and experimenter were blinded as to whether the target number of chews was baseline levels or a reduction from the individual's baseline. Furthermore, participants were not informed that an aim of the study was to investigate behavior modification, but rather were informed that a sensor system was being evaluated.

In addition to collecting sensor data, participants rated the food palatability and their satiety using a visual analog scale (Couper, Tourangeau, & Conrad, 2006).

The total food mass consumed was significantly lower in the 25% reduction group (median 10.1% lower) compared to both the baseline and the 100% groups. On the other hand, the food mass consumed during the 100% target meal was not significantly different from the quantity of food consumed at baseline. While the length of the meal was not significantly different in the 100% compared to the baseline meal, the reduced chew meal was significantly shorter in duration. There were no statistically different changes in food palatability and satiety scores across meals.

Strengths and Weaknesses

Farooq, et al. (2017) effectively used a chewing sensor to modify behavior. The study also leveraged novel information from wearable eating sensors to produce an unbiased and quantitative assessment of food intake while providing the subjects with real-time feedback to modify behavior. For example, the chewing sensor can detect meal duration automatically. In fact, most of the chewing sensors also automatically detect the timing of eating episodes. That is, the sensor can automatically detect when an individual starts eating and when they end.

While the preliminary study results are promising, the intervention was performed in a laboratory setting. It is unknown how the results will transfer to free-living individuals. Will individuals be compliant and wear the device, integrated into eyeglasses, at all meals? Will the individual feel comfortable wearing the device in public restaurant settings? Future work should attempt to overcome these limitations through device design changes to meet the needs of a broader population using the sensors in their own environment.

A Smartphone-Based Gestational Weight Gain Intervention

In 2009, the Institute of Medicine (IOM) compiled a comprehensive list of quality research studies evaluating pregnancy weight gain and pregnancy outcomes (Rasmussen, Yaktine, & Institute of Medicine (U.S.). Committee to Reexamine IOM Pregnancy Weight Guidelines, 2009). The IOM review led to a pre-pregnancy, ***body mass index (BMI)***–specific set of ***gestational weight gain (GWG)*** recommendations, which have been validated by prospective studies. Gaining weight within the guidelines leads to positive pregnancy outcomes, while gaining outside the guidelines is associated with adverse outcomes (Asvanarunat, 2014; Siegel, Tita, Machemehl, Biggio, & Harper, 2017; Yee, Cheng, Inturrisi, & Caughey, 2011). Unfortunately, studies show that two-thirds of women exceed the IOM guidelines for weight gain during pregnancy (Rasmussen, et al., 2009). In addition, women with overweight and obesity factors are most at risk for exceeding *GWG* guidelines. Since nearly two-thirds of women of reproductive age are either overweight or obese (*At A Glance, 2016 Women's Reproductive Health Improving the Health of Women and Families*), a reliably accurate, feasible, and scalable method to facilitate behavior modification and adherence to target dietary goals is important.

The SmartMoms intervention program enrolled 54 pregnant, overweight, and/or obese women between the ages of 18 and 40, with the goal of keeping women within the IOM gestational guidelines during pregnancy. Three groups were designated for this study. The first group, the intervention SmartMoms group, was treated remotely using smartphones that recorded daily weights when participants stood on a scale equipped with wireless technology. These weights were then superimposed on graphs of the IOM guidelines. A validated differential equation model (D. M. Thomas, Navarro-Barrientos, Rivera, Heymsfield, Bredlau, Redman, et al., 2012) was programmed into the smartphones to assign dietary intake recommendations and objectively monitor energy intake during pregnancy. The model was not developed using data as in statistically derived models, but instead relied on a law of physics: the first law of thermodynamics. When the first law of thermodynamics is applied to humans, it reduces to the energy balance equation, where the rate of energy stored is equal to the rate of energy consumed minus the rate of energy expended. Physical activity was measured using a step counter, or ***pedometer***. The weight graphs could also be accessed by counselors, and deviations from acceptable ranges set by the IOM guidelines resulted in real-time, personalized feedback and treatment recommendations.

SmartMoms in two intervention groups were trained by counselors on how to adjust their energy intake or physical activity to remain within the IOM guidelines. The training consisted of 18 lessons on behavior modification strategies. An example of training included appropriate goal setting, like setting a 500-calorie dinner goal instead of simply eating too much. Other examples included tips to modify diet, for example, receiving home delivery of groceries or consuming the clinic's provided foods. In addition, the SmartMoms participants received behavior modification counseling weekly between their first and second trimester and then biweekly thereafter until delivery.

Two other groups were measured: a usual-care control group that received no intervention and an in-person clinic group that received the weight graphs and guidance in person as opposed to remote delivery. The training materials for in-person interventions were identical to those for the Smart-Moms group delivered remotely. Outcome measures included the proportion of women that met the IOM GWG guidelines, adherence to the program, and costs to participants.

A lower proportion of women in both intervention groups (SmartMoms delivered in person and SmartMoms delivered remotely; 56% and 58%, respectively) recorded weight gains in excess of the IOM *GWG* guidelines compared to the usual or normal standard-of-care group (85%)—a difference that was statistically significant. Total costs were also tabulated for each participant. This included travel to and from the clinic, time spent with the counselor, interventionist time, and special equipment (scale, *pedometer*). Costs for the remote intervention group participants were substantial compared to in-person intervention expenses. The remote group also reported higher adherence to the program than the in-person group: 77% versus 61%, respectively.

Strengths and Weaknesses

The smartphone-delivered intervention to guide GWG to meet the IOM guidelines was an affordable and effective intervention compared to both in-person guidance and usual care. Because the feedback from electronic scales and the weight graphs were accomplished daily, women tended to adhere more to the remotely delivered program. This smartphone-based intervention is also scalable to larger population sizes.

The main limitation of any intervention during pregnancy is that low-income women receive pregnancy care at lower rates. Women in lower socioeconomic strata are less likely to be able to afford or own their own weight scale, to know their weight from routine physicals, or to seek clinical care early in gestation (Olson, Strawderman, & Graham, 2017). These circumstances could be changed with community-wide interventions like the B'More for Healthy Babies program ("B'More for Healthy Babies").

The B'More Healthy Babies program is a Baltimore-based, city-wide initiative that was started in response to the recognition of Baltimore's infant mortality public health crisis of 2009 (Truiett-Theodorson, Tuck, Bowie, Summers, & Kelber-Kaye, 2015). The B'More Healthy Babies program, led by the Baltimore City Health Department, assembled a coalition of community organizations to deliver evidence-based interventions that targeted the causes of infant mortality rates, one of them being maternal obesity. Currently, there are freely available weight management programs to help women enter pregnancies at a healthy *BMI*, but no interventions in the program target excessive GWG. Remote technologies like SmartMoms would fill this gap, are affordable, and could scale well within a community intervention like B'More Healthy Babies. Future work should evaluate the capacity of SmartMoms to be used in a large-scale community intervention. Specifically, research should focus on whether smartphone delivery is a viable option for low-income communities. More importantly, it should examine how intervention and technology design should be modified to optimize intervention outcomes for diverse populations.

School-Based Obesity Prevention Intervention

In response to an alarming increase in childhood obesity prevalence rates (Ogden, Carroll, Kit, & Flegal, 2014), there have been concerted efforts to implement school-based nutrition and physical activity intervention programs (Atkinson & Nitzke, 2002; Neumark-Sztainer, Story, Hannan, & Re, 2003). To evaluate program efficacy, administrators have relied on outcome data, such as *BMI-z* scores (Bogart, Elliott, Cowgill, Klein, Hawes-Dawson, Uyeda, et al., 2016); however, *BMI-z* scores provide no information about changes in children's nutrition and overall food choices. Similarly, self-reported food diaries are poor measures. They are unfeasible in children and typically are reported by parents or guardians (Yonemori, Ennis, Novotny, Fialkowski, Ettienne, Wilkens, et al., 2017). Recently, Louisiana employed a semi-automatic procedure to estimate energy intake. The goal was to design an objective measure of food intake for children (Hawkins, Burton, Apolzan, Thomson, Williamson, & Martin, 2018) to evaluate the efficacy of a program to reduce sugar and sodium consumption in children's school lunches.

The Louisiana (LA) Healthy study was a randomized, cluster-controlled, school-based intervention trial designed to promote healthy eating and improve physical activity over 28 months. Thirty-three elementary schools, consisting of 1,626 students in Louisiana, participated in the program from 2006 to 2009, with the goal of inhibiting inappropriate weight gain in children from fourth through sixth grades. Over the course of the program, students were followed up in sixth through eighth grades.

The program was delivered in two components: a primary component targeting changes in the school environment to promote healthy eating and increased physical activity for all students and a secondary component (i.e., the intervention arm), delivered to a segment of students using computer modules designed to improve healthy eating and physical activity through behavior modification (Gabriele, Stewart, Sample, Davis, Allen, Martin, et al., 2010). The education modules differed based on student weight status. Normal-weight children received education on weight maintenance, while overweight children received education on weight loss. The computer modules also included age-appropriate links to a lesson of the week, games and activities, and the ability to chat with or email their internet counselor. For example, lessons included choosing healthy items to place into a grocery cart or selecting healthy snacks. If an internet counselor in the LA Healthy program was online, the students could chat directly with the counselor. Students could also send and receive emails with an internet counselor if they desired.

Children's food selection, consumption, plate waste, sodium, and sugar were measured in control and intervention arms for three continuous days using a ***digital food photography*** method at baseline, 18 months, and 28 months. The digital photography method first obtains digital images of food selected and placed on a plate immediately before and again after eating using two digital video cameras (Sony DCR-TRV22; Sony Electronics). One camera was used to photograph the selected food at the beginning of the meal, and the second camera was used to photograph the outgoing trays, which represented food waste. Differences between food selections and plate waste defined food intake. Digital photographs of selected food and waste were analyzed by a computer program developed to estimate food portions from digital photographs. The computer program allowed raters to simultaneously compare a reference portion for each food with the food selected and with plate waste. Two raters independently estimated what percentage of the reference portion appeared in each photograph by 10% increments. The rater's estimates were input into another computer program called the Remote Food Photography Method that estimates food composition using the Pennington Biomedical Research Center nutrient database. This method of digital assessment has been demonstrated to reliably and accurately classify the type of foods selected, measure portion size, and estimate caloric content (Rose, Streisand, Aronow, Tully, Martin, & Mackey, 2018).

Findings from this study revealed that both treatment and duration of study (18 months vs. 28 months) affected food selection and consumption. By month 18, sodium consumption decreased by approximately 206 mg per lunch in the intervention group compared to controls. Moreover, added sugar consumption decreased by 3.7 tsp per lunch. At month 28, there were significant differences in energy consumption with a greater reduction in the intervention arm.

Strengths and Weaknesses

Digital food photography presents an accurate and objective measurement of total energy intake, food selection, and composition of nutrients that replaces the need for food questionnaires. A limitation of the method is that it requires a ruler to be placed next to the plate to estimate portion size and to enable identification of individuals enrolled in the study. Individuals also know that their food is being photographed and may choose to modify their behavior as a result. However, inclusion of a control group that is also undergoing digital food photography minimizes the intervention effect in this study. Finally, the algorithm is also not completely automated. The method requires human evaluation combined with a computer algorithm. Despite these limitations, the digital food method offers a strong alternative to evaluate not only energy intake but also food choices made by individuals.

Novel Biochemical Analysis of Food Intake and Energy Expenditure

The two modifiable components of energy balance, energy intake and energy expenditure, can be measured using biochemical analysis. With an emerging focus on obesity treatments altering *macronutrient* composition of diets (Razmpoosh, Zare, Fallahzadeh, Safi, & Nadjarzadeh, 2020; Witjaksono, Jutamulia, Annisa, Prasetya, & Nurwidya, 2018; Wright, Zhou, Sayer, Kim, & Campbell, 2018), objectively tracing total energy (Schoeller & van Santen, 1982), protein (Bingham, 2003), and carbohydrate intake (Schoeller, 2013) is critical. The use of chemical labels to track compounds as they enter a chemical reaction, are acted upon, and are changed by enzymes and cofactors was a key method used in dissecting the complex network of coupled chemical reactions involved in human metabolism. While a plethora of useful and unique types of chemical labels such as fluorophores and nuclear spin-labeled molecules exists, the gold standard in characterizing biochemical pathways over the past 80 years has been the use of *stable isotopes*, such as carbon, nitrogen, oxygen, or hydrogen atoms, with additional neutrons allowing the detection of that specific atom and where it resides in the metabolic line from precursor compound to a variety of products. Compounds such as *amino acids*, the monomer building blocks of proteins, contain all four elements and have the capacity to be labeled at one or more sites on each molecule. Herein we describe three stable isotopic labeling tools relied on by many biochemical research teams (Wilkinson, 2018). While the cost of implementing biochemical labeling tools may have previously seemed out of reach, increased collaboration across disciplines is making it possible to include biochemical analysis within obesity interventions to guide participants accurately and to evaluate adherence post-hoc.

The Doubly Labeled Water Method

Water, or *dihydrogen monoxide*, is a molecule of one oxygen atom and two hydrogen atoms. The addition of a single neutron to the complement of protons in the nuclei of each of these atoms (termed isotopes of neutron-free versions of the same atoms) increases the mass of the molecule without changing the bulk characteristics of water or how this *DLW* is used in the human metabolic cycles involving energy, regeneration, and normal cellular and tissue maintenance. Yet *DLW* is chemically distinct enough from natural water to allow for precise chemical quantitation using standard mass spectrometer techniques. In short, the heavy *hydrogen isotope* leaves the body as water, whereas the heavy *oxygen isotope* leaves the body as both water and carbon dioxide. In collecting and analyzing the isotopic content of the water in subjects' urine, the isotopic fraction distributed across water and carbon dioxide is determined and the energetic expenditure is calculated based on that value. The experiment relies on expensive reagents, requires strict subject compliance with the experimental protocol, and demands a mass spectrometer capable of isotopic analysis (Westerterp, 2017). The financial cost per study participant is approximately $450 for the *DLW* dose and $150 for subsequent chemical analysis. Despite these challenges, the *DLW* method remains the gold standard for estimating energy intake by summing *DLW* measured energy expenditure with changes in body energy stores (Gilmore, Ravussin, Bray, Han, & Redman, 2014; Heymsfield, Peterson, Thomas, Hirezi, Zhang, Smith, et al., 2017).

A Carbon Isotope to Estimate Sugar Intake

Current nutrition research has focused on sugar intake (Bray & Popkin, 2014a, 2014b; Malik, Popkin, Bray, Despres, & Hu, 2010; Yang, Zhang, Gregg, Flanders, Merritt, & Hu, 2014). Therefore, nutrition interventions that aim to decrease participant sugar intake require objective knowledge of a participant's sugar consumption. Given the interrelated nature of the networks of genes and small-molecule metabolites in the energy production and storage pathways, it should come as no surprise that a common metabolite like a free amino acid could be used as a gauge to assess the amount and direction of energy processed through the network. An isotopically labeled carbohydrate (sugar) in a subject's food source could be tracked by analyzing the isotopic content of ***alanine*** in blood or urine, which reflects the energetic pathway as a part of the shunting mechanism between glycolysis and the production of acetyl-CoA. The isotopic analysis of *alanine* in biospecimens using a mass spectrometer provides a quantitative assessment of energy expenditure (Schoeller, 2013).

Protein Intake From Nitrogen Balance

Dietary interventions that increase protein intake have also received ongoing attention (Drummen, Tischmann, Gatta-Cherifi, Fogelholm, Raben, Adam, et al., 2020; Sousa, Ribeiro, Pinto, Sanches, da Silva, Coelho, et al., 2018; Wright, et al., 2018). Similar to tracking sugar intake, supplementing a subject's diet with excess natural or isotopically labeled *amino acids* provides a direct supply of the monomer building blocks of proteins to the subject. Excess *amino acids* will then be metabolized and used by several other circuits. The nitrogen-labeled *amino acids* can be assessed as proteins, ammonia, and other nitrogen-containing biomolecules using standard chemical separation techniques coupled with mass spectrometry (Smith, Arteaga, & Heymsfield, 1982).

To assess the food consumption and exertion of a study subject, one or more types of biospecimens must be collected, including urine, blood, or saliva. The different biospecimens must be handled and processed appropriately to ensure the chemical quantitation and identification techniques are able to measure the molecules of interest within these very complex mediums; these involved methodologies are described elsewhere. Should the experiment involve isotopically labeled consumables, the heavy carbon, nitrogen, oxygen, or hydrogen atoms can be separated chemically to identify the intermediate or product species into which they have been transferred. The mass spectrometer will then provide the abundance of each isotope of that element embedded within a particular molecule. For example, a ***13C-labeled carboxy*** terminus of a ***lysine molecule*** as a reactant at the outset of an experiment may end up in a *different amino acid* or another class of molecule altogether, depending on the needs of the cell and tissue. The tracing of these labeled molecules occurs by collecting biospecimens like serum, chemically or physically separating the targeted class of biomolecule (in this case, *amino acids*) from the others in the complex ensemble of molecules in the sample, and then quantifying the abundance of the isotope label within all *lysine molecules* captured in the sample.

The biospecimen collected at time points following the pulse of the isotopically labeled metabolite will reflect the kinetics of the processing of that metabolite, which is completely dependent upon the consumption of food and the activity intensity and duration during the experiment. As the isotope ratio returns to the pre-pulse levels or as the isotope is chemically transferred to a product compound, these data will reflect the temporal response of the metabolic networks, and a quantitative assessment of exertion and food consumption is determined.

Strengths and Weaknesses

For studies involving biochemical analysis of consumption and exertion, the use of isotopically labeled biomolecules allows for the participants to engage in routine daily lives outside the laboratory over the duration of the experiment. Similar to the sensor studies, the data obtained from biochemical analyses are objective. The limitation of biochemical methods includes the reliance on a laboratory and chemical analysis expertise, which may not be readily available in a nutrition or psychology department. Therefore, the cost of performing biochemical studies will also include laboratory equipment and external expertise. However, with strong interdisciplinary teams and recognition that self-reported data are not without cost, biochemical analyses can fill a gap needed for rigorous and objective data in nutrition and obesity studies where one can draw scientific conclusions.

Conclusion

Developing interventions for obesity treatment requires precise and reliable knowledge of two components of energy balance: energy intake and energy expenditure. For decades, investigators and clinicians relied on self-report surveys such as 24-hour recall, food frequency questionnaires, and physical activity questionnaires. With the advent of the biochemical *DLW* method, self-reported energy intake and energy expenditure have been deemed unreliable for developing accurate energy intake and energy expenditure targets for behavioral interventions (Dhurandhar, et al., 2015; Schoeller, Thomas, Archer, Heymsfield, Blair, Goran, et al., 2013). However, recent advances in novel, wearable sensor technology and biochemical analysis are transforming the field, offering affordable and reliable alternatives to measuring critical components of energy balance required to guide patients with obesity to healthy weight status. We propose that multidisciplinary teams with expertise in both biochemical and wearable device science are poised to provide accurate and quantitative data guiding the future of obesity and nutrition research.

References

Asvanarunat, E. (2014). Outcomes of gestational weight gain outside the Institute of Medicine Guidelines. *Journal of the Medical Association of Thailand*, *97*(11), 1119–1125.

At a glance 2016 women's reproductive health improving the health of women and families. Retrieved from www.cdc.gov/chronicdisease/resources/publications/aag.htm

Atkinson, R. L., & Nitzke, S. A. (2002). Randomized controlled trial of primary-school based intervention to reduce risk factors for obesity. *Journal of Pediatrics*, *140*(5), 633–634.

Benedict, F. G., Goodall, H. W., Ash, J. E., Langfeld, H. S., Kendall, A. I., & Higgins, (1915). *A study of prolonged fasting*. Washington, DC: Carnegie Institution of Washington.

Bingham, S. A. (2003). Urine nitrogen as a biomarker for the validation of dietary protein intake. *Journal of Nutrition*, *133 Suppl 3*(3), 921S–924S. doi:10.1093/jn/133.3.921S

B'More for healthy babies. Retrieved from https://health.baltimorecity.gov/maternal-and-child-health/bmore-healthy-babies

Bogart, L. M., Elliott, M. N., Cowgill, B. O., Klein, D. J., Hawes-Dawson, J., Uyeda, K., et al. (2016). Two-year BMI outcomes from a school-based intervention for nutrition and exercise: A randomized trial. *Pediatrics*, *137*(5). doi:10.1542/peds.2015-2493

Bond, D. S., Thomas, J. G., Raynor, H. A., Moon, J., Sieling, J., Trautvetter, J., et al. (2014). B-MOBILE: A smartphone-based intervention to reduce sedentary time in overweight/obese individuals: A within-subjects experimental trial. *PLoS One*, *9*(6), e100821. doi:10.1371/journal.pone.0100821

Bray, G. A., & Popkin, B. M. (2014a). Dietary sugar and body weight: Have we reached a crisis in the epidemic of obesity and diabetes? Health be damned! Pour on the sugar. *Diabetes Care*, *37*(4), 950–956. doi:10.2337/dc13-2085

Bray, G. A., & Popkin, B. M. (2014b). Sugar consumption by Americans and obesity are both too high: Are they connected? Response to letter by John White, PhD. *Pediatric Obesity*, *9*(5), e78–79. doi:10.1111/ijpo.214

Burn, N., Norton, L. H., Drummond, C., & Ian Norton, K. (2017). Changes in physical activity behaviour and health risk factors following a randomised controlled pilot workplace exercise intervention. *AIMS Public Health*, *4*(2), 189–201. doi:10.3934/publichealth.2017.2.189

Chaput, J. P., Barnes, J. D., Tremblay, M. S., Fogelholm, M., Hu, G., Lambert, E. V., et al. (2018). Thresholds of physical activity associated with obesity by level of sedentary behaviour in children. *Pediatric Obesity*. doi:10.1111/ijpo.12276

Couper, M. P., Tourangeau, R., & Conrad, F. G. (2006). Evaluating the effectiveness of visual analog scales: A web experiment. *Social Science Computer Review, 24*(2), 227–245.

Dhurandhar, N. V., Schoeller, D., Brown, A. W., Heymsfield, S. B., Thomas, D., Sorensen, et al. (2015). Energy balance measurement: When something is not better than nothing. *International Journal of Obesity (London), 39*(7), 1109–1113. doi:10.1038/ijo.2014.199

The Diabetes Prevention Program. Design and methods for a clinical trial in the prevention of type 2 diabetes. (1999). *Diabetes Care, 22*(4), 623–634. doi:10.2337/diacare.22.4.623

Drummen, M., Tischmann, L., Gatta-Cherifi, B., Fogelholm, M., Raben, A., Adam, T. C., et al. (2020). High compared with moderate protein intake reduces adaptive thermogenesis and induces a negative energy balance during long-term weight-loss maintenance in participants with prediabetes in the postobese state: A PREVIEW study. *Journal of Nutrition, 150*(3), 458–463. doi:10.1093/jn/nxz281

Farooq, M., McCrory, M. A., & Sazonov, E. (2017). Reduction of energy intake using just-in-time feedback from a wearable sensor system. *Obesity (Silver Spring), 25*(4), 676–681. doi:10.1002/oby.21788

Gabriele, J. M., Stewart, T. M., Sample, A., Davis, A. B., Allen, R., Martin, C. K., et al. (2010). Development of an internet-based obesity prevention program for children. *J Diabetes Sci Technol, 4*(3), 723–732. doi:10.1177/193229681000400328

Gilmoreou, L. A., Ravussin, E., Bray, G. A., Han, H., & Redman, L. M. (2014). An objective estimate of energy intake during weight gain using the intake-balance method. *American Journal of Clinical Nutrition, 100*(3), 806–812. doi:10.3945/ajcn.114.087122

Grande, F. (1968). Energetics and weight reduction. *American Journal of Clinical Nutrition, 21*(4), 305–314. doi:10.1093/ajcn/21.4.305

Hawkins, K. R., Burton, J. H., Apolzan, J. W., Thomson, J. L., Williamson, D. A., & Martin, C. K. (2018). Efficacy of a school-based obesity prevention intervention at reducing added sugar and sodium in children's school lunches: The LA Health randomized controlled trial. *International Journal of Obesity (London), 42*(11), 1845–1852. doi:10.1038/s41366-018-0214-y

Hermsen, S., Frost, J. H., Robinson, E., Higgs, S., Mars, M., & Hermans, R. C. (2016). Evaluation of a smart fork to decelerate eating rate. *Journal of the National Academy of Nutrition and Dietetics, 116*(7), 1066–1068. doi:10.1016/j.jand.2015.11.004

Heymsfield, S. B., Peterson, C. M., Thomas, D. M., Hirezi, M., Zhang, B., Smith, S., et al. (2017). Establishing energy requirements for body weight maintenance: Validation of an intake-balance method. *BMC Res Notes, 10*(1), 220. doi:10.1186/s13104-017-2546-4

Jasper, P. W., James, M. T., Hoover, A. W., & Muth, E. R. (2016). Effects of bite count feedback from a wearable device and goal setting on consumption in young adults. *Journal of the National Academy of Nutrition & Dietetics, 116*(11), 1785–1793. doi:10.1016/j.jand.2016.05.004

Kelley, D. E. (2002). Action for health in diabetes: The look AHEAD clinical trial. *Current Diabetes Report, 2*(3), 207–209.

Klenk, J., Dallmeier, D., Denkinger, M. D., Rapp, K., Koenig, W., Rothenbacher, et al. (2016). Objectively measured walking duration and sedentary behaviour and four-year mortality in older people. *PLoS One, 11*(4), e0153779. doi:10.1371/journal.pone.0153779

Lichtman, S. W., Pisarska, K., Berman, E. R., Pestone, M., Dowling, H., Offenbacher, E., et al. (1992). Discrepancy between self-reported and actual caloric intake and exercise in obese subjects. *New England Journal of Medicine, 327*(27), 1893–1898. doi:10.1056/NEJM199212313272701

Little, R. J., D'Agostino, R., Cohen, M. L., Dickersin, K., Emerson, S. S., Farrar, J. T., et al. (2012). The prevention and treatment of missing data in clinical trials. *New England Journal of Medicine, 367*(14), 1355–1360. doi:10.1056/NEJMsr1203730

Malik, V. S., Popkin, B. M., Bray, G. A., Despres, J. P., & Hu, F. B. (2010). Sugar-sweetened beverages, obesity, type 2 diabetes mellitus, and cardiovascular disease risk. *Circulation, 121*(11), 1356–1364. doi:10.1161/CIRCULATIONAHA.109.876185

Neumark-Sztainer, D., Story, M., Hannan, P. J., & Rex, J. (2003). New moves: A school-based obesity prevention program for adolescent girls. *Preventive Medicine, 37*(1), 41–51.

Nunez, C., Nair-Shalliker, V., Egger, S., Sitas, F., & Bauman, A. (2018). Physical activity, obesity and sedentary behaviour and the risks of colon and rectal cancers in the 45 and up study. *BMC Public Health, 18*(1), 325. doi:10.1186/s12889-018-5225-z

Ogden, C. L., Carroll, M. D., Kit, B. K., & Flegal, K. M. (2014). Prevalence of childhood and adult obesity in the United States, 2011–2012. *JAMA, 311*(8), 806–814. doi:10.1001/jama.2014.732

Olson, C. M., Strawderman, M. S., & Graham, M. L. (2017). Association between consistent weight gain tracking and gestational weight gain: Secondary analysis of a randomized trial. *Obesity (Silver Spring), 25*(7), 1217–1227. doi:10.1002/oby.21873

Passmore, R. (1963). The composition of weight gains and weight losses. *Annals of the New York Academy of Science, 110*, 675–678.

Patterson, R., McNamara, E., Tainio, M., de Sa, T. H., Smith, A. D., Sharp, S. J., et al. (2018). Sedentary behaviour and risk of all-cause, cardiovascular and cancer mortality, and incident type 2 diabetes: A systematic review and dose response meta-analysis. *Eur J Epidemiol, 33*(9), 811–829. doi:10.1007/s10654-018-0380-1

Rasmussen, K. M., Yaktine, A. L., & Institute of Medicine (U.S.). Committee to Reexamine IOM Pregnancy Weight Guidelines. (2009). *Weight gain during pregnancy: Teexamining the guidelines*. Washington, DC: National Academies Press.

Razmpoosh, E., Zare, S., Fallahzadeh, H., Safi, S., & Nadjarzadeh, A. (2020). Effect of a low energy diet, containing a high protein, probiotic condensed yogurt, on biochemical and anthropometric measurements among women with overweight/obesity: A randomised controlled trial. *Clinical Nutrition ESPEN, 35*, 194–200. doi:10.1016/j.clnesp.2019.10.001

Rose, M. H., Streisand, R., Aronow, L., Tully, C., Martin, C. K., & Mackey, E. (2018). Preliminary feasibility and acceptability of the remote food photography method for assessing nutrition in young children with type 1 diabetes. *Clinical Practice in Pediatric Psychology, 6*(3), 270–277. doi:10.1037/cpp0000240

Ross, R., Hudson, R., Day, A. G., & Lam, M. (2013). Dose-response effects of exercise on abdominal obesity and risk factors for cardiovascular disease in adults: Study rationale, design and methods. *Contemporary Clinical Trials, 34*(1), 155–160. doi:10.1016/j.cct.2012.10.010

Sazonov, E., Schuckers, S., Lopez-Meyer, P., Makeyev, O., Sazonova, N., Melanson, E. L., et al. (2008). Non-invasive monitoring of chewing and swallowing for objective quantification of ingestive behavior. *Physiological Measurements, 29*(5), 525–541. doi:10.1088/0967-3334/29/5/001

Schoeller, D. A. (2013). A novel carbon isotope biomarker for dietary sugar. *Journal of Nutrition, 143*(6), 763–765. doi:10.3945/jn.113.177345

Schoeller, D. A., Thomas, D., Archer, E., Heymsfield, S. B., Blair, S. N., Goran, M. I., et al. (2013). Self-report-based estimates of energy intake offer an inadequate basis for scientific conclusions. *American Journal of Clinical Nutrition, 97*(6), 1413–1415. doi:10.3945/ajcn.113.062125

Schoeller, D. A., & van Santen, E. (1982). Measurement of energy expenditure in humans by doubly labeled water method. *Journal of Applied Physiology: Respiratory, Environmental and Exercise Physiology, 53*(4), 955–959. doi:10.1152/jappl.1982.53.4.955

Shields, M., & Tremblay, M. S. (2008). Sedentary behaviour and obesity. *Health Reports, 19*(2), 19–30.

Siegel, A. M., Tita, A. T., Machemehl, H., Biggio, J. R., & Harper, L. M. (2017). Evaluation of institute of medicine guidelines for gestational weight gain in women with chronic hypertension. *AJP Rep, 7*(3), e145–e150. doi:10.1055/s-0037-1604076

Smith, J. L., Arteaga, C., & Heymsfield, S. B. (1982). Increased ureagenesis and impaired nitrogen use during infusion of a synthetic amino acid formula: A controlled trial. *New England Journal of Medicine, 306*(17), 1013–1018. doi:10.1056/NEJM198204293061702

Song, B., & Thomas, D. M. (2007). Dynamics of starvation in humans. *Journal of Mathematical Biology, 54*(1), 27–43. doi:10.1007/s00285-006-0037-7

Sousa, R. M. L., Ribeiro, N. L. X., Pinto, B. A. S., Sanches, J. R., da Silva, M. U., Coelho, C. F. F., et al. (2018). Long-term high-protein diet intake reverts weight gain and attenuates metabolic dysfunction on high-sucrose-fed adult rats. *Nutrition & Metabolism (London), 15*, 53. doi:10.1186/s12986-018-0290-y

Thomas, D. M., Navarro-Barrientos, J. E., Rivera, D. E., Heymsfield, S. B., Bredlau, C., Redman, et al. (2012). Dynamic energy-balance model predicting gestational weight gain. *American Journal of Clinical Nutrition, 95*(1), 115–122. doi:10.3945/ajcn.111.024307

Thomas, J. G., & Bond, D. S. (2015). Behavioral response to a Just-in-Time Adaptive Intervention (JITAI) to reduce sedentary behavior in obese adults: Implications for JITAI optimization. *Health Psychology, 34S*, 1261–1267. doi:10.1037/hea0000304

Truiett-Theodorson, R., Tuck, S., Bowie, J. V., Summers, A. C., & Kelber-Kaye, J. (2015). Building effective partnerships to improve birth outcomes by reducing obesity: The B'more Fit for healthy babies coalition of Baltimore. *Evaluation Program Planning, 51*, 53–58. doi:10.1016/j.evalprogplan.2014.12.007

University of Minnesota. Laboratory of Physiological Hygiene, & Keys, A. B. (1950). *The biology of human starvation*. Minneapolis, MN: University of Minnesota Press.

Westerterp, K. R. (2017). Doubly labelled water assessment of energy expenditure: Principle, practice, and promise. *European Journal of Applied Physiology, 117*(7), 1277–1285. doi:10.1007/s00421-017-3641-x

Wilkinson, D. J. (2018). Historical and contemporary stable isotope tracer approaches to studying mammalian protein metabolism. *Mass Spectrometry Reviews, 37*(1), 57–80. doi:10.1002/mas.21507

Witjaksono, F., Jutamulia, J., Annisa, N. G., Prasetya, S. I., & Nurwidya, F. (2018). Comparison of low calorie high protein and low calorie standard protein diet on waist circumference of adults with visceral obesity and weight cycling. *BMC Res Notes, 11*(1), 674. doi:10.1186/s13104-018-3781-z

Wright, C. S., Zhou, J., Sayer, R. D., Kim, J. E., & Campbell, W. W. (2018). Effects of a high-protein diet including whole eggs on muscle composition and indices of cardiometabolic health and systemic inflammation in older adults with overweight or obesity: A randomized controlled trial. *Nutrients, 10*(7). doi:10.3390/nu10070946

Yang, Q., Zhang, Z., Gregg, E. W., Flanders, W. D., Merritt, R., & Hu, F. B. (2014). Added sugar intake and cardiovascular diseases mortality among US adults. *JAMA Intern Med, 174*(4), 516–524. doi:10.1001/jamainternmed.2013.13563

Yee, L. M., Cheng, Y. W., Inturrisi, M., & Caughey, A. B. (2011). Effect of gestational weight gain on perinatal outcomes in women with type 2 diabetes mellitus using the 2009 Institute of Medicine guidelines. *American Journal of Obstetrics & Gynecology, 205*(3), 257 e251–256. doi:10.1016/j.ajog.2011.06.028

Yonemori, K. M., Ennis, T., Novotny, R., Fialkowski, M. K., Ettienne, R., Wilkens, L. R., et al. (2017). Collecting wrappers, labels, and packages to enhance accuracy of food records among children 2–8 years in the Pacific region: Children's Healthy Living Program (CHL). *Journal of Food Composition & Analysis, 64*(Pt 1), 112–118. doi:10.1016/j.jfca.2017.04.012

13

SOCIAL NETWORKS, DEPRESSION, AND STRESS

Rachel Kramer

Overview

Major depressive disorder (MDD) is a widespread psychological disorder, with a lifetime prevalence rate of 16.6% and a median age of onset of 30 years (Kessler, Berglund, Demler, Jin, Merikangas, & Walters, 2005). Further, MDD is a public health concern that predicts suicidal ideation and completion and is a leading cause of death among a variety of age groups (Johnson, Hayes, Brown, Hoo, & Ethier, 2014; Bostwick & Pankratz, 2000). The World Health Organization ranks MDD as one of the top five causes of disability and is associated with chronic medical conditions, including arthritis (Dickens, McGowan, Clark-Carter, & Creed, 2002), chronic pain (Munce, Stansfeld, Blackmore, & Stewart, 2007), and hypertension (Rubio-Guerra, Rodriguez-Lopez, Vargas-Ayala, Huerta-Ramirez, Serna, & Lozano-Nuevo, 2013).

The deleterious effects of MDD on individual and global health have stimulated research on predictive and maintenance factors, assessment, and development of evidence-based treatments of MDD (Wong & Licinio, 2001). Assessment and diagnosis of MDD are conducted through a variety of methods. More stringent approaches use structured or semi-structured interviews (e.g., the Structured Clinical Interview for DSM [SCID]; First, Gibbon, Spitzer, & Williams, 1995) for adults or the Kiddie Schedule for Affective Disorders and Schizophrenia (K-SAD-S); Kaufman, Birmaher, Brent, Rao, Flynn, Moreci, et al., 1997) for children and teens. While structured interviews are considered gold standards for conferring MDD and other diagnoses (American Psychiatric Association, 2013), structured interviews can be lengthy and arduous for participants, are costly, and require advanced training to conduct (Segal, Coolidge, O'Riley, & Heinz, 2006).

Less intensive and time-consuming methods (i.e., self-report questionnaires) have been introduced to assess depression. Common questionnaires for depression include the Beck Depression Inventory-II (BDI-II; Beck, Steer, & Brown, 1996) and Center for Epidemiological Studies Scale for Depression (CES-D; Radloff, 1977) for adults and the Children's Depression Inventory (CDI; Kovacs, 1981) for children. These surveys use Likert scales with face validity (e.g., asking how sad or irritable an individual feels), take less time to complete, and are normed on a variety of populations (Crawford, Cayley, Lovibond, Wilson, & Hartley, 2011; Hamilton, 1967). While some argue depression exists on a continuum (Angst & Merikangas, 2001), relying on self-reports alone cannot confer diagnosis. As with any self-report questionnaire, those assessing MDD may lack sensitivity and/or specificity and, consequently, may not reliably or accurately identify patients who are depressed or at risk for depression (Zimmerman & Coryell, 1994). However, self-report questionnaires may facilitate understanding the severity of MDD, enabling researchers and clinicians to compare individuals and assess changes in depression over time.

To further understand and prevent MDD, researchers have been examining risk factors associated with its development. Life stressors are frequently cited risk factors for depression (Brown & Harris, 1989). Other research suggests that MDD may have psychobiological roots. For instance, the *diathesis–stress model of MDD* posits an individual may have a genetic predisposition (Kendler, Neal, Kessler, Heath, & Eaves, 1993) but may not develop a depressive episode without experiencing a life stressor. Other models evaluating the relationship between stress and MDD include the *stress sensitization hypothesis*, which postulates that less stress is required to induce the recurrent onset of MDD, and the *stress generation hypothesis*, which proposes that individuals with MDD may experience greater stress related to its symptoms and associated behaviors (e.g., ruminative thinking and affected social ties). Researchers also propose a reciprocal relationship between stress and MDD (Hammen, 2006), making it difficult to understand the directionality of the relationship.

Another concern with valid research methodology involves how stress is assessed; stress is often correlated with outcome (Hammen, 2005). Researchers originally measured stress using self-report checklists; however, participants may respond to such checklists ideologically (e.g., what stresses one person may not affect another individual; Kessler, 1997) and based on their current emotional state. Brown and Harris (1989) have created assessments adjusting for context and duration of the stressor. Further, researchers may rely on biological markers of stress not addressed in this chapter (see Rohleder, Nater, Wolf, Ehlert, & Kirschbaum, 2004).

Researchers have argued that many factors explain or moderate the relationship between stress and depression; social support has been identified as one of these factors (Cohen & Wills, 1985). Many models have been evaluated. For instance, the *buffering model* asserts social support will decrease the impact of stress, depressive symptomatology, and health risk (Cassel, 1976). The *main effect model* emphasizes that social networks are protective (Hammer, 1981), and larger social networks are associated with lower risk of depression. Both the *main effect* and *buffering effect models* have been supported, but assessment methodology may affect results (Cohen & Wills, 1985). Indeed, social networks and social support have been assessed numerous ways (e.g., the number and types of social supports as in instrumental, emotional, perceived support, and frequency of contact; O'Reilly, 1988).

This chapter will address questions of how social networks and support relate to stress and depression by presenting different studies assessing *diathesis-stress*, *buffering*, and *main effect models* and the link between social networks, stress, and depression. It also features diverse, novel, and effectively designed studies. Specific methodologies employed include ecological momentary assessment, participatory action research, cross-sectional, and longitudinal designs.

Research in Practice

Gene by Environment (Stress Buffering)

A frequently cited study by Caspi, Sugden, Moffitt, Taylor, Craig, Harrington, et al. (2003) examines the link between stress and depressive symptoms. This prospective longitudinal study evaluated the *diathesis-stress* (gene by environment; G × E) risk of depression by having a total of 1,037 participants between three and 26 years old provide data at ten separate times. While experiencing life stress is considered a universal experience, not everyone who experiences stress develops depression. The discipline of behavioral genetics serves as a modality to explore and test the *diathesis-stress model* of depression (Monroe & Simons, 1991). One relevant biological factor is *serotonin*, a neurotransmitter that has been implicated in depression. Indeed, *serotonin reuptake–inhibitor* medications have successfully treated depression (Jakobsen, Katakam, Schou, Hellmuth, Stallknecht, Leth-Møller, et al., 2017). As such,

Caspi, et al. (2003) examined the ***5HTTLPR genotype***, a genotype strongly linked with *serotonin*, to assess how significant, stressful life events and the G × E interaction might predict MDD. They hypothesized that the recessive ***s allele (s/s)*** versus the dominant long ***l allele (l/l)*** would be associated with greater MDD risk given the *s allele* is associated with lower transcriptional efficacy of *serotonin* compared to the *l allele* (Lesch, Bengel, Heils, Sabol, Greenberg, Petri, et al., 1996). While the *5HTTLPR* gene does not predict depression directly (Plomin, DeFries, Craig, & McGuffin, 2003), Caspi, and colleagues (2003), hypothesized genes and life stress would interact to predict depression. Indeed, Caspi, et al. (2003) found participants with an *s allele* who experienced life stress reported greater incidences of MDD and suicide attempts even after controlling for prior MDD.

Several follow-up studies have been conducted to expand on Caspi, and colleagues' (2003) landmark study (Wankerl, Wüst, & Otte, 2010). Kilpatrick, Koenen, Ruggiero, Acierno, Galea, and Resnick (2007) also examined the *5-HTTLPR* G × E interaction by specifically looking at MDD and post-traumatic stress disorder (PTSD) diagnosis occurring after hurricane exposure. On top of assessing the G × E relationship with MDD, the authors also evaluated the association between social support and risk for development of MDD and PTSD (although only data on MDD will be presented).

While Kilpatrick, and colleagues (2007) used a cross-sectional design, researchers randomly sampled community members in Florida affected by a devastating hurricane in the area. The study recruited 589 participants who provided saliva samples to assess *5-HTTLPR* genotype and responded to standardized questionnaires assessing PTSD and MDD (Robins, Cottler, Bucholz, Compton, North, & Rourke, 2000). Genotyping was completed using polymerase chain reaction after size fractionation was completed (Gelernter, Kranzler, & Cubells, 1997). Kilpatrick, et al. (2007) also assessed different aspects of social support six months prior to the hurricane using the Medical Outcomes Study Social Support Survey (MOS; Sherbourne & Stewart, 1991). The MOS assesses support by summing perceived support on three domains, including emotional (e.g., having someone available to support one's emotions), appraisal (e.g., advicet), and instrumental (pragmatic and action-based) support. Kilpatrick, and colleagues (2007) also measured degree of impact of the hurricane (low, medium, and high) based on economic, safety, and related stressors.

Using logistic regression analysis controlling for sex, age, and ancestral proportion to evaluate the odds of a diagnosis of MDD, Kilpatrick, et al. (2007) noted an incidence rate of 5.6% for MDD. Interestingly, low social support was not directly related to MDD (while PTSD was), nor were there interactions between 5-*HTTLPR* genotypes and degree of hurricane exposure or social support on odds for MDD diagnosis. However, three-way interactions indicated that among participants with high hurricane exposure and low social support, individuals with the *s allele* were 21.5 times more likely to be diagnosed with MDD than those with the *l allele*.

This study demonstrates many strengths, including the use of validated assessment measures. Specifically, the MOS scale (Sherbourne & Stewart, 1991) assesses perceived quality versus quantity of social support. Cohen and Wills's (1985) ***buffering model of social support on depression*** emphasizes that the quality of social support should be considered versus the number of social supports. Furthermore, Kilpatrick, and colleagues (2007) utilized a representative sample experiencing one specific stressful life event, thus controlling for confounds (e.g., differences in experience of life events; Wankerl, et al., 2010).

There are a few limitations to this study, including the use of retrospective reports of social support, since retrospective accounts of social support may be biased (Hammen, 2005). Individuals who are depressed likely perceive less social support (Cohen, Towbes, & Flocco, 1988) and report less accurate negative affect (Telford, McCarthy-Jones, Corcoran, & Rowse, 2011), limiting interpretation. Since the three categories of social support were summed, it is also unclear what category of social support was most beneficial or impactful to MDD diagnosis. Additionally, there was no assessment of whether participants had a current or lifetime history of MDD prior to the hurricane, increasing the potential of confounds, including the kindling effect (i.e., less stress needed for relapse for MDD; Monroe & Harkness, 2005). Greater frequency of stressful life events has been associated with increased PTSD risk (Nooner, Linares, Batinjane, Kramer, Silva, & Cloitre, 2012). This was also not directly assessed during the research study.

Targeted Rejection

As researchers have examined the impact of specific stressors on depression, there is growing support for interpersonal stressors catalyzing the development of MDD (Paykel, 2003; Slavich, Thornton, Torres, Monroe, & Gotlib, 2009), given that social connectedness is considered to be pivotal to survival and development (e.g., Ainsworth, 1978; Bolby, 1969). As such, Slavich, and colleagues (2009) examined how interpersonal life stressors influence the development of MDD. The researchers were specifically interested in how MDD may be predicted by the perceived rejection by a peer: ***targeted rejection* (TR)**. *TR* occurs when an individual is the sole target of rejection and they perceive a loss of social status. An example of *TR* is a nonmutual breakup with a romantic partner.

To assess this, Slavich, et al. (2009) used responses from 27 adults (*M*age = 32.67). Most participants were female (85%), Asian (44.44%) or Caucasian (40.74%), and well-educated. Despite the small sample size, a strength of the study was the use of validated and reliable assessment measures. To assess current and lifetime depression history, the researchers used the SCID (First, et al. 1995) with at least two raters' responses reviewed to check for reliability.

To assess life stress, Slavich, and colleagues (2009) employed the Life Events and Difficulties Schedule (LEDS; Brown & Harris, 1989), which assesses severe life events occurring within one year of the assessment. The LEDS enables researchers to understand the event's context and the individual's biographical circumstances. To conduct the LEDS, a two-hour semi-structured interview assessed types of life stress and then a panel of raters judged the severity of the stressor. During this study, events rated as severe were further coded into *TR* events and *non-TR* events, as well as coded into three domains, specifically work, school, or relationship. On top of being highly reliable assessments, the LED and SCID utilize calendars, which enabled the researchers to measure the outcome variable of time related to depression onset.

Cox regression survival analyses were run to evaluate differences in time of onset to depression for participants with a severe *TR* or *non-TR*. Hypotheses that *TR* events would lead to earlier onset of MDD were supported; *TR* led to onset of MDD significantly sooner than *non-please delete space here TR* events. On average, *TR* events were associated with onset of MDD at 30.4 days compared to 101.4 days for *non-TR* events. Another strength of the study was the assessment of alternative explanations. Slavich, and colleagues (2009) assessed whether life domain (e.g. school, work, or relationship) related to differences in MDD onset, since all life events were coded as severe. There were no differences related to the life domain. They also assessed the stress sensitization model of MDD, which suggests that previous MDD diagnoses may require less severe stress events to predict recurrence of MDD. This relationship was not supported, however. Further, the stress generation model asserts that a history of depression predicts greater social distress and potentially *TR*. Researchers actually noted history of MDD predicted more *non-TR* than *TR*, contradicting the *stress generation model*.

Despite some of the study's strengths, a larger sample would have been beneficial in supporting the findings. It would have also been interesting to assess the length of time for remission of MDD. Further, the study only assessed severe life stress; it would be interesting to assess a continuum of life stressors to further evaluate *TR* on MDD risk. Indeed, further research supports *TR* in the risk of depression (see Slavich, Tartter, Brennan, & Hammen, 2014).

Participatory Action Research

While researchers originally favored lab-controlled studies to control for confounds and find causal relationships, researchers have started to develop greater diversity in research methodology. First, there is concern about how results might replicate outside of the lab setting (Reis, 2012). Further, participants in studies are often recruited "willingly," but often based upon convenience (e.g., college student samples). Participants may not represent the populations that research questions are asking about (Peterson & Merunka, 2014). As such, other methodologies have been developed to increase ecological validity and to include actual participants of interest.

Participatory action research (PAR) is one form of qualitative research that addresses such concerns. PAR, originally developed by Kurt Lewin (1946) with his research on societal segregation and minority assimilation, has several aims. With roots in feminist and postmodern research theory (Kelly, 2005), PAR equalizes the roles of the community (participants) and researchers; participants are given equal say in the research aims. Further, PAR aims to engender social change through this shared collaboration (Chataway, 1997; Mason & Boutilier, 1996). Thus participants are willing and the studies are interpretable beyond the lab setting.

One study evaluating the link between social networks, stress, and depression using PAR was conducted in Canada by Ross, Ali, and Toner (2009) recruiting young women ranging between ages 16 and 22. The study was intended to increase researchers' understanding of how young women define depression. It highlighted the best preventative measures against depression and incorporated perspectives from individuals with and without a history of depression. This study incorporated many tenets of PAR across multiple phases and included "team" member input in designing focus questions and collaborating in discussions (MacDonald, 2012). Participants were recruited through multiple avenues, including but not limited to posters and flyers in neighborhoods, schools (e.g., flyers, morning announcements), ads in the newspaper, and invitations from researchers. The diverse group of 48 young women then formed a Youth Advisory Team (YAT), which met with a project coordinator to develop the focus of the research project on depression, including focus group questions intended to increase knowledge of depression in their community. The team worked together to recruit from populations that they felt would benefit, including adolescent mothers, individuals with diverse sexual orientations, and ethnicities/races from rural and urban regions in Ontario.

Once the study was designed, researchers trained the YAT in group facilitation; two YAT leaders then co-facilitated focus groups of four to eight participants. The sessions were audiotaped, and participants completed surveys after each focus group. Researchers were thoughtful in theme identification and establishing reliability—two independent coders examined agreement in the themes identified (a third rater mitigated discrepancies, as needed). Ultimately, the group collaboratively narrowed the study aim to one of understanding and helping young women with depression.

Five major themes were identified through the focus groups on depression, including 1) signs and symptoms, 2) contributing factors, 3) factors that help individuals with MDD with depression, 4) prevention, and 5) barriers to obtaining help. Several points emerging from these five themes highlighted the relationship between stress, depression, and social networks. Specifically, participants identified pressures from family, society, and interpersonal conflict to be contributing factors to depression. Further, having to assimilate to a different culture and experiencing lower social support from family and peers was also considered influential in depression risk. Improvements in depression were associated with involvement in one's social network. Lastly, perceived support from friends and family members, *especially* mothers, and other socially driven resources (e.g., support groups, telephone hotlines, and psychologists) were beneficial in decreasing depression.

This study demonstrated many strengths. For one, Ross, and colleagues (2009) worked to decrease any power differential between researchers and participants by using only female research staff and having researchers disclose their experience working with depressed individuals or with depression themselves. *PAR* is most effective when it includes three methods of obtaining data to reduce limitations resulting from relying on one single qualitative method (MacDonald, 2012). Ross, et al. (2009) achieved this through including surveys, focus groups, observations, and recordings of each group. Ross, and colleagues (2009) also created an action plan to facilitate change in the community, another integral element of *PAR* research (MacDonald, 2012). The YAT held a well-received, province-wide conference, where the teens presented information on their own experiences with and about depression generally.

Some limitations to the current *PAR* include some of the common limitations identified for *PAR* generally (MacDonald, 2012). For one, Ross, et al. (2009) reported that focus groups had divergent opinions that were sometimes difficult to account for but were likely related to different social and demographic backgrounds (e.g., sexual identities, life experiences). Further, at times, some of the methodology appeared vague; it was unclear how focus groups were assigned. Likely a limitation of many *PAR* studies, replication would be difficult, given the method used. Regardless, this study significantly contributes to understanding the impact of social networks on stress and depression and supports the use of qualitative methods in examining the connection between social support (or lack thereof), stress, and depression.

Ecological Momentary Assessment

Independent of the factors that cause and sustain MDD, research suggests that MDD is associated with poor emotion regulation (Forbes & Dahl, 2005), especially among children and adolescents. For instance, depressed youth experience **negative affect (NA)** with increased intensity (lability) and length of time (Silk, Steinberg, & Morris, 2003). Relatedly, depressed youth experience decreased **positive affect** (**PA**; Forbes & Dahl, 2005). Looking at *NA* and *PA* is imperative, since they are considered orthogonal processes (Rafaeli & Revelle, 2006).

When conceptualizing MDD as a disorder of affect regulation, researchers argue that assessing emotions retrospectively hinders valid results (Stone, Schwartz, Neale, Shiffman, Marco, Hickcox, et al., 1998). Depressed individuals exhibit poorer recall of *NA* and *PA* and remember severe events versus recent ones (Ben-Zeev & Young, 2010; Stone, et al., 1998). To address such concerns, lab studies have assessed affect in depression (e.g., Jazbec, McClure, Hardin, Pine, & Ernst, 2005; Pine, Lissek, Klein, Mannuzza, Moulton, Guardino, et al., 2004). Although they provide more accurate assessment of emotional experiences, they possess low ecological validity (Stone, et al., 2007) and may not adequately or ethically induce events prompting affective responses (especially interpersonal stressors). Bearing such concerns in mind, researchers have attempted to understand how social environments and moment-to-moment emotions affect depression (Telford, et al., 2011).

As such, Silk, Forbes, Whalen, Jakubcak, Thompson, and Ryan (2011) employed **ecological momentary assessment (EMA)** to assess how affect varies between depressed and nondepressed youth and how social context affects affective variability and range. *EMA* was a fitting choice; it provides insight into emotions in the real world, reduces memory bias, evaluates behavior outside of controlled environments (e.g., a lab), and improves the generalizability of research results.

Utilizing a complex design, Silk, and colleagues (2011) recruited controls and youth suffering from major depressive disorder (CON and MDD, respectively). The researchers used a cell phone *EMA* protocol conducted over eight weeks. Participants were called 12 times on weeks zero, one, three, five, and seven. Due to limitations related to school attendance, research assistants called participants from Friday afternoon through Monday evening. Participants were diagnosed with MDD using the K-SADS-PL (Kaufman, et al., 1997), a validated and structured assessment. Depressed youth received selective *serotonin reuptake inhibitors* and/or **cognitive behavioral therapy**. Silk, and colleagues (2011) were mindful to control for many confounding variables among groups, including history of bipolar disorder, medical conditions or other extreme health concerns, IQ, and family history of MDD among CON.

During each call, participants were asked to rate their current emotion on four *NA* and *PA* scales of the Positive and Negative Affect Schedule for Children (PANAS-C; Laurent, Catanzaro, Joiner, Rudolph, Potter, Lambert, et al., 1999). Participants were also asked open-ended questions about social context (i.e., activity [solitary or recreational activities], locations, who they were with [alone, friends, or family]). The four *NA* scales were sad, angry, nervous, and upset, summed to create a total negative affect score (Global *NA*). The four *PA* subscales were happy, joyful, excited, and energetic, also summed for an overall positive affect score (Global *PA*). A ratio of global *PA* and *NA* (*PA:NA*) was also computed by dividing the Global *PA* by Global *NA*. Lastly, Silk, and colleagues (2011) computed lability scores for Global *NA* and the four *NA* scales by computing the standard deviation for each emotion across calls. Inter-rater reliability was calculated for the content on social context, yielding an acceptable statistic (*k* = .85 to .98).

Most analyses were conducted per recommendations (Nezlek, 2012) using repeated measures linear mixed effects models to account for the nesting of assessments across time and within participants. Independent variables included within subject (time), between subject (diagnostic group: MDD versus CON), and the interaction between time and diagnostic group. Dependent variables included Global *NA* and *PA* and all affect ratings, *PA:NA*, *NA* variability, social context, and activity type. The researchers also controlled for many confounds, including age, race, gender, and baseline *NA*, as MDD were hypothesized to have higher *NA* given their diagnosis.

Overall, a total of 79 youth (61% female) ages seven to 17 years old (*Mage* = 12.6) participated. There were 47 MDD participants and 32 CON. Results suggested that, overall, MDD endorsed greater Global *NA*, sadness, anger, nervousness, and a lower ratio of *PA:NA* than CON. Further, MDD, but not CON, reported decreases in overall Global *NA*, sadness, and anger (and lability of all three *NA*) but no change in the ratio of *PA:NA* over time. While Silk, and colleagues (2011) did not note any changes over time in social interactions among MDD despite the changes in Global *NA*, sadness, anger, and nervousness, Global *NA* was highest for both groups when peers were alone or with family. Adolescents had the highest ratio of *PA:NA* when alone or with friends. Solitary activities were also associated with greater sadness.

This study makes many contributions, including addressing how affect, social support, and depression are associated in the natural environment through sound statistical and research design and reduce concerns with recall bias and concerns with ecological validity, as participants were at home. However, there are a few limitations. For instance, perceived stress and perceived quality of relationships were not assessed during this study. These differences may explain some of the differences in participants' emotions. Additionally, while not possible to obtain, it would be helpful to assess affect during other contexts and stress levels (e.g., school, exams). Given concerns with recall bias in depression, it may have been interesting to utilize an ***event-contingent EMA protocol*** (responding when a specific event occurs) versus a ***signal contingent protocol*** (responding when a researcher assistant calls). Further, *EMA* may be burdensome to use, difficult to interpret due to multiple measurements (Nezlek, 2012), and subject to demand characteristics, threatening validity (Gunthert & Wenze, 2012).

Social Networking Sites and Depression

The development and expansion of the internet, specifically websites and applications available to consumers, also play a role in our understanding of the interaction of social networks, depression, and stress. For better or worse, ***social networking sites (SNS)*** are pervasive in society. For instance, 75% of individuals who have Facebook report using the application every day (Smith & Anderson, 2018), with about 68% of adults in the United States possessing a Facebook account.

At face value, these sites can expand social connections and opportunities to engage with family and friends. Indeed, some studies suggest *SNS* like Facebook can be beneficial (Ryan & Xenos,

2011). However, research is also suggesting there may be harmful effects of *SNS* use. For instance, Twenge, Joiner, Rogers, & Martin (2017) noted a significant positive relationship between depressive symptoms, suicidality, and screen time. A few models have been developed to explain how this relationship may work. Some argue that Facebook increases social comparison (Appel, Gerlach, & Crusius, 2016) and loneliness (Song, Zmyslinski-Seelig, Kim, Drent, Victor, Omori, et al., 2014).

Some of the complexities in understanding the link between *SNS* use and depression relates to study methodology. While the methodology was appropriate for initial research, studies were cross-sectional, limiting the understanding of causality (Kross, Verduyn, Demiralp, Park, Lee, Lin, et al., 2013). To look beyond, other methods have been used. For instance, Kross, and colleagues (2013) employed a prospective longitudinal design and recruited 82 participants with a Facebook account to respond to questions over a 14-day period about mood, loneliness, depression, self-esteem, and Facebook use and found that Facebook use was associated with worse affect and life satisfaction.

Experimental studies, which allow for greater causal explanations, also support the association between *SNS* and depression. For instance, Tromholt (2016) found that when participants did not use Facebook for a week, they reported improved satisfaction and affect compared to individuals using Facebook as usual. However, Hunt, Marx, Lipson, and Young (2018) argue against the feasibility of abstaining from Facebook use. Active participation on Facebook is also associated with less envy and impact on well-being compared to individuals passively using Facebook (Verduyn, Lee, Park, Shablack, Orvell, Bayer, et al., 2015).

Other methodological concerns exist regarding studies examining the relationship between stress, depression, and *SNS*. For instance, research on *SNS* relies on participants' recall, the amount of time, and how they use *SNS* (Lup, Trub, & Rosenthal, 2015). As such, one study by Hunt, and colleagues (2018) addressed previous concerns with internal and external validity examining the impact of *SNS* use, social connection, and depression. The study was run for three weeks (one week of baseline data) and asked participants in the experimental condition (*SNS* limiting) to limit time on Facebook, Instagram, and Snapchat to ten minutes per platform. Another group was given no instructions to use *SNS* differently (control). The researchers assessed experimental changes over a longer period of time compared to previous research (Kross, et al., 2013; Verduyn, 2015) and was more realistic in asking participants to limit time on each *SNS* versus requiring complete abstinence (Tromholt, 2016).

In conducting their research, Hunt and colleagues (2018) assessed subjective well-being from a measure of perceived social support using the Interpersonal Support and Evaluation List (Cohen & Hoberman, 1983); perceived loneliness using a well-validated measure, the UCLA Loneliness Scale (Russell, Peplau, & Cutrona, 1980); state anxiety (Spielberger State-Trait Anxiety Inventory; Spielberger, Gorsuch, Lushene, Vagg, & Jacobs, 1983); depression (Beck Depression Inventory-II [BDI-II]; Beck, et al., 1996); self-esteem (Rosenberg Self-Esteem Scale; Rosenberg, 1979); and well-being (Ryff Psychological Well-Being Scale; Ryff, 1995). To ensure the accurate reporting of time spent on *SNS*, participants shared, using their phone, the total screen time of each *SNS* used for the first three weeks of the study.

Contrary to other studies, Hunt and colleagues (2018) reported no correlation between any of their dependent variables and *SNS* use. Even when assessing baseline objective use, *SNS* use did not relate to self-reported severity of MDD. Further, Hunt, et al. (2018) examined the correlation between reported and *actual* (as recorded by participants' phones) *SNS* use, a relatively novel approach, given that most studies only assess *SNS* use via self-reported estimates. They noted a moderate correlation ($r = .31$, $p = .01$) between actual and self-reported use—a concerning result because many studies simply employ self-reported *SNS* use.

Findings indicated participants in the *SNS*-limiting group reported lower loneliness compared to controls at the end of the intervention. Furthermore, regardless of baseline depression, depression symptoms did not significantly change among controls. However, significant changes in depression symptoms were noted for the SNS-limiting group, especially among individuals endorsing clinical levels of depression at baseline (scoring above the clinical cutoff of 14 on the BDI-II), who reported MDD scores nearly below the clinical cutoff (*M* = 14.5) at the end of the intervention. This suggests the intervention was particularly beneficial for individuals high in baseline depression.

While this study was novel and featured an improvement in methods, there are several considerations for future research. One includes limiting *SNS* use on all technology beyond mobile phone use. Further, repeated measures analyses of covariance (ANCOVAs) may have also been a more statistically appropriate method of data analysis, as they account for within- and between-subject variance (Schneider, Avivi-Reich, & Mozuraitis, 2015).

Even though researchers attempted to obtain data a month after the study, there was considerable attrition and the sample was too small to evaluate further. Future studies should examine whether type of posts or engagement in *SNS* relates to depression. Mediation and moderation would also be important to assess (e.g., do decreases in perceived loneliness explain changes in depressive symptoms observed in the experimental group?). However, perhaps *SNS* use relates to depression in even more complex ways.

Strengths and Limitations

In all, these studies examined the link between social networks, stress, and depression using a variety of methodologies, each carrying strengths and limitations. To address concerns with assessment of life stress (Brown & Harris, 1989), the validated scales employed in the studies presented account for the idiographic and subjective impact of life stressors on individuals (Kilpatrick, et al. 2007; Slavich, et al. 2009). Likewise, all studies used empirically validated measures to assess MDD symptoms and for diagnostic purposes. Although the assessment of social support can be nuanced, researchers utilized theoretically informed assessments (e.g., assessment of types of social support for the buffering hypothesis; Cohen & Wills, 1985; Hunt, et al., 2018; Kilpatrick, et al., 2007).

In addition, all of the studies recruited participants *relevant* to the research questions, rather than recruiting a convenience sample (Hunt, et al. 2018; Kilpatrick, et al., 2007; Ross, et al., 2009; Silk, et al., 2011; Slavich, et al., 2009). Diversity and inclusion and exclusion parameters were addressed thoughtfully, too (Ross, et al. 2009; Silk, et al., 2011). In addition, the relationships between modern technology, social networks, stress, mood, and depression were explored with a particular emphasis on resolving the issue of recall bias (Hunt, et al., 2018; Silk, et al., 2011). Researchers also tried to examine the impact of life context (e.g., engagement with social networks, surviving a hurricane, depression as a teenager) beyond understanding behavior in a lab setting (Hunt, et al., 2018; Ross, et al., 2009; Silk, et al., 2011).

However, there are some limitations to the studies, including small sample size (Slavich, et al., 2009), inability to assume causal relationships and to understand how other factors such as previous diagnosis of MDD affects stress and MDD symptomology (Kilpatrick, et al., 2007), and replicability (Ross, et al. 2009). Further, some studies may have benefited from a greater focus on perceived social support, stress (Silk, et al., 2011), or considered other statistical analyses (Hunt, et al., 2018).

Conclusion

The current chapter is limited in presenting all of the methods and theories relevant to the topic. For instance, researchers have noted chronic stress, particularly interpersonal chronic stress, increases the risk for MDD (Sheets & Craighead, 2014). There are also other theories examining the link between social networks, stress, and coping—for instance, the interpersonal life stress model of depression (Hammen, 2006). Other methodologies, including studies evaluating the treatment of depression (e.g., randomized controlled designs or effectiveness trials), would have been interesting to evaluate; many evidence-based treatments focus on improving social networks to reduce symptoms of depression (Frank & Spanier, 1995; Martell, Dimidjian, & Herman-Dunn, 2013). The measurement of stress has also expanded beyond self-report questionnaires to biological measures (Baum & Grunberg, 1997). This chapter does not assess how biological markers of stress are affected by social networks, nor does it present data linking the explored relationships directly to health. Several other studies, however, suggest evidence of this relationship (Robles, Glaser, & Kiecolt-Glaser, 2005).

Future studies should address concerns raised in the chapter, including ecological validity, behavioral, biological, and related assessments of stress and depression. Included in this list is being thoughtful about recall biases among individuals with MDD (Ben-Zeev & Young, 2010), properly operationalizing social support (Cohen & Wills, 1985), and understanding the context and ideographic features relevant to participants' report of stress (Brown & Harris, 1989; Hammen, 2005). Regardless, research continues to support social networks as an essential factor in predicting and explaining the relationship between stress and depression (Cohen & Wills, 1985; Hammen, 2005). While research methodology has significantly progressed, continued utilization of technology, examination of the biological and psychological interactions among variables, evaluation of modern social networks (e.g., *SNS*), and research focused on ecological and internal validity are recommended.

References

Ainsworth, M. D. S. (1978). The Bowlby-Ainsworth attachment theory. *Behavioral and Brain Sciences*, *1*(3), 436–438. doi:10.1017/S0140525X00075828

American Psychiatric Association. (2013). *Diagnostic and statistical manual of mental disorders* (5th ed.). Arlington, VA: American Psychiatric Publishing. doi:10.1176/appi.books.9780890425596

Angst, J., & Merikangas, K. R. (2001). Multi-dimensional criteria for the diagnosis of depression. *Journal of Affective Disorders*, *62*(1–2), 7–15. doi:10.1016/S0165-0327(00)00346-3

Appel, H., Gerlach, A. L., & Crusius, J. (2016). The interplay between Facebook use, social comparison, and depression. *Current Opinion in Psychology*, *9*, 44–49. doi:10.1016/j.copsyc.2015.10.006

Baum, A., & Grunberg, N. (1997). Measurement of stress hormones. In S. Cohen, R. C. Kessler, & L. U. Gordon (Eds.), *Measuring stress: A guide for health and social scientists* (pp. 175–192). New York, NY: Oxford University Press.

Beck, A. T., Steer, R. A., & Brown, G. K. (1996). *Manual for the beck depression inventory-II*. San Antonio, TX: Psychological Corporation. doi:10.1037/t00742-000

Ben-Zeev, D., & Young, M. A. (2010). Accuracy of hospitalized depressed patients' and healthy controls' retrospective symptom reports. *Journal of Nervous and Mental Disease*, *198*(4), 280–285. doi:10.1097/NMD.0b013e3181d6141f

Bolby, J. (1969). *Attachment and loss: Volume 1*. Attachment. New York, NY: Basic Books.

Bostwick, J. M., & Pankratz, V. S. (2000). Affective disorders and suicide risk: A reexamination. *American Journal of Psychiatry*, *157*(12), 1925–1932. doi:10.1176/appi.ajp.157.12.1925

Brown, G. W., & Harris, T. O. (Eds.). (1989). *Life events and illness*. New York, NY: The Guilford Press.

Caspi, A., Sugden, K., Moffitt, T. E., Taylor, A., Craig, I. W., Harrington, H., et al. (2003). Influence of life stress on depression: Moderation by a polymorphism in the 5-HTT gene. *Science*, *301*(3531), 386–389. doi:10.1126/science.1083968

Cassel, J. (1976). The contribution of the social environment to host resistance. *American Journal of Epidemiology*, *104*(2), 107–123. doi:10.1093/oxfordjournals.aje.a112281

Chataway, C. J. (1997). An examination of the constraints on mutual inquiry in a participatory action research project. *Journal of Social Issues*, *53*(4), 747–765. doi:10.1111/j.1540-4560.1997.tb02459.x

Cohen, L. H., Towbes, L. C., & Flocco, R. (1988). Effects of induced mood on self-reported life events and perceived and received social support. *Journal of Personality and Social Psychology*, *55*(4), 669–679. doi:10.1037/0022-3514.55.4.669

Cohen, S., & Hoberman, H. M. (1983). Positive events and social supports as buffers of life change stress 1. *Journal of Applied Social Psychology*, *13*(2), 99–125. doi:10.1111/j.1559-1816.1983.tb02325.x

Cohen, S., & Wills, T. A. (1985). Stress, social support, and the buffering hypothesis. *Psychological Bulletin, 98*(2), 310–357. doi:10.1037/0033-2909.98.2.310

Crawford, J., Cayley, C., Lovibond, P. F., Wilson, P. H., & Hartley, C. (2011). Percentile norms and accompanying interval estimates from an Australian general adult population sample for self-report mood scale BAI, BDI- CRSD, CES-D, DASS, DASS-21, STAI-X, STAI-Y, SRDS, and SRAS). *Australian Psychologist, 46*(1), 3–14. doi: 10.1111/j.1742-9544.2010.00003.x

Dickens, C., McGowan, L., Clark-Carter, D., & Creed, F. (2002). Depression in rheumatoid arthritis: A systematic review of the literature with meta-analysis. *Psychometric Medicine, 64*(1), 52–60. doi:10.1097/00006842-200201000-00008

First, M. B., Gibbon, M., Spitzer, R. L., & Williams, J. B. W. (1995). User's guide for the structured clinical interview for DSM—IV Axis I disorders (SCID-I, Version 2.0). *Unpublished Manuscript, Biometrics Research Department, New York State Psychiatric Institute.* doi:10.1037/t07827-000

Forbes, E. A., & Dahl, R. E. (2005). Neural systems of positive affect: Relevance to understanding child and adolescent depression? *Development and Psychopathology, 17*(3), 827–850. doi:10.1017/S095457940505039X

Frank, E., & Spanier, C. (1995). Interpersonal psychotherapy for depression: Overview, clinical efficacy, and future directions. *Clinical Psychology: Science and Practice, 2*(4), 349–369. doi:10.1111/j.1468-2850.1995.tb00048.x

Gelernter, J., Kranzler, H., & Cubells, J. F. (1997). Serotonin transporter protein (SLC6A4) allele and haplotype frequencies and linkage disequilibria in African-and European-American and Japanese populations and in alcohol-dependent subjects. *Human Genetics, 101*(2), 243–246. doi:10.1007/s004390050624

Gunthert, K. C., & Wenze, S. J. (2012). Daily diary methods. In M. R. Mehl & T. S. Conner (Eds.), *Handbook of research methods for studying daily life* (pp. 144–159). New York, NY: The Guilford Press.

Hamilton, M. (1967). Development of a rating scale for primary depressive illness. *British Journal of Social and Clinical Psychology, 6*(4), 278–296. doi:10.1111/j.2044-8260.1967.tb00530.x

Hammen, C. (2005). Stress and depression. *Annual Review of Clinical Psychology, 1,* 293–319. doi: 10.1146/annurev.clinpsy.1.102803.143938

Hammen, C. (2006). Stress generation in depression: Reflections on origins, research, and future directions. *Journal of Clinical Psychology, 62*(9), 1065–1082. doi:10.1002/jclp.20293

Hammer, M. (1981). "Core" and "extended" social support networks in relation to health and illness. *Social Science and Medicine, 17*(7), 405–411. doi: 10.1016/0277-9536(83)90344-1

Hunt, M. G., Marx, R., Lipson, C., & Young, J. (2018). No more FOMO: Limiting social media decreases loneliness and depression. *Journal of Social and Clinical Psychology, 37*(10), 751–768. doi:10.1521/jscp.2018.37.10.751

Jakobsen, J. C., Katakam, K. K., Schou, A., Hellmuth, S. G., Stallknecht, S. E., Leth-Møller, K., et al. (2017). Selective serotonin reuptake inhibitors versus placebo in patients with major depressive disorder: A systematic review with meta-analysis and Trial Sequential Analysis. *BMC Psychiatry, 17*(1), 58. doi:10.1186/s12888-016-1173-2

Jazbec, S., McClure, E., Hardin, M., Pine, D. S., & Ernst, M. (2005). Cognitive control under contingencies in anxious and depressed adolescents: An antisaccade task. *Biological Psychiatry, 58*(8), 632–639. doi:10.1016/j.biopsych.2005.04.010

Johnson, N. B., Hayes, L. D., Brown, K., Hoo, E. C., & Ethier, K. A. (2014). CDC national health report: Leading causes of morbidity and mortality and associated behavioral risk and protective factors-United States, 2005–2013. *WMWR, 64,* Supplement. Retrieved from https://stacks.cdc.gov/view/cdc/25809

Kaufman, J., Birmaher, B., Brent, D., Rao, U. M. A., Flynn, C., Moreci, P., et al. (1997). Schedule for affective disorders and schizophrenia for school-age children-present and lifetime version (K-SADS-PL): Initial reliability and validity data. *Journal of the American Academy of Child & Adolescent Psychiatry, 36*(7), 980–988. doi:10.1097/00004583-199707000-00021

Kelly, P. J. (2005). Practical suggestions for community interventions using participatory action research. *Public Health Nursing, 22*(1), 65–73. doi:10.1111/j.0737-1209.2005.22110.x

Kendler, K. S., Neal, M. C., Kessler, R. C., Heath, A. C., & Eaves, L. J. (1993). The lifetime history of major depression in women: Reliability of diagnosis and heritability. *Archives of General Psychiatry, 50*(11), 863–870. doi:10.1001/archpsyc.1993.01820230054003

Kessler, R. C. (1997). The effects of stressful life events on depression. *Annual Review of Psychology, 48*(1), 191–214. doi:10.1146/annurev.psych.48.1.191

Kessler, R. C., Berglund, P., Demler, O., Jin, R., Merikangas, K. R., & Walters, E. E. (2005). Lifetime prevalence and age-of-onset distributions of DMS-IV disorders in the National Comorbidity Survey Replication. *Archives of General Psychiatry, 62*(6), 593–602. doi:10.1001/archpsyc.62.6.593

Kilpatrick, D. G., Koenen, K. C., Ruggiero, K. J., Acierno, R., Galea, S., & Resnick, H. S. (2007). The serotonin transporter genotype and social support and moderation of posttraumatic stress disorder and depression in hurricane-exposed adults. *American Journal of Psychiatry, 164*(11), 1693–1699. doi:10.1176/appi.ajp.2007.06122007

Kovacs, M. (1981). Rating scales to assess depression in school-aged children. *Acta Paedopsychiatry*, *46*, 305–315. Retrieved from https://psycnet.apa.org/record/1981-31663-001

Kross, E., Verduyn, M. P., Demiralp, E., Park, J., Lee, D. S., Lin, N., et al. (2013). Facebook use predicts decline in subjective well-being in young adults. *PLos One*, *8*, e698441.

Laurent, J., Catanzaro, S. J., Joiner, T. E., Jr., Rudolph, K. D., Potter, K. I., Lambert, S., et al. (1999). A measure of positive and negative affect for children: Scale development and preliminary validation. *Psychological Assessment*, *11*(3), 326–338. doi:10.1037/1040-3590.11.3.326

Lesch, K. P., Bengel, D., Heils, A., Sabol, S. Z., Greenberg, B. D., Petri, S., et al. (1996). Association of anxiety-related traits with a polymorphism in the serotonin transporter gene regulatory region. *Science*, *274*(5292), 1527–1531. doi:10.1126/science.274.5292.1527

Lewin, K. (1946). Action research and minority problems. *Journal of Social Issues*, *2*(4), 34–46. doi:10.1111/j.1540-4560.1946.tb02295.x

Lup, K., Trub, L., & Rosenthal, L. (2015). Instagram #instasad? Exploring associations among Instagram use, depressive symptoms, negative social comparison, and strangers followed. *Cyberpsychology Behavior and Social Networking*, *18*(5), 247–252. doi:10.1089/cyber.2014.0560

MacDonald, C. (2012). Understanding participatory action research: A qualitative research methodology option. *Canadian Journal of Action Research*, *13*(2), 34–50. doi:10.33524/cjar.v13i2.37

Martell, C. R., Dimidjian, S., & Herman-Dunn, R. (2013). *Behavioral activation for depression: A clinician's guide*. New York, NY: The Guilford Press.

Mason, R., & Boutilier, M. (1996). The challenge of genuine power sharing in participatory research: The gap between theory and practice. *Canadian Journal of Community Mental Health*, *15*(2), 145–152. doi:10.7870/cjcmh-1996-0015

Monroe, S. M., & Harkness, K. L. (2005). Life stress, the "kindling" hypothesis, and the recurrence of depression: Considerations from a life stress perspective. *Psychological Review*, *112*(2), 417. doi:10.1037/0033-295X.112.2.417

Monroe, S. M., & Simons, A. D. (1991). Diathesis-stress theories in the context of life stress research: Implications for the depressive disorders. *Psychological Bulletin*, *110*(3), 406–425. doi:10.1037/0033-2909.110.3.406

Munce, S. E., Stansfeld, S. A., Blackmore, E. R., & Stewart, D. E. (2007). The role of depression and chronic pain conditions in absenteeism: Results from a national epidemiologic survey. *Journal of Occupational and Environmental Medicine*, *49*(11), 1206–1211. doi:10.1097/JOM.0b013e318157f0ba

Nezlek, J. B. (2012). Multilevel modeling analyses of diary-style data. *Handbook of Research Methods for Studying Daily Life*, 357–383.

Nooner, K. B., Linares, L. O., Batinjane, J., Kramer, R. A., Silva, R., & Cloitre, M. (2012). Factors related to posttraumatic stress disorder in adolescence. *Trauma, Violence, & Abuse*, *13*(3), 153–166. doi:10.1177/1524838012447698

O'Reilly, P. (1988). Methodological issues in social support and social network research. *Social Science & Medicine*, *26*(8), 863–873. doi:10.1016/0277-9536(88)90179-7

Paykel, E. S. (2003). Life events and affective disorders. *Acta Psychiatrica Scandinavica*, *108*, 61–66. doi:10.1034/j.1600-0447.108.s418.13.x

Peterson, R. A., & Merunka, D. R. (2014). Convenience samples of college students and research reproducibility. *Journal of Business Research*, *67*(5), 1035–1041. doi:10.1016/j.jbusres.2013.08.010

Pine, D. S., Lissek, S., Klein, R. G., Mannuzza, S., Moulton, J. L., III, Guardino, M., et al. (2004). Face-memory and emotion: Associations with major depression in children and adolescents. *Journal of Child Psychology and Psychiatry*, *45*(7), 1199–1208. doi:10.1111/j.1469-7610.2004.00311.x

Plomin, R. E., DeFries, J. C., Craig, I. W., & McGuffin, P. E. (2003). *Behavioral genetics in the postgenomic era*. American Psychological Association. doi:10.1037/10480-000

Radloff, L. S. (1977). The CES-D scale: A self-report depression scale for research in the general population. *Applied Psychological Measurement*, *1*(3), 385–401. doi:10.1177/014662167700100306

Rafaeli, E., & Revelle, W. (2006). A premature consensus: Are happiness and sadness truly opposite affects? *Motivation and Emotion*, *30*(1), 1–12. doi:10.1007/s11031-006-9004-2

Reis, H. T. (2012). Why researchers should think "real world": A conceptual rationale. In M. R. Mehl & T. S. Conner (Eds.), *Handbook of research methods for studying daily life* (pp. 144–159). New York, NY: The Guilford Press.

Robins, L. N., Cottler, L. B., Bucholz, K. K., Compton, W. M., North, C. S., & Rourke, K. M. (2000). *Diagnostic interview schedule for the DSM-IV (DIS-IV)*. St. Louis, MO: Washington University School of Medicine.

Robles, T. F., Glaser, R., & Kiecolt-Glaser, J. K. (2005). Out of balance: A new look at chronic stress, depression, and immunity. *Current Directions in Psychological Science*, *14*(2), 111–115. doi:10.1111/j.0963-7214.2005.00345.x

Rohleder, N., Nater, U. M., Wolf, J. M., Ehlert, U., & Kirschbaum, C. (2004). Psychosocial stress-induced activation of salivary alpha-amylase: An indicator of sympathetic activity? *Annals of the New York Academy of Sciences*, *1032*(1), 258–263. doi:10.1196/annals.1314.033

Rosenberg, M. (1979). *Conceiving of the self.* New York, NY: Basic Books.

Ross, E., Ali, A., & Toner, B. (2009). Investigating issues surrounding depression in adolescent girls across Ontario: A participatory action research project. *Canadian Journal of Community Mental Health, 22*(1), 55–68. doi:10.7870/cjcmh-2003-0004

Rubio-Guerra, A. F., Rodriguez-Lopez, L., Vargas-Ayala, G., Huerta-Ramirez, S., Serna, D. C., & Lozano-Nuevo, J. J. (2013). Depression increases the risk for uncontrolled hypertension. *Experimental & Clinical Cardiology, 18*(1), 10–12. Retrieved from www.ncbi.nlm.nih.gov/pmc/articles/PMC3716493/

Russell, D., Peplau, L. A., & Cutrona, S. C. E. (1980). The revised UCLA Loneliness Scale: Concurrent and discriminant validity evidence. *Journal of Personality & Social Psychology, 39*(3), 472–480.

Ryan, T., & Xenos, S. (2011). Who uses Facebook? An investigation of the relationship between the Big Five, shyness, narcissism, loneliness, and Facebook usage. *Computers in Human Behavior, 27*(5), 1658–1664. doi:10.1016/j.chb.2011.02.004

Ryff, C. D. (1995). Psychological well-being in adult life. *Current Directions in Psychological Science, 4*, 99–104.

Schneider, B. A., Avivi-Reich, M., & Mozuraitis, M. (2015). A cautionary note on the use of the Analysis of Covariance (ANCOVA) in classification designs with and without within-subject factors. *Frontier in Psychology, 6*, 474. doi:10.3389/fpsyg.2015.00474

Segal, D. L., Coolidge, F. L., O'Riley, A., & Heinz, B. A. (2006). Structured and semistructured interviews. In *Clinician's handbook of adult behavioral assessment* (pp. 121–144). Academic Press.

Sheets, E. S., & Craighead, W. E. (2014). Comparing chronic interpersonal and noninterpersonal stress domains as predictors of depression recurrence in emerging adults. *Behavior Research and Therapy, 63*, 36–42. doi:10.1016/j.brat.2014.09.001

Sherbourne, C. D., & Stewart, A. L. (1991). The MOS social support survey. *Social Science & Medicine, 32*(6), 705–714. doi:10.1016/0277-9536(91)90150-B

Silk, J. S., Forbes, E. E., Whalen, D. J., Jakubcak, J. L., Thompson, W. K., & Ryan, N. D. (2011). Daily emotional dynamics in depressed youth: A cell-phone ecological momentary assessment study. *Journal of Experimental Child Psychology, 110*(2), 241–257. doi:10.1016/j.jecp.2010.10.007

Silk, J. S., Steinberg, L., & Morris, A. S. (2003). Adolescents' emotion regulation in daily life: Links to depressive symptoms and problem behavior. *Child Development, 74*(6), 1869–1880. doi:10.1046/j.1467-8624.2003.00643.x

Slavich, G. M., Tartter, M. A., Brennan, P. A., & Hammen, C. (2014). Endogenous opioid system influences depressive reactions to socially painful targeted rejection life events. *Psychoneuroendocrinology, 49*, 141–149. doi:10.1016/j.psyneuen.2014.07.009

Slavich, G. M., Thornton, T., Torres, L. D. Monroe, S. M., & Gotlib, I. H. (2009). Targeted rejection predicts hastened onset of major depression. *Journal of Social and Clinical Psychology, 28*(2), 223–243. doi:10.1521/jscp.2009.28.2.223

Smith, A., & Anderson, M. (2018). Social media use in 2018. *Pew Research Center.* Retrieved from http://pewinterent.org/2018/03/01/social-media-use-in-2018/

Song, H., Zmyslinski-Seelig, A., Kim, J., Drent, A., Victor, A., Omori, K., et al. (2014). Does Facebook make you lonely? A meta analysis. *Computers in Human Behavior, 36*, 446–452. doi:10.1016/j.chb.2014.04.011

Spielberger, C. D., Gorsuch, R. L., Lushene, R., Vagg, P. R., & Jacobs, G. A. (1983). *Manual for the state-trait anxiety inventory.* Palo Alto, CA: Consulting Psychologists Press.

Stone, A. A., Schwartz, J. E., Neale, J. M., Shiffman, S., Marco, C. A., Hickcox, M., et al. (1998). A comparison of coping assessed by ecological momentary assessment and retrospective recall. *Journal of Personality and Social Psychology, 74*(6), 1670–1680. doi:10.1037/0022-3514.74.6.1670

Stone, A. A., Shiffman, S., Atienza, A. A., Nebeling, L., Stone, A., Shiffman, et al. (2007). Historical roots and rationale of ecological momentary assessment (EMA). In *The science of real-time data capture: Self-reports in health research.* New York, NY: Oxford University Press.

Telford, C., McCarthy-Jones, S., Corcoran, R., & Rowse, G. (2011). Experience sampling methodology studies of depression: The state of the art. *Psychological Medicine, 42*(6), 1119–1129. doi:10.1017/S0033291711002200

Tromholt, M. (2016). The Facebook experiment: Quitting Facebook leads to high levels of well-being. *Cyberpsychology, Behavior, and Social Networking, 19*(11), 661–666. doi:10.1089/cyber.2016.0259

Twenge, J. M., Joiner, T. E., Rogers, M. L., & Martin, G. N. (2017). Increases in depressive symptoms, suicide-related outcomes, and suicide rates among U.S. adolescents after 2010 and links to increased new media screen time. *Clinical Psychological Science, 6*(1), 3–17. doi:10.1177/2167702617723376

Verduyn, P., Lee, D. S., Park, J., Shablack, H., Orvell, A., Bayer, J., et al. (2015). Passive Facebook usage undermines affective well-being: Experimental and longitudinal evidence. *Journal of Experimental Psychology: General, 144*(2), 480–488. doi:10.1037/xge0000057

Wankerl, M., Wüst, S., & Otte, C. (2010). Current developments and controversies: Does the serotonin transporter gene-linked polymorphic region (5-HTTLPR) modulate the association between stress and depression? *Current Opinion in Psychiatry, 23*(6), 582–587. doi:10.1097/YCO.0b013e32833f0e3a

Wong, M., & Licinio, J. (2001). Research and treatment approaches to depression. *Nature Reviews, 2*(5), 343–351. doi:10.1038/35072566

Zimmerman, M., & Coryell, W. (1994). Screening for major depressive disorder in the community: A comparison of measures. *Psychological Assessment, 6*(1), 71–74. doi:10.1037/1040-3590.6.1.71

14
DON'T SWEAT IT! NEUROIMAGING STUDIES OF STRESS

Ayesha Khan and Sukhvinder S. Obhi

In his best-selling book, *Why Zebra Don't Get Ulcers* (1998), neurobiologist Robert Sapolsky asks the reader to imagine the following scenario:

> It's two o'clock in the morning, and you're lying in bed. You have something immensely important and challenging to do the next day—a critical meeting, a presentation, an exam. You have to get a decent night's rest, but you're still wide awake. You try different strategies for relaxing, take deep breaths, try to imagine restful mountain scenery, but instead you lie there more tense by the second.
>
> *(p. 1)*

The situation describes a unique aspect of contemporary life. Most of the challenges experienced by people no longer are related to physical threats like war, drought, famine, parasites or defending against wild animals; instead, the vast majority of issues we deal with are largely psychosocial in nature. Giving a public presentation, meeting a deadline, or planning a wedding can be classified as emotionally charged experiences because they may lead to failure, social defeat or disappointment. What results is a complex array of behavioral, cognitive and physiological processes that help us successfully cope with both the actual and perceived stressors of life (see review in Schneiderman, Ironson, & Siegel, 2005).

This chapter begins with a historical, scientific overview of one element of our daily experience: psychological stress. We then discuss the underlying biological mechanisms that mediate the human stress response, especially the roles played by our endocrine system. As this field encompasses a broad range of theoretical and methodological approaches, we acknowledge that our work is not a full review of the neuroimaging research on stress. Rather, we focus on key electrophysiological and neuroimaging studies currently used to study the stress responses in humans.

Research in Practice

"Stress in health and disease is medically, sociologically, and philosophically the most meaningful subject for humanity that I can think of."

—Hans Selye (1907–1982)

The term "stress" is a derivative of the Latin verb, *"strictus,"* which means, "to draw tight" (Strictus, n.d.). Its use in Middle English denoted "hardships or forces exerted on a person" (Stress, n.d.).

Although modern stress research largely focuses on the cognitive processes that contribute to the occurrence and management of commonplace and extraordinary experiences of stress, much of the history of stress research is rooted in medicine. The French experimental physiologist Claude Bernard was one of the earliest figures to study stress through empirical work. Bernard suggested that physiological systems are constantly working to maintain a *milieu intérieur*, or a "constancy of the internal environment"; simply put, Bernard recognized that the body strives to maintain balance (Gross, 1998). Walter B. Canon would later formalize Bernard's observation by coining the term **homeostasis** to describe an organism's tendency to maintain internal balance (Cannon, 1963).

The Hungarian Canadian endocrinologist Hans Selye gained large-scale recognition through his work on *chronic* stress by establishing a relationship between ongoing stress and disease. Selye's work expanded upon Canon's conception of stress, which primarily focused on a subject's acute response to an immediate threat, more commonly known as a **fight-or-flight** state. Selye observed that laboratory rats exhibited a multi-stage physiological response to stress, later to be formalized in Selye's General Adaptation Syndrome. Specifically, Selye's experiments revealed that the rats exhibited a three-phase response when they were subjected to ongoing stress in the form of either temperature fluctuations, surgical injury or excessive exercise. Phase 1, an **alarm reaction**—wherein the *fight-or-flight* system is activated—occurs in response to an immediate threat to the body. If the stressor is not abated, then the body engages in **resistance** (Phase 2), wherein various internal networks, such as the immune system, are recruited for assistance. The final stage, **exhaustion** (Phase 3), brings, as the name implies, exhaustion, illness, and eventual death, as the subject has little capacity to cope with the stressor due to depleted bodily resources. Prolonged stress produced the same physiological result in all of Selye's subjects: pathology of the adrenal glands, atrophy in the lymphatic system, and peptic ulcers (Tan & Yip, 2018).

In their seminal paper *Stress and the Individual* (1993), Bruce McEwen and Eliot Stellar reinterpreted Selye's work by presenting a modified conceptualization of stress formation and the associated processes that may lead to disease. According to this adapted model, the original concept of **homeostasis** was limited because it did not consider real-world conditions wherein one's physiology is constantly responding to changing environmental conditions. As such, McEwen and Stellar reintroduced the concept of **allostasis**—as defined by Sterling and Eyer (1988)—literally meaning to achieve stability through change (McEwen, 2007). It may be more useful to think about the body as operating within a range of functions. This range is dynamic and varies depending on age and health status. For example, younger people and those with greater levels of health are more able to cope with stressors than those who are older or in poorer health (Lipsitz & Goldberg, 1992; Naliboff, Benton, Solomon, Morley, Fahey, Bloom, et al., 1991; Sterling & Eyer, 1988). **Allostatic load** occurs due to ongoing wear and tear on the body from either chronic overactivity or inactivity of physiological systems that are normally involved in responding to environmental challenges (McEwen & Stellar, 1993). Equally important, a person's life history can influence their perception of a stressor in unique and unexpected ways. One's reaction to physical and psychological stressors, or the extent to which the body experiences *allostatic load*, is determined by several factors, including the social context in which the stressor occurs, genetic makeup, psychological history, social history, and the health-damaging and health-promoting behaviors of the individual (McEwen, 1998; McEwen & Stellar, 1993).

The Brain–Body Connection: The Hypothalamic-Pituitary-Adrenal Axis

There is a strong consensus that both immediate and long-term stress activate a wide range of bodily responses (see review in Yaribeygi, Panahi, Sahraei, Johnston, & Sahebkar, 2017). An emergency reaction causes the sympathetic nervous system to release **peripheral hormones**, such as epinephrine and norepinephrine, to increase blood pressure and heart rate in order to redistribute blood to the muscles. The response to an ongoing stressor is somewhat different. The **hypothalamic-pituitary-adrenal (HPA) axis** is activated during emergency responses. In such instances, stressors lasting longer than a few minutes will lead to increased production of the metabolic hormone, cortisol (see review in Sapolsky, Romero, & Munck, 2000). The **HPA axis** functions via a feedback loop that tells the structures in the central nervous system, such as the hypothalamus and the pituitary gland, to release the neurohormones **corticotropin-releasing hormone** (**CRH**; from the paraventricular nucleus of hypothalamus) and **adrenocorticotropic hormone** (**ACTH**; from the anterior portion of the pituitary gland) into the bloodstream. Once *CRH* releases from the hypothalamus, its effects occur on the nearby pituitary gland to release *ACTH*, which then travels in the blood to the adrenal glands located atop of the kidneys to secrete the hormone cortisol (Figure 14.1).

Once cortisol is released from the adrenal glands, it circulates in the blood, affecting most tissues of the body. When present in high concentrations, *cortisol* exerts a negative-feedback effect that causes *CRH* and *ACTH* production in the hypothalamus and pituitary gland to be suppressed. On the other hand, *CRH* and *ACTH* production increases when blood cortisol levels fall below an

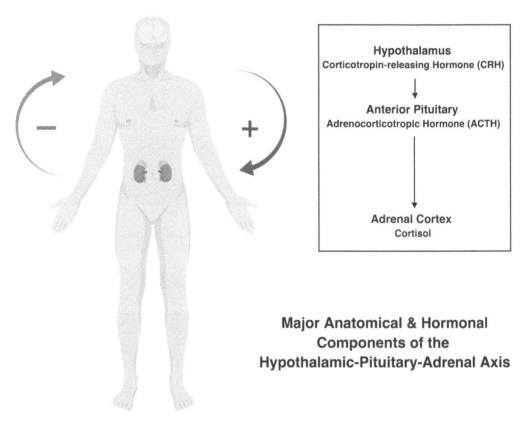

Major Anatomical & Hormonal Components of the Hypothalamic-Pituitary-Adrenal Axis

Figure 14.1 Hypothalamic hormones travel through a capillary system to the inferior portion of the anterior pituitary gland, where they stimulate neurons to produce and secrete hormones. The releasing hormone in the hypothalamic-pituitary-adrenal axis is the corticotropin-releasing hormone (CRH). CRH acts on the anterior pituitary to release adrenocorticotropic hormone (ACTH), which travels in the blood to the adrenal cortex of the adrenal glands, located atop of the kidneys, to secrete cortisol in humans. Most cells in the body have cortisol receptors resulting in wide-reaching effects such as those involved in energy metabolism, immune functioning, cardiovascular responses, and reproduction. A negative-feedback loop decreases hormone secretion in the brain after reaching a target concentration. Positive feedback can stimulate the production of both CRH and ACTH.

Created with Biorender.com

optimal level. Stress may override this system, however, as it can disrupt the *HPA axis's* response to the typical pattern of negative feedback. The *HPA axis* is activated during stressful situations, leading to the increased secretion of ACTH and cortisol. If the stressful situation persists, levels of *ACTH* and cortisol may reach abnormally high concentrations (see review in Spencer & Deak, 2017). *HPA* activation results in increased glucose in the blood and the suppression of major systems, such as those involved in immune functions, digestive and cardiovascular responses, and, potentially, reproduction (Joseph & Whirledge, 2017; Schneiderman, et al., 2005; Whirledge & Cidlowski, 2010).

Under unstressed conditions, however, the *HPA* system exhibits a classic circadian rhythm. In a hallmark study, when blood cortisol levels were measured across seven 24-hour periods in healthy subjects, a temporal pattern was observed. The highest cortisol release occurred in the morning, and lowest at night just prior to sleeping (Weitzman, Fukushima, Nogeire, Howard, Gallagher, & Hellman, 1971). Indeed, the **cortisol awakening response**—in which blood levels are highest within the first hour of waking—is now used as a proxy to assess the integrity of the *HPA axis* (see review in Chida & Steptoe, 2009).

It is important to appreciate that stress has been studied by researchers in multiple disciplines. Earlier, we sketched a brief overview of core concepts derived from the fields of medicine and biology. Next, we highlight the key contributions made by psychologists in our understanding of stress in humans.

A Brief History of Psychological Approaches to Understanding Stress in Humans

World War II provided the impetus for research into stress due to combat. In the post-war era, it became obvious that many life events could also induce psychological and emotional effects similar to those experienced in combat. Given that early interest in stress arose during the reign of behaviorism in psychology, initial attempts to understand stress were characterized by an "input-output" worldview. There was no consideration of mental processes; rather, researchers attempted to understand the relationships between certain classes of input and corresponding behavioral output.

A shift in our conceptualization of stress came when **stimulus-organism-response (S-O-R)** models emerged. Landmark work by Richard Lazarus showed that stress responses varied across people, with some showing strong stress responses and others showing no response at all (Lazarus & Eriksen, 1952). Thus, individual differences play a crucial role in intervening between a potential stressor and the organism's response. This intervening stage is termed "appraisal" and involves a set of cognitive processes that differ across people and situations.

Early psychological work on stress often involved exposing individuals to stressors in the laboratory (e.g., watching stressful videos) and measuring the physiological and subjective psychological responses to those experiences. Researchers showed that by inducing specific psychological states in participants before watching stressful videos, psychological and physiological responses were modulated. For example, inducing beliefs that the videos (often horrific scenes of injury/harm) were staged lowered both subjective measures of distress and autonomic nervous responses. In contrast, when participants focused on threats, pain and suffering, subjective and physiological measures of stress increased (Lazarus & Alfert, 1964; Speisman, Lazarus, Davison, & Mordkoff, 1964). Efforts to deal with a stressor are referred to as *coping* (Lazarus, 1993a, 1993b). (There are different styles of coping, including **problem-focused** and **emotion-focused**, but space limitations preclude a fuller treatment of these coping styles). Stress can induce positive or negative emotions, depending on both individual variables (motives, beliefs, etc.) and environmental context.

Psychological work on stress has helped shape our conceptual understanding of the topic and helped carve out research questions. Building on this, cognitive neuroscientists have studied stress using multiple methods, but given the breadth of the literature, comprehensive coverage of these studies of stress is beyond the scope of this chapter. Instead, we present a selective review of studies using a range of methods, including but not limited to *electroencephalography (EEG)* and *functional magnetic resonance imaging (fMRI)*. In the next section, we will highlight a small subset of studies that have used *EEG* to examine how asymmetry in frontal cortical activity relates to individual responses to stressful situations. These studies are built upon the important finding that *frontal EEG asymmetry* correlates with stress in non-human primates—in particular, right *frontal EEG* activity has been found to be positively related to high concentrations of *CRH* in rhesus monkeys (Kalin, Shelton, & Davidson, 2000; Kline, Allen, & Schwartz, 1998). We first introduce the concept of *frontal EEG asymmetry* and then consider how it has been used in stress research.

Multiple studies have established that asymmetries in *EEG* activity in the frontal cortex are associated with emotion (Davidson, Schwartz, Saron, Bennett, & Goleman, 1979; Ahern & Schwartz, 1985; Davidson, Schaffer, & Saron, 1985; Tucker, 1981). These asymmetries appear to comprise trait-like properties (e.g., resting state measures) and show state-dependent effects (e.g., modulation in specific tasks; Coan & Allen, 2004; Smith, Hendrick, Smith, Bateman, Moffatt, Rathleff, et al., 2017). *Frontal EEG asymmetry* is often measured as activity in the alpha range (typically 8 to 13 Hz) of the EEG signal. Given that alpha activity is inversely related to underlying cortical processing, lower levels of alpha are taken to indicate greater brain activity. Often, frontal alpha asymmetry is reported as a difference score between right and left frontal alpha (Coan & Allen, 2004; Smith, et al., 2017; Galang & Obhi, 2018; for a recent detailed methods paper see Smith, et al., 2017).

To date, research suggests that relatively greater frontal left cortical activity is associated with approach motivation (Harmon-Jones, Peterson, & Harris, 2009; Harmon-Jones & Sigelman, 2001; Smith, et al., 2017; De Pascalis, Cozzuto, Caprara, & Alessandri, 2013; see also Davidson, 1998). Greater relative right frontal cortical activity, however, is associated with withdrawal (e.g., Coan, Allen, & Harmon-Jones, 2001; Tullet, Harmon-Jones, & Inzlicht, 2012; Carver & White, 1994; Gray, 1987; Coan & Allen, 2003a, 2003b; Harmon-Jones & Allen, 1997).

Stress researchers use both naturalistic studies in which the stressor is a real-life circumstance and laboratory studies that allow the stressor to be manipulated. The obvious benefit of naturalistic approaches is ecological validity, whereas a benefit of laboratory approaches is experimental control. In this section, we describe noteworthy studies that have employed *EEG* measures of frontal brain activity to understand the stress response in humans (see Figure 14.2 for an overview of an approach to studying human stress with *EEG*).

Lewis, Weekes, and Wang (2007) investigated how naturalistic stressors affect frontal alpha asymmetry, cortisol levels and measures of subjective wellbeing. These authors based their work on studies showing that increased activity in the right frontal cortex is related to increased stress and decreased immune functioning (Davidson, Coe, Dolski, & Donzella, 1999; Kang, Davidson, Coe, Wheeler, Tomarken, & Ershler, 1991; see also Barneoud, Neveu, Vitiello, & LeMoal, 1987; Neveu, 1988, 1993; Quaranta, Siniscalchi, Frate, & Vallotigara, 2004). Specifically, the authors asked whether exposure to a naturalistic stressor would elevate cortisol and psychological stress levels and whether this would be associated with increased right frontal activity and negative health symptoms.

The experiment involved participants visiting the lab during the school year in a week when they had no examinations/assignments due and again during a week when they had multiple exams/assignments due. Psychological stress was measured using the Perceived Stress Scale (Cohen, Kamarch, & Mermelstein, 1983) and additional state and trait anxiety measures (Speilberger, Gorsuch, Lushene, Vagg, & Jacobs, 1983). Health status was assessed via the Health Symptoms Inventory (Weekes, Lewis, Patel, Garrison-Jakel, Berger, & Lupien, 2006). Salivary cortisol was used as an index of *HPA axis* activity, and frontal alpha asymmetry was measured. Upon arrival at the lab, participants completed the scale measures and provided a salivary sample. *EEG* data were then collected during eight one-minute blocks when eyes were either opened or closed. Immediately afterwards, participants

Don't Sweat It!

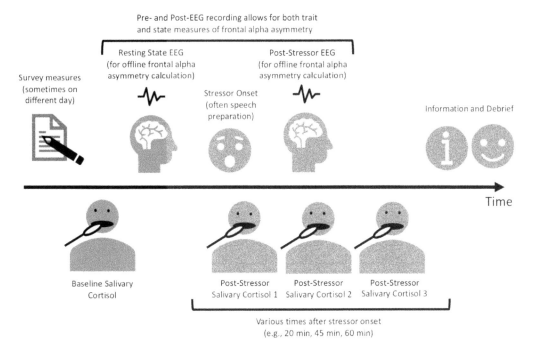

Figure 14.2 Overview of possible experimental approach to studying the human stress response using EEG frontal alpha asymmetry, self-report and salivary cortisol measures.

provided a second salivary sample. The order of low- and high-stress conditions was counterbalanced across participants.

Perceived stress was greater during high-stress compared to low-stress periods, confirming that the conditions were meaningfully different to participants. Despite this change in subjective stress, there was no change in cortisol across the two periods. There was, however, a shift from relatively greater left frontal activity in the low-stress period to relatively greater right frontal activity in the high-stress period. Furthermore, there was a correlation between right frontal activity and negative health symptoms in the high examination stress period. There was no relationship between changes in right frontal activity (between the low-stress and high-stress conditions) and changes in either psychological stress or *HPA* activity.

The study by Lewis, and colleagues (2007) is noteworthy for a number of reasons. First, it involves assessment of multiple measures of stress during a naturally high-stress versus low-stress time period. Second, it demonstrated that changes in psychological stress and frontal alpha asymmetry are possible in the absence of changes in cortisol and that right frontal activity is positively associated with negative health symptoms. These results underscore the complexity of links between subjective and objective measures. This study prompts two questions: Are there positive associations between *EEG* frontal asymmetry, cortisol and subjective stress, and if so, when do they occur?

As alluded to earlier, a key aim for researchers is to understand why the stress response differs across individuals. The next study we discuss evaluated the effects of individual differences in **action orientation** (i.e., those who are prone to respond quickly, being high in action orientation, and those who are prone to engage in cognitive perseveration, being low in action orientation) on the relationship between cortisol and relative left frontal brain activity (again using *EEG*). In contrast to the previous study, this study involved inducing stress using the Trier Social Stress Test (Kirschbaum, Pirke, & Hellhammer, 1993).

189

The Trier Social Stress Test

The Trier Social Stress Test (TSST), introduced in 1993, is a means to induce psychosocial stress in laboratory settings. Recall that in an influential meta-analysis of lab studies of acute psychological stressors, Dickerson and Kemeny (2004) found that cortisol responses are higher when situational demands are uncontrollable, when participants are unable to avoid negative outcomes and when participants are subjected to social evaluative threat wherein others can judge an individual's performance negatively. The meta-analysis concluded that the TSST is one of the few available stress protocols that satisfies these criteria (Kudielka, Hellhammer, & Kirschbaum, 2007). The TSST is relatively simple. It consists of a short preparation period of a few minutes (often three to four), followed by a test period in which the participant has to deliver a speech for five minutes and perform mental arithmetic in front of an audience (for a detailed description of the procedure see Kirschbaum, et al., 1993; Kudielka, et al., 2007).

In their study, Düsing, Tops, Radtke, Kuhl, and Quirin (2016) highlight that individuals are known to differ in the extent to which they can initiate actions in social contexts. For example, someone at risk of negative social evaluation or social rejection may initiate action to protect or maintain social inclusion. However, it is also possible that an individual faced with the same threat of social evaluation and rejection may hesitate and engage in extended planning or rumination prior to initiating action. Thus, individuals differ in the extent to which they are action oriented. Düsing and colleagues wanted to establish whether differences in *action orientation* influence the association between the cortisol response to social evaluative threat and relative left frontal cortical activity, which is an indicator of approach motivation (Harmon-Jones, Gable, & Peterson, 2010). The authors further surmised that being stuck in a mode of cognitive perseveration would be associated with higher levels of cortisol compared to being engaged in active coping via the initiation of action. Thus, the authors predicted that individuals low in *action orientation* would show a positive relationship between cortisol levels and relative left frontal activity. In contrast, they predicted that individuals who were able to engage in active coping via action initiation (i.e., those individuals who were high in *action orientation*) would not show the association between stress-related cortisol elevation and relative left frontal activity.

To test these predictions, the authors used a variant of the TSST in which participants were told they would be making a speech within a job interview context that would be video-recorded for later analysis. Prior to the stress manipulation, participants completed a resting-state *EEG* session in which *EEG* data were collected during eight one-minute periods of eyes open or eyes closed. Participants then completed another *EEG* recording session 20 minutes after the onset of the stressor. Before arriving for the main experiment, participants had already completed a measure of *action orientation*, using the "demand related *action orientation* scale"—a scale that asks about demanding everyday situations and classifies participants as high or low in action orientation (Kuhl, 1994a). Salivary cortisol measures were taken immediately before introducing the stressor and then at three subsequent times (20, 45 and 60 minutes after the stressor).

The authors sought to determine whether the change in frontal cortical activity (from pre-stressor to post-stressor) was related to the cortisol response to the stressor. In accordance with their hypothesis, they found that stronger cortisol response was related to increased relative left frontal activation only for participants low in *action orientation*. The authors interpreted this finding to mean that individuals deal with threat through active coping—which requires approach-motivated action and which is associated with relatively greater left frontal activity. However, they suggest that some individuals have difficulty translating increased approach motivation into action and that such individuals may be susceptible to remaining in a state of cognitive perseveration and worry (i.e., being preoccupied with a future event and being engaged in some form of planning to deal with it). The study by Düsing, and colleagues (2016) provides a nice example of how researchers examine the effects of individual difference variables on the relationship between asymmetry in frontal activity and *HPA* activity. This is an important endeavor, as there are presumably a host of individual difference variables that influence an individual's stress response.

As we alluded to earlier, patterns of frontal asymmetry may relate to stress in both a trait-like and state-like manner—possibilities that are captured in so-called ***dispositional models*** that estimate a person's general tendency for approach/avoidance and ***capability models*** that measure the combined effects of emotional demands and an individual's ability to regulate affect (Coan, Allen, & McKnight, 2006).

In the final study to be discussed, researchers compared *dispositional* and *capability models* by assessing patterns of frontal alpha asymmetry at baseline and while preparing to give a speech, as well as the change from baseline to preparation for the speech. Rather than assessing the potential relationship between frontal alpha asymmetry and cortisol elevation in response to stress, the researchers examined the relationship between patterns of frontal alpha asymmetry and attentional bias toward emotional faces. Pérez-Edgar, Kujawa, Nelson, Cole, and Zapp (2013) used the Emotional Picture Dot Probe Task, which involves the simultaneous presentation of two faces, one emotional and one neutral, and the subsequent appearance of a cue in either location. Participants respond to the cue with a pre-instructed response. The logic of the task is that if attention is drawn to the emotional face, response times will be fast when the cue appears in a location congruent with the emotional face. Participants performed the Dot Probe Task and underwent resting-state *EEG* recording and *EEG* recording during preparation for a speech (stressor). The results showed that increases in right frontal alpha asymmetry between baseline and post-stressor stages were associated with attentional bias toward angry faces and avoidance of happy faces. Importantly, only the change in asymmetry (i.e., becoming more right sided) between baseline and post-stressor stages of the experiment was associated with attentional bias. Pérez-Edgar and colleagues (2013) interpret their findings as consistent with the capability model in that shifts in frontal alpha asymmetry, but not resting frontal alpha asymmetry per se, seem to be important in an individual's response to a mild stressor. Studies of the human stress response using *EEG* asymmetry represent a tiny fraction of the cognitive neuroscience of stress. Next, we highlight some examples of research using other neuroimaging approaches. To preview, the studies we highlight underscore the complexities of doing stress-related research using scanning methods and the challenges involved in interpreting data across multiple studies.

The Montreal Imaging Stress Task

Neuroimaging studies that aim to identify the neural correlates of the *HPA* stress response in humans are challenging for a number of reasons. For instance, identifying the specific psychological stressors capable of activating the stress system in a controlled and time-sensitive manner while in a scanning environment presents a formidable challenge. There are also inconsistent findings regarding the effects of various psychological stressors on cortisol activity. One meta-analysis found that tasks that are performance based and characterized by social-evaluative threat may induce similar changes in cortisol release. This finding indicates that *HPA* responsiveness could be measured through experimental paradigms that incorporate a perceived social threat to the participant (see review in Dickerson & Kemeny, 2004).

The Montreal Imaging Stress Task (MIST) was developed specifically to enable researchers to induce psychosocial stress in a scanning environment. Here we describe the MIST procedure developed by Dedovic, Renwick, Mahani, Engert, Lupien, and Pruessner (2005) to study individual differences in the brain's response to stress. The protocol typically begins with a training session outside of the scanner. Here, the researchers determine the length of time it takes for each participant to solve mental arithmetic problems of varying difficulty under no time constraints. During an experimental condition, participants are instructed to solve mental math problems presented on a computer screen (e.g., $2 + 9 - 7$ being the easiest and $12 * 12 / 16$ being the more difficult problem) and to indicate their answers by using a mouse to select a number from a rotary dial. To induce a high rate of failure, a time limit is enforced. If the participant incorrectly answers three consecutive times, an algorithm increases the time limit by 10% until the participant is able to answer the questions correctly. Participants receive feedback in the form of one-word responses such as "correct," "incorrect," or "timeout." Two indicators, one for individual performance and one for a mock average group performance, are shown to the participant throughout this condition. Between experimental runs, the researcher reminds the participant that, on average, their peers correctly answered 80% to 90% of the questions. The participant also is told that their performance must be in line with the group average if their data are to be included in the study. To further induce social-evaluative threat, participants are reminded that members of the research team are monitoring their answers. In a control condition, the arithmetic problems are presented using the same format, level of difficulty, and frequency, but without a time restriction. Neither the participant's performance nor the group average is displayed. Feedback is still shown after each task, but because of the absence of a time limit, average performance increases to about 90%. In between runs, the investigator tells the participant to try to perform the task as quickly and accurately as possible, but they do not provide any evaluation. A rest condition records baseline brain activity where participants view a screen without performing any task (Dedovic, et al.,2005).

In one experiment, Pruessner, Dedovic, Khalili-Mahani, Engert, Pruessner, Buss, et al. (2008) used the MIST procedure along with *fMRI* (*n* = 40) and **15OH20 positron emission tomography** (**PET**; *n* = 10) to study neuronal activation in a group of healthy young male and female participants. Their specific question concerning the psychosocial response of the limbic system in the MIST was motivated in part by findings from the animal literature in which limbic system activity plays an important role in regulating the response to a stressor. To link cortisol response to brain activity, saliva samples were collected from participants before and after the experimental, control and rest conditions in the PET portion of the study. Predictably, cortisol levels were highest in the experimental condition and lowest in the rest condition. In the *fMRI* portion of the study, several saliva samples were obtained starting from 50 minutes before the onset of MIST until 50 minutes after. Here, saliva was also collected on a separate, non-testing day upon awakening and 15, 30, 45 and 60 minutes afterwards. Similar to the PET study, cortisol levels increased after the experience of psychosocial stress. Due to a large heterogeneity between cortisol responses, the researchers reviewed the data in more detail. An interesting pattern emerged: Roughly half of the participants decreased their production of cortisol over the course of the *fMRI* experiment. Nonetheless, these participants (classified as "non-responders") did not exhibit a lower cortisol awakening response.

When brain activity was assessed, aside from increased activation in the brain regions typically involved with mental arithmetic (e.g., the occipital parietal and motor cortex and the cerebellum), there was a reduction in cerebral blood flow of suspected stress-network areas in relation to social-evaluative stress. There was also deactivation in key structures such as the hippocampus, amygdala, hypothalamus, medial orbitofrontal cortex and cingulate cortices. Importantly, the researchers also observed that an increased cortisol response to the MIST was related to decreased limbic system activity. However, this finding was limited to the participants classified as "responders." For example, a higher percentage of deactivation in the hippocampus was associated with a stress-related increase in cortisol. The researchers concluded that the reduction in activity of significant limbic system structures such as the hippocampus might be essential to psychosocial stress. And the degree of deactivation, particularly in key limbic structures, is associated with the cortisol response. Although this study demonstrated similar brain region activity to that documented in animal-based studies, the exact control mechanism related to psychological stress in humans remains elusive.

In another study using the MIST, Boehringer, Tost, Haddad, Lederbogen, Wüst, Schwarz, et al. (2015) were interested in the role of the **perigenual division** of the **anterior cingulate cortex (pACC)** in potentially regulating the *HPA axis*. As this region has been implicated in the pathophysiology of depression (Pezawas, Meyer-Lindenberg, Drabant, Verchinski, Munoz, Kolachana, et al., 2005), the researchers combined multimodal structural and functional imaging to study anatomical and functional connectivity between the *pACC* and the hypothalamus in a group of healthy men (*n* = 11) and women (*n* = 14). A major additional aim of this study was to assess whether the cortisol awakening response was related to activity in the *pACC* and to the experience of social-evaluative stress.

In order to quantify basal *HPA* activity, participants were asked to provide saliva samples upon waking and then 30 minutes, eight hours and 14 hours afterwards (Day 1). On a different day, brain function was studied using the MIST and *fMRI* (Day 2). The ***structural magnetic resonance imaging (MRI)*** scan was conducted before the start of the stress test, and saliva cortisol was measured at multiple points in time, such as after rest, before entering the scanner, after the anatomical scan, after MIST runs and after leaving the scanner. Heart rate was measured continuously during the experiment, and participants used a Likert scale to quantify subjective stress levels prior to and following stress induction. The social-evaluative portions of the *fMRI* experiment led to increases in salivary cortisol, heart rate, blood pressure and feelings of stress, thus indicating that stress was induced in the scanner. Interestingly, the basal cortisol levels measured on a different day prior to the experiment were found to predict cortisol levels before participants entered the scanner, indicating that pre-stress baseline values on both days were comparable. However, the cortisol awakening response on Day 1 was not predictive of the stress-induced cortisol values on Day 2 of the experiment. These data indicate that in comparison to activity in the *HPA axis* that occurs at the time of waking, psychosocial stressors might affect *HPA* functioning in a different manner. There was, however, a significant inverse relationship between the cortisol awakening response and stress-related activity in the *pACC*. That is, individuals with a higher cortisol awakening response showed lower *pACC* brain activity in relation to the stress-inducing task. This is consistent with the hypothesis that the *anterior cingulate cortex* plays a role in *HPA axis* inhibition. Furthermore, *pACC* activity increased during stress across participants. The researchers reasoned that if the *pACC* was involved in the regulation of the *HPA axis*, then it should also functionally interact with the hypothalamus. Functional connectivity analysis revealed that both the *pACC* and hypothalamus were positively connected during stress, indicating communication between the two structures. Interestingly, individuals with a higher cortisol awakening response exhibited decreased functional connectivity between these two brain regions. These data support a link between the *pACC* and the cortisol awakening response and between *pACC* activity and the functioning of the *HPA axis*.

A recent study investigated what is known as the ***cross-stressor adaptation hypothesis***—that physical training lowers physiological and psychological responses to stress—using the MIST procedure (Zschucke, Renneberg, Dimeo, Wüstenberg, & Ströhle, 2015). In this experiment, participants were divided into two groups: men who exercised less than once a week (sedentary; ***SED***) and men who trained in an endurance sport such as running, cycling, swimming or rowing (highly trained; ***HT***) at least three times a week. Each group contained 20 participants, with all participants being between the ages of 20 and 30 years old. Prior to the start of the experiment, all participants were fitness tested and their ***VO2 max values*** (a measurement of the maximum amount of oxygen that is utilized during intensive exercise) were recorded. The participants also completed various questionnaires related to their levels of stress and anxiety. Both categories of participants (*SED* and *HT*) were divided into moderate aerobic exercise groups (***HT_AER*** and ***SED_AER***) and placebo exercise groups (***HT_PLAC*** and ***SED_PLAC***).

The *AER* groups walked or ran on a treadmill for 30 minutes at 60% to 70% of their individual VO_2 *max*, while the *PLAC* groups engaged in light exercises. Following the completion of their respective tasks, participants were asked to complete the same stress and anxiety questionnaires before undergoing several *fMRI* tasks (see Bothe, Zschucke, Dimeo, Heinz, Wüstenberg, & Ströhle, 2013; Knutson, Westdorp, Kaiser, & Hommer, 2000), including the MIST protocol. After completing the MIST procedure (roughly 90 minutes after exercise or placebo treatment), the participants were asked to provide answers to the same questionnaires once again. Saliva samples were taken at different time points throughout the experiment, including arrival in the test room (Baseline 1); after the completion of questionnaires (Baseline 2; Pre-exercise); after the exercise treatment (Post-exercise); before entering the scanner (Pre-MRI); after the first task (MRI +20); after the second task (MRI +35); after the structural MRI (Pre-MIST); directly after the MIST (+1); and after the subjects left the scanner (MIST +10, +20, +30 and +45 min). Samples were analyzed for cortisol and *α–amylase*, a marker of sympathetic nervous system arousal.

Across the whole sample, subjective stress and negative affect were lower after the exercise treatment. Not surprisingly, exercise induced nervous system activation as the levels of α-amylase increased after exercise, and exercise-related changes were positively correlated between cortisol and α-amylase. As expected, participants reported higher state anxiety, negative affect, subjective stress and lower positive affect after the MIST. As per the *cross-stressor adaptation hypothesis*, cortisol responses to the MIST were lower in the *AER* group than in the *PLAC* group. In particular, participants in the *AER* treatment showed a higher brain response in the hippocampus and lower response in the prefrontal cortex. In contrast to the Pruessner, et al. (2008) results described earlier, the current study did not show a deactivation of the hippocampus. The researchers speculate that this may be due to their modification of the fMRI protocol. Nevertheless, as the hippocampus and the prefrontal cortex are implicated in the regulation of the *HPA axis*, these findings point to a possible role of these structures on the buffering effects of exercise on stress.

Conclusion

The neuroimaging work discussed points to the involvement of limbic and frontal structures in the regulation of the stress response. Yet the precise nature of activity among the various brain regions is yet to be fully determined. Protocols such as the MIST have been effective in identifying a number of the main structures involved in the stress response, including the hippocampus, parahippocampus, amygdala, insula, pre-frontal and frontal and cingulate cortices (Boehringer et al., 2015; Pruessner, et al., 2008; Zschucke, et al., 2015). However a number of limitations remain. These include the fact that some participants do not respond to stressors (i.e., non-responders), the role of possible gender differences (e.g., Bangasser & Valentino, 2014) and differences in experimental approaches and tasks. These limitations pertain to all types of stress research in cognitive neuroscience—in which researchers attempt to elucidate the brain correlates of the stress response. Overall, the study of stress in humans encompasses a broad range of approaches, and the focus of this chapter is necessarily narrow. Given this, to gain a more comprehensive perspective, we encourage the reader to seek out other examples of stress-related studies in cognitive neuroscience, using different paradigms and approaches. Doing so will provide a broader appreciation of the variation in approaches and the range of experimental questions being asked. As the studies we reviewed show, results do not always paint a clear picture of underlying mechanisms. Thus, we underscore that a key challenge for brain and behavioral scientists interested in stress is to integrate seemingly disparate data into a coherent theoretical perspective.

References

Ahern, G. L., & Schwartz, G. E. (1985). Differential lateralization for positive and negative emotion in the human brain: EEG spectral analysis. *Neuropsychologia*, *23*(6), 745–755. https://doi.org/10.1016/0028-3932(85)90081-8

Bangasser, D. A., & Valentino, R. J. (2014). Sex differences in stress-related psychiatric disorders: Neurobiological perspectives. *Frontiers in Neuroendocrinology*, *35*(3), 303–319. https://doi.org/10.1016/j.yfrne.2014.03.008

Barneoud, P., Neveu, P. J., Vitiello, S., & LeMoal, M. (1987). Functional heterogeneity of the right and left cerebral neocortex in the modulation of the immune system. *Physiology and Behavior*, *41*, 525–530. https://doi.org/10.1016/0031-9384(87)90306-4

Boehringer, A., Tost, H., Haddad, L., Lederbogen, F., Wüst, S., Schwarz, E., et al. (2015). Neural correlates of the cortisol awakening response in humans. *Neuropsychopharmacology*, *40*(9), 2278–3385. https://doi.org/10.1038/npp.2015.77

Bothe, N., Zschucke, E., Dimeo, F., Heinz, A., Wüstenberg, T., & Ströhle, A. (2013). Acute exercise influences reward processing in highly trained and untrained men. *Medicine & Science in Sports & Exercise*, *45*(3), 583–591. https://doi.org/10.1249/MSS.0b013e318275306f

Cannon, W. B. (1963). *The wisdom of the body*. New York, NY: Norton.

Carver, C. S., & White, T. L. (1994). Behavioral inhibition, behavioral activation, and affective responses to impending reward and punishment: The BIS/BAS scales. *Journal of Personality and Social Psychology*, *67*(2), 319–333. https://doi.org/10.1037/0022-3514.67.2.319

Chida, Y., & Steptoe, A. (2009). Cortisol awakening response and psychosocial factors: A systematic review and meta-analysis. *Biological Psychology*, *80*(3), 265–278. https://doi.org/10.1016/j.biopsycho.2008.10.004

Coan, J. A., & Allen, J. J. B. (2003a). Frontal EEG asymmetry and the behavioral activation and inhibition systems. *Psychophysiology*, *40*(1), 106–114. https://doi.org/10.1111/1469-8986.00011

Coan, J. A., & Allen, J. J. B. (2003b). The state and trait nature of frontal EEG asymmetry in emotion. In K. Hugdahl & R. J. Davidson (Eds.), *The asymmetrical brain* (pp. 565–615). Cambridge, MA: MIT Press.

Coan, J. A., & Allen, J. J. B. (2004). Frontal EEG asymmetry as a moderator and mediator of emotion. *Biological Psychology*, *67*(1–2), 7–50. https://doi.org/10.1016/j.biopsycho.2004.03.002

Coan, J. A., Allen, J. J. B., & Harmon-Jones, E. (2001). Voluntary facial expression and hemispheric asymmetry over the frontal cortex. *Psychophysiology*, *38*(6), 912–925. https://doi.org/10.1111/1469-8986.3860912

Coan, J. A., Allen, J. J. B., & McKnight, P. E. (2006). A capability model of individual differences in frontal EEG asymmetry. *Biological Psychology*, *72*(2), 198–207. https://doi.org/10.1016/j.biopsycho.2005.10.003

Cohen, S., Kamarch, T., & Mermelstein, R. (1983). A global measure of perceived stress. *Journal of Health & Social Behavior*, *24*(4), 385–396.

Davidson, R. J., Coe, D. D., Dolski, I., & Donzella, B. (1999). Individual differences in prefrontal activation asymmetry predict natural killer cell activity at rest and in response to challenge. *Brain, Behavior, and Immunity*, *13*(2), 93–108. https://doi.org/10.1006/brbi.1999.0557

Davidson, R. J. (1998). Anterior electrophysiological asymmetries, emotion, and depression: Conceptual and methodological conundrums. *Psychophysiology*, *35*(5), 607–614. https://doi.org/10.1017/s0048577298000134

Davidson, R. J., Schaffer, C. E., & Saron, C. (1985). Effects of lateralized presentations of faces on self-reports of emotion and asymmetry in depressed and non-depressed subjects. *Psychophysiology*, *22*(3), 353–364. https://doi.org/10.1111/j.1469-8986.1985.tb01615.x

Davidson, R. J., Schwartz, G. E., Saron, C., Bennett, J., & Goleman, D. J. (1979). Frontal versus parietal EEG asymmetry during positive and negative affect. *Psychophysiology*, *16*, 202–203.

Dedovic, K., Renwick, R., Mahani, N. K., Engert, V., Lupien, S. J., & Pruessner, J. C. (2005). The montreal imaging stress task: Using functional imaging to investigate the effects of perceiving and processing psychosocial stress in the human brain. *Journal of Psychiatry and Neuroscience*, *30*(5), 319–325. Retrieved from www.ncbi.nlm.nih.gov/pmc/articles/PMC1197276/pdf/20050900s00003p319.pdf

De Pascalis, V., Cozzuto, G., Caprara, G. V., & Alessandri, G. (2013). Relations among EEG-alpha asymmetry, BIS/BAS, and dispositional optimism. *Biological Psychology*, *94*(1), 198–209. https://doi.org/10.1016/j.biopsycho.2013.05.016

Dickerson, S. S., & Kemeny, M. E. (2004). Acute stressors and cortisol responses: A theoretical integration and synthesis of laboratory research. *Psychological Bulletin*, *130*(3), 355. https://doi.org/10.1037/0033-2909.130.3.355

Düsing, R., Tops, M., Radtke, E. L., Kuhl, J., & Quirin, M. (2016). Relative frontal brain asymmetry and cortisol release after social stress: The role of action orientation. *Biological Psychology*, *115*, 86–93. https://doi.org/10.1016/j.biopsycho.2016.01.012

Galang, C. M., & Obhi, S. S. (2018). Social power and frontal alpha asymmetry. *Cognitive Neuroscience*, *10*(1), 44–56. https://doi.org/10.1080/17588928.2018.1504763

Gray, J. A. (1987). *Problems in the behavioural sciences, vol. 5: The psychology of fear and stress* (2nd ed.). New York, NY: Cambridge University Press.

Gross, C. G. (1998). Claude Bernard and the constancy of the internal environment. *The Neuroscientist*, *4*(5), 380–385. https://doi.org/10.1177/107385849800400520

Harmon-Jones, E., & Allen, J. J. (1997). Behavioral activation sensitivity and resting frontal EEG asymmetry: Covariation of putative indicators related to risk for mood disorders. *Journal of Abnormal Psychology*, *106*(1), 159–163. https://doi.org/10.1037/0021-843X.106.1.159

Harmon-Jones, E., Gable, P. A., & Peterson, C. K. (2010). The role of asymmetric frontal cortical activity in emotion-related phenomena: A review and update. *Biological Psychology*, *84*(3), 451–462. https://doi.org/10.1016/j.biopsycho.2009.08.010

Harmon-Jones, E., Peterson, C. K., & Harris, C. R. (2009). Jealousy: Novel methods and neural correlates. *Emotion*, *9*(1), 113–117. Retrieved from http://charris.ucsd.edu/articles/HarmanPetersonHarris_2009.pdf

Harmon-Jones, E., & Sigelman, J. (2001). State anger and prefrontal brain activity: Evidence that insult-related relative left-prefrontal activation is associated with experienced anger and aggression. *Journal of Personality and Social Psychology*, *80*(5), 797–803. https://doi.org/10.1037/0022-3514.80.5.797

Joseph, D., & Whirledge, S. (2017). Stress and the HPA axis: Balancing homeostasis and fertility. *International Journal of Molecular Sciences*, *18*(10), 2224. https://doi.org/10.3390/ijms18102224

Kalin, N. H., Shelton, S. E., & Davidson, R. J. (2000). Cerebrospinal fluid corticotrophin-releasing hormone levels are elevated in monkeys with patterns of brain activity associated with fearful temperament. *Biological Psychiatry*, *47*(7), 579–585. https://doi.org/10.1016/S0006-3223(99)00256-5

Kang, D. H., Davidson, R. J., Coe, C. L., Wheeler, R. E., Tomarken, A. J., & Ershler, W. B. (1991). Frontal brain asymmetry and immune function. *Behavioral Neuroscience*, *105*(6), 860–869. Retrieved from https://centerhealthyminds.org/assets/filespublications/KangFrontalBehavioralNeuroscience.pdf

Kirschbaum, C., Pirke, K. M., & Hellhammer, D. H. (1993). The "trier social stress test": A tool for investigating psychobiological stress response in a laboratory setting. *Neuropsychobiology*, *28*(1–2), 76–81. https://doi.org/10.1159/000119004

Kline, J. P., Allen, J. J., & Schwartz, G. E. (1998). Is left frontal brain activation in defensiveness gender specific? *Journal of Abnormal Psychology*, *107*, 149–153. https://doi.org/10.1037/0021-843X.107.1.149

Knutson, B., Westdorp, A., Kaiser, E., & Hommer, D. (2000). FMRI visualization of brain activity during a monetary incentive delay task. *NeuroImage*, *12*(1), 20–27. https://doi.org/10.1006/nimg.2000.0593

Kudielka, B. M., Hellhammer, D. H., & Kirschbaum, C. (2007). Ten years of research with the trier social stress test revisited. In E. Harmon-Jones & P. Winkielman (Eds.), *Social neuroscience* (pp. 56–83). New York, NY: The Guilford Press.

Kuhl, J., & Kazen, M. (1994). Self-discrimination & memory: state orientation & false self-ascription of assigned activities. *Journal of Personality & Social Psychology, 66* (6), 1103.

Lazarus, R. S. (1993a). Coping theory and research: Past, present, and future. *Psychosomatic Medicine*, *55*(3), 234–247. https://doi.org/10.1097/00006842-199305000-00002

Lazarus, R. S. (1993b). From psychological stress to the emotions: A history of changing outlooks. *Annual Review of Psychology*, *44*, 1–21. https://doi.org/10.1146/annurev.ps.44.020193.000245

Lazarus, R. S., & Alfert, E. (1964). Short-circuiting of threat by experimentally altering cognitive appraisal. *The Journal of Abnormal and Social Psychology*, *69*(2), 195–205. https://doi.org/10.1037/h0044635

Lazarus, R. S., & Eriksen, C. W. (1952). Effects of failure stress upon skilled performance. *Journal of Experimental Psychology*, *43*(2), 100–105. https://doi.org/10.1037/h0056614

Lewis, R. S., Weekes, N. Y., & Wang, T. H. (2007). The effect of a naturalistic stressor on frontal EEG asymmetry, stress, and health. *Biological Psychology*, *75*(3), 239–247. https://doi.org/10.1016/j.biopsycho.2007.03.004

Lipsitz, L. A., & Goldberger, A. L. (1992). Loss of complexity and aging. *JAMA*, *267*(13), 1806–1809. doi:10.1001/jama.1992.03480130122036

McEwen, B. S. (1998). Stress, adaptation, and disease: Allostasis and allostatic load. *Annals of the New York Academy of Sciences*, *840*(1), 33–44. https://doi.org/10.1111/j.1749-6632.1998.tb09546.x

McEwen, B. S. (2007). Physiology and neurobiology of stress and adaptation: Central role of the brain. *Physiological Reviews*, *87*(3), 873–904. https://doi.org/10.1152/physrev.00041.2006

McEwen, B. S., & Stellar, E. (1993). Stress and the individual: Mechanisms leading to disease. *Archives of Internal Medicine*, *153*(18), 2093–2101. doi:10.1001/archinte.1993.00410180039004

Naliboff, B. D., Benton, D., Solomon, G. F., Morley, J. E., Fahey, J. L., Bloom, E. T., et al. (1991). Immunological changes in young and old adults during brief laboratory stress. *Psychosomatic Medicine*, *53*(2), 121–132. https://doi.org/10.1097/00006842-199103000-00002

Neveu, P. J. (1988). Cerebral neocortex modulation of immune functions. *Life Science*, *42*(20), 1917–1923. https://doi.org/10.1016/0024-3205(88)90490-0

Neveu, P. J. (1993). Brain lateralization and immunomodulation. *International Journal of Neuroscience*, *70*(1–2), 135–143. https://doi.org/10.3109/00207459309000569

Pérez-Edgar, K., Kujawa, A., Nelson, S. K., Cole, C., & Zapp, D. J. (2013). The relation between electroencephalogram asymmetry and attention biases to threat at baseline and under stress. *Brain and Cognition*, *82*(3), 337–343. https://doi.org/10.1016/j.bandc.2013.05.009

Pezawas, L., Meyer-Lindenberg, A., Drabant, E. M., Verchinski, B. A., Munoz, K. E., Kolachana, B. S., et al. (2005). 5-HTTLPR polymorphism impacts human cingulate-amygdala interactions: A genetic susceptibility mechanism for depression. *Nature Neuroscience*, *8*(6), 828. https://doi.org/10.1038/nn1463

Pruessner, J. C., Dedovic, K., Khalili-Mahani, N., Engert, V., Pruessner, M., Buss, C., et al. (2008). Deactivation of the limbic system during acute psychosocial stress: Evidence from positron emission tomography and functional magnetic resonance imaging studies. *Biological Psychiatry*, *63*(2), 234–240. https://doi.org/10.1016/j.biopsych.2007.04.041

Quaranta, A., Siniscalchi, M., Frate, A., & Vallotigara, G. (2004). Paw preference in dogs: Relations between lateralized behaviour and immunity. *Behavioral Brain Research*, *153*(2), 521–525. https://doi.org/10.1016/j.bbr.2004.01.009

Sapolsky, R. M. (1998). *Why zebras don't get ulcers: The acclaimed guide to stress, stress-related diseases, and coping-now revised and updated.* Holt Paperbacks.

Sapolsky, R. M., Romero, L. M., & Munck, A. U. (2000). How do glucocorticoids influence stress responses? Integrating permissive, suppressive, stimulatory, and preparative actions. *Endocrine Reviews*, *21*(1), 55–89. https://doi.org/10.1210/edrv.21.1.0389

Schneiderman, N., Ironson, G., & Siegel, S. D. (2005). Stress and health: Psychological, behavioral, and biological determinants. *Annual Review of Clinical Psychology*, *1*, 607–628. https://doi.org/10.1146/annurev.clinpsy.1.102803.144141

Smith, B. E., Hendrick, P., Smith, T. O., Bateman, M., Moffatt, F., Rathleff, M. S., et al. (2017). Should exercise be painful in the management of chronic musculoskeletal pain? *British Journal of Sports Medicine*, *51*(23), 1679–1687. https://doi.org/10.1136/bjsports-2016-097383

Speilberger, C. D., Gorsuch, R. L., Lushene, R., Vagg, P. R., & Jacobs, G. A. (1983). *Manual for the state-trait anxiety inventory.* Palo Alto, CA: Consulting Psychologists Press.

Speisman, J. C., Lazarus, R. S., Davison, L., & Mordkoff, A. M. (1964). Experimental analysis of a film used as a threatening stimulus. *Journal of Consulting Psychology*, *28*(1), 23–33. https://doi.org/10.1037/h0047028

Spencer, R. L., & Deak, T. (2017). A users guide to HPA axis research. *Physiology & Behavior*, *178*, 43–65. https://doi.org/10.1016/j.physbeh.2016.11.014

Sterling, P., & Eyer, J. (1988). Allostasis: A new paradigm to explain arousal pathology. In S. Fisher & J. Reason (Eds.), *Handbook of life stress, cognition, and health.* Oxford, England: John Wiley & Sons Inc.

Stress. (n.d.). *In Oxford dictionary online.* Retrieved from www.oxforddictionaries.com/us/definition/american_english/stress

Strictus. (n.d.). *In Latin-dictionary online.* Retrieved from www.latindictionary.org/strictus

Tan, S. Y., & Yip, A. (2018). Hans Selye (1907–1982): Founder of the stress theory. *Singapore Medical Journal*, *59*(4), 170–171. https://doi.org/10.11622/smedj.2018043

Tucker, D. M. (1981). Lateral brain function, emotion, and conceptualization. *Psychological Bulletin*, *89*(1), 19–46. https://doi.org/10.1037/0033-2909.89.1.19

Tullett, A. M., Harmon-Jones, E., & Inzlicht, M. (2012). Right frontal cortical asymmetry predicts empathic reactions: Support for a link between withdrawal motivation and empathy. *Psychophysiology*, *49*(8), 1–9. https://doi.org/10.1111/j.1469-8986.2012.01395.x

Weekes, N. Y., Lewis, R. S., Patel, F. R., Garrison-Jakel, J., Berger, D., & Lupien, S. J. (2006). Validation of examination stress as an ecological inducer of cortisol and psychology responses to stress controlling for sex, time of day and seasonal effects. *Stress*, *9*(4), 199–206. https://doi.org/10.1080/10253890601029751

Weitzman, E. D., Fukushima, D., Nogeire, C., Howard, R., Gallagher, T. F., & Hellman, L. (1971). Twenty-four hour pattern of the episodic secretion of cortisol in normal subjects. *The Journal of Clinical Endocrinology & Metabolism*, *33*(1), 14–22. https://doi.org/10.1210/jcem-33-1-14

Whirledge, S., & Cidlowski, J. A. (2010). Glucocorticoids, stress, and fertility. *Minerva Endocrinol. 35*(2), 109–125. Retrieved from www.ncbi.nlm.nih.gov/pmc/articles/pmc3547681/pdf/nihms403039.pdf/?tool=ebi

Yaribeygi, H., Panahi, Y., Sahraei, H., Johnston, T. P., & Sahebkar, A. (2017). The impact of stress on body function: A review. *EXCLI Journal*, *16*, 1057–1072. https://doi.org/10.17179/excli2017-480

Zschucke, E., Renneberg, B., Dimeo, F., Wüstenberg, T., & Ströhle, A. (2015). The stress-buffering effect of acute exercise: Evidence for HPA axis negative feedback. *Psychoneuroendocrinology*, *51*, 414–425. https://doi.org/10.1016/j.psyneuen.2014.10.019

PART IV

Population Demographics

15

NEIGHBORHOOD STUDIES OF ADOLESCENT HEALTH

Deborah Fish Ragin, Yasmin M. Hussein, Kheyyon Parker, and Veronica Julien

Overview

Several chapters in this handbook address adolescent health issues. This may reflect, in part, the enormous amount of work in the field, a myriad of unaddressed questions, or other more compelling reasons. Research suggests that not only are adolescents a less healthy cohort than their younger counterparts but the risky health behaviors they engage in may have long-lasting consequences, well into adulthood.

Adolescents, defined here as ages 15 to 24, number more than 1.2 billion, over 16% of the world's population (United Nations Department of Economic and Social Affairs, 2019). From 2000 to 2012, the World Health Organization (WHO) reported an impressive 12% decline in mortality rates for adolescents (WHO, 2020). But this compares unfavorably to mortality rates for children 14 years of age or younger for the period 1998–2018, which show a 53% reduction in mortality rates for children under five and a 59% reduction in the same for children ages five to 14 (Kleinert, 2007; United Nations Inter-Agency Group, 2019). A number of factors may account for the differences in mortality rates between children under 14 and adolescents. For the under-14 cohort, advances in neonatal care and expanded access to vaccines against childhood diseases significantly improved viability. For adolescents, however, internal factors, here meaning biological (puberty) and childhood development, as well as social determinants, shape health behaviors that, in turn, contribute to health outcomes (Sawyer, Afifi, Bearinger, Blakemore, Dick, Ezeh, et al., 2012). Research suggests that the combined impact of these internal and external (social) factors result in high-risk behaviors that negatively affect health (Hertzman, 1999; Patton & Viner, 2007; Sawyer, et al., 2012; Viner, Ozer, Denny, Marmot, Resnick, Fatusi, et al., 2012). Not surprisingly, then, some researchers employ an ecological approach to study adolescent health. This approach, they believe, more accurately captures the numerous simultaneous internal and external influences on adolescents that can lead to negative health outcomes that continue even into adulthood (Gold, Kawachi, Kennedy, Lunch, & Connell, 2001; Kulbok & Cox, 2002; Sawyer, et al., 2012; Ragin, 2018).

Ecological models examine the multilevel influences of the environment on an individual's behavior and explore the interactions within and across the intrapersonal (biological, psychological, lifestyle choices), interpersonal (social, cultural), and environmental levels (Stokols, 1996). Consistent with this view, some researchers have re-examined the role of the neighborhood and neighborhood characteristics on adolescent outcomes. The point here is that all individuals live in a context, adolescents included. Thus, using a contextual and multilevel view of development, consistent with Bronfenbrenner's ecological systems analysis (1979), seems appropriate when examining health outcomes. Such an approach enables researchers to distinguish neighborhood effects from familial factors (see Sellstrom & Bremberg, 2006). Indeed, the neighborhood appears to be a particularly important factor for this age group. Researchers must use caution, however, when using multilevel study designs to draw inferences about health outcomes (Diez-Roux, 1998), and we explore these concerns after reviewing a sample of neighborhood studies.

In general, researchers employ one of four basic study designs when examining the impact of neighborhood characteristics on health outcomes: ***national or multisite studies of individuals/families, city/regional studies, neighborhood studies,*** or ***empirical studies*** (Leventhal & Brooks-Gunn, 2000). Briefly, *national/multisite studies* sample a few individuals from a wide range of neighborhoods and ***socioeconomic status (SES)***. While Leventhal and Brooks-Gunn (2000) note that such a design yields stronger and more consistent effects of neighborhood than city or regional designs, *national/multisite studies* select small clusters of individuals from a wide range of neighborhoods. This limited number of individuals per neighborhood results in an underestimation of the local effects that inform the area's characteristics.

City/regional studies, as the name suggests, select participants from a defined city or metropolitan area. This may capture neighborhood effects from a narrower socioeconomic or ethnic range, depending on the composition of the city or metropolitan area captured (Leventhal & Brooks-Gunn, 2000). In such studies, neighborhood may also be defined by school attendance. Yet school attendance is an imprecise measure of the area's characteristics. As Saporito and Sohoni (2007) show, school attendance may inaccurately represent the socioeconomic or ethnic composition of a neighborhood, since it assumes that all children in the school catchment area attend the local public school. Such assumptions are not accurate in school districts in the United States, for example, where White children often attend private schools while living in racially diverse neighborhoods or school catchment areas.

Neighborhood-based designs select specific neighborhoods but add to this cohort a range of areas that also capture the target population. Unlike the *national/multisite studies*, this method ensures that sufficient numbers of individuals per neighborhood are included to allow for multilevel, hierarchical linear regression (Leventhal & Brooks-Gunn, 2000). This approach accommodates the assumption that individuals are nested within specific locations. It also assumes that neighborhoods are more heterogeneous, showing more variability within than across the area (Leventhal & Brooks-Gunn, 2000).

Finally, *empirical studies* represent a "gold standard" among many researchers but is not always achievable. Such studies entail random assignment of families to specific neighborhoods. This approach may work well when cities are under mandated desegregation orders, as happened in Yonkers, New York (United States v. Yonkers Bd. Of Education, 1985), or voluntarily relocating from selected public housing projects, as happened in Chicago, Illinois. In these and other cases, however, the desegregation orders that reassigned families to other neighborhoods occurred because of either court-mandated decrees or local policy ordinances. When available, such events present researchers with a textbook-like, quasi-experimental design opportunity to study the impact of the new neighborhoods' characteristic on the health and well-being of the relocated families.

Of the four neighborhood designs highlighted, we focus here on studies employing either *neighborhood-based* or *empirical designs* as best practices when examining the relationship between environmental factors and adolescent health outcomes.

Neighborhood-Based Studies

Adolescence and Obesity

The Centers for Disease Control and Prevention (CDC) reported that high school–aged adolescents in the United States were less likely to engage in alcohol or cigarette use in 2017, behaviors thought to contribute to the leading causes of death, disability, or social problems in the United States (CDC, 2019). But according to the same data, other adolescent health behaviors, such as poor nutritional habits leading to obesity, marijuana use, video gaming, and suicide behaviors, have held either steady or increased in frequency when compared to adolescents in the previous two decades (CDC, 2019). Multilevel systems studies with a *neighborhood-based* design may help explain these changes.

To be sure, several studies of the social health determinants of obesity in adolescents find that individual and family-level variables contribute significantly to obesity in teens. **Obesity**, here meaning abnormal or excessive fat accumulation that poses a health risk, is most commonly describe in terms of **body mass index (BMI)**, expressed as **kg/m₂**, where *kg* = weight in kilograms and m_2 = height in meters, squared. Research suggests that lifestyle behaviors, the environment, and structural factors are all risk factors for obesity, and perhaps even more so for adolescents. For example, studies by Salvy, Feda, Epstein, and Roemmich (2017) suggest that the best predictor of **BMI-z** scores for adolescents is not their birthweight, but rather the *BMI-z* of their best friend, an environmental factor. Similarly, research by Li, Liu, Haynie, Gee, Chairasia, and Seo (2016) show that adolescents are more likely to meet the recommended levels of moderately vigorous physical activity if peers and/or family members also met these same standards, lifestyle, and share environmental factors.

Indeed, family characteristics is one of several factors considered in multilevel studies of neighborhood characteristics. Other studies examine the relationship between a neighborhood's built environments (e.g., parks and recreational spaces, retail outlets offering healthy foods) and obesity (Huang, Moudon, Cook, & Drewnowski, 2014; Salois, 2012; Xu & Wang, 2015). Specifically, they examine neighborhood structural disadvantages, such as the presence of convenience stores in the area in lieu of supermarkets or minimal or inadequate physical recreation areas; environmental factors that contribute to obesity, especially in low-income, minority neighborhoods (Gordon-Larsen, Nelson, Page, & Popkin, 2006; Slater, Bowen, Corsini, & Gardner, 2010). Not surprisingly, studies show a relationship between the low-income or minority neighborhood's structural or built environment and obesity. Yet the presence of supermarkets in low-income and minority neighborhoods in itself may not ensure access to healthier food options. Additional research by Ragin and colleagues (unpublished data) reveals that while supermarkets in low-income neighborhoods exist within walking distance for many residents, they were less likely to stock healthier food options, such as lean ground beef (93% lean) or larger quantities (half-gallon or gallon containers) of low-fat or skim milk, healthy items in quantities affordable to low-income families.

A thorough study by Rossen (2014) examines the relationship between demographic and neighborhood-level socioeconomic risk factors and obesity, using a multilevel technique to separate neighborhood effects from family influence (Sellstrom & Bremberg, 2006). Rossen used a retrospective, *neighborhood-based* design to analyze data collected in two existing databases. First, using the National Health and Nutrition Examination Survey (NHANES) database, Rossen obtained direct and indirect measures of health on over 17,000 children, ages two to 18. The Mobile Examination Component (MEC) of NHANES uses a multistage probability sampling design (oversampling low-income and minority groups) to select eligible participants in the United States for home interviews and physical exams (Rossen, 2014). Using continuous, two-year survey cycles, NHANES obtains demographic, socioeconomic, dietary, and health-related information on participating families. It provides verified information on a participant's mental, dental, and physiological health as well as prevalence of chronic conditions, such as obesity (Centers for Disease Control & Prevention, 2017).

Rossen examined five survey cycles of NHANES data, collected between 2001 and 2010, resulting in 10 years of data. The researchers computed age-specific and sex-specific *BMI* for children ages two to 18. Children with age- and sex-specific *BMI*s in excess of 95% were classified as obese, and those with *BMI*s between 85% and 95% were considered overweight. Other family demographics extracted for this study included age, age squared, sex, race, family household–to–poverty index, caregiver's highest level of education, and marital status.

Second, Rossen used the US Census 2000 Summary File 3 to obtain sociodemographic and economic characteristics for the selected NHANES sample (Rossen, 2014). Using the NHANES restricted database, Rossen obtained the geographic identifiers needed to match children in the sample to their census track. The census track data yielded an income-to-poverty (PIR) ratio, percentage of adults 25 years of age or older without a high school diploma, percentage of unemployed men over age 16, percentage of families below the federal poverty threshold and percentage receiving public assistance, proportion of single-family households, and mean household income (Rossen, 2014).

As anticipated, Rossen found higher levels of obesity among non-Hispanic Black and Mexican American children (21%) than among non-Hispanic White children (15%). But when adjusting for various individual-level and neighborhood-level socioeconomic status variables, this association was attenuated by 74% for non-Hispanic Black vs. non-Hispanic White children and by 49% for Mexican American vs. non-Hispanic Whites. When examining risk factors and resiliency for obesity, however, Rossen's findings present a conundrum. They reveal that minority children raised in families with higher individual incomes (i.e., above the poverty threshold) but living in low-deprivation neighborhoods are at lower risk of developing obesity. In contrast, Black families with higher family incomes who reside in high-deprivation neighborhoods (here meaning poorer infrastructure/facilities) are at greater risk of becoming obese than are White children with the same profile (Rossen, 2014). Her findings might suggest that at least two system-level factors, family income and neighborhood deprivation, interact with race to create a different risk profile for obesity for minority versus White children.

Research by Goodman, Slap, and Huang (2003) yields similar outcomes when using ***population attributable risk (PAR)***. This measure, first introduced by Levin (1953), measures the portion of disease cases that would be prevented if the risk factor were removed. Goodman and colleagues examined the effects of one family-level variable (parental education) and one neighborhood-level variable (*SES*) on an adolescent's risk of depression and obesity.

Using data from the National Longitudinal Study of Adolescent Health (ADD-Health), Goodman and colleagues' retrospective study of approximately 15,000 adolescents (grades 7 to 12) analyzed the impact of parental education and household income on self-reported height, obesity (weight), and depression, assessed using the Centers for Epidemiologic Study Depression Scale (CES-D). All ADD-Health data were collected during interviews with parents and children. Results from this study suggest that lower household income and low parental education were associated with depression and obesity for approximately one-third of the sample.

Findings from both Goodman's and Rossen's studies illustrate the value of using existing and detailed databases along with family- and neighborhood-level data to understand the multilevel effects of neighborhoods on child and adolescent obesity. Rossen's focus on neighborhood-level factors and deprivation builds upon earlier work suggesting that neighborhood structural factors such as poverty, single-parent households, institutional resources, community social organizations (including role models), and community deprivation are important characteristics that influence children and adolescent behaviors and outcomes (Jencks & Mayer, 1990; Leventhal & Brooks-Gunn, 2000; Wilson, 1987).

Substance Use

Marijuana use among adolescents has remained constant or increased over the past several decades (CDC, 2019). This may come as no surprise, as indeed, adolescence is a developmental period that may entail experimentation and an increased risk of substance use regardless of the adolescent family's *SES* (Bachman, O'Malley, Johnston, Schulenberg, & Wallace, Jr., 2011; Hanson & Chen, 2007; Pampel, Krueger, & Denney, 2010; Zucker, 2008). Studies show that higher *SES* teens appear to report more cigarette, alcohol, and drug use than low *SES* teens, in part because of greater disposable income (Hanson & Chen, 2007). The research also suggests that additional factors may differentiate adolescents when it comes to substance use.

One individual factor that appears to influence substance use among adolescents is their legal status in the United States. Studies of adolescents by Gfroerer and Tan (2003) and of adults by Reingle, Caetano, Mills, and Vaeth (2014) suggest that the immigration status and length of time of Mexicans in the United States is linked to the amount and frequency of substance use. A study by Borges, Cherpitel, Orozco, Zenmore, Wallesch, Medina-Mora, et al. (2016) offers a compelling methodological approach to examining the impact of both immigration and environment on substance use with their sample of 18- to 65-year-old Mexican immigrants. Therefore, we choose this study to evaluate with the caveat that the age cohort includes adults.

Borges et al.'s prospective, *neighborhood-based*, cross-sectional study conducted face-to-face, computer-assisted interviews with over 2,300 Mexicans living in three border towns in Texas and approximately 2,400 Mexicans living in "sister cities" in Nuevo Leon and Tamaulipas, Mexico. They chose these border and sister cities to increase the homogeneity of comparisons (Borges, et al., 2016).

The researchers used a multistage, random cluster sampling procedure to recruit participants in each country. In the United States, Borges and colleagues first selected census block groups with a Hispanic population of at least 70%. In the second stage, researchers randomly selected from each block three households with eligible participants, here meaning residents between 18 and 65 years old and of Mexican origin. Similarly, in Mexico, the researchers first used the census basic geostatistical areas (similar to census block groups in the United States), followed by a random selection of three households per area with residents 18 to 65 years of age (Borges, et al., 2016). Each household was surveyed three times on three different days of the week and times of day.

In addition to demographic variables, including gender, age, marital status, and border vs. non-border city, researchers collected information on substance use, here meaning alcohol or drugs, and immigration status or efforts of the interviewee and their parents to immigrate. Substance use information gathered included lifetime and past-year alcohol use and alcohol use disorder, as defined by the *Diagnostic and Statistics Manual of Mental Disorders* (*DSM-IV*; Borges, et al., 2016). Drug use data included all prescription drugs, including pain relievers, sedatives, illicit drugs (e.g., marijuana, cocaine, heroin, and methamphetamines), and two measures from the *DMS-IV* to assess drug use disorders: persistent but unsuccessful efforts to reduce drug use and use in physically dangerous situations, such as driving an automobile (Borges, et al., 2016). Immigration status was determined from six questions. If living in the United States, participants were asked if they were born in Mexico, at what age they arrived in the United States (before or after age 13), whether one parent was born in the United States, or whether neither parent was born in the United States. If living in Mexico, participants' status was determined by asking whether they ever migrated to the United States, or if they have a family member living in the United States. Finally, Borges and colleagues assessed the participant's mobility through questions that measured whether participants ever visited the other country, whether they were native to their current city of residence or, if not, whether they lived there since their arrival to the country.

Results from Borges et al.'s study suggest that multilevel, individual, and environmental factors, including acculturation to and amount of time in the United States, language, social relations and assimilation changes, alcohol and drug norms, and greater availability to substances in the United States all contribute to higher levels of drug and alcohol use or abuse by immigrant Mexicans. This outcome was more pronounced in younger immigrants, those who left Mexico for the United States before age 13.

At first glance, Borges et al.'s findings appear to emphasize the role of non-neighborhood factors, such as immigration status, acculturation, language and social relations, and greater access to drugs or alcohol on substance use. A closer examination of this study, however, reveals that neighborhood characteristics include not only the structural components but the social environment as well. Thus, the degree to which a person has "acculturated" to the new country or their social relations would speak to a person's sense of community and social support; in other words, the social characteristics of neighborhood (Jun, Jivraj, & Taylor, 2020). As such, Borges et al.'s study demonstrates the important role of a neighborhood's social characteristic on health behaviors.

Hybrid City-Regional and Neighborhood-Based Studies

Neighborhood-based studies, when combined with a *city-regional study design*, offer another multilevel analysis providing additional insights into influences on health behaviors. Henrikson, Feighery, Schleicher, Coviling, Kline, Fortmann, et al.'s (2008) study of adolescent smoking behaviors is a prime example. Their examination of density of tobacco outlets and advertisements in walking distance of regional high schools in California suggests that several factors, including the proximity of retail smoking outlets to high schools, affects adolescents' likelihood to smoke. They categorized neighborhoods into three groups: urban, consisting of large and mid-size cities; suburban, including the urban fringes of large and mid-sized cities as well as large towns; and rural, incorporating small town and rural areas. Then, using a blended *city/ regional* and *neighborhood-based* design, Henrikson and colleagues culled multiple data sources to measure the likely impact of regional and neighborhood characteristics on student smoking. First, they obtained student smoking prevalence data within the last 30 days from the California Student Tobacco Survey (CTS) for approximately 25,000 students in 135 randomly selected high schools. Included in these data were estimates of the number of cigarettes students smoked in the last 30 days.

Next, to determine the density of tobacco outlets, Henrikson and colleagues obtained the addresses and unique postal codes of the tobacco outlets within a half-mile radius of each of the 135 selected schools using California's retailer-licensing database. A half-mile marker was selected based on the CDC's estimate that 0.5 miles represents an average walking distance for transportation studies to and from schools (Henrikson, et al., 2008). The number of tobacco outlets within the 0.5-mile distance around the school provided the measure of outlet density.

Third, in 28 randomly sampled neighborhoods, trained observers counted the total number of cigarette advertisements in retail establishments within the half-mile marker. Advertisements included signs, displays, and branded items like shopping carts or clocks. In neighborhoods with six or fewer outlets, observers counted the total number of advertisements in all six or fewer stores. In neighborhoods with more than six stores, observers noted the number of ads in six or 50% of the stores, whichever yielded the higher number. All observations occurred proximal to the survey administration, generally within two to 12 weeks of administration.

Finally, to ensure no overlap of neighborhood school districts, Henrikson et al. used Topologically Integrated Graphical Encoding & Referencing (TIGER) and Census 2000 track data to compare the half-mile boundary around each school. Census track data were also used to define the race, ethnicity, population density, and median household income of neighborhoods, while the California Basic Educational Data System was used to characterize the race, ethnicity, and proportion of students in each school who qualified for free lunch (Henrikson, et al., 2008). This study's hybrid approach to a neighborhood study of tobacco outlets and their effects on smoking prevalence among high school students provides a novel way to use city/regional and school attendance data, refined by neighborhood characteristics, to address the question of the effects of neighborhood characteristics on students' smoking behaviors.

Their findings suggest that the prevalence of current smoking among students was highest in the schools embedded in neighborhoods with the highest density of smoking outlets. Similarly, the density of smoking ads was also associated with school smoking prevalence. Perhaps unsurprisingly, the highest concentration of smoking outlets was located in Hispanic and commercially disadvantaged neighborhoods. Yet the prevalence of smoking appears highest in suburban areas.

Empirical Studies

Mental Health

Mental health is yet another issue that, if originating in adolescence, may result in a negative trajectory well into adulthood (Ingoldsby & Shaw, 2002). There are a host of conditions that amply fit under the heading of mental health. Here, we choose to focus on the more general description of a condition that affects a person's thinking, mood, or feeling (Shelter & Young, 1979); one that will affect how a person engages socially, environmentally, emotionally, mentality, and physically.

Ample research suggests that both internal (intrapersonal) and external (environmental) factors can affect mental health (Kling, Liebman, & Katz, 2007; Mulvey, 2002). One such environmental factor appears to be neighborhood characteristics, although there is considerable disagreement about which neighborhood factors are most influential (Macintyre, Ellaway, & Cummins, 2002). Consistent with our focus on *neighborhood-based* research, Schmidt, Glymour, and Osypuk (2017) examine the effects of neighborhood characteristics on the mental health of adolescent males and females, using an *empirical design*. Recall that, as noted earlier, Leventhal and Brooks-Gunn (2000) identified this method as one of two strong designs for examining the impact of neighborhood characteristics on health outcomes. The limitation here is that this design is usually dependent on an event or occurrence outside of the researchers' control, such as a court-mandated or federal/regional policy that implements reassignments of neighborhood residence.

Schmidt, et al.'s study (2017) examined the mental health effects of an experimental housing mobility program in five major cities in the United States, sponsored by the US Department of Housing and Urban Development (U.S. Department of Housing & Urban Development [HUD], 1996). In the original HUD experiment, known as **Moving to Opportunity for Fair Housing (MTO)**, the program identified low-income families residing in public housing units who voluntarily agreed to relocate to "higher-opportunity" neighborhoods. HUD defined "higher-opportunity" neighborhoods as residences within metropolitan areas that contained 1) low concentrations of persons living in poverty, 2) better housing, and 3) better educational and employment opportunities (U.S. Department of Housing and Urban Development (HUD), 1996). Approximately 4,600 families who met the eligibility requirements (current residents of public housing or housing projects with children 17 years of age or younger and who qualified for rental assistance) were placed on waiting lists for further screening. Additional screening included regional evaluations (conducted by the participating city), a baseline survey, signed formal agreements to participate, and informed consent to participate in the study. The approximately 4,600 eligible families were randomly assigned to one of three conditions. Just under one-fourth (1,037) were enrolled in the "low-poverty" experimental condition (E1), here meaning receipt of a **Section 8 housing voucher** for relocation to higher-opportunity neighborhoods (less than 10% poverty level per census track) with full support services (individual counselors, training workshops) and counselors who accompanied them on their housing "shops." The remaining 3,563 families were placed randomly in either the second experimental condition (E2), the *Section 8 housing voucher* for rental assistance redeemable in any neighborhood but no additional services, or the control condition (C), including families who could remain in public assistance but who received no additional support services (US Department of Housing and Urban Development, 1996).

Schmidt et al.'s study of the mental health of adolescents whose families participated in this HUD study extracted data from two surveys conducted by HUD: a baseline survey prior to the move and an interim survey approximately 3 to 5 years post-move. HUD surveys were administered in person to the head of the family and up to two children per household. Approximately 89% of adolescents (2,829) were interviewed in the interim survey. Eligible adolescents were 12 to 19 years of age.

Schmidt et al.'s study analyzed adolescents' self-reported data collected on six dimensions from the interim survey: past-month psychological distress, past six-month behavioral problems, lifetime substance use, past 30-day alcohol/cigarette/marijuana use, social connectedness, and maternal mental health. The past-month psychological distress scale included six items (depressed, nervous, restless or fidgety, hopeless, everything was an effort, and worthless) measured using a five-point Likert scale ("none of the time" to "all of the time"). The Behavioral Problem Index included 11 items to assess behavioral problems in the last six months, including "trouble concentrating," "lie or cheat," and "tease others." Adolescents rated themselves on these items using a three-point Likert scale, ranging from "not true" to "often true." Substance use information in the past 30 days was measured by teen self-report of smoking or drinking (yes/no) and the number of days of each. Similarly, cigarette use information also for the past 30 days was assessed, reporting the number of cigarettes consumed rather than number of days they smoked. Lifetime use of alcohol, marijuana, or cigarettes similarly was measured on a "never" or "ever" scale (Schmidt, et al., 2017).

The social connectedness scale assessed teens' network of adults or other teens. For adults, respondents indicated the number of adults available to confide in or rely on for help. For teens, participants reported on the number of friends (<3, <5) and the location of these friends (from original neighborhood). This measure also included a peer deviance measure to assess whether participants had friends involved in problem behaviors, including gang membership, carrying weapons, or using drugs (Schmidt, et al., 2017).

Finally, a maternal mental health measure was included to assess the mental stability of the primary caregiver for over 90% of these adolescents. Measures included lifetime major depressive disorder, past-year generalized anxiety disorder, psychological distress or not feeling calm or peaceful within the last 30 days (Schmidt, et al., 2017).

Schmidt and colleagues' results were both expected and surprising. They report that for adolescent girls in the *MTO* experimental group (E1), this program improved many of the mediating and main effects of depression compared with the control group (C), the group that remained in public housing. Thus, girls in E1 reported a decrease in 30-day and lifetime substance use, improved social connectedness, and a decrease in psychological distress. On the other hand, the *MTO* program increased substance use, behavioral problems, and psychological distress for males in E1, while improving their social connectedness when compared with the control group (C). That is to say, males reported fewer friends in the old neighborhood. This differential impact by gender is puzzling. The researchers suggest that reliance on substance use to address problems may be a more common coping strategy for males than females. This begs the question: Are there different problems encountered by males and females when participating in such a program?

Strengths and Limitations of Neighborhood-Based and Empirical Studies

Research on the effects of low-income, under-resourced neighborhoods on behavior yields neither new nor surprising findings (Shaw & McKay, 1942; Wilson, 1987). When coupled with theories of development, such as that proposed by Bronfenbrenner (1979), and social ecological theories which stress the role of context and multilevel systems, neighborhood characteristics become an important factor in health outcomes. As such, it is not surprising that researchers look beyond the individual and family-level variables to examine the role of this environmental determinant on health, writ large. Reid (2010/2011) notes that environmental factors account for fully 60% of health behaviors and outcomes. The question remains, however, which factors, and more specifically, which neighborhood characteristics are most instrumental in shaping health behaviors and outcomes.

The research studies presented here aim to measure individual, family, and neighborhood characteristics, attempting to separate the neighborhood effect from the family and individual influences. This is not always successful. Schmidt and colleagues' *MTO* study, the empirical study of the impact of moving to "higher-opportunity" neighborhoods on adolescent mental and psychological health, presents both strengths and limitations. The goal was to measure the effects of moving to a higher-resourced community on adolescent mental health. However, several methodological issues limit its success here. While this study is characterized as an "empirical" study, it is more accurately described as quasi-experimental. Researchers were not able to control many of the design elements. For example, Schmidt, et al. (2017) acknowledge that they were not able to actually measure the effect of the move for over 50% of the E1 group. Their study took place when only half of the E1 group had moved to their new neighborhoods. In effect, they measured the impact on 50% the E1 group who were offered vouchers to move. This might explain some of the interesting but confusing gender differences on behavioral health and substance use.

Additionally, the researchers note that theirs was not a clean measure of effect of neighborhood on behavioral and psychological health. Rather, this study measures the combined effects of neighborhood, mobility (willingness of families to move), and housing. It may be unlikely that the opportunity to move to a new neighborhood occasioned by a court-ordered mandate or public policy will be free of the confounding factor of mobility or housing.

Finally, this study is policy dependent. That is to say, the ability to conduct a quasi-experimental design with a control and experimental group to test the effects of the neighborhood characteristics of a new, highly resourced neighborhood on psychological and behavioral health is constrained by government policy or court mandates, an uncommon occurrence.

By contrast, research by Henrikson et al. examining smoking behaviors as a function of density of tobacco outlets and ads or by Borges et al. examining the effects of immigration status and acculturation on substance use has no such limitations. These studies are designed using naturally occurring phenomenon. They contribute to the field of *neighborhood-based* and *city/region studies* by demonstrating how to construct or use finely calibrated measures that identify and characterize critical neighborhood factors. Henrikson et al. focus on the structural features of the neighborhood (e.g., tobacco outlets, number of ads) and their interaction with demographic factors at the neighborhood and school level. By comparison, Borges et al. integrate the individual- and family-level variables (e.g., immigration status, family immigration status, length of residence, substance use) with social and structural neighborhood characteristics (neighborhood demographics, country and geographic location) to illustrate the influence of social factors (e.g., acculturation) on health behaviors.

Finally, combining factors on several levels, Rossen examines the impact of individual-level *(BMI)* and family-level demographics with neighborhood characteristics to examine their combined effects on an adolescent's obesity outcomes. Her findings, however, reveal the complex relationship between race/ethnicity and neighborhood resources. It illustrates the difficulty of fully separating the effects of family characteristics from neighborhood factors.

One final factor complicates the interpretation of all such studies. As Diez-Roux (1998) notes, such studies must be cognizant of two major fallacies: the ***ecological fallacy***, a tendency to draw inferences at the individual level based on group-level data, and the ***atomistic fallacy***, drawing inferences at the group level based on individual-level data. Such fallacies are possible when interpreting the findings from each of these studies. As Rossen illustrates, the data indicating higher levels of obesity for African American and Hispanic children may be true at the group level, but the parent's income level and individual-level variables mitigate against the likelihood of obesity among these minority groups: an example of the *ecology fallacy*. Researchers will need to consider these factors carefully when interpreting their findings.

Conclusion

The studies presented here encourage researchers to consider health research designs that assess an individual's behaviors or outcomes in light of their context. This is not to suggest that cognitive decision-making factors are irrelevant. Rather, these studies demonstrate the wealth of information structural and social neighborhood factors may provide when attempting to explain health outcomes. The challenge here is identifying best practices for selecting and measuring the neighborhood characteristics. The *neighborhood-based* and *empirical study designs*, with their limitations, appear to represent best practices for multilevel studies of adolescent health outcomes.

References

Bachman, J. G., O'Malley, P. M., Johnston, L. D., Schulenberg, J. E., & Wallace, J. M., Jr. (2011). Racial/ethnic differences in the relationship between parental education and substance use among U. S. 8th-, 10th-, and 12th-grade students: Findings from the monitoring the future project. *Journal of Studies on Alcohol and Drugs*, *72*, 279–285. https://doi.org/10.15288/jsad.2011.72.279

Borges, G., Cherpitel, C. J., Orozco, R., Zenmore, S. E., Wallesch, L., Medina-Mora, M.-E., et al. (2016). Substance use and cumulative exposure to American society: Finding from both Sides of the US-Mexico Border region. *American Journal of Public Health*, *106*(1), 119–127.

Bronfenbrenner, U. (1979). *The ecology of human development: Experiments by nature and design.* Cambridge, MA: Harvard University Press.

Centers for Disease Control & Prevention (CDC). (2017). *About the national health and nutrition examination survey, national centers for health statistics.* Retrieved February 20, 2020, from www.cdc.gov/nchs/nhanes/about_nhanes.htm

Centers for Disease Control & Prevention (CDC). (2019). *Adolescent and school health: Trends in the prevalence of tobacco use national YRBS: 1991–2017.* Retrieved August 10, 2020, from https://www.cdc.gov/healthyyouth/data/yrbs/factsheets/2017_tobacco_trend_yrbs.htm

Diez-Roux, A. V. (1998). Bringing context back into epidemiology: Variables & fallacies in multilevel analyses. *American Journal of Public Health*, *88*(2), 216–222.

Gfroerer, J. C., & Tan, L. L. (2003). Substance use among foreign-born youths in U.S.: Does length of residence matter? *American Journal of Public Health*, *93*(11), 1892–1895.

Gold, R., Kawachi, I., Kennedy, B. P., Lunch, J. W., & Connell, F. A. (2001). Ecological analysis of teen birth rates: Association with community income & income inequality. *Maternal & Child Health*, *5*, 161–167. https://doi.org/10.1023/A:1011343817153

Goodman, E., Slap, G. B., & Huang, B. (2003). The public health impact of socioeconomic status on adolescent depression and obesity. *American Journal of Public Health*, *93*(11), 1844–1850.

Gordon-Larsen, P., Nelson, P. C., Page, P., & Popkin, B. M. (2006). Equality in the built environment underlies key health disparities in physical activity & obesity. *Pediatrics*, *117*(2), 417–424.

Hanson, M. D., & Chen, E. (2007). Socioeconomic status and substance use behaviors in adolescents: The role of family resources versus family social status. *Journal of Health Psychology*, *12*(1), 32–35. https://doi.org/10.1177%2F1359105306069073

Henrikson, L., Feighery, E. C., Schleicher, N. C., Coviling, D. W., Kline, R. S., & Fortmann, S. P. (2008). Is adolescent smoking related to the density & proximity of tobacco outlets and retail cigarette advertising near schools? *Preventive Medicine*, *47*, 210–214. https://doi.org/10.1016/j.ypmed.2008.04.008

Hertzman, C. (1999). The biological embedding of early experiences & its effects on health in adulthood. *Annals of the New York Academy of Science*, *896*, 85–95. https://doi.org/10.1111/j.1749-6632.1999.tb08107.x

Huang, R., Moudon, A. V., Cook, A. J., & Drewnowski, A. (2014). The spatial clustering of obesity: Does the built environment matter? *Journal of Human Nutrition & Dietetics*, *28*(6), 604–612. https://doi.org/10.1111/jhn.12279

Ingoldsby, E. M., & Shaw, D. S. (2002). Neighborhood contextual factors & early-starting Antisocial pathways. *Clinical Child & Family Psychology Review*, *5*(1), 21–55. https://doi.org/10.1111/jhn.12279

Jencks, C., & Mayer, S. (1990). The social consequences of growing up in a poor neighborhood. In L. E. Lynn & McGeary, M. F. H. (Eds.). *Inner-city poverty in the United States.* (pp. 111–186). Washington, DC: National Academies Press.

Jun, J., Jivraj, S., & Taylor, K. (2020). Mental health & ethnic density among adolescents in England: A cross-sectional study. *Social Science & Medicine*, *244*, article #112569. https://doi.org/10.1016/j.socscimed.2019.112569

Kleinert, S. (2007, March 31). Adolescent health: An opportunity not to be missed. *The Lancet*, *369*, 1057–1058.

Kling, J. R., Liebman, J. B., & Katz, L. F. (2007). Experimental analysis of neighborhood effects. *Econometrica*, *75*(1), 83–119. https://doi.org/10.1111/j.1468-0262.2007.00733.x

Kulbok, P. A., & Cox, C. L. (2002). Dimensions of adolescent health behavior. *Journal of Adolescent Health*, *31*, 394–400. https://doi.org/10.1016/S1054-139X(02)00422-6

Leventhal, T., & Brooks-Gunn, J. (2000). The neighborhoods they live in: The effects of Neighborhood residence on child and adolescent outcomes. *Psychological Bulletin*, *126*(2), 309–337. https://psycnet.apa.org/doi/10.1037/0033-2909.126.2.309

Levin, M. L. (1953). The occurrence of lung cancer in man. *Acta-Unio Internationalis Contra Cancrum*, *9*(3), 531–541.

Li, K., Liu, D., Haynie, D., Gee, B., Chairasia, A., & Seo, D.-C. (2016). Individual, social & environmental influences on the transitions in physical activity among emerging adults. *BMC Public Health*, *16*, 682. https://doi.org/10.1186/s12889-016-3368-3

Macintyre, S., Ellaway, A., & Cummins, S. (2002). Place effects on health: How can we, conceptualize, operationalize and measure them? *Social Science & Medicine*, *55*(1), 125–139. https://doi.org/10.1016/S0277-9536(01)00214-3

Mulvey, A. (2002). Gender, economic context & perception of safety & quality of life: A case study of Lowell, Massachusetts USA 1982–96. *Journal of Community Psychology*, *30*(5), 655–679. https://doi.org/10.1023/A:1016321231618

Pampel, F. C., Krueger, P. M., & Denney, J. T. (2010). Socioeconomic disparities in health behaviors. *Annual Reviews of Sociology*, *36*, 349–370. https://doi.org/10.1146/annurev.soc.012809.102529

Patton, G. C., & Viner, R. (2007). Pubertal transitions in health. *Lancet*, *369*, 1130–1139. https://doi.org/10.1016/S0140-6736(07)60366-3

Ragin, D. F. (2018). *Health psychology: An interdisciplinary approach* (3rd ed.). New York, NY: Routledge/Taylor & Francis Group.

Reid, C. (2010/2011). Building communities and improving health: Finding new solutions to an old problem. *Community Investments: Health and Community Development*, *22*(3), 2–10.

Reingle, J. M., Caetano, R., Mills, B. A., & Vaeth, P. A. (2014). The role of immigration age on alcohol & drug use among border & non-border Mexican Americans. *Alcoholism: Clinical Experimental Research*, *38*(7), 2080–2086. https://doi.org/10.1111/acer.12440

Rossen, L. M. (2014). Neighborhood economic deprivation explains racial/ethnic disparities in overweight and obesity among children and adolescents in the USA. *Journal of Epidemiology & Community Health*, *68*(2), 123. http://dx.doi.org/10.1136/jech-2012-202245

Salois, M. J. (2012). Obesity & diabetics, the built environment & the local food economy in the United States 2007. *Economics & Human Biology*, *10*(1), 35–42. https://doi.org/10.1016/j.ehb.2011.04.001

Salvy, S.-J., Feda, D. M., Epstein, L. H., & Roemmich, J. N. (2017). Friends & social contexts as unshared environments: A discordant sibling analysis of obesity & health-related behaviors in young adolescents. *International Journal of Obesity*, *41*, 569–575. www.nature.com/articles/ijo2016213#citeas

Saporito, S., & Sohoni, D. (2007). Mapping educational inequality: Concentrations of poverty Among poor & minority students in public schools. *Social Forces*, *85*(3), 1227–1253. https://doi.org/10.1353/sof.2007.0055

Sawyer, S. M., Afifi, R. A., Bearinger, L. H., Blakemore, S.-J., Dick, B., Ezeh, A. C., et al. (2012). Adolescent Health 1: Adolescence: A foundation for future health. *The Lancet*, *379*, 1630–1640.

Schmidt, N. M., Glymour, M. M., & Osypuk, T. L. (2017). Housing mobility and adolescent mental health: The role of substance use, social networks, and family mental health in the moving to opportunity study. *SSM- Population Health*, *3*, 318–325. https://doi.org/10.1016/j.ssmph.2017.03.004

Sellstrom, E., & Bremberg, S. (2006). The significance of neighborhood context to child & adolescent health & well-being: A systematic review of multi-level studies. *Scandinavian Journal of Public Health*, *34*, 544–554. https://doi.org/10.1080%2F14034940600551251

Shaw, C., & McKay, H. (1942). *Juvenile delinquency and urban areas*. Chicago, IL: University of Chicago Press.

Shelter, H., & Young, B. (1979). *National alliance on mental illness*. Retrieved March 30, 2020, from www.nami.org/

Slater, A., Bowen, J., Corsini, N., & Gardner, C. (2010). Understanding parents' concerns about children's diet, activity & weight status: An important step towards effective obesity prevention interventions. *Public Health Nutrition*, *13*(8), 1221–1228. https://doi.org/10.1017/S1368980009992096

Stokols, D. (1996). Translating social ecological theory into guidelines for community health promotion. *American Journal of Health Promotion*, *10*(4), 282–298. https://doi.org/10.4278%2F0890-1171-10.4.282

United Nations Department of Economic and Social Affairs. (2019). *Ten key messages: International youth day, 12 August 2019*. Retrieved February 3, 2020, from www.un.org/development/desa/youth/wp-content/uploads/sites/21/2019/08/WYP2019_10-Key-Messages_GZ_8AUG19.pdf

United Nations Inter-agency Group for Child Mortality Estimation. (2019). *Levels & trends in child mortality: Report 2019: Estimates developed by the UN inter-agency group for child mortality estimates*. New York, NY: United Nations Children's Fund.

United States v. Yonkers Bd. of Education. (1985). *No. 80 CIV 6761 (LBS), 611 F. Supp.* Retrieved March 3, 2020, from www.leagle.com/decision/19851341611fsupp73011221

U.S. Department of Housing & Urban Development. (1996). Expanding housing choices for HUD-Assisted families: Moving to opportunity. *First Biennial Report to Congress, Moving to Opportunity for Fair Housing*

Demonstration Program. Retrieved March 11, 2020, from www.huduser.gov/portal/publications/affhsg/expand/toc.html

Viner, R. M., Ozer, R. M., Denny, S., Marmot, M., Resnick, M., Fatusi, A., et al. (2012). Adolescent health 2: Adolescence & the social determinants of health. *Lancet, 379,* 1641–1652. https://doi.org/10.1016/S0140-6736(12)60149-4

WHO. (2020). *Maternal, newborn, child & adolescent health: Adolescent health epidemiology.* Retrieved February 3, 2020, from www.who.int/maternal_child_adolescent/epidemiology/adolescence/en/

Wilson, W. J. (1987). *The truly disadvantaged: The inner-city, the underclass, and public policy.* Chicago, IL: University of Chicago Press.

Xu, Y., & Wang, F. (2015). Built environment & obesity by urbanicity in the U.S. *Health & Place, 34,* 19–29. https://doi.org/10.1016/j.healthplace.2015.03.010

Zucker, R. A. (2008). Anticipating problem alcohol use developmentally from childhood into middle adulthood: What have we learned? *Addiction, 103,* 100–108. https://doi.org/10.1111/j.1360-0443.2008.02179.x

16

RE-EVALUATING THE SOCIAL GRADIENT

Alan Marshall and Valeria Skafida

Overview

A wide body of literature has regularly identified stark inequalities in various health outcomes according to social class and the characteristics of the places in which people live. Such health inequalities are persistent over time, with those in lower social classes living shorter lives in poorer health than their counterparts in higher social classes. The mechanisms that cause health inequality and their relative importance remain very much contested. In this chapter, we focus on how innovative and theoretically informed quantitative research designs drawing on increasingly sophisticated longitudinal social surveys can provide deeper understandings of health inequality drivers. In a period where much attention is being given to big data, "data science", and machine learning techniques, we join others in arguing that smart research design and theoretically informed analysis of longitudinal and interdisciplinary social survey data ought not be neglected (Norman, Marshall, & Lomax, 2017).

All of the studies presented involve observational data, but several draw on forms of natural experiment, exploiting policy changes or national comparison, to provide more convincing evidence of causal claims around drivers of health inequality. We define a natural experiment as a situation where the exposure of individuals to an event of interest is out of a researcher's control, but the process that determines the exposure is random, or "as if" random (Dunning, 2012; Craig, Katikireddi, Leyland, & Popham, 2017). Thus, theoretically informed multivariate analysis is required to control for any lingering socio-economic and demographic differences between exposed and unexposed groups.

Research in Practice

Case Study 1. Accelerated Longitudinal Design: How Are Health Inequalities Changing Over Time and Across Cohorts?

A key question in many societies concerns how trends in population health are evolving in the context of increasing life expectancies. Most national populations are becoming increasing elderly in age structure, bringing concerns for the capacity of societies to meet the associated and expected increases in health care costs. Improvements in health offer the potential for savings in the costs associated with population ageing, and are one of a number of valuable arguments that challenge pessimistic views of population ageing (Spijker & Macinnes, 2012; Sanderson & Scherbov, 2010).

Long-term increases in life expectancies have prompted the development of two theories relating trends in population health to trends in life expectancy. Societies may experience a ***compression*** *of morbidity* in which the onset of poor health is delayed so that as life expectancy increases, people spend fewer years of their life in poor health (Fries, 1980). More pessimistically, an **expansion of morbidity**, is where the age of poor health onset remains constant, or worse, moves to younger ages, so that gains in life expectancy are composed of increasing years spent with chronic health problems (Gruenberg, 1976). Accurately capturing trends in population health across cohorts is crucial to evaluate the plausibility of the previously mentioned theories, which may vary according to socio-economic position.

Some studies use repeated cross-sectional data to explore trends in health across cohorts (Martin, Schoeni, Andresk, & Jagger, 2011). Yet a weakness of such approaches is that analysis of cross-sectional data is problematic in terms of separating age and cohort effects. A major strength of longitudinal data is that we can model how health outcomes *evolve* over time for particular cohorts, including stratification by socio-economic characteristics. Here we describe an **accelerated longitudinal design** from a study that compares cohort-specific trajectories of frailty among older adults in England using the English Longitudinal Study of Ageing (ELSA; Marshall, Nazroo, Tampubolon, & Vanhoutte, 2015a).

ELSA is an observational study comprising a representative sample of the English population who are aged over 50 and living within private households. The study commenced in 2002 with a sample of 11,391 people and is a particularly rich data source for those interested in exploring health inequalities in later life, since it contains an extensive diversity of health measures as well as a range of information on socio-economic and demographics characteristics, life events (such as retirement), histories, biomarkers, and social participation. The survey is repeated every two years, and the frailty study described makes use of five waves of data covering the period 2002 to 2010. Cheshire, Hussey, & Phelps (2012) provide further details on ELSA.

The outcome of interest in this study is **frailty**, a key concept within geriatric clinical practice that is generally agreed to be a non-specific health state reflecting age-related decline in multiple systems. There are a number of instruments through which *frailty* is operationalized, but here a **frailty index** proposed by Rockwood and colleagues (Searle, Mitnitski, Gahbauer, Gill, & Rockwood, 2008) is adopted. The *frailty index* is calculated based on the proportion of a wide range of "deficits" or health problems that are held by an individual (Searle, et al., 2008). Deficits are coded to a 0 to 1 scale, with 1 indicating a person has a particular deficit and 0 the opposite, and the proportion of deficits held by an individual is taken as the value of the *frailty index*, which can vary from 0 (least frail) to 1 (most frail). In the case study presented here, Marshall, and colleagues (2015a) use 60 deficits covering a range of domains, including activities of daily living (e.g., climbing several flights of stairs without resting); cognitive function (e.g., ability to recall words immediately and after delay); falls and fractures; joint replacement; and self-reported measures of vision, hearing, chronic diseases, cardiovascular diseases, and depression. The particular value of the ELSA frailty index is that it gives an indication of an individual's capacity for independent living and the risk of suffering an event (such as a fall).

Multilevel growth curve models are used to model the level of frailty in 2002 and the change in frailty over the next four waves of data to 2010. Multilevel models are useful in situations where there is structure in the observed data stemming from an underlying hierarchy or clustering (Snijders & Bosker, 2011). Here the structure is embedded within the longitudinal nature of the data; repeated observations of frailty are nested within individuals. The value of multilevel models in this context is that the technique offers one approach to deal with the non-independence of repeated measures of frailty within an individual. An individual's frailty score is modeled as a function of time (wave), age cohort, and their interaction, enabling us to model a separate trajectory of frailty with time for each age cohort

The modeled frailty trajectories are illustrated in Figure 16.1(a–c). A number of points emerge. First, there are higher levels of frailty among women and with declining wealth. The extent of inequality in frailty by wealth is stark; the level and change in frailty for an individual in the richest tertile at age 80 (from 2002) are comparable to that observed in an individual at age 70 in the poorest tertile. Thus, we see a 10-year gap in the experience of frailty across the wealth distribution in England. A further result of concern is the lack of evidence for improvements in frailty in those later-born cohorts compared to earlier-born cohorts, which, in the context of rising life expectancy, suggests an expansion of morbidity. The longer lives of earlier-born compared to later-born cohorts are likely composed of additional years in a frail state. Further examination shows that the cohort

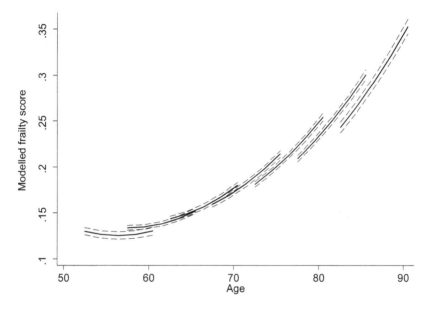

Figure 16.1a   Frailty trajectories: all people (aged 50+)*

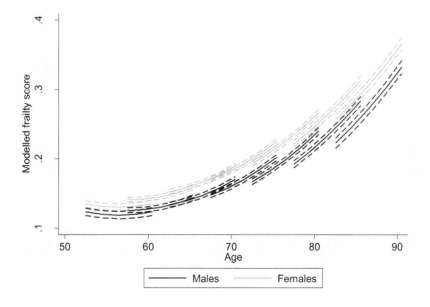

Figure 16.1b   Frailty trajectories: by gender*
Continued overleaf

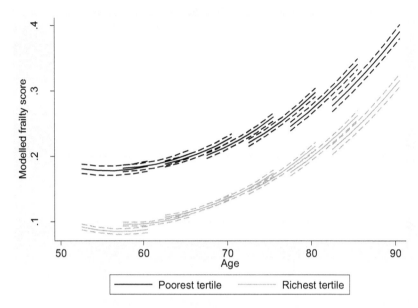

Figure 16.1c Frailty trajectories: by wealth*

Note: *The solid lines indicate the level and change in frailty for each age cohort between 2002 (start of the line) and 2010 (end of each line). The dotted lines show the confidence intervals around the modeled frailty estimates.

difference in observed frailty occurs for cohorts aged over 70 in 2002 and particularly for those in the poorest tertiles. Overlapping frailty trajectories among the most affluent indicate no such cohort differences in frailty across cohorts for this group, and so a widening in frailty inequalities by wealth occurred in England from 2002 to 2010. Marshall et al. (2015a) consider a number of possible drivers of this result with one potential theory relating to rising inequality from the 1980s that has been subsequently sustained (Shaw, Davey Smith, & Dorling, 2005) and thought to carry harmful health consequences (Shaw, Dorling, Gordon, & Smith, 1999).

A couple of weaknesses of this modelling strategy should be considered. First, ELSA, like other longitudinal studies, is subject to non-random attrition due to mortality and non-response. Analysis of attrition reveals this group is more likely to be frail, male, older, and poor. Might attrition account for the substantive findings reported earlier? It would seem unlikely for a couple of reasons. First, sensitivity analysis using longitudinal weights to account for attrition and the sample of respondents who responded to all five waves reveals similar results to those reported. Second, the patterns of attrition would suggest steeper frailty trajectories from the same starting point, particularly for older and poorer cohorts, strengthening the cohort differences that are reported in the paper. A more challenging weakness relates to the impossibility of separating age, period, and cohort effects, which is well documented in the literature (Bell & Jones, 2014). In particular, the cohort differences that we see in frailty for those aged over 70 in 2002 may be attributable to a period effect, although the relatively short period of the study (2002–2010) would suggest such a period effect is perhaps less plausible.

Case Study 2: Using Cohort Data to Explore Changes in Social Inequalities in Infant Feeding Patterns

Understanding health inequalities within a life-course perspective entails also paying attention to the very start of life and the infant years. A large body of literature has focused on infant nutrition and on how social inequalities in infant feeding correlate with subsequent health outcomes, including cognitive (Horta, Loret de Mola, & Victora, 2015) and more general health outcomes (Zalewski, Patro, Veldhorst, Kouwenhoven, Crespo Escobar, & Calvo Lerma, 2017). Within the United Kingdom, Scotland has historically stood out as the nation with some of the lowest breastfeeding rates. In Scotland, significant investment in maternity services, as well as changes in Scottish legislation (Skafida, 2014; Wood, Stockton, & Brown, 2012), have taken place over the years to improve breastfeeding practices. Scotland collects a variety of data on infant feeding that can be used. These include government-funded infant feeding surveys as well as administrative data on infant feeding routinely collected by health visitors. The limitations of these data sources are discussed later. Social surveys, which collect data on, among other things, infant feeding, are a third source of data, and this brings us to the focus of this case study.

This case study examines research published by Skafida (2014) that showcases how a repeated cross-sectional survey design can be used to understand complex and changing patterns of social inequality in infant feeding habits within the context of change in breastfeeding support services and policy. In Scotland, from 2005 onwards, maternity provision moved from a model of universalism towards progressive universalism, where more support was offered to more vulnerable mothers (Wood, et al., 2012). This change in provision creates opportunity for a "natural experiment" (Craig, et al., 2017; Dunning, 2012; Petticrew, Cummins, Ferrell, Findlay, Higgins, Hoy, et al., 2005) where policy changes are rolled out on a national level, offering a unique opportunity for analysis using a before-and-after comparison. This case study uses data from the Growing Up in Scotland (GUS) longitudinal survey. The survey tracks two separate nationally representative cohorts of babies born in Scotland in 2004–05 and 2010–11 (samples of 5,030 and 5,838, respectively). Interviews were carried out predominantly with the mothers of the study children (children aged c.10 months) in the homes of the participants. While each cohort was interviewed again annually, this study uses a **repeated cross-sectional longitudinal design**—a design where identical questions are being asked of two separate cohorts at two different time points and where the cohorts can be directly compared to each other.

Mothers were asked whether they had ever breastfed their child and how old the child was when last breastfed (the survey asks both about exclusive and mixed breastfeeding). The GUS survey also collected data on a broad range of independent variables known from the literature to be related to breastfeeding, such as socio-economic characteristics and employment-related factors. A range of such variables were controlled for in the analysis: an occupation-based social class indicator, maternal education, equivalized household income, maternal age, family composition, mother's ethnicity, whether a language other than English is spoken at home, maternal employment status, and whether paid or unpaid maternity leave was taken. The study used multivariate binary logistic regression and **proportional hazards regression** (also known as survival analysis). Many studies using regression analyses fail to report analysis of interaction effects (Vatcheva, Lee, McCormick, & Rahbah, 2016), neglecting the possibility that association between an independent and dependent variable varies across the distribution of another independent variable. This study tested and found significant interaction effects between time and educational qualifications, which brought to light some of the most important findings of this research.

This research reported a small (3%), non-significant increase in breastfeeding initiation for the 2010–11 cohort compared to the 2004–05 cohort. A key finding was a significant interaction between time and maternal educational qualifications. Among mothers who breastfed, the magnitude of the difference in breastfeeding durations between different groups of mothers changed with the passing of weeks and months. There was no significant difference in breastfeeding duration between cohorts of mothers who were educated at or above the university undergraduate degree level. However, mothers with no educational qualifications in the 2010–11 cohort were far more likely to continue breastfeeding until six months compared with mothers with no qualifications in the 2004–05 cohort (hazard ratio of breastfeeding cessation 0.37:1 for the 2010–11 cohort compared to the 2004–05 cohort). These findings suggest that the "progressive universalism" adopted from 2005 onwards (Wood, et al., 2012) may have been partly responsible for the positive change in breastfeeding habits among less advantaged mothers.

A key strength of this case study is that the data were used both in comparison to other data sources and across time in relation to policy change. Compared to the 2017 Scottish Infant Feeding Survey, which had a response rate of 30% (Scottish Government, 2018), GUS had much better response rates at 80% for the 2004–05 cohort and 65% for the 2010–11 cohort. A high response rate and a representative sample are of key importance to fully understand social inequality, especially since respondents from disadvantaged backgrounds are far less likely to respond to any type of survey (Fowler, 2009). Administrative health data may have a larger sample size, but are limited in that they 1) only count those who use particular services, 2) are prone to changes in collection procedure that hamper time series analysis, and 3) usually lack variables to inform a meaningful analysis of either social stratification of feeding habits or of how infant feeding relates to subsequent outcomes in children. A number of other studies have looked at local area-based, work-based, or hospital-based breastfeeding interventions (Abdulwadud & Snow, 2007; Gau, 2004; Kelaher, Dunt, Feldman, Nolan, & Raban, 2009; Labbok, 2013). This case study's key strength over such research is that it assesses change in feeding habits at a national level following a period of universal policy change in Scotland with regard to legislation and maternity services. The case study is able to compare habits before and after a policy change using rich and high-quality data from a nationally representative, longitudinal, social survey for two birth cohorts. Neither administrative health data nor other health surveys would have been able to provide similar insights on the stratification of infant feeding practices and the changes that have occurred over time.

All studies suffer from limitations. In this case, breastfeeding variables relied on maternal recall at 10 months postpartum. By only having data for two birth cohorts, it is not clear if there were prior upward trends in breastfeeding initiation and duration before 2004–05 unrelated to the policy changes. Data from an Infant Feeding Survey in 2000 and 2005 point to an increase in breastfeeding initiation between 2000 and 2005 (Bolling & BMRB Social Research, 2007), but actual figures are not comparable with those in our case study due to methodological differences between surveys. The case study presented here assumed that change in breastfeeding trends that are not explained by independent variables are explained by a period rather than a cohort effect. However, it remains difficult to state with certainty that changes in maternity care prolonged breastfeeding duration among less educated mothers in the later cohort or whether this might be linked to other period effects. For example, high media coverage of breastfeeding issues in later years or the promotion of breastfeeding in public discourse have made breastfeeding more culturally acceptable.

This case study highlights the utility of longitudinal social surveys that are repeated across birth cohorts, particularly when it comes to understanding complex and changing patterns of social stratification of infant feeding habits and the impact of policy change.

Case Study 3: Hypertension Care Outcomes in the United States and England

The methodological perspective of this third case study is on the use of an international comparison to test the performance of different health care systems on care outcomes (Marshall, Nazroo, Feeney, Lee, Vanhoutte, & Pendleton, 2015b). Such a comparison is useful in that we might expect social inequalities in health to be influenced through the way in which health care provision is organized.

The case study we draw on is from Marshall, and colleagues (2015b) and involves a comparison of hypertension (or high blood pressure) care outcomes among older people in the United States and England. The United States and England offer a valuable comparison since they have very different health care systems. In England, health care is predominantly publicly funded, with its National Health Service providing a comprehensive range of health services, largely free to those using them. In contrast, health care in the United States has long been dominated by the private sector. Marshall and colleagues (2015b) compare care outcomes in 2008, thus providing a comparison of two health systems with different funding models. Hypertension care outcomes offer an interesting perspective. The condition is asymptomatic, providing a role for screening, particularly since interventions are cheaper than dealing with subsequent health problems (WHO, 2013). The population with hypertension is increasing due to population ageing, population growth, and the rise of unhealthy lifestyle choices related to diet and sedentary living (Fields, Burt, Cutler, Hughes, Roccellam, & Sorlie, 2004). Hypertension is a major risk factor for cardiovascular disease (WHO, 2013) a condition that, like other health outcomes, follows a strong social gradient

The study draws on the Health and Retirement Study (HRS; Karp, 2002) in the United States and the ELSA (as described in Case Study 1) with all data relating to 2008. ELSA was set up, in part, to offer a comparative study to the HRS and contained harmonized variables facilitating the comparison of outcomes across countries. Both ELSA and HRS collect social and biomedical data, both of which are used here to select a sub-sample of respondents who have any previously diagnosed hypertension or measured high blood pressure during a visit by a medical professional as part of the data collection process. Using this sub-sample, three care outcomes are distinguished and form the dependent variables for the study:

- *Hypertension-controlled*—diagnosed with hypertension in the past but has normal measured blood pressure in the nurse visit.
- *Hypertension-uncontrolled*—diagnosed with hypertension in the past but has high measured blood pressure in the nurse visit.
- *Hypertension-undiagnosed*—never been diagnosed with hypertension in the past but has high measured blood pressure in the nurse visit.

The "good" care outcome here is *hypertension-controlled*, since hypertension has been identified and is being successfully managed. Both other categories can be considered "poor" outcomes where hypertension was either not controlled or has not been previously diagnosed.

A key question here concerns the thresholds used in the diagnosis and treatment of high blood pressure in the United States and England, since these thresholds have the potential to influence results and conclusions. Documentation in each country suggests a formal threshold of a systolic blood pressure of 140/90 *mm Hg*. However, there is strong evidence of more aggressive diagnosis and treatment in the United States compared to England, where the Quality Outcomes Framework suggests a threshold of 150/90 *mm Hg* is used in practice (NICE, 2006; U.S. DHSS, 2004; Banks & Smith, 2011; Wolf, Cooper, Kramer, Banegas, Giampaoli, & Joffres, 2004). The main analysis of the case study uses a measured blood pressure of 140/90 *mm Hg* as the threshold for identification of hypertension, but in sensitivity analysis, a threshold of 150/90 *mm Hg* is used for England, reflecting its less aggressive diagnosis and treatment of hypertension.

Three multinomial logistic regression models are fitted:

- *Base model*—with independent variables comprising country (United States/England), age, sex, body mass index (BMI), ethnicity (white, US non-white, England non-white).
- *Health insurance model*—country/insurance status (England, US private insurance, US government insurance) and all the variables of the base model.
- *Wealth inequality model*—all the variables of the base model and wealth quintiles.

All models were fitted separately for ages 50 to 64 and age 65 and older, reflecting the very different nature of health care provision in the United States at these ages. In the United States in 2008, there were two main government health insurance schemes. Medicaid provided health insurance coverage to a relatively small group comprising the poor, disabled, and those with specific health problems. Medicare covered all US citizens (or permanently resident in the United States for at least five years) aged over 65.

The base model reveals that *controlled hypertension* is more common in the United States compared to England. For example, in the United States at age 50 to 64, 53% (confidence interval [CI] 50% to 57%) of the hypertensive population have *controlled hypertension* compared to 45% (CI 42% to 48%) in England. This result is driven entirely by lower levels of *undiagnosed hypertension* in the United States than in England. For example, in the United States, at age 50 to 64, 18% (CI 15% to 21%) of the population have *undiagnosed hypertension* compared to 26% (CI 24% to 29%) in England. Levels of *uncontrolled hypertension* are comparable in the United States and England. These broad results hold for sample members above and below age 65. To a large degree, we might view the differences in care outcomes as a function of the more aggressive diagnosis and treatment of hypertension in the United States. The sensitivity testing in which the threshold for measured high blood pressure is set at the auditing level in the English Quality Outcomes Framework (150/90 *mm Hg*) reveals that the cross-national differences in care outcomes are not significant except for persisting (but attenuated) lower levels of *undiagnosed hypertension* in the United States at the very oldest ages.

The health insurance model reveals very low levels of undiagnosed hypertension for those in the United States aged 60 to 64 who hold government insurance compared to those with private insurance. Hypertension care outcomes are strikingly similar for those with government insurance compared to private insurance for those aged over 65. In sum, there is no evidence to suggest that private health care in the United States offers better care outcomes compared to state provision through Medicare and Medicaid. The group in the United States with the poorest health care outcomes are, not surprisingly, those who hold no health insurance, although the small samples in this group are likely to be the reason why the differences fail to reach statistical significance.

Finally, the wealth model demonstrates stronger inequality in health care outcomes in the United States compared to England. For example, in the United States (age 60 to 64) the levels of *uncontrolled hypertension* decline with wealth, with no such gradient present in England. An unexpected result that emerges from the wealth model is that *undiagnosed hypertension increases* in prevalence with increasing wealth in both the United States and England. One theory for this is that the result stems from greater contact with medical services and opportunity for blood pressure tests among poorer groups, who tend to have generally poorer health than more affluent groups.

A key strength of this study is that it tests the success of two different health care systems in managing a health condition (hypertension) that is on the increase. The inclusion of *undiagnosed hypertension* is a particular contribution in this paper neglected in other research. There are weaknesses that ought to be taken into account, however. Whilst differences in care outcomes are attributed to the nature of health service provision (public versus private), it cannot be discounted that alternative explanations might exist. For example, the United States is known to have a more specialized health service than England, with a higher ratio of specialists to generalists and greater sums of money (per capita) invested in health care in the United States.

Case Study 4: Life Events and the Social Gradient

This fourth case study is based on a paper (Finney & Marshall, 2018) that explores how the event of moving home in later life affects subsequent wellbeing and the extent to which motivations for moving may influence wellbeing. The methodological framework involves restructuring data around the event of moving home and the use of a ***spline model*** that comprises two linear regressions that capture trajectories, or change, in wellbeing prior to and then following a move.

The paper uses the ELSA, described in the first case study, but here the focus is on a sub-sample (*n* = 1,387) who moved home during the period 2002 to 2012 for which six waves of ELSA data are available. The data are restructured around a ***time to move*** variable that records the number of years prior to and after a move of home. The *time to move* variable assigns negative values prior to the move of home and positive values afterwards. In the study, the time to move variable takes values that range from −10 to +10.

Wellbeing can be conceptualized in different ways. For example, **hedonic wellbeing** refers to happiness stemming from increased pleasure and decreased pain, whilst **eudaimonic wellbeing** is defined by fulfilment in life that stresses aspects such as autonomy and self-actualization (Vanhoutte, 2014). This case study adopts the Control, Autonomy, Self-Realization and Pleasure (CASP)-19 scale, which includes 19 questions that tap into several concepts of wellbeing relating to each of the earlier domains (Wiggins, Netuveli, Hyde, Higgs, & Blane, 2007). The CASP-19 score is derived by summing the score of the 19 Likert-scale questions to give a continuous measure of wellbeing in which higher scores indicate higher levels of wellbeing.

The key independent variable is the (self-reported) motivation for a move of home based upon a question posed to all those who moved home during the ELSA period of the study. The research divides moves of home into two categories, distinguishing those moves that are "voluntary" and those that are "involuntary." Voluntary moves include responses such as "moved to a better " or "moved to be nearer friends or family." Involuntary moves include responses such as "moved for health reasons" or "moved due to a split from partner." The guiding principle is to categorize as voluntary those reasons for a move that imply increased social networks. Additional independent variables are included in models to capture key correlates of wellbeing from the literature, including age, sex, wealth (quintiles), economic activity, self-reported illness, and cohabitation that might confound any relationship between reason for a move and wellbeing.

The models that investigate how wellbeing changes throughout a move use repeated measures and a linear regression model, fitted using the generalized estimating equations method, which accommodates the autoregressive correlation between an individual's wellbeing scores across time (Lipsitz, Kim, & Zhao, 1994). A *spline model* with a knot at the time of move is used to accommodate different trajectories in wellbeing scores in the lead up to and following a move. The *spline model* quantifies the trajectory (or change) in wellbeing over time, distinguishing separate terms for the rate of change in wellbeing prior to and after a move of home. This enables assessment of whether the rate of change in wellbeing score alters as populations experience a move. Interactions between motivation for move (voluntary and involuntary) and each of the pre- and post-move of home slopes are included in the models, providing flexibility for a different trajectory of wellbeing before and after a move, depending on whether that move is defined as voluntary or involuntary.

The findings suggest that there does appear to be a difference in the trajectories of wellbeing prior to and after a move rooted in the reason for that move. Compared to those who moved for voluntary reasons, involuntary movers experienced a steeper decline in wellbeing prior to a move that levelled off after the move. Thus, for involuntary movers, there appears to be evidence of a difference in the slope of wellbeing between time prior to and after the event of moving home. For those who move for voluntary reasons, the rate of decline in wellbeing is identical before and after a move, suggesting that a move of home does not influence broader trends in wellbeing at later life. The above results hold after including the set of socioeconomic and demographic controls mentioned earlier. Predicted wellbeing scores are illustrated in Figure 16.2. The steep decline in wellbeing among involuntary movers prior to a move of home may reflect difficulties in circumstances that are alleviated by the move, thereby reducing the inequalities observed in wellbeing between involuntary and voluntary movers (at eight years after a move).

Methodologically, the case study adds to an emerging body of research (e.g., Nowak, Van Ham, Findlay, & Gayle, 2013) demonstrating that longitudinal data with migration and the reason for a move can give a greater understanding of migration as a process of selection and social inequalities. ELSA's rich details on why people move demonstrates the point often made theoretically, but seldom shown empirically: it is essential to know the reason for a residential move in order to understand the experience of migration and its consequences. Finally, the study demonstrates how life events, here meaning internal migration, can contribute towards understanding subsequent inequality in health and other outcomes by giving greater attention to drivers of life events (e.g., moving home) and the related inequalities in choices and constraints. As noted in the previous case studies, although results

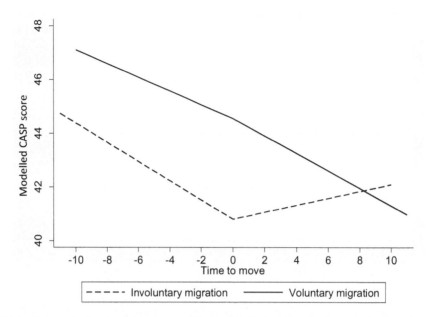

Figure 16.2 Trajectories (or change) in mean wellbeing (CASP-19) scores before and after a residential move. Model wellbeing scores relate to age (in wave prior to move) of 50 and the reference category of all other independent variables.

Note: The model controls for economic activity, tenure, marital status, wealth, age and sex (for all these variables we take the value immediately prior to the move).

hold after inclusion of weights designed to correct for attrition, we cannot discount the possibility that conclusions might have differed with a full sample.

Case Study 5: Area Health Effects: Is Urbanization Good for Health?

The final case study adopts a natural experiment to consider whether urbanization in the Chinese context brings health benefits (Hou, Nazroo, Banks, & Marshall, 2019). This research fits within a broader literature on area health effects that proposes that the characteristics of an area influence health outcomes over and above the individual characteristics (Manley, Van Ham, Bailey, Simpson, & Maclennan, 2013). A number of pathways have been suggested for ways in which an area can affect health (Galster, 2012). For example, one explanation proposes that living in a deprived neighborhood is more stressful than living in an affluent area and that such stresses accumulate over time to harm health either directly or through a mediator such as increasing the prevalence of health-harming lifestyle choices (Diez Roux & Mair, 2010).

In developing countries, a particular question of interest concerns whether there is an area health effect connected to living in an urban area. The question is contested, in that, on the one hand, urban areas bring improved infrastructure, economic opportunity, and access to health services that are associated with better health outcomes compared to rural areas (Godfrey & Julien, 2005; Leon, 2008). Yet on the other hand, and particularly in the context of rapid and unplanned urbanization, urban areas in developing countries have been linked to other factors that are harmful to health, including poorer air quality and other forms of pollution, increases in unhealthy lifestyle choices around sedentary living, diet, smoking, alcohol consumption, and road traffic accidents. (For a fuller review, see Eckhert & Kohler, 2014.)

One of the many challenges for research on area health effects is the issue of dealing with health-selective migration (or immobility) between areas (van Ham & Manley, 2012). Migration is known to be health selective; the propensity to either migrate or remain in particular areas is associated with a set of socio-economic characteristics that are also correlated with health outcomes. The poorer health observed in some areas may stem from health-selective migration comprising out-migration of those pre-disposed to better health outcomes and immobility, or in-migration, of individuals at greater risk of experiencing poor health. It is the spatial sorting of residents according to socio-economic circumstances that results from health-selective migration, rather than any impact of area, that determines the inequalities in health observed across neighborhoods. Area effects studies have attempted to deal with the issue of selection through multilevel models that enable separation of variability in health outcomes to individual and area levels after controlling for the characteristics of individuals that predict both health and health-selective migration. In such models, area effects tend to be small, but are often statistically significant and are queried by critics who observe that some characteristics that correlate with both selection and health outcomes are either unobserved or unmeasured. However, if such characteristics were included in models, then any area health effect would become insignificant (Cheshire, 2009).

This case study examines a paper that assesses whether living in an urban area brings health benefits in a Chinese context (Hou, et al., 2019). The research design of the study exploits a natural experiment to overcome the issue of selection that hampers studies examining area health effects. The dataset used in the study is the Chinese Health and Retirement Longitudinal Study (CHARLS). The key to the natural experiment that forms the research design is the speed, scale, and planned nature of migration in China that enables three groups to be identified:

1. ***The in situ urbanized-rural population***: this group grew up in a rural area that became urban due to the expansion of a nearby urban center. The scale of urbanization in China is sufficient to yield a sample that is large enough for analytic purposes.
2. ***The urban population***—comprising those who have always lived in an urban area.
3. ***The rural population***—comprising those who have always lived in a rural area.

These groups are determined using three sources of information collected within CHARLS: respondents' ***Hukou status***, an urban/rural classification of their current residence, and details of their migration history. The *Hukou* system in China can be viewed as a form of internal passport used to control migration within the country. There are two types of *Hukou*: one that distinguishes birth in an agricultural rural area (rural) or in a non-agricultural (urban) area. CHARLS also captures information on whether a respondent's current residence is rural or urban, based on a classification developed by the National Bureau of Statistics and details on lifetime migration history. These three variables enable a sample of non-migrants to be extracted. A comparison of *Hukou status* and the urban/rural classification variables for each individual distinguishes the three groups.

Two health outcomes are modeled in this paper: self-rated health and depression. Self-rated health is based upon a survey question that asks the respondent to evaluate their health on a scale from 1 (poor) to 5 (excellent). The measure of depression is operationalized using the 10-item Center for Epidemiological Studies Depression Scales (CES-D) (Radloff, 1977). Waist circumference is also modeled as an indicator of obesity, reflecting the claims in the literature about unhealthy lifestyle choices around diet and sedentary living in urban areas.

An ordinary least squares regression model is used to predict the self-rated health score, the CES-D depression score, and waist circumference. Sensitivity testing using a multinomial logistic regression to predict self-reported health did not alter any substantive findings. For each health outcome, a set of five models is developed in which independent variables are progressively added in as blocks, reflecting theoretically proposed differences in health outcomes in urban and rural areas.

The sequential modelling framework is as defined as follows:

- *Demographic model*—age and sex.
- *Early life model*—age, sex, and indicators of early life circumstances, including education, first job, and lower leg length (to knee height) as an objective measure of youth and childhood health and socioeconomic circumstances.
- *Socioeconomic model*—age, sex, indicators of early life circumstances, and current socio-economic circumstances, including expenditure, tenure, economic activity, and others.
- *Lifestyle choices model*—age, sex, indicators of early life circumstances, current socio-economic circumstances, and lifestyle choices (exercise).
- *Infrastructure model*—age, sex, indicators of early life circumstances, current socio-economic circumstances, lifestyle choices, and infrastructure (no toilets in the household, non-flushable toilets, and flushable toilets).

The self-rated health models reveal poorer self-rated health among those in rural areas compared to the reference category of urbanized-rural across all five models. In the *demographic model*, the self-rated health score for those in rural areas is higher than for those in urbanized-rural areas by a score of 0.165, indicating that, on average, people in rural areas rate their health as being poorer than their urbanized-rural counterparts. Interestingly, there is little attenuation in this differential across the early life; the *socio-economic model* and *lifestyle choice model* suggesting that these factors do not contribute to the differential observed in self-rated health between the urbanized-rural and rural populations. In the final *infrastructure model*, there is some attenuation in the differential, which drops by 18% to 0.121, suggesting that poorer infrastructure in rural areas may account for part of the poorer self-rated health observed in rural areas. Turning to urban populations, the initial *demographic model* suggests no evidence of difference in self-rated health compared to the urbanized-rural population. However, after controlling for early life circumstances, scores of self-reported health appear higher in the urban population (by 0.096), indicating poorer health among urban compared to urbanized-rural dwellers. This result can be explained by the observation that the urbanized-rural population is known to have spent their childhood in rural areas and to have experienced more challenging early life circumstances compared to those who have always lived in urban areas. After we account for this disadvantage, the health advantage of the urbanized-rural group relative to the urban population emerges.

The results for depression are similar to those for self-rated health. There are higher CES-D scores in rural compared to urbanized-rural populations across all models, indicating higher levels of depression in rural areas. Similarly, the strongest attenuation in this differential occurs between the *lifestyle choice* and *infrastructure model*, indicating aspects of improved infrastructure in cities are likely relevant to depression in rural compared to urbanized-rural populations. In the *demographic model*, the urban population has a lower mean depression score than the urbanized-rural population. However, similar to the results for self-rated health, once early life circumstances are included in the model, levels of depression are observed to be higher in urban compared to urbanized-rural populations.

The models for the final outcome, waist circumference, reveal lower waist circumferences in rural populations compared to urbanized-rural populations, a result that holds across all models. In the *demographic model*, the average waist circumference of the rural population is 2.6 cm less than that of the urbanized-rural population. The strongest attenuation in the differential between rural and urbanized-rural populations comes after inclusion of socio-economic controls, resulting in the differential falling from 2.7 cm in the *early life model* to 2.0 cm in the *socio-economic model*. The urban group has a 2.2 cm larger waist circumference than the urbanized-rural population in the *demographic model*. After controlling for socio-economic factors, however, there is no evidence of a statistically significant difference in waist circumference between the urban and urbanized-rural populations.

The overarching conclusion that emerges from this analysis is that planned urbanization in the Chinese context appears to bring health benefits associated with living in an urban area. Infrastructure appears to be a key factor, explaining the health advantages that urban areas confer. Those who lived in rural areas that became urbanized experience improved health outcomes compared to populations who have always lived in urban areas, once differences in early life circumstances are controlled for. Urbanization does appear to be associated with larger waist circumferences, and improvements in socio-economic circumstances are likely a contributory factor.

The key strength of this paper is the identification of a group that experienced urbanization *in situ*, thus overcoming the issue of the health-selective nature of migration to urban areas in other national contexts. A key weakness of the research is that it examines fairly broad indicators of health, while other more specific indicators might reveal different patterns, particularly those that are influenced by factors such as air pollution, which is known to be worse in Chinese urban areas compared to rural areas.

Conclusion

In this chapter, we presented five case studies containing empirical evidence on the complex drivers of social and spatial health inequalities. We describe concerning evidence of an expansion of morbidity among older, poorer adults in England. We illustrate the importance of policy on health-related outcomes through a policy-related reduction in the inequalities in breastfeeding duration in Scotland. Furthermore, we examined the role of the health care system on the greater inequalities in hypertension care outcomes in the United States compared to England. We show how the reason for a move of home in later life, itself socially structured, can influence trajectories of wellbeing. We provide evidence to support the health benefits of urbanization in the Chinese context, separate from any effect of health-selective migration. The insights derived flow from theoretically informed research designs combined with improvements in social survey data collection, including harmonized national datasets, interdisciplinary forms of data combining medical and social information, and the maturation of longitudinal studies such the ELSA and the HRS. We expect further progress as interdisciplinary teams of researchers increasingly combine social, biological, and life-course data to understand how life "gets under the skin" to determine the stark and persistent social inequalities in health outcomes and the ways in which they might be addressed.

We conclude that research which uses robust methodological approaches to capitalize on natural experiment settings can yield highly insightful and policy-relevant findings. We encourage researchers to identify and take advantage of such research opportunities.

References

Abdulwadud, O. A., & Snow, M. E. (2007). Interventions in the workplace to support breastfeeding for women in employment. *Cochrane Database of Systematic Reviews, 3*, CD006177. https://doi.org/10.1002/14651858. CD006177.pub2

Banks, J., Marmot, M., Oldfield, Z., et al. (2006). Disease and disadvantage in the United States and in England. *JAMA, 295*(17), 2037–2045. https://doi.org/10.1001/jama.295.17.2037

Banks, J., & Smith, J. P. (2011). International comparisons in health economics evidence from aging studies. *Annual Review of Economics, 4*, 57–81. https://doi.org/10.1146/annurev-economics-080511-110944

Bell, A., & Jones, K. (2014). Another "futile quest"? A simulation study of Yang and Land's hierarchical age-period-cohort mode. *Demographic Research, 30*, 333–360. doi:10.4054/DemRes.2014.30.11

Bolling, K., & BMRB Social Research. (2007). *Infant feeding survey 2005: A survey conducted on behalf of the Information Centre for Health and Social Care and the UK Health Departments.* London: Great Britain. Department of Health.

Cheshire, H., Hussey, D., Phelps, A., et al. (2012). Methodology. In J. Banks, J. Nazroo, & A. Steptoe (Eds.), *Dynamics of ageing: Evidence from the English longitudinal study of ageing* (pp. 183–213). London: The Institute for Fiscal Studies.

Cheshire, P. (2009). Policies for mixed communities: Faith-based displacement activity? *International Regional Science Review, 32*(3), 343–375. https://doi.org/10.1177/0160017609336080

Craig, P., Katikireddi, S., Leyland, A., & Popham, F. (2017). Natural experiments: An overview of methods, approaches, and contributions to public health intervention research. *Annual Review of Public Health, 38*, 39–56. https://doi.org/10.1146/annurev-publhealth-031816-044327

Diez Roux, A. V., & Mair, C. (2010). Neighborhoods and health. *Annals of the New York of Sciences, 1186*, 125–145. https://doi.org/10.1111/j.1749-6632.2009.05333.x

Dunning, T. (2012). *Natural experiments in the social sciences: A design-based approach.* Cambridge, MA: Cambridge University Press.

Eckhert, S., & Kohler, S. (2014). Urbanization and health in developing countries: A systematic review. *World Health & Population, 15*(1), 7–20. https://doi.org/10.12927/whp.2014.23722

Fields, L. E., Burt, V. L., Cutler, J. A., Hughes, J., Roccella, E. J., & Sorlie, P. (2004). The burden of adult hypertension in the United States 1999 to 2000: A rising tide. *Hypertension, 44*, 398–404. https://doi.org/10.1161/01.hyp.0000142248.54761.56

Finney, N., & Marshall, A. (2018). Is migration in later life good for wellbeing? A longitudinal study of ageing and selectivity of internal migration. *Area, 50*(4), 492–500. https://doi.org/10.1111/area.12428

Fowler. (2009). *Survey research methods* (4th ed.). London, UK: Sage Publications.

Fries, J. (1980). Aging, natural death, and the compression of morbidity. *New England Journal of Medicine, 303*(3), 130–135. https://doi.org/10.1056/nejm198007173030304

Galster, G. (2012). The mechanism(s) of neighborhood effects: Theory, evidence and policy implications. In M. van Ham, D. Manley, N. Bailey, L. Simpson, & D. Maclennan (Eds.), *Neighbourhood effects research: New perspectives.* London, UK: Springer.

Gau, M. L. (2004). Evaluation of a lactation intervention program to encourage breastfeeding: A longitudinal study. *International Journal of Nursing Studies, 41*(4), 425–435. https://doi.org/10.1016/j.ijnurstu.2003.11.002

Godfrey, R., & Julien, M. (2005). Urbanisation and health. *Clinical Medicine, 5*(2), 137–141. https://doi.org/10.7861/clinmedicine.5-2-137

Gruenberg, E. M. (1976). The failure of success. *Milbank Quarterly, 55*(1), 3–24. https://doi.org/10.1111/j.1468-0009.2005.00400.x

Horta, B. L., Loret de Mola, C., & Victora, C. G. (2015). Breastfeeding and intelligence: A systematic review and meta-analysis. *Acta Paediatrica, 104*(467), 14–19. https://doi.org/10.1111/apa.13139

Hou, B., Nazroo, J., Banks, J., & Marshall, A. (2019). Are cities good for health? A study of the impacts of planned urbanisation in China. *International Journal of Epidemiology, 48*(4), 1083–1090. https://doi.org/10.1093/ije/dyz031

Karp, F. (2002). *Growing older in America: The health and retirement study.* National Institute on Aging/National Institutes of Health/US Department of Health and Human Services. Retrieved from www.nia.nih.gov/sites/default/files/2017-06/health_and_retirement_study_0.pdf

Kelaher, M., Dunt, D., Feldman, P., Nolan, A., & Raban, B. (2009). The effect of an area-based intervention on breastfeeding rates in Victoria, Australia. *Health Policy, 90*(1), 89–93. https://doi.org/10.1016/j.healthpol.2008.08.004

Labbok, M. H. (2013). Breastfeeding: Population-based perspectives. *Pediatric Clinics of North America, 60*(1), 11–30. https://doi.org/10.1016/j.pcl.2012.09.011

Leon, D. A. (2008). Cities, urbanization and health. *International Journal of Epidemiology, 37*(1), 1, 4–8. https://doi.org/10.1093/ije/dym271

Lipsitz, S. R., Kim, K., & Zhao, L. (1994). Analysis of repeated categorical data using generalized estimating equations. *Statistical Medicine, 13*(11), 1149–1163. https://doi.org/10.1002/sim.4780131106

Manley, D., Van Ham, M., Bailey, N., Simpson, L., & Maclennan, D. (Eds.). (2013). *Neighbourhood effects or neighbourhood-based problems? A policy context.* London: Springer Publisher.

Marshall, A., Nazroo, J., Feeney, K., Lee, J., Vanhoutte, B., & Pendleton, N. (2015b). Comparison of hypertension health care outcomes among older people in the USA and England. *Journal of Epidemiology and Community Health, 70*(3), 264–270. https://doi.org/10.1136/jech-2014-205336

Marshall, A., Nazroo, J., Tampubolon, G., & Vanhoutte, B. (2015a). Cohort differences in the levels and trajectories of frailty among older people in England. *Journal of Epidemiology and Community Health, 69*, 316–321. https://doi.org/10.1136/jech-2014-204655

Martin, L., Schoeni, R., Andreski, P., & Jagger, C. (2011). Trends and inequalities in late-life health and functioning in England. *Journal of Epidemiology and Community Health, 66*(10), 874–880. Retrieved from https://jech.bmj.com/content/66/10/874.info

National Institute for Clinical Excellence (NICE). (2006). *Management of hypertension of adults in primary care.* National Institute for Clinical Excellence Guideline, 34, 2006. Retrieved August 10, 2020, from http://www.nice.org.uk/guidance/cg34

Norman, P., Marshall, A., & Lomax, N. (2017). Data analytics: On the cusp of using new sources? *Radical Statistics*, *115*, 19–30. https://orcid.org/0000-0002-6211-1625

Nowak, B., Van Ham, M., Findlay, A., & Gayle, V. (2013). Does migration make you happy? A longitudinal study of internal migration and subjective wellbeing. *Environment and Planning A*, *45*(4), 986–1002. Retrieved from http://citeseerx.ist.psu.edu/viewdoc/download?doi=10.1.1.418.7894&rep=rep1&type=pdf

Petticrew, M., Cummins, S., Ferrell, C., Findlay, A., Higgins, C., Hoy, C., et al. (2005). Natural experiments: An underused tool for public health? *Public Health*, *119*(9), 751–757. https://doi.org/10.1016/j.puhe.2004.11.008

Radloff, L. S. (1977). The CES-D scale: A self-report depression scale for research in the general population. *Applied Psychological Measurement*, *1*(3), 385–401. https://doi.org/10.1177/014662167700100306

Sanderson, W. C., & Scherbov, S. (2010). Demography: Remeasuring aging. *Science*, *329*(5997), 1287–1288. https://doi.org/10.1126/science.1193647

Scottish Government. (2018, February). *Scottish maternal and infant nutrition survey* (2017). Edinburgh: Scottish Government. Retrieved from www.gov.scot/binaries/content/documents/govscot/publications/statistics/2018/02/scottish-maternal-infant-nutrition-survey-2017/documents/00531610-pdf/00531610-pdf/govscot%3adocument/00531610.pdf

Searle, S., Mitnitski, A., Gahbauer, E., Gill, T. M., & Rockwood, K. (2008). Standard procedure for creating a frailty index. *BMC Geriatrics*, *8*(24), 1–10. https://doi.org/10.1186/1471-2318-8-24

Shaw, M., Davey Smith, G., & Dorling, D. (2005). Health inequalities and new labour: How the promises compare with real progress. *BMJ*, *330*, 1016–1021. https://doi.org/10.1136/bmj.330.7498.1016

Shaw, M., Dorling, D., Gordon, D., & Smith (1999). *The widening gap: Health inequalities and policy in Britain*. Bristol, England: Policy Press.

Skafida, V. (2014). Change in breastfeeding patterns in Scotland between 2004 and 2011 and the role of health policy. *The European Journal of Public Health*, *24*(6), 1033–1041. https://doi.org/10.1093/eurpub/cku029

Snijders, T., & Bosker, R. (2011). *Multilevel analysis: An introduction to basic and advanced multilevel modelling* (2nd ed.). London: Sage Publications.

Spijker, J., & MacInnes, J. (2012). Population ageing: The time bomb that isn't? *BMJ*, *347*, f6598, 20–22. https://doi.org/10.1136/bmj.f6598

U.S. Department of Health and Human Services (DHSS). (2004). *The Seventh Report of the Joint National Committee on Prevention, Detection, Evaluation, and Treatment of High Blood Pressure*. NIH Publication No. 04-5230. Retrieved April 29, 2020, from www.nhlbi.nih.gov/files/docs/guidelines/jnc7full.pdf

van Ham, M., & Manley, D. (2012). Neighbourhood effects research at a crossroads: Ten challenges for future research. *Environment and Planning*, *44*(12), 2787–2793. Retrieved from www.econstor.eu/handle/10419/75321

Vanhoutte, B. (2014). The multidimensional structure of subjective well-being in later life. *Journal of Population Ageing*, *7*(1), 1–20. https://doi.org/10.1007/s12062-014-9092-9

Vatcheva, K., Lee, M., McCormick, J., & Rahbah, M. (2016). The effect of ignoring statistical interactions in regression analyses conducted in epidemiologic studies: An example with survival analysis using Cox proportional hazards regression model. *Epidemiology*, *6*(1), 216. Retrieved from https://doi.org/10.4172/2161-1165.1000216

Wiggins, R. D., Netuveli, G., Hyde, M., Higgs, P., & Blane, D. (2007). The evaluation of a self-enumerated scale of quality of life (CASP-19) in the context of research on ageing: A combination of exploratory and confirmatory approaches. *Social Indicators Research*, *89*(1), 61–77.

Wolf-Maier, K., Cooper, R. S., Kramer, H., Banegas, J. R., Giampaoli, S., Joffres, M. R., et al. (2004). Hypertension treatment and control in five European countries, Canada, and the United States. *Hypertension*, *43*(1), 10–17. https://doi.org/10.1161/01.HYP.0000103630.72812.10

Wood, R., Stockton, D., & Brown, H. (2012). Moving from a universal to targeted child health programme: Which children receive enhanced care? A population-based study using routinely available data: Targeting child health programme support. *Child: Care, Health and Development*, *39*(6), 772–781. https://doi.org/10.1111/j.1365-2214.2012.01423.x

World Health Organisation. (2013). *A global brief on hypertension: Silent killer, global public health crisis*. Geneva, Switzerland: World Health Organization. Retrieved from https://apps.who.int/iris/bitstream/10665/79059/1/WHO_DCO_WHD_2013.2_eng.pdf

Zalewski, B. M., Patro, B., Veldhorst, M., Kouwenhoven, S., Escobar, P. C., Lerma, J. C., et al. (2017). Nutrition of infants and young children (one to three years) and its effect on later health: A systematic review of current recommendations (Early Nutrition project). *Critical Reviews in Food Science and Nutrition*, *57*(3), 489–500. https://doi.org/10.1080/10408398.2014.888701

17
CHRONIC ILLNESS
The Case of Chronic Fatigue Syndrome-Myalgic Encephalomyelitis

Leonard A. Jason, Joseph Cotler, Shaun Bhatia,
and Madison Sunnquist

Overview

Chronic fatigue syndrome (**CFS**) and *myalgic encephalomyelitis* (**ME**) affect approximately 1 million Americans (Jason, Richman, Rademaker, Jordan, Plioplys, Taylor, et al., 1999a); while some individuals believe that *CFS* and *ME* refer to the same illness, others characterize *ME* as a more severe, neurological disorder that is discrete from *CFS* (Twisk, 2015). This controversy will be reviewed in detail. The widespread, debilitating symptoms of the illnesses include but are not limited to feeling sick after activity (known as post-exertional malaise), memory and concentration problems, and unrefreshing sleep (IOM, 2015).

Some researchers suggest that *ME* and *CFS* were first conceptualized under the diagnostic label "*neurasthenia*," defined as a neurological disease characterized by muscle weakness or fatigue. Notably, *neurasthenia* was one of the most frequently diagnosed illnesses in the late nineteenth century. However, use of this term had substantially decreased by the mid-twentieth century (Wessely, 1994).

Throughout the twentieth century, several outbreaks of idiopathic, fatigue-related illnesses occurred, including "atypical poliomyelitis" at Los Angeles County Hospital in 1934 (Meals, Hauser, & Bower, 1935), "encephalomyelitis" at the Royal Free Hospital in London in 1955 (Crowley, Nelson, & Stovin, 1957), and "chronic mononucleosis–like syndrome" in Lake Tahoe, Nevada, in 1984 (Barnes, 1986). After the Lake Tahoe outbreak, national attention began to focus on this illness (Wessely, 1994), and in 1988, it was named *chronic fatigue syndrome* by the Centers for Disease Control and Prevention (CDC; Holmes, Kaplan, Gantz, Komaroff, Schonberger, Straus, et al., 1988). For over two decades, the case definition that the CDC developed (Fukuda, Straus, Hickie, Sharpe, Dobbins, & Komaroff, 1994) has been prominently used in research and clinical practice; however, the Institute of Medicine (IOM) recently developed an updated clinical case definition (IOM, 2015).

The annual direct and indirect costs of *ME* and *CFS* in the United States are estimated to be between $19 and $24 billion (Jason, Benton, Johnson, & Valentine, 2008). Individuals with ME and *CFS* have an increased risk of cardiovascular-related mortality and a lower mean age of death by suicide and cancer in comparison to the general US population (McManimen, Devendorf, Brown, Moore, Moore, & Jason, 2016). In addition, arthritis, high blood pressure, fibromyalgia, and multiple chemical sensitivities are commonly comorbid (Jason, Porter, Hunnell, Brown, Rademaker, & Richman, 2011). Although no virus has been identified as the cause of *ME* and *CFS*, the immune system may be overactive (Fischer, William, Strauss, Unger, Jason, Marshall, et al., 2014), and there is evidence that *ME* and *CFS* may be caused by, or associated with, immune and/or brain dysfunction (Jason, Zinn, & Zinn, 2015).

Our chapter focuses on the best methods that have been implemented in *ME* and *CFS* research. We provide insights about why certain procedures were used in order to guide other investigators who are conceptualizing and implementing their research in similar or overlapping areas. The next section begins with a discussion of the challenges faced by patients, particularly given the stigma associated with *ME* and *CFS* (Jason, Holbert, Torres-Harding, & Taylor, 2004). The section after that describes existing case definitions for *ME* and *CFS*, highlighting their limitations and the resulting methodological complications for researchers and clinicians. Subsequent sections review the prevalence of *ME* and *CFS*, innovative research in immunology, and approaches to *ME* and *CFS* treatment. Finally, we conclude with a summary of the strengths and limitations of current research and suggests areas for future research.

Research in Practice

Stigma Associated With the Name

Prior to the CDC's decision to name the illness "*CFS*" due to the ubiquity of fatigue among those diagnosed (Holmes, Kaplan, Gantz, Komaroff, Schonberger, Strauss, et al., 1988), clinicians in England were referring to the same constellation of symptoms as "*ME*" (Ramsay, 1988). Many patients and patient advocacy groups expressed dissatisfaction with this name change, noting that "chronic fatigue syndrome" trivializes the seriousness of the illness (Blease & Geraghty, 2018), given that patients' experiences could be misconstrued as everyday tiredness. Moreover, the term selected to characterize an illness during initial observation or exploratory analysis can influence how patients are perceived and treated by medical personnel, family members, and work associates.

In 1998, a patient contacted the first author and suggested a study to experimentally document how the name of this illness might influence attributions. With input from this patient, the DePaul University research team launched a study to evaluate whether different names for this illness influenced attributions regarding its cause, nature, severity, contagion, and prognosis. In this study, medical trainees were provided with a case description of a patient with prototypic symptoms of *ME* and *CFS*. Trainees were randomly assigned to different experimental conditions (i.e., the diagnostic label used for the illness). While 41% of medical trainees believed patients would recover when referring to the illness as *CFS*, only 16% believed the patient condition would improve when referring to the illness as *ME*. Additionally, medical trainees were more likely to attribute the illness to medical causes when referring to the illness as *ME* (Jason, Taylor, Plioplys, Stepanek, & Shlaes, 2002).

These results indicate a stereotyping effect among medical practitioners when a chronic illness's name is characterized by a single, commonly experienced symptom (chronic fatigue), as opposed to a name that uses medical terminology (*ME*). These findings were consistent with existing evidence that the term *CFS* contributed to negative attitudes among health care providers toward those with this syndrome (Green, Romei, & Natelson, 1999). Furthermore, studies have demonstrated that renaming stigmatized conditions to reflect a wider spectrum of symptoms has led to an overall decrease in negative stereotyping for some patients (Koike, Yamaguchi, Ojio, Shimada, Watanabe, & Ando, 2015). Early missteps in condition naming can unwittingly result in patient stigmatization. In fact, many individuals now refer to this illness as either *ME* or *ME/CFS*.

Case Definition

A ***case definition*** is a set of criteria used to classify whether a person has a particular disease, syndrome, or other health condition (CDC, 2012). *Case definitions* should be clear, simple, and reliable, allowing them to be easily and accurately applied to a population. *Case definitions* are used for a variety of functions, such as clinical diagnosis or routine population screening (Bassil, 2016). The use of an agreed-upon *case definition* ensures that the morbidity of a disease is captured with a high degree of specificity and sensitivity so that disease trends can be compared over time, place, and other factors (CDC, 2012). As such, from a methodological perspective, it is essential that the *case definition* identify as homogenous of a disease entity as possible (Hennekens & Buring, 1987); unfortunately, regarding *ME* and *CFS*, there are 20 different case definitions (Brurberg, Fonhus, Larun, Flottorp, & Malterud, 2014), and individuals given a diagnosis of *ME* or *CFS* have varied symptomatology.

As mentioned earlier, the term *CFS* was first used by the CDC, along with a *case definition* that required eight or more symptoms (Holmes, et al., 1988). However, this definition was criticized for its large symptom requirement that could increase clinicians' propensity to misdiagnosis *CFS* among individuals with somatization disorder, a diagnosis that similarly requires eight unexplained symptoms. Consequently, the CDC revised the case definition in 1994 to reduce the number of symptoms required. This *case definition* is referred to as Fukuda, Straus, Hickie, Sharpe, Dobbins, and Komaroff's (1994) *CFS* criteria; patients must experience four of eight possible symptoms in order to receive a diagnosis. Despite this improvement, the *case definition* remained polythetic: patients could fulfill Fukuda, et al.'s (1994) criteria without core symptoms, such as post-exertional malaise. The Canadian Clinical Consensus (CCC) criteria (Carruthers, Jain, De Meirleir, Peterson, Klimas, Lerner, et al., 2003) corrected this issue; individuals must report several cardinal symptoms of the illness in order to be diagnosed, including post-exertional malaise, memory and concentration problems, and unrefreshing sleep (Carruthers, et al., 2003; Jason, Torres-Harding, Jurgens, & Helgerson, 2004).

In 2011, the *ME* International Consensus Criteria (ME-ICC) were developed; these criteria were significant due to their use of the term "*ME*" instead of "*CFS*," as well as the removal of fatigue as a symptom criterion. However, these criteria again increased the number of required symptoms to eight (Carruthers, van de Sande, De Meirleir, Klimas, Broderick, Mitchell, et al., 2011), similar to the earlier Holmes, et al. (1988) criteria, and individuals who met the ME-ICC demonstrated increased rates of psychiatric comorbidity compared to those who met Fukuda et al.'s (1994) criteria (Brown, Jason, Evans, & Flores, 2013). Most recently, the IOM (IOM, 2015) released an updated clinical *case definition*; however, it broadened the scope of acceptable comorbid medical and psychiatric conditions, and therefore, it is less likely to identify a homogenous group of patients for research purposes (Jason, Fox, & Gleason, 2018).

These *ME* and *CFS case definitions* have created considerable methodological problems for researchers because if different *case definitions* are used by investigators, it is more difficult to compare participants in *ME* and *CFS* studies. Heterogeneity across research samples limits researchers' ability to replicate findings related to potential illness etiologies, biomarkers, and treatments. For example, a study by Johnston, Brenu, Hardcastle, Huth, Staines, and Marshall-Gradisnik (2014) compared healthy controls to two patient groups: a group who met the Fukuda, et al. (1994) *CFS* criteria and a group who met the ME-ICC criteria (Carruthers, et al., 2011). They found significant differences in general health and disability scores, as well as differences in hemoglobin, hematocrit, and red cell count, with the ME-ICC criteria identifying a more impaired group. Establishing a consensus on a research *case definition* remains one of the most significant challenges for researchers in this field.

To contribute to the development of a sensitive, specific *case definition*, numerous studies have attempted to identify which characteristic symptoms can differentiate *ME* and *CFS* from other chronic illnesses, indicating that these symptoms should be required by *case definitions*. In one innovative study, researchers compared the presence or absence of 26 "unspecific" symptoms in outpatients with severe fatigue who had either *ME* or *CFS*, systemic lupus erythematosus, or fibromyalgia (Linder, Dinser, Wagner, Krueger, & Hoffmann, 2002). These investigators generated classification criteria to differentiate patients with *ME* and *CFS* from those with lupus and fibromyalgia using regression tree analysis and artificial neural network analysis, composed of computer-based models used to evaluate complex correlations. The patients were randomly divided into two groups. One group served to derive classification criteria sets by sophisticated procedures, including artificial neural networks in parallel. These criteria were then validated with the second group. Symptoms that best differentiated patients with *ME* and *CFS* from the other patients were acute onset of fatigue and sore throat. Additionally, a recent study highlighted that the duration of post-exertional malaise symptoms can distinguish *ME* and *CFS* from other chronic illnesses (Cotler, Holtzman, Dudun, & Jason, 2018). The lesson that is apparent from this section is that it is essential for a consensus on a *case definition* among investigators for establishing a solid empiric foundation in any illness or disease.

Community-Based Epidemiology

Prevalence is used to estimate the magnitude of a health problem (Szklo & Nieto, 2007) in order to determine the type and quantity of services required to address an illness. Government organizations like the National Institutes of Health (NIH) benefit from having standardized measurements of disease burden to inform funding decisions (Best, 2012; NIH, 2017). Numerous *ME* and *CFS prevalence* studies have been published since the release of the first case definitions, but estimates vary widely due to differences in recruitment methodology and inclusion criteria (Johnston, Brenu, Staines, & Marshall-Gradisnik, 2013).

An initial point *prevalence* estimate of *ME* and *CFS* ranged from 4.0 to 8.7 per 100,000 persons (Reyes, Gary, Dobbins, Randall, Steele, Fukuda, et al., 1997), suggesting that there were fewer than 20,000 affected individuals in the United States. This study used a case ascertainment method whereby physicians identified patients who presented with unexplained fatigue and referred them for a medical examination to determine whether they met criteria for *CFS*. Of note, this methodology excludes individuals with limited access to health care. Moreover, physicians who doubted the existence of *CFS* would be less likely to refer patients to this study. Findings from this study contributed to beliefs that *ME* and *CFS* were relatively rare and primarily affected white, middle-class women.

A subsequent *prevalence* study by Jason, et al. (1999a) corrected the recruitment limitations of the prior study through screening a random, community-based sample of 18,675 individuals for *ME* and *CFS* symptomatology. In other words, any individual with a phone number was eligible for inclusion in this study, regardless of access to health care. Those who endorsed *ME*- or *CFS*-like symptoms during an initial telephone interview were invited to participate in a comprehensive medical and psychiatric evaluation. Approximately 0.42% of the sample met Fukuda, et al.'s (1994) *CFS* criteria, indicating that approximately 1 million people in the United States had this illness. Findings contradicted the perception that *ME* and *CFS* primarily affected Caucasian women of higher socioeconomic status; in contrast to this belief, higher *prevalence* rates were found among individuals of lower socioeconomic status and those who identified as Latinx. Furthermore, about 90% of participants who fulfilled *CFS* criteria had not been previously diagnosed by a physician prior to participation in the study (Jason, et al., 1999a). These findings highlight the limitations of *ME* and *CFS* epidemiological studies that rely upon physician referrals.

Between 2003 and 2007, CDC estimates of the percentage of individuals who fulfilled the Fukuda, et al. *CFS* criteria (1994) in the United States increased tenfold, from 0.24% (Reyes, Nisenbaum, Hoaglin, Unger, Emmons, Randall, et al., 2003) to 2.54% (Reeves, Jones, Maloney, Heim, Hoaglin, Boneva, et al., 2007). It is unlikely that the *prevalence* of this illness exponentially grew during this time period. Rather, this dramatic increase likely resulted from a broader operationalization of Fukuda, et al.'s *CFS* criteria (1994) that may have included individuals with primary affective disorders, specifically, major depressive disorder (Jason, et al., 2018).

The aforementioned studies demonstrate how recruitment methodology and case definition application can substantially affect prevalence estimates; these issues must be considered when interpreting *ME* and *CFS* study results (Jason, et al., 2018). The lesson for researchers studying community-based samples is that those participants might have characteristics very different from participants in more tertiary-care settings. Epidemiological approaches that use methods that select samples unbiased by care-seeking characteristics are more likely to accurately describe generalizable and representative features of samples.

Network Analysis of Cytokines

Researchers have incorporated methods pioneered by immunologists to examine potential biomarkers using multiplex assays identifying **cytokines** (small proteins that are involved in cell signaling) previously too small and localized to evaluate effectively (Hamblin, 1993; Broderick Katz, Fernandes, Fletcher, Klimas, Smith, et al., 2012). Incorporating a new methodology is partly due to new technologies in the field of immunology, which have only been available with greater precision in recent decades. Using these new methods, several studies have identified a significant association between the release of pro-inflammatory *cytokines* and experiences of fatigue (e.g., Paulsen, Laird, Aass, Lea, Fayers, Kaasa, et al., 2017; Raudonis, Kelley, Rowe, & Ellis, 2017; Tripp, Tarn, Natasari, Gillespie, Mitchell, Hackett, et al., 2016). Natelson, Tseng, and Ottenweller (2005) found increases in *cytokines* in the cerebrospinal fluid of patients with *ME* and *CFS*, supporting the hypothesis that symptoms may be due to immune dysfunction within the central nervous system. However, measurements of *cytokine* concentrations in blood samples from patients with *ME* and *CFS* have produced inconsistent results. For example, some studies have demonstrated greater concentrations of pro-inflammatory *cytokines* in patients compared to healthy blood samples (Gaab, Rohleder, Heitz, Engert, Schad, Schürmeyer, et al., 2005), while other studies observed a greater concentration of anti-inflammatory *cytokines* present in patients with *ME* and *CFS* (Ter Wolbeek, Doornen, Kavelaars, Putte, Schedlowski, & Heijnen, 2007). Differences in *cytokine* findings may be explained by methodological inconsistencies and focusing on only a few *cytokines* at a time. What is needed is more systems-oriented network research, which has been used to understand disorders in the field of psychopathology (Borsboom, 2017).

Some of the most promising network research (Broderick, et al., 2012) has examined *cytokine* expression among youth who had experienced infectious mononucleosis (IM), posited as an infectious trigger of *ME* and *CFS*. Results indicated that 24 months following IM diagnosis, levels of **interleukin-2 (IL-2**; a protein that activates the immune system to shrink tumors) and **interleukin-8 (IL-8**; a key mediator associated with inflammation) were significantly higher in youth who had developed *ME* and *CFS* than youth who did not develop *ME* and *CFS* following IM. In addition, youth who developed *ME* and *CFS* had lower levels of **interleukin-5 (IL-5**; proteins that stimulate immune responses, such as inflammation) and **interleukin-23 (IL-23**; a member of the family of *cytokines* with pro-inflammatory properties). Broderick, et al. (2012) then applied linear discriminant classification analysis to the *cytokines* and retrospectively classified the youth based on levels of IL-2, 6, 8, 23, and **IFN-γ** (interferon gamma) into the patient or recovered control group with a specificity of 88% and a sensitivity of 94%. This research suggests that *cytokine* networks, rather than individual *cytokine* levels, should be examined to better understand dysfunction within the immune system. In Broderick, Fuite, Kreitz, Vernon, Klimas, and Fletcher (2010), such analysis indicated that **interleukin-10** (a protein with potent anti-inflammatory properties) had weak overall relationships in healthy controls but had strong associations to multiple other *cytokines* in patients with *ME* and *CFS*. This observation of differences in network importance would not have been possible if researchers had attenuated their focus to examine individual correlations as opposed to correlations as part of a wider system.

By examining *cytokines* as interconnected clusters, not isolated quantities, we might better identify abnormalities in the immune response demonstrated by patients with *ME* and *CFS*. A similar challenge to this area of research, however, is that findings might be dependent on which *case definition* is used, as well as differences in the methods of sampling and analysis (Maher, Klimas & Fletcher, 2003).

Treatment

As variation in case definition application has limited the field's search for biomarkers and effective treatments for *ME* and *CFS*, clinicians and researchers have developed and tested several nonpharmacological treatments. The most commonly applied psychological treatments for patients with *ME* and *CFS* include **cognitive behavioral therapy (CBT)** and **graded exercise therapy (GET)**. These interventions have been implemented with the following underlying assumptions: while a virus or other pathogen might have precipitated the illness, fatigue and physical impairment were now being maintained by lack of activity (i.e., deconditioning), and patients' focus on physical symptoms further increased their perception of the severity of their illness (Vercoulen, Swanink, Galama, Fennis, Jongen, Hommes, et al., 1998). These types of psychological interventions may contribute to the stigmatization of *ME* and *CFS*, as they reject any biological illness etiologies and suggest that patients' symptoms result from their own thoughts and behaviors (Geraghty, 2016). Furthermore, many patients note that such interventions do not respect their experiences. For example, patients are often instructed by physicians to increase their activity level, despite resulting symptoms of exacerbation. Self-reports of the patient experience in response to *CBT* and *GET* have been decidedly mixed, with many patients describing a worsening of symptoms and dissatisfaction following *CBT* and *GET* intervention (ME Association, 2010; Action for M.E., 2010).

A recent study by Sunnquist and Jason (2018) found that the **psychogenic** (having a psychological cause) **model** proposed by Vercoulen, Swanink, Galama, Fennis, Jongen, Hommes, et al. (1998) was not supported when more rigorous *case definitions* were employed. In addition, Price, Mitchell, Tidy, and Hunot (2008) reviewed studies of *CBT* with a total of 1,043 *CFS* participants; although 40% of the sample showed clinical improvement by treatment's end, this improvement was not maintained at one- to seven-month follow-ups when including patients who had dropped out in outcome analyses. Another study that generated considerable controversy by White, Goldsmith, Johnson, Potts, Walwyn, DeCesare, and colleagues (2011) suggested that these types of interventions helped many patients both improve and recover their functioning. However, when data from the randomized trial ultimately was made available for re-analysis, recovery rates in the *GET* and *CBT* groups were low and not significantly higher than in the control group (Wilshire, Kindlon, Courtney, Matthees, Tuller, Geraghty, et al., 2018).

The psychogenic model of *ME* and *CFS* is further challenged by evidence that the psychological profiles of patients with *ME* and *CFS* do not differ from those of healthy individuals. For example, Camacho and Jason (1998) found that patients with *ME* and *CFS* do not have significantly different levels of optimism, stress, and social support compared to healthy controls. Furthermore, the *GET*-induced symptom exacerbation reported by patients with *ME* and *CFS* may have a physiological basis. Incremental exercise has been associated with oxidative stress and marked alterations of muscle membrane excitability (Jammes, Steinberg, Mambrini, Bregeon, & Delliaux, 2005). While behavioral activation strategies improve mood and reduce fatigue among individuals with primary depression (Cuijpers, van Straten, & Warmerdam, 2007), gradual increases in daily activity worsen mood, muscle pain intensity, and time spent each day with fatigue among individuals with *ME* and *CFS* (Black, O'Connor, & McCully, 2005).

As an alternative approach to *CBT* and *GET*, the "**energy envelope theory**" was developed and implemented in the 1990s (Jason, Melrose, Lerman, Burroughs, Lewis, King, et al., 1999b; King, Jason, Frankenberry, Jordan, & Tryon, 1997). Rather than gradually increasing patient activity without regard to symptom intensification, the *energy envelope theory* suggests that by maintaining expended energy levels within the "envelope" of perceived available energy levels, individuals with *ME* and *CFS* would be able to better sustain physical and mental functioning while reducing symptom severity and the frequency of relapses (Jason, Brown, Brown, Evans, Flores, Grant-Holler, et al., 2013). Over time, patients could learn to assess their perceived available daily energy levels and use that level to monitor their energy expenditures. There is some empirical support that by engaging in this type of energy maintenance, patients with *ME* and *CFS* have been able to reduce fatigue severity and increase vitality (Jason, Roesner, Porter, Parenti, Mortensen, & Till, 2010).

The "***pacing***" approach in the treatment of *ME* and *CFS* may be viewed as compatible with the *energy envelope theory*; patients are encouraged to be as active as possible within the limits imposed by their illness, but are encouraged to ignore symptoms that do not make them feel unwell (Goudsmit, 1996; Goudsmit, Jason, Nijs, & Wallman, 2012). In contrast to *CBT* and *GET*, patients are instructed to either rest or change to an activity involving different muscles when more serious symptoms occur, an indication that their "limits" have been exceeded (Goudsmit & Howes, 2008). This pacing approach was used in a 12-week program that encouraged symptom-contingent graded exercise; increases in activity were advised only when patients felt comfortable maintaining their current levels of activity (Wallman, Morton, Goodman, Grove, & Guilfoyle, 2004). Outcomes of this study indicated that none of the patients felt that the program made them worse, and 91% of the participants rated their overall health as "better."

Pacing and *energy envelope theory* interventions represent alternative approaches for improving the quality of life of individuals with *ME* and *CFS*. These programs help patients better monitor energy levels and stay within their energy envelopes by encouraging lifestyle changes that may involve reprioritizing activities, such as better balancing work and leisure time (Goudsmit, et al. 2012). Though these types of interventions often result in better health-related quality of life among patients with *ME* and *CFS* (Taylor, Jason, Shiraishi, Schoeny, & Keller, 2006), it is important to emphasize that these approaches should be combined with a comprehensive, tailored, and multidisciplinary treatment plan that accounts for patients' medical needs (Jason, et al., 2013). Most importantly, from a methodological perspective, if individuals are not accurately diagnosed, incorrect treatments can be applied to these patients, causing further harm and stigma.

Strengths and Limitations

Despite inconclusive evidence, individuals with *ME* and *CFS* continue to be referred for psychological treatments, such as *CBT* and *GET* that presume a psychogenic illness etiology. This issue may result, in part, from the dearth of training offered in medical schools related to this illness (Peterson, Peterson, Emerson, Regalbuto, Evans, & Jason, 2013). Many health care professionals lack the training to adequately evaluate and treat *ME* and *CFS* (Jason, et al., 2002). Given the limited number of physicians with *ME* and *CFS* expertise, patients have difficulty finding knowledgeable and sympathetic doctors (Tidmore, Jason, Chapo-Kroger, So, Brown, & Silverman, 2015). In the United States, more than 50% of patients have not seen an *ME* or *CFS* specialist for treatment due to geographic or financial barriers (Sunnquist, Nicolson, Jason, & Friedman, 2017). Furthermore, as appointments with specialists are scarce, patients may wait months or years to obtain a diagnosis or access adequate health care. Given these challenges, individuals with *ME* and *CFS* often experience high levels of anger and feelings of estrangement (Green, et al., 1999; McManimen, Stoothoff, McClellan, & Jason, 2018). Health care providers should be cognizant of the barriers faced by those with *ME* and *CFS* and understanding of any frustration that patients express.

The name of the illness is another contributor to frustration within the patient community. As indicated in the previous sections, stakeholders (including patient advocacy groups, researchers, and clinicians) lack consensus regarding the appropriate terminology for *ME* and *CFS*. Some prefer the term *ME*, others *ME/CFS*, and still others *CFS* (Blease & Geraghty, 2018; Twisk, 2018). Those interested in working with individuals who have *ME* or *CFS* should be mindful to use their preferred term for the illness, as disregarding this preference could cause tension.

In addition to divergent opinions about the appropriate illness name, the field has yet to agree on which case definition to use in research and practice. Without a commonly agreed-upon research case definition, laboratory settings will collect heterogeneous samples, leading to difficulty in replicating studies and discovering biological markers. As with many other diseases, until biological markers of *ME* and *CFS* are identified, many will continue to doubt the legitimacy of this illness, and this skepticism contributes to the stigma that patients experience when interacting with health care professionals.

Despite these limitations, important progress has occurred over the past 30 years. For example, in the 1990s, the illness had been commonly referred to as the "yuppie flu" (Friedberg & Jason, 1998). This controversial and stigmatizing label resulted from flawed epidemiology that suggested those with the illness were primarily White, upper-middle-class women. Results of community-based studies revealed that the majority of patients were not "yuppies," but were from less privileged socioeconomic backgrounds (Jason et al, 1999a; Jason, et al., 2011). In addition, while some still attribute the fatigue experienced by patients with *ME* and *CFS* to psychiatric issues, more recent research has shown that those with solely a major depressive disorder can be accurately distinguished from those with *ME* and *CFS* (Hawk, Jason, & Torres-Harding, 2006). Finally, while there are no concrete biological markers, promising research is being conducted examining network-based biological markers, such as *cytokines*, which will hopefully provide a clearer understanding of the physiological aspects of *ME* and *CFS* (Broderick, et al., 2010). Although often misunderstood and mischaracterized, the perceptions towards those with this illness has begun to change in positive ways to reduce stigmatization of the patient community.

Recommendations for Future Research

In this final section, we return to one of the central issues that researchers and clinicians confront when engaging in work in this area, and that involves the failure to reach a consensus regarding a research *case definition*. As spotlighted, lack of *case definition* uniformity has caused methodological challenges for investigators. The ability to replicate findings related to potential illness etiologies and courses of treatments and establish consistent prevalence estimates are challenging, in part, due to the heterogeneity caused by multiple *case definitions*.

Unfortunately, those engaged in work in the *ME* and *CFS* fields are continuing to deal with this lack of consensus on such critical issues as the *case definition*. For example, when the IOM (2015) recommended a clinical *case definition*, their recommendations were largely kept secret until publication of the full report. The lack of transparency and the criticism that followed were further examples of a patient community that has long felt disempowered, excluded, and ignored (Jason, Sunnquist, Brown, McManimen, & Furst, 2015). In addition, as this IOM clinical *case definition* has received considerable attention, it is important to recognize that it lacks, for the most part, exclusionary criteria, which exist in other *case definitions* (e.g., Carruthers, et al., 2003, Fukuda, et al., 1994). Proponents of the IOM criteria contend their criteria were deliberately broad, as they were to be used for clinical rather than research purposes. Yet in the absence of a research *case definition*, some investigators have already begun to use these clinical criteria as a research *case definition* (Chu, Norris, Valencia, & Montoya, 2017), and if this occurs, then the *case definition* will not identify a homogeneous group of patients across research settings (Jason, Sunnquist, Gleason, & Fox, 2017). Fluctuating prevalence and disease burden estimates, difficulties in finding biological markers, and problems in interpreting the results of treatment trials are by-products of multiple *case definitions*.

In addition to proposing a new *case definition*, the IOM (2015) recommended a name change for this illness to **systemic exertion intolerance disease (SEID)**. The recommendation sparked a divisive debate between *ME* and *CFS* stakeholders. Similar to the shift from the name "*myalgic encephalomyelitis*" to "*chronic fatigue syndrome*," many patients felt that the name *SEID* trivialized their experiences by focusing on a singular symptom (exertion intolerance) to characterize their overall experience (Jason, Sunnquist, Brown, McManimen, & Furst, 2015). Supported by patient opinion research (Jason, Taylor, Stepanek, & Plioplys, 2001; Jason, Nicolson, & Sunnquist 2016), many patients have stressed the desire to have a more medically driven name, such as "*myalgic encephalomyelitis*." While hybrid names (e.g., *ME/CFS*) have garnered support and exposure, developing a new name without feedback from and contact with key constituents will likely engender mixed reactions (Jason, Sunnquist, Brown, McManimen, & Furst, 2015). Moving forward with issues like the *case definition* and naming convention, more input is needed from the patient community on these types of critical decisions that affect the *ME* and *CFS* field.

It might be useful to consider a shift away from strictly consensus-based *case definitions* to a more empirically driven approach in establishing a *case definition* for *ME* and *CFS* (Jason, 2015). Recently, representatives from the federal government, including the CDC and NIH, as well as scientists and patient groups, have focused their efforts on the development of common data elements, which involves developing consensus on what instruments to use for assessing patients (CFSAC, 2015). As an example, one such instrument is the DePaul Symptom Questionnaire, which assesses *ME* and *CFS* symptoms and severity (Jason & Sunnquist, 2018). Hopefully, future efforts will involve an international consensus regarding a research *case definition* using available evidence and collecting data to support evidence-based decisions (Jason, et al., 2018). In addition, there is a need to develop a consensus on other *critical case definition* criteria, for example, identifying what frequency and severity thresholds should be used to determine whether symptoms count toward meeting criteria and operationalizing critical terms within *case definitions*, such as a "substantial reduction" in functioning, "lifelong fatigue," "fatigue not substantially alleviated by rest," and "fatigue that is the result of excessive exertion" (Jason, et al., 2018, p. 55).

The controversy that emerged between patient groups and gatekeepers after the release of the IOM report regarding *ME* and *CFS* case definitions and the illness's name are only recent examples of this illness's complicated historical narrative. We believe that to change this narrative, participatory mechanisms that are vetted by stakeholders at all levels are necessary for ongoing data collection and interactive feedback (Jason, Sunnquist, Brown, McManimen, & Furst, 2015). As an exemplar, the International Encephalitis Consortium was a working group started in 2010 with the aim of advancing encephalitis research. During their meeting in 2012, they clearly outlined objectives to facilitate advancement in their field, which strongly paralleled the needs of the *ME* and *CFS* community: standardization of a *case definition* and development of diagnostic algorithms to support patient evaluation (Venkatesan, Tunkel, Bloch, Lauring, Sejvar, Bitnun, et al., 2013). This consortium represents a model for organization and mobilization that the *ME* and *CFS* field could replicate. Groups like the Chronic Fatigue Syndrome Advisory Committee and/or the International Association of *ME/CFS* could appoint similar working groups to tackle the *case definition* and name-change issues. These working groups could engage in a process of polling patients and scientists; collecting and summarizing data; sharing the results with large constituencies; and maintaining a process that is collaborative, open, interactive, and inclusive. Key gatekeepers, including patients, scientists, clinicians, and government officials, could work collaboratively and transparently to build a consensus for change, and most critically, to ensure that all parties are involved in decision-making processes (Jason, Sunnquist, Brown, McManimen, & Furst, 2015).

Conclusion

As important as it is to find a consensus on a *case definition*, equally critical is sensitizing the health care community to the unique needs of this vulnerable group and developing treatment centers for appropriate diagnosis and rehabilitation. Clinical centers of excellence would allow for the evaluation of pharmacological treatments, which could engender a paradigm shift away from psychogenic interventions. In such treatment rehabilitation settings, it might be possible to identify appropriate treatments for different subtypes of *ME* and *CFS* (Huber, Sunnquist, & Jason, 2018), as those with more severe symptoms or those with orthostatic and gastrointestinal manifestations of this illness might require specific tailored and focused treatment options.

The *ME* and *CFS* community has been vociferous in their advocacy efforts for increased funding for research, the creation of centers for clinical excellence, and the establishment of a research *case definition*. It is clear that policy makers are more likely to be receptive to these issues if patients act collectively and forcefully (Best, 2012), as occurred within the area of HIV/AIDS. Yet the patient community continues to remain divided regarding the most basic issues, such as what to call their illness, and this division complicates the formation of collective efforts of activism that are needed to accomplish many of the necessary goals of this patient movement.

References

Action for M.E. (2010). *Severely neglected: M.E. in the U.K.-membership survey.* Retrieved from www.actionforme.org.uk/Resources/Action%20for%20ME/Documents/get-informed/Severely%20Neglected%202001.pdf

Barnes, D. M. (1986). Mystery disease at Lake Tahoe challenges virologists and clinicians. *Science, 234*(4776), 541–542. doi:10.1126/science.3020689

Bassil, K. (2016, August 1). *Encyclopedia Britannica: Case definition.* Retrieved May 17, 2018, from www.britannica.com/science/case-definition

Best, R. K. (2012). Disease politics and medical research funding: Three ways advocacy shapes policy. *American Sociological Review, 77*(5), 780–803. https://doi.org/10.1177/0003122412458509

Black, C. D., O'Connor, P. J., & McCully, K. K. (2005). Increased daily physical activity and fatigue symptoms in chronic fatigue syndrome. *Dynamic Medicine, 4*(3). https://doi.org/10.1186/1476-5918-4-3

Blease, C., & Geraghty, K. J. (2018). Are ME/CFS patient organizations "militant"? *Journal of Bioethical Inquiry.* https://doi.org/10.1007/s11673-018-9866-5

Borsboom, D. (2017). A network theory of mental disorders. *World Psychiatry, 16*(1), 5–13. https://doi.org/10.1002/wps.20375

Broderick, G., Fuite, J., Kreitz, A., Vernon, S. D., Klimas, N., & Fletcher, M. A. (2010). A formal analysis of cytokine networks in chronic fatigue syndrome. *Brain, Behavior, and Immunity, 24*(7): 1209–1217. https://doi.org/10.1016/j.bbi.2010.04.012

Broderick, G., Katz, B. Z., Fernandes, H., Fletcher, M. A., Klimas, N., Smith, F. A., et al. (2012). Cytokine expression profiles of immune imbalance in post-mononucleosis chronic fatigue. *Journal of Translational Medicine, 10*(191). https://doi.org/10.1186/1479-5876-10-191

Brown, A. A., Jason, L. A., Evans, M. A., & Flores, S. (2013). Contrasting case definitions: The ME International Consensus Criteria vs. the Fukuda et al. CFS criteria. *North American Journal of Psychology, 15*(1), 103–120. Retrieved from www.ncbi.nlm.nih.gov/pmc/articles/PMC4215640/

Brurberg, K. G., Fonhus, M. S., Larun, L., Flottorp, S., & Malterud, K. (2014). Case definitions for Chronic Fatigue Syndrome/Myalgic Encephalomyelitis (CFS/ME): A systematic review. *BMJ Open, 4*(2). https://doi.org/10.1136/bmjopen-2013-003973

Camacho, J., & Jason, L. A. (1998). Psychosocial factors show little relationship to chronic fatigue syndrome recovery. *Journal of Psychology and the Behavioral Sciences, 12*, 60–70. Retrieved from https://view2.fdu.edu/academics/becton-college/psychology-and-counseling/jpbs/1998/

Carruthers, B. M., Jain, A. K., De Meirleir, K. L., Peterson, D. L., Klimas, N. G., Lerner, A. M., et al. (2003). Myalgic encephalomyelitis/chronic fatigue syndrome. *Journal of Chronic Fatigue Syndrome, 11*(1), 7–115. https://doi.org/10.1300/J092v11n01_02

Carruthers, B. M., van de Sande, M. I., De Meirleir, K. L., Klimas, N. G., Broderick, G., Mitchell, T., et al. (2011). Myalgic encephalomyelitis: International consensus criteria. *Journal of Internal Medicine, 270*(4), 327–338. https://doi.org/10.1111/j.1365-2796.2011.02428.x

Centers for Disease Control and Prevention. Principles of Epidemiology in Public Health Practice, Third Edition: An Introduction to Applied Epidemiology and Biostatistics. (2012, May 18). Retrieved May 17, 2018, from www.cdc.gov/ophss/csels/dsepd/ss1978/lesson1/section5.html

CFSAC Recommendations and agency responses. (2015, August 18–19). Revised responses added March 8, 2016. Retrieved from www.hhs.gov/ash/advisory-committees/cfsac/recommendations/2015-08-18/cfsac-recommendations-and-agency-responses/index.html

Chu, L., Norris, J. L., Valencia, I. J., & Montoya, J. G. (2017). Patients diagnosed with myalgic encephalomyelitis/chronic fatigue syndrome also fit systemic exertion intolerance disease criteria. *Fatigue, 5*(2), 114–128.

Cotler, J., Holtzman, C., Dudun, C., & Jason, L. (2018). A brief questionnaire to assess post-exertional malaise. *Diagnostics, 8*(3), 66. https://doi.org/10.3390/diagnostics8030066

Crowley, N., Nelson, M., & Stovin, S. (1957). Epidemiological aspects of an outbreak of encephalomyelitis at the Royal Free Hospital, London, in the summer of 1955. *Epidemiology & Infection, 55*(1), 102–122. https://doi.org/10.1017/s0022172400061295

Cuijpers, P., van Straten, A., & Warmerdam, L. (2007). Behavioral activation treatments of depression: A meta-analysis. *Clinical Psychology Review, 27*(3), 318–326. https://doi.org/10.1016/j.cpr.2006.11.001

Fischer, D. B., William, A. H., Strauss, A. C., Unger, E. R., Jason, L., Marshall, G. D., Jr., et al. (2014). Chronic fatigue syndrome: The current status and future potentials of emerging biomarkers. *Fatigue, 2*(2), 93–109. https://doi.org/10.1080/21641846.2014.906066

Friedberg, F., & Jason, L. A. (1998). *Understanding chronic fatigue syndrome: An empirical guide to assessment and treatment.* Washington, DC: American Psychological Association.

Fukuda, K., Straus, S. E., Hickie, I., Sharpe, M. C., Dobbins, J. G., & Komaroff, A. (1994). The chronic fatigue syndrome: A comprehensive approach to its definition and study: International chronic fatigue syndrome study group. *Annual Internal Medicine, 121*(12), 953–959. https://doi.org/10.7326/0003-4819-121-12-199412150-00009

Gaab, J., Rohleder, N., Heitz, V., Engert, V., Schad, T., Schürmeyer, T. H., et al. (2005). Stress-induced changes in LPS-induced pro-inflammatory cytokine production in chronic fatigue syndrome. *Psychoneuroendocrinology, 30*(2), 188–198. https://doi.org/10.1016/j.psyneuen.2004.06.008

Geraghty, K. (2016). "PACE-Gate": When clinical trial evidence meets open data access. *Journal of Health Psychology.* Retrieved from https://doi.org/10.1177/1359105316675213

Goudsmit, E. M. (1996). *The psychological aspects and management of chronic fatigue syndrome.* London: Brunel University. Retrieved from https://bura.brunel.ac.uk/bitstream/2438/4283/1/FulltextThesis.pdf

Goudsmit, E. M., & Howes, S. (2008). Pacing: A strategy to improve energy management in chronic fatigue syndrome. *Health Psychology Update, 17*(1), 46. https://doi.org/10.3109/09638288.2011.635746

Goudsmit, E. M., Jason, L. A., Nijs, J., & Wallman, K. E. (2012). Pacing as a strategy to improve energy management in myalgic encephalomyelitis/chronic fatigue syndrome: A consensus document. *Disability and Rehabilitation, 34*(13), 1140–1147. https://doi.org/10.3109/09638288.2011.635746

Green, J., Romei, J., & Natelson, B. J. (1999). Stigma and chronic fatigue syndrome. *Journal of Chronic Fatigue Syndrome, 5*, 63–75. https://doi.org/10.1300/J092v05n02_04

Hamblin, A. S. (1993). *Cytokines and cytokine receptors.* Oxford, England: IRL Pr.

Hawk, C., Jason, L. A., & Torres-Harding, S. (2006). Differential diagnosis of chronic fatigue syndrome and major depressive disorder. *International Journal of Behavioral Medicine, 13*(3), 244–251. https://doi.org/10.1207/s15327558ijbm1303_8

Hennekens, C. H., & Buring, J. E. (1987). *Epidemiology in medicine* (1st ed.). Boston: Little, Brown and Company.

Holmes, G. P., Kaplan, J. E., Gantz, N. M., Komaroff, A. L., Schonberger, L. B., Straus, S. E., et al. (1988). Chronic fatigue syndrome: A working case definition. *Ann Intern Med, 108*(3), 387–389. https://doi.org/10.7326/0003-4819-108-3-387

Huber, K. A., Sunnquist, M., & Jason, L. A. (2018). Latent class analysis of a heterogeneous international sample of patients with myalgic encephalomyelitis/chronic fatigue syndrome. *Fatigue: Biomedicine, Health & Behavior, 6*(3), 163–178. https://doi.org/10.1080/21641846.2018.1494530

IOM (Institute of Medicine). (2015). *Beyond myalgic encephalomyelitis/chronic fatigue syndrome: Redefining an illness.* Washington, DC: National Academies Press.

Jammes, Y., Steinberg, J. G., Mambrini, O., Bregeon, F., & Delliaux, S. (2005). Chronic fatigue syndrome: Assessment of increased oxidative stress and altered muscle excitability in response to incremental exercise. *Journal of Internal Medicine, 257*(3), 299–310. https://doi.org/10.1111/j.1365-2796.2005.01452.x

Jason, L. A. (2015, March 4). *IOM's effort to dislodge chronic fatigue syndrome.* Oxford, England: Oxford University Press Blog. Retrieved from http://oxford.ly/18LEEiQ

Jason, L. A., Benton, M., Johnson, A., & Valentine, L. (2008). The economic impact of ME/CFS: Individual and societal level costs. *Dynamic Medicine, 7*(6). https://doi.org/10.1186/1476-5918-7-6

Jason, L. A., Brown, M., Brown, A., Evans, M., Flores, S., Grant-Holler, E., et al. (2013). Energy conservation/envelope theory interventions to help patients with myalgic encephalomyelitis/chronic fatigue syndrome. *Fatigue, 1*(1–2), 27–42. https://doi.org/10.1080/21641846.2012.733602

Jason, L. A., Fox, P. A., & Gleason, K. D. (2018). The importance of a research case definition. *Fatigue: Biomedicine, Health & Behavior, 6*(1), 52–58. https://doi.org/10.1080/21641846.2018.1389336

Jason, L. A., Holbert, C., Torres-Harding, S., & Taylor, R. R. (2004). Stigma and the tern chronic fatigue syndrome: Results of surveys on changing the name. *Journal of Disability Policy Studies, 14*(4), 222–228. https://doi.org/10.1177/10442073040140040401

Jason, L. A., Melrose, H., Lerman, A., Burroughs, V., Lewis, K., King, C. P., et al. (1999b). Managing chronic fatigue syndrome: Overview and case study. *AAOHN Journal*, *47*(1), 17–21. https://doi.org/10.1177/216507999904700104

Jason, L. A., Nicolson, L., & Sunnquist, M. (2016). Patient perceptions regarding possible changes to the name and criteria for chronic fatigue syndrome and myalgic encephalomyelitis. *Journal of Family Medicine and Community Health*, *3*(4), 1090. Retrieved from https://pdfs.semanticscholar.org/ccfb/c70dd5743168048afa410beef526e198af38.pdf

Jason, L. A., Porter, N., Hunnell, J., Brown, A., Rademaker, A., & Richman, J. A. (2011). A natural history study of chronic fatigue syndrome. *Rehabilitation Psychology*, *56*(1), 32–42. https://doi.org/10.1037/a0022595

Jason, L. A., Richman, J. A., Rademaker, A. W., Jordan, K. M., Plioplys, A. V., Taylor, R. R., et al. (1999a). A community-based study of chronic fatigue syndrome. *Archives of Internal Medicine*, *159*, 2129–2137. https://doi.org/10.1001/archinte.159.18.2129

Jason, L. A., Roesner, N., Porter, N., Parenti, B., Mortensen, J., & Till, L. (2010). Provision of social support to individuals with chronic fatigue syndrome. *Journal of Clinical Psychology*, *66*(3), 249–258. https://doi.org/10.1002/jclp.20648

Jason, L. A., & Sunnquist, M. (2018). The development of the DePaul Symptom Questionnaire: Original, expanded, brief and pediatric versions. *Frontiers in Pediatrics*, *6*, 330. https://doi.org/10.3389/fped.2018.00330

Jason, L. A., Sunnquist, M., Brown, A., McManimen, S., & Furst, J. (2015). Reflections on the Institute of Medicine's systemic exertion intolerance disease. *Polskie Archiwum Medycyny Wewnetrznej*, *125*(7–8), 576–581. https://doi.org/10.20452/pamw.2973

Jason, L. A., Sunnquist, M., Gleason, K., & Fox, P. (2017). Mistaken conclusion that Systemic Exercise Intolerance Disease is comparable to research case definitions: A rebuttal to Chu et al. *Fatigue: Biomedicine, Health & Behavior*, *5*, 231–238. https://doi.org/10.1080/21641846.2017.1362780

Jason, L. A., Taylor, R. R., Plioplys, S., Stepanek, Z., & Shlaes, J. (2002). Evaluating attributions for an illness based upon the name: Chronic fatigue syndrome, myalgic encephalopathy and Florence Nightingale disease. *American Journal of Community Psychology*, *30*(1), 133–148. https://doi.org/10.1023/A:1014328319297

Jason, L. A., Taylor, R. R., Stepanek, Z., & Plioplys, S. (2001). Attitudes regarding chronic fatigue syndrome: The importance of a name. *Journal of Health Psychology*, *6*(1), 61–71. https://doi.org/10.1177/135910530100600105

Jason, L. A., Torres-Harding, S. R., Jurgens, A., & Helgerson, J. (2004). Comparing the Fukuda et al. criteria and the Canadian case definition for chronic fatigue syndrome. *Journal of Chronic Fatigue Syndrome*, *12*(1), 37–52. https://doi.org/10.1300/J092v12n01_03

Jason, L. A., Zinn, M. L., & Zinn, M. A. (2015). Myalgic encephalomyelitis: Symptoms and biomarkers. *Current Neuropharmacology*, *13*(5), 701–734. https://doi.org/10.2174/1570159x13666150928105725

Johnston, S. C., Brenu, E. W., Hardcastle, S. L., Huth, T. K., Staines, D. R., & Marshall-Gradisnik, S. M. (2014). A comparison of health status in patients meeting alternative definitions for Chronic Fatigue Syndrome/Myalgic Encephalomyelitis. *Health and Quality of Life Outcomes*, *12*, 64. https://doi.org/10.1186/1477-7525-12-64

Johnston, S. C., Brenu, E. W., Staines, D. R., & Marshall-Gradisnik, S. (2013). The adoption of Chronic Fatigue Syndrome/Myalgic Encephalomyelitis case definitions to assess prevalence: A systematic review. *Annals of Epidemiology*, *23*(6), 371–376. https://doi.org/10.1016/j.annepidem.2013.04.003

King, C. P., Jason, L. A., Frankenberry, E. L., Jordan, K. M., & Tryon, W. (1997). Think inside the envelope. *CFIDS Chronicle, Fall*, 10–14.

Koike, S., Yamaguchi, S., Ojio, Y., Shimada, T., Watanabe, K., & Ando, S. (2015). Long-term effect of a name change for schizophrenia on reducing stigma. *Social Psychiatry and Psychiatric Epidemiology*, *50*(10), 1519–1526. https://doi.org/10.1007/s00127-015-1064-8

Linder, R., Dinser, R., Wagner, M., Krueger, G. R., & Hoffmann, A. (2002). Generation of classification criteria for chronic fatigue syndrome using an artificial neural network and traditional criteria set. *In Vivo*, *16*(1), 37–43.

Maher, K., Klimas, N. G., & Fletcher, M. A. (2003). Immunology. In L. A. Jason, P. A. Fennell, & R. R. Taylor (Eds.), *Handbook of chronic fatigue syndrome* (pp. 124–151). Hoboken: John Wiley & Sons.

McManimen, S. L., Devendorf, A. R., Brown, A. A., Moore, B. C., Moore, J. H., & Jason, L. A. (2016). Mortality in patients with Myalgic Encephalomyelitis and Chronic Fatigue Syndrome. *Fatigue: Biomedicine, Health & Behavior*, *4*(8), 195–207. https://doi.org/10.1080/21641846.2016.1236588

McManimen, S. L., Stoothoff, J., McClellan, D., & Jason, L. A. (2018). Effects of unsupportive social interactions, stigma, and symptoms on patients with Myalgic Encephalomyelitis and Chronic Fatigue Syndrome. *Journal of Community Psychology*, *46*(8), 959–971. https://doi.org/10.1002/jcop.21984

Meals, R. W., Hauser, V. F., & Bower, A. G. (1935). Poliomyelitis: The Los Angeles epidemic of 1934: Part I. *California and Western Medicine*, *43*(2), 123–125. Retrieved from www.ncbi.nlm.nih.gov/pmc/articles/PMC1753530/pdf/calwestmed 00402-0020.pdf

M.E. Association. (2010). *M.E. association*. Retrieved from www.meassociation.org.uk/

Natelson, B. H., Tseng, C.-L., & Ottenweller, J. E. (2005). Spinal fluid abnormalities in patients with chronic fatigue syndrome. *Clinical and Diagnostic Laboratory Immunology, 12*, 53–55. https://doi.org/10.1128/CDLI.12.1.52-55.2005

National Institutes of Health. (2017). *NIH announces centers for myalgic encephalomyelitis/chronic fatigue syndrome research*. Retrieved from www.nih.gov/news-events/news-releases/nih-announces-centers-myalgic-encephalomyelitis-chronic-fatigue-syndrome-research

Paulsen, Ø., Laird, B., Aass, N., Lea, T., Fayers, P., Kaasa, S., et al. (2017). The relationship between pro-inflammatory cytokines and pain, appetite and fatigue in patients with advanced cancer. *PloS One, 12*(5). https://doi.org/10.1371/journal.pone.0177620

Peterson, M. T., Peterson, T. W., Emerson, S., Regalbuto, E., Evans, M. A., & Jason, L. A. (2013). Coverage of CFS within U.S. medical schools. *Universal Journal of Public Health, 1*(4), 177–179. doi:10.13189/ujph.2013.010404

Price, J. R., Mitchell, E., Tidy, E., & Hunot, V. (2008). Cognitive behaviour therapy for chronic fatigue syndrome in adults. *Cochrane Database of Systematic Review*, (3), Cd001027. https://doi.org//10.1002/14651858.CD001027.pub2

Ramsay, M. A. (1988). *Myalgic encephalomyelitis and postviral fatigue states: The saga of royal free disease* (2nd ed.). London: Gower.

Raudonis, B. M., Kelley, I. H., Rowe, N., & Ellis, J. (2017). A pilot study of proinflammatory cytokines and fatigue in women with breast cancer during chemotherapy. *Cancer Nursing, 40*(4), 323–331. https://doi.org/10.1097/ncc.0000000000000406

Reeves, W. C., Jones, J. F., Maloney, E., Heim, C., Hoaglin, D. C., Boneva, R. S., et al. (2007). Prevalence of chronic fatigue syndrome in metropolitan, urban, and rural Georgia. *Population Health Metrics, 5*(5). https://doi.org/10.1186/1478-7954-5-5

Reyes, M., Gary, H. E., Jr., Dobbins, J. G., Randall, B., Steele, L., Fukuda, K., et al. (1997, February 21). Descriptive epidemiology of chronic fatigue syndrome: CDC surveillance in four cities. *Morbidity and Mortality Weekly Report Surveillance Summaries, 46*(No. SS-2), 1-13.

Reyes, M., Nisenbaum, R., Hoaglin, D. C., Unger, E. R., Emmons, C., Randall, B., et al. (2003). Prevalence and incidence of chronic fatigue syndrome in Wichita, Kansas. *Arch Intern Med, 163*(13), 1530–1536. https://doi.org/10.1001/archinte.163.13.1530

Sunnquist, M., & Jason, L. A. (2018). A reexamination of the cognitive behavioral model of chronic fatigue syndrome. *Journal of Clinical Psychology, 74*(7), 1234–1245. https://doi.org/10.1002/jclp.22593

Sunnquist, M., Nicolson, L., Jason, L., & Friedman, K. J. (2017). Access to medical care for individuals with myalgic encephalomyelitis and chronic fatigue syndrome: A call for centers of excellence. *Modern Clinical Medicine Research, 1*(1), 28–35. https://doi.org/10.22606/mcmr.2017.11005

Szklo, M., & Nieto, F. J. (2007). *Epidemiology: Beyond the basics* (K. G. McNeill, 2nd ed.). Sudbury, MA: Jones and Bartlett Publishers.

Taylor, R. R., Jason, L. A., Shiraishi, Y., Schoeny, M. E., & Keller, J. (2006). Conservation of resources theory, perceived stress, and chronic fatigue syndrome: Outcomes of a consumer-driven rehabilitation program. *Rehabilitation Psychology, 51*, 157–165. https://doi.org/10.1037/0090-5550.51.2.157

Ter Wolbeek, M. T., Doornen, L. J., Kavelaars, A., Putte, E. M., Schedlowski, M., & Heijnen, C. J. (2007). Longitudinal analysis of pro- and anti-inflammatory cytokine production in severely fatigued adolescents. *Brain, Behavior, and Immunity, 21*(8), 1063–1074. https://doi.org/10.1016/j.bbi.2007.04.007

Tidmore, T., Jason, L. A., Chapo-Kroger, L., So, S., Brown, A., & Silverman, M. (2015). Lack of knowledgeable healthcare access for patients with neuro-endocrine-immune diseases. *Frontiers in Clinical Medicine, 2*(2), 46–54. Retrieved from www.researchgate.net/profile/Leonard_Jason/publication/269096352_Lack_of_knowledgeable_healthcare_access_for_patients_with_neuro-endocrine-immune_diseases/links/547f700080cf2ccc7f8b92142/lack-of-knowledgeable-healthcare-access-for-patients-with-neuro-endocrine-immune-diseases.pdf

Tripp, N. H., Tarn, J., Natasari, A., Gillespie, C., Mitchell, S., Hackett, K. L., et al. (2016). Fatigue in primary Sjögren's syndrome is associated with lower levels of proinflammatory cytokines. *RMD Open, 2*(2). https://doi.org/10.1136/rmdopen-2016-000282

Twisk, F. N. M. (2015). Commentary on Jason et al. (2015): Towards separate empirical case definitions of myalgic encephalomyelitis and chronic fatigue syndrome. *Health Psychology and Behavioral Medicine, 3*(1). https://doi.org/10.1080/21642850.2015.1027705

Twisk, F. N. M. (2018). Myalgic encephalomyelitis, chronic fatigue syndrome, and systemic exertion intolerance disease: Three distinct clinical entities. *Challenges, 9*(1), 19. https://doi.org/10.3390/challe9010019

Venkatesan, A., Tunkel, A. R., Bloch, K. C., Lauring, A. S., Sejvar, J., Bitnun, A., et al. (2013). Case definitions, diagnostic algorithms, and priorities in encephalitis: Consensus statement of the international encephalitis consortium. *Clinical Infectious Diseases, 57*(8), 1114–1128. https://doi.org/10.1093/cid/cit458

Vercoulen, J. H., Swanink, C. M., Galama, J. M., Fennis, J. F., Jongen, P. J., Hommes, O. R., et al. (1998). The persistence of fatigue in chronic fatigue syndrome and multiple sclerosis: Development of a model. *Journal of Psychosomatic Research*, *45*(6), 507–517. https://doi.org/10.1016/S0022-3999(98)00023-3

Wallman, K. E., Morton, A. R., Goodman, C., Grove, R., & Guilfoyle, A. M. (2004). Randomised controlled trial of graded exercise in chronic fatigue syndrome. *Medical Journal of Australia*, *180*, 444–448. https://doi.org/10.5694/j.1326-5377.2004.tb06019.x

Wessely, S. (1994). The history of chronic fatigue syndrome. In S. E. Straus (Ed.), *Chronic fatigue syndrome* (pp. 2–44). Boca Raton, FL: CRC Press (1887).

White, P. D., Goldsmith, K. A., Johnson, A. L., Potts, L., Walwyn, R., DeCesare, J. C., et al. (2011). Comparison of adaptive pacing therapy, cognitive behaviour therapy, graded exercise therapy, and specialist medical care for chronic fatigue syndrome (PACE): A randomised trial. *Lancet*, *377*(9768), 823–836. https://doi.org/10.1016/s0140-6736(11)60096-2

Wilshire, C., Kindlon, T., Courtney, R., Matthees, A., Tuller, D., Geraghty, K., et al. (2018). Rethinking the treatment of chronic fatigue syndrome: A reanalysis and evaluation of findings from a recent major trial of graded exercise and CBT. *BMC Psychology*, *6*(1), 6. https://doi.org/10.1186/s40359-018-0218-3

18

GENDER AND AGING RESEARCH METHODS

Sabihah Moola and Christo P. Cilliers

Overview

This chapter on gender and aging offers a gendered perspective of the aging of the population, a factor of interest to many health psychologists. This is related to health psychology, explaining how the population is expected to age from the perspectives of both males and females. Women tend to live longer than men and are usually the caregivers of the family (Arber, 1991; HelpAge International, 2002). Women and men differ with regard to their physical, psychological, emotional, and social aging processes (HelpAge International, 2002). However, for both genders, from a social perspective, it seems that society forgets the aged. Vulnerability exists socially in both genders as they age, since women are more likely to become widows or divorcees, while some men who age can no longer work and support their families. This has a negative effect on both genders (HelpAge International, 2002).

Culture has stereotyped women to play different roles, such as "family roles," "care-givers," and "career-quitters," among other labels, as they age in relation to men (Arber, 1991). From a cultural perspective, women experience changes as they age; however, aging research should not only focus on the negative features of aging. The notion of "social gerontology" emerges where women experience different reactions to aging. Some become socially empowered by partaking in activities such as prayer groups, dancing, or physical activity to empower themselves (Wray, 2003). In these activities, women can socially engage and become self-developed. With a healthy body and mind, women are able to maintain relationships and practice their religious beliefs more easily (Wray, 2003). In comparison to women, men tend to feel socially cut off from society after retirement, as they are less engaged with work, a core aspect of masculinity. They can experience an identity crisis as they feel functionless within the notion of aging (Russell, 2007).

Trends in gender and aging research, as will be discussed in this chapter, include active aging in terms of physical and mental health, gender differences in relation to how men and women age or accept aging as a process, and the different roles that men and women are categorized into as they age. Productivity in terms of age and retirement can give rise to economic issues. The aspect of quality of individual life and family life as one ages changes as well. The concern of physical health and well-being, including the cost of healthcare as well as cultural groundings that contribute to aging in different genders, similarly are affected (Andrews, Sidorenko, Gutman, Gray, Anisimov, Bezrukov, et al., 2006).

This chapter approaches the topic of gender and aging in the following manner: the different methodologies are listed, and research conducted using these methods are explained and applied to gender research from a psychological healthcare perspective, where applicable. Thereafter, the strengths and weakness of the methodologies are outlined, and finally, highlights for best practices for emerging scholars are explained.

Research in Practice

Case Study 1: Qualitative Research Design

Qualitative research is a method used to collect data and analyze situations on an in-depth level (du Plooy, 2009). This approach works well with research on gender and aging in health psychology, as it caters to the individual's perspective or opinion. Either gender has an opportunity to voice their personal opinion whether in interviews, focus groups, or observational analysis. Bryman (2012) confirms also that because qualitative research does not rely on numbers per se, it can focus on the actual details. Qualitative research aims to analyze the social context of a situation. Therefore, this methodology is appropriate in helping to unpack different perspectives.

Triangulation is a process whereby different data collection methods are used to collect data in qualitative studies in order to verify the data collected (du Plooy, 2009). With the aged, interviews as well as focus groups can obtain personal data from these participants in a one-on-one format. A general example here is if one is conducting research with aged males and females, their actual voice can be obtained by individually interviewing each participant of the selected sample. Then, a focus group can follow up in order to understand common beliefs of the audience, here meaning older persons. Last, these formats can be followed by observations at a care center for the aged to watch for and observe the factors introduced in the previous methods in order to triangulate findings and ensure credibility is obtained with a qualitative research design.

Bryman (2012) claims that inductively, there is a relationship between theory and research whereby the relationship is generated from the theory. When one follows an *epistemological* (interpretivistic) *approach*, the focus is on understanding the social world through an investigation of that world by its participants. If one considers an *ontological* (constructionist) *approach*, the focus is on interactions between individuals and not on the "out there phenomena" in social dimensions. Through the process of *triangulation*, both these approaches can be used in order to verify data.

Qualitative research as a strategy means that researchers have the ability to say interesting and important things about the social world around us and engage with the evidence to support the rationale (Gilbert & Stoneman, 2016). Qualitative research findings are communicated through narratives, such as research reports that deliver representations of the social world. The process of reflexivity allows the researcher to engage with the entire research process and therefore be able to validate and authenticate the findings.

Methodology, Instruments, Outcomes, and Results of the Qualitative Studies

In different countries, a variety of research has been executed qualitatively with the aged in relation to health psychology. From a health perspective, Venn and Arber (2012) assert that older people believe that as they age, their sleep patterns are affected negatively. A qualitative study was conducted using 62 in-depth interviews with older men and women who lived in their own homes in England. The study aimed to research sleeping medication and the decisions taken by the aged in relation to not consuming pills to sleep better. The study pointed out that research was lacking related to older people who try to cope by themselves, as opposed to seeking professional or medical assistance to sleep better. This entire research project formed part of a larger study where in this phase (phase 2) semi-structured interviews were used to understand "the meanings and experiences of poor sleep for older people living in their own homes and the strategies they used to improve their sleep" (Venn

& Arber, 2012, p. 1217). A qualitative approach was selected in order to gain an understanding into the significance of sleep or the lack thereof in the lives of the aged. The results from this study indicated that older people did not view poor sleep as a health issue, but rather as a process of normality in aging. The participants also claimed that they did not consume sleeping pills, as they felt they were addictive and feared that they might lose control. Control was a core aspect in this study, since older people felt that they could go about their daily lives and function in society even with a lack of sleep. Consuming sleeping pills, they felt, could make them lose control of their lives. The aspect of vulnerability and dependability is rife in aged men and women (Andrews, et al., 2006). Out of the sample of 62 senior men and women only nine were using sleeping pills, yet all of the participants experienced sleeping problems. However, they believed, psychologically, that lack of sleep comes with age (Venn & Arber, 2012).

Knodel and Ofstedal (2003) emphasize that in the developing world, due to life circumstances and socioeconomic situations, among other factors, women live longer than men and generally age as widows, making them economically vulnerable. However, they point out that "older women are universally more vulnerable to social, economic, and health disadvantages than older men" (Knodel & Ofstedal, 2003, p. 677). Some women give up their careers to raise their children, and as they age, they are affected psychologically and financially by this sacrifice. On the other hand, many men are financial caretakers of their families, and as they age and retire, they are affected by a lack of ability to be financially independent.

Jankowski, Diedrichs, Williamson, Harcourt, and Christopher (2016) emphasize that aging affects both men and women differently from the perspective of body image. This study notes that sociocultural pressures can affect body changes in older people. In a United Kingdom (UK) study with a sample of British and South Asian older adults (65 to 92 years of age), six focus groups were conducted between March and June 2012 to explore how body image and aging affect individuals in a culturally diverse setting. The focus groups were conducted as follows: nine support organizations for the aged from the southwest of England were approached to obtain permission for research to be conducted on body image, aging, and society. Only three organizations granted permission, enabling one of the researchers to be able to attend the session meeting and recruit participants for this study. The focus groups consisted of "4–6 participants, with four single-sex groups (two groups of males, two groups of females) and two mixed-sex groups" (Jankowski, et al., 2016, p. 552).

As people age, their physical appearance changes and health often deteriorates. This can negatively affect a person's psychological state of mind. Results from this study indicated that older people felt that the effects of aging on physical ability were more distressing than such effects on appearance, since lack of mobility leads to loss of identity, self-sufficiency, and independence (Jankowski, et al. 2016). However, participants here were of the opinion that physical beauty was more of a concern for women compared to men. It needs to be noted that the study alerts us to the fact that preoccupations about body image can also lead to health concerns and affect one's psychological mind-set, since people can engage in eating disorders or become depressed. Social pressures also work against the aged, since many sociocultural practices dictate that the ideals of image and beauty reside in the young (Jankowski, et al., 2016).

Russell (2007) emphasizes an interesting point on qualitative research, which is that it allows the aged to speak or have a voice of their own, rather than adhere to generalizations or stereotypes from statistics. Older people can experience an identity crisis because they are segregated from social life. Psychologically they can be affected by compulsory retirement, and the loss of work can affect negatively on both genders. Older people tend to become emotionally attached to spaces, especially workspaces. Medically, men receive far less attention, becoming almost "invisible," since overall their lifespan is shorter when compared to women (Russell, 2007).

A qualitative research framework caters to an in-depth, personal account of gender and aging from a psychological health perspective (Russell, 2007). The fieldwork method of data collection enables research to be conducted in a naturalistic, real-world setting where data can be induced and themes or patterns can be developed from original sources (Patton, 2005).

A weakness is that sample sizes in qualitative research designs are much smaller than quantitative research designs, and therefore findings cannot be generalized. However, the counter argument to this weakness is that with qualitative research designs, an in-depth analysis is conducted with a smaller sample to better understand phenomena (Kumar, 2011).

Highlights for Best Practices for Current and Emerging Scholars

One of the best research practices is to immerse oneself in the research setting, using different qualitative research methods to "unpack" stories from the aged. This allows the individual's personal experience of aging to come to the front. Perhaps a salient best practice is the use of triangulation (where the researcher makes use of different data sources) to ensure reliability and validity during the fieldwork process (Frankel & Devers, 2000).

Case Study 2: Intervention Research

Examples in ***intervention research*** include social and emotional behavior that can be assessed or explained in order to solve a problem (Bryman, 2012; du Plooy, 2009). Such processes can occur within both qualitative and quantitative research designs. An ***intervention behavior*** needs to be identified, which can help solve the problem within its context (examples include social, environment, political, and/or religious; du Plooy, 2009).

Methodology, Instruments, Outcomes, and Results of Intervention Studies

Intervention studies were conducted in relation to social isolation that occurs in the aged due to various social aspects that lead older people to become lonely. A study conducted by Bartlett, Warburton, Lui, Peach, and Carroll (2013) researched social isolation in older people in Queensland, Australia. Three pilot projects were conducted at different social settings in Queensland to evaluate the risk of isolation in older people. This research formed part of the cross-government projects to reduce social isolation in Queensland (CGPRSIOP). Validated psychological measures were used to evaluate the effect of the interventions. The methodology adhered to using pre- and post-test surveys, as well as social isolation scales, which were used to evaluate programs. The research was conducted in five locations. At each site researchers employed a community development approach, designing and implementing group activities that doubled as services and that allowed social networks to evolve from the programs designed. The results indicated that programs were beneficial for reducing loneliness and promoting social support in the aged. The study provided "new insights into evaluating interventions for reducing social isolation" (Bartlett, et al., 2013, p. 1167). Interventions were put in place to try to overcome loneliness in older people; however, the measurement of these were challenging due to methodological and practical issues. The study concluded that more research is required in this field (Bartlett, et al., 2013).

Intervention studies are usually longitudinal in nature and therefore can assist in solving problems over longer periods of time or during different interventions. In relation to health psychology and the aged, long-term care, quality of life, and nutrition in older people can be assessed more reliably, However, *intervention studies* that have methodological limitations, such as small samples and lack of sufficient time between the intervention and the actual research, can affect the results (Bartlett, et al., 2013).

Highlights for Best Practices for Current and Emerging Scholars

This research methodology can be adapted to either a qualitative or quantitative research design as it aims to solve problems. It therefore lends itself for use to examine different research questions in the context of gender and aging.

Case Study 3: Ecological Momentary Assessment

Shiffman, Stone, and Hufford (2008) postulate that **ecological momentary assessment (EMA)** as a research methodology aims to study "a very wide range of behaviors, experiences, and conditions" (p. 5). Thus, this is not a single research method, but a combination of different data collection methods. *EMA* works well with individual-based health and psychological research, since individual experiences can be measured over time (i.e., between the different stages of assessments from start to relapse; Shiffman, et al., 2008).

When linked to gender and aging, *EMA* can be considered appropriate, since the process or stages of aging can be studied at different moments, and the gradual process of either aging positively or negatively can be explored from a psychological perspective. Lastly, *EMA* aims "to address questions about individual differences, about particular episodes or situations, about unfolding of processes over time, and about the interactions among these factors" (Shiffman, et al., 2008, p. 3).

Methodology, Instruments, Outcomes, and Results of the EMA Studies

EMA can be used to study behavioral changes regarding mood disorders and depression, among other psychological illnesses (aan het Rot, Hogenelst, & Schoevers, 2012). Dunton, Atienza, Castro, and King (2009) used *EMA* to study how "cognitive, social, affective, contextual and physiological" aspects influence elderly people's physical activity (p. 249). Study participants recorded in real time their level of physical activity using electronic diaries. Reminders were set on electronic handheld devices, which were used as diaries, to alert the elderly to make recordings over a two-week period, four times a day. The reminders were set as prompts (morning, midday, afternoon, and evening) in order to alert them to record the activity timely. An auditory signal reminded them to key in the information; however, if they did not respond a second signal was sent as a further reminder. A 45-minute period was provided to complete each assessment, after which the time lapsed until the next scheduled assessment. The study included 23 adults, aged between 50 and 76 years, with 70% of the sample being female. Aspects such as "self-efficacy, positive and negative effect, control, demand, fatigue, energy, social interactions and stressful events were assessed during each sequence" (Dunton, et al., 2009, p. 249). The outcomes of the study indicated that "greater self-efficacy and control predicted greater moderate-to-vigorous physical activity" between each assessment of physical activity between the prompts (p. 249). Enhanced social interaction also contributed positively to physical activity overall in the sample.

Smyth and Stone (2003) claim that behavioral research can be appropriately monitored or assessed using *EMA* methodology, since it caters to "psychological, behavioral, and physiological processes in the natural environment" (p. 35). Unpacked, this means that *momentary* data is collected in real time in a natural setting, whereas physiological and psychological data is collected and evaluated in stages or with follow-up research.

EMA gathers data in real time from personal experiences. Specific behavioral and contextual experiences are collected from individuals as they occur in the real-world context (Cain, Depp, & Jeste, 2009). In research on gender and aging, behavioral characteristics can be analyzed from the actual experience in a given context. Shiffman, et al. (2008) note that the strengths of this methodology occur because data is collected in the moment, from the real world, with a possibility of repeat assessments to analyze behavioral changes.

One could argue a possible weakness is that reactivity can occur when a person's behavior is being monitored or assessed by himself or herself, since a person can alter his or her behavior when assessing it alone. Another point to note is that compliance with diary recording, for example, can tire the individual, or they can forget and then later, when they do a recording, bias can occur in the information being captured (Shiffman, et al., 2008).

Highlights for Best Practices for Current and Emerging Scholars

With this methodology, data collected in real-life contexts, from actual people, allows for a variety of data collection methods to be used. Behavioral research can be tracked and individualized accordingly.

Case Study 4: Participatory Research

Participatory research is a social approach in the right direction, rather than using it as a discipline or methodology. Several terms are used interchangeably to refer to participatory social research, but the foci are different. Some of these are *participant research, participatory research, action research, partnership research, practitioner research, emancipatory research*, and *collaborative research* (Gilbert & Stoneman, 2016). Therefore, in considering the mentioned terms, it is vital to focus on the extent to which action, participation, or both action and participation are used.

Participatory research is also involved in psychology social/health research and contributes to an acknowledgement of a reaction against traditional forms of research. Traditionally, the researcher was seen as the expert bringing his or her knowledge to the research setting, while those being researched played a passive role, not being involved once the initial research contact happened. In contrast, participatory forms of research see the active involvement of participants in the research process as crucial and valuable. Conducting research is not only *for* but also *by* the participants; it is an acknowledgement of and reaction against the inequality of power between the researcher and participants. Lastly, it is a way of recognizing that theory and practice in research are both important (Gilbert & Stoneman, 2016).

Methodology, Instruments, Outcomes, and Results of Participatory Research Studies

Statistics South Africa (StatsSA) defines the General Household Survey (GHS) as "an annual household survey which measures the living circumstances of South African households. The GHS collects data on education, health and social development, housing access to services and facilities, food security, and agriculture" (Statistics South Africa, 2012, datalog.worldbank.org.)

Makiwane, Ndinda, and Botsis (2012) explore the intersection between gender, race, and aging in South Africa using the GHS data (2010), conducted annually (since 2002) by StatsSA. The main goal of the study was to analyze the position of the elderly, with a specific focus on women, observing sex ratios, education, marriage, and employment (income) indicators in South Africa.

In South Africa, there are nine provinces. The GHS research uses a multistage stratified sample to proportionally represent the nine different provinces where citizens of South Africa reside. The sample selected is proportional to the citizen population. This means stratifying the population by provinces and selecting a systematic sample from the nine strata (Bryman, 2012). In the GHS (2010), a representative sample of 25,653 households were interviewed, using a multistage stratified sample by provinces.

Makiwane, Ndinda, and Botsis (2012) claim that between 2000 and 2030 the number of persons older than 60 will double because of a noticeable drop in fertility. For Africans, this means that a larger ratio of women are reaching old age as compared to men. The latter means that young men who have a better chance of employment and education are generally heading smaller households, while less educated older women (the majority outside employment) head larger households.

Research has shown that often the elderly—as the major caregivers—supply the main sources of income for a variety of generations in one household by using their social grants (these refer to pensions paid on a monthly basis by the state to senior citizens over the age of 60 years) to maintain the whole household. Furthermore, the results showed that when it came to aged females, six out of ten women in South Africa lived longer than men and therefore bore a larger dependency and care burden in the households they headed (Makiwane, et al., 2012).

White men and White women have higher percentages of employment and are earning a larger income in their old age, as compared to other races in South Africa, due to the injustices of the apartheid political system. The higher skill and income levels amongst Whites comes from the apartheid era in South Africa, where Whites were privileged in all aspects and Blacks/African (including Indians and Colored) were disadvantaged. These data reflect social discrimination mostly in educational attainment and marriage rates. Additionally, the income-earning levels of African women are worse than any other elderly group (Makiwane, et al., 2012).

In contrast to African research related to gender and aging, in the UK a study explored how older women used visuals to express their process of aging, as will be discussed next.

Research by Hogan and Warren (2012) consisted of four projects with women 65 years and older in Britain (UK) using visuals (pictures/images) to empower women to express their experiences of aging and to produce different images of aging. For this study, a team of researchers from diverse disciplines, all interested in gender and aging, came together for the Representing Self-Representing Aging initiative. Aging is significant to older women because their understanding of aging and ageism is intensely deep-rooted in appearance. Age changes the way women feel about the aging process, and poverty during old age is one of the structural inequalities that needs emphasis. Groundbreaking innovative methods used by these researchers, with a variety of participatory methods, included photo diaries, phototherapy, film booths, and art elicitation.

The project was launched at a women's-only film screening session of Deirdre Fishel's *Still Doing It: The Intimate Lives of Women Over 65*. After the screening, the audience could talk to a camera in a private booth about their views on the representation of late-in-life sexuality. Two other groups were organized—one group was from a underprivileged area in Green Estate in Sheffield. The famous photographer, Laura Pannak, was assigned to this group, where individuals were photographed in a variety of settings—reinterpreting mundane scenes (Hogan & Warren, 2012).

A second group was recruited from an extra-care scheme in a sheltered housing project in Guildford Grange. A fine-art photographer, Monica Fernandez, was assigned to work with participants. At exhibitions, some of the visuals from Guilford Grange were uncomfortable to view and juxtapositions thereof were disturbing. Other visuals, however, captured liveliness and flamboyance in subjects with which viewers visiting the exhibition could identify. There were also opposing opinions—some viewers felt it lowered women as it was not age-suitable behavior. Audience feedback was captured at two of the three exhibition venues (Hogan & Warren, 2012).

The last group was Rosy Martin's six days of intense phototherapy workshops (42 hours of group work). Participants had to keep a photo dairy in which women study and reframe their own age and aging narratives. Women worked in pairs and took turns being client/performer and photographer. Using counseling techniques and gestalt psychotherapy, woman explored their journeys through photographed intervals (Hogan & Warren, 2012).

Interviews took place before and after the four corresponding groups. Playing a major role in this study is the key difference between participatory and conventional methodologies that lies in the power of the research process. "Participatory approaches are those that broadly recognize the 'particular expertise' of people within particular circumstances" (Hogan & Warren, 2012, p. 335). From a research viewpoint, the four separate projects produced diverse insights and brought issues for investigation to the fore. In a way, the use of visual images produced a parallel discourse to the written text. This can be seen as active co-research between researchers and participants. A disadvantage was that different members of the research team had different understandings of the term participatory.

As many countries in Africa are moving and working towards decolonial education, *participatory research* is probably one of the better research methods to use while working in intercultural health settings. The focus of decolonial research is mainly to separate and untie the production of knowledge from a primarily Eurocentric episteme by doing research with indigenous communities that foreground indigenous epistemologies and voices. Furthermore, it is moving away from what is seen as the perceived universality and superiority of Western knowledge and culture (Zavala, 2013). *Participatory research* is used in the fields of psychology, communication, and social/health research, and in this way contributes to an acknowledgement of and reaction against traditional forms of research. Such an example of ***decolonial participatory research*** is a way of contributing positively to aged research from the participants' perspective and reposition participants and the researcher in all aspects of the research activities (Datta, 2018). The strength of the stratified random sampling in the GHS ensured that the sample was distributed "in the same way as the population in terms of the stratifying criterion" (Bryman, 2012).

Highlights for Best Practices for Current and Emerging Scholars

Datta (2018) asserts that in Africa, it is essential that both the research and researcher require decolonization to enhance research in order to create a positive impact on ethical research and participants in the community. Therefore, research needs to include critical perspectives on environmental justice, anti-racist theory, practice, land-based education, and cross-cultural research methodology. In addition, research related to the health and well-being of the aged should focus on aspects of social justice and human rights from an indigenous, decolonial perspective (Datta, 2018).

Indigenous healthcare treatment options contribute to a process of decolonization and anti-colonial struggles, as it honors approaches of knowing the social reality of the other (Datta, 2018). Health research needs to consider herbal remedies that the aged can use to treat different illnesses. Cultural beliefs require the acknowledgement of herbal remedies for treatment and cure (Moola, 2015).

According to Rodriguez and Inturias (2018), modernity includes psychological harm for indigenous people, as it affects their cultural identity, self-respect, freedom of choice, and overall well-being. From an indigenous perspective, research related to the aged of both genders can harm their psychological state, since mental and physical harm is perpetuated on three levels, namely, power, knowledge, and the self.

Agboka (2014) claims "the way in which scientific research is implicated in the worst excesses of colonialism remain a powerfully remembered history for many of the world's colonized peoples" (p. 297). A variety of postmodern challenges arises when it comes to postcolonial methodologies and social justice perspectives: issues of ideology, power, social justice, and global tensions. Traditionally, the researcher was seen as the expert bringing his or her knowledge to the research setting, while those being researched play a passive role, not being involved once the initial research contact happened. Therefore, *participatory (action)* is a form of decolonial research that can help address emerging issues of social justice and knowledge investigation, especially when it comes to power (i.e., researcher–participant symmetry) relations in many postcolonial disenfranchised sites (Agboka, 2014).

The main advantage of *participatory research* is that it underscores the active involvement of participants in the research process as crucial and valuable. In African countries, the agenda of decolonization and social justice is important to "reveal the ways that colonialism continues to operate and to affect lives in new and innovative ways as well as to show the unmitigated damage implicated by past colonial practices" (Agboka, 2014, p. 298). Conducting research is not only for but also by the participants; it is an acknowledgement of and reaction against the inequality of power between the researcher and participants, and lastly it is a way of recognizing that theory and practice in research are both important (Gilbert & Stoneman, 2016).

Case Study 5: Cohort Studies

When one investigates the course of diseases, it is mainly to establish links between risk factors and health outcomes. In this context, an ideal method to use is cohort studies. **Cohort studies** is a category of longitudinal research designs. Some authors will also view this design as a form of a longitudinal study that samples a group of people who share a defining characteristic. Scholars such as Keyton (2011) and Bryman (2012) argue that *cohort studies* is a "little-used design" in social research, claiming that we use it mostly as an extension of survey research. Bryman (2012) asserts that we typically find this research in social science fields such as human geography, social policy, and sociology. In addition, Bryman (2012) distinguishes between *cohort* and **panel studies** falling within longitudinal designs, while Keyton (2011) also adds that **trend studies** is a series of longitudinal studies.

Trend studies measure the same items over a period of time, drawing different samples at each time, while the survey research questions stay the same. *Panel studies*, on the other hand, sample and recruit groups of people, and the same people answer the same questions over the selected time period. As *cohort studies* look at groups of people, research "can be forward-looking (prospective) or backward looking (retrospective;" MacGill, 2018, p. 1). The focus of this section is on *cohort studies*, and the most typical example of a *cohort study* is found in the work of Hamilton, Lane, Gaston, Patton, MacDonald, Simpson, et al. (2013), where 4,709 patients have a shared event in common, such as a patient satisfaction survey in total joint replacements over a four-year period (January 2006 to December 2010).

Methodology, Instruments, Outcomes, and Results of the Cohort Studies

In the study by Hamilton, et al. (2013), researchers investigated the factors that influence patient satisfaction with surgical services (2,462 hip and 2,247 total knee replacements).

The outcomes of the research was that three

> factors broadly determine the patient's overall satisfaction following lower limb joint arthroplasty; meeting preoperative expectations, achieving satisfactory pain relief, and a satisfactory hospital experience. Pain relief and expectations are managed by clinical teams; however, a fractured access to surgical services impacts on the patient's hospital experience which may reduce overall satisfaction. In the absence of complications, how we deliver healthcare may be of key importance along with the specifics of what we deliver, which has clear implications for units providing surgical services.
>
> *(Hamilton, et al., 2013, p. 1)*

They also explored the relationship between overall satisfaction, satisfaction with specific aspects of outcome, and measured clinical outcomes. Satisfaction (mostly used in marketing and communication) is a performance indicator for healthcare surgery in the UK, Europe (cancer), and the United States (cosmetic actions). Besides the effective surgical procedure, there were a variety of other aspects that influenced a patient's total satisfaction. These include if the procedure was explained beforehand, giving information at the admission and discharge of patients, and the speediness of responses by the ward (Hamilton, et al., 2013). Patients completed questionnaires before the operations (mostly to get information on population parameters). The research team recorded the patient's length of stay upon discharge.

Patients rated "their overall satisfaction with their operated hip or knee" after 12 months by selecting one of the four scales, namely, "very satisfied, satisfied, unsure or dissatisfied" (Hamilton, et al., 2013, p. 1). The main strength of this patient satisfaction study is that it benefits from a large prospective patient *cohort* at a single National Health Service (NHS) orthopedic center with multiple surgeons. Most patients report high satisfaction with joint arthroplasty, but the researchers report that they need to take care in the use of a typical instrument—as it can be prejudiced for measuring satisfaction. One can assume the generalizability of this study, but cannot confirm it (Hamilton, et al., 2013).

In another *cohort study*, Hasse, Ledergerber, Furrer, Battlegay, Hirschel, Cavassini, et al. (2011) argue that life expectancy among human immunodeficiency virus (HIV)–infected individuals has increased, while quality of life has improved with antiretroviral therapy (ART). Patterns of morbidity and mortality among HIV-infected individuals taking ART are changing as an effect of improved immune systems and better survival. The Swiss HIV Cohort Study (SHCS) explored the influence of aging on the epidemiology of non-AIDS diseases.

The forthcoming and observational SHCS started in 1998 with nonstop enrollment. The SHCS study regulated the frequency of clinical events where 8,844 (96%) of 8,848 participants added to 40,720 cohort visits, from January 2008 to December 2010. A reported 2,223 (26.4%) were aged 50 to 64 years, and 450 (5.3%) were aged 65 years and older. The average period of HIV infection was 15.4 years, while 23.2% had earlier clinical AIDS. The researchers observed 994 incidents of non-AIDS–related illnesses in the reference period: cases of bacterial pneumonia, myocardial infarctions, strokes, cases of diabetes mellitus, trauma-associated fractures, fractures without ample trauma, and non-AIDS malignancies. Multivariable threat ratios for stroke, myocardial infarction, diabetes mellitus, and bone fractures without adequate trauma, osteoporosis, and non-AIDS–defining malignances were elevated for persons aged 65 years and older (Hasse, et al., 2011).

Across groups, differences were probed, using Cox regression, adjusted for CD4-cell count, viral load, injection drug use, sex, years of HIV infection, and smoking (Hasse, et al., 2011). Results from Hasse, et al. (2011) show that comorbidity and "multimorbidity because of non-AIDS diseases, particularly diabetes mellitus, cardiovascular disease, non-AIDS-defining malignancies, and osteoporosis, become more important in care of HIV-infected persons and increase with older age" (p. 1132).

The strengths of *cohort studies* include that researchers are able to track attitudes and behavior over a long-term period, which results in data that is more authentic. This contributes to observing large groups of individuals and recording their exposure to certain risk factors. Finding exposure to these risk factors leads to discovering clues of the possible cause for diseases.

When it comes to weaknesses, the limitations of missing data loom large. Researchers cannot afterwards gather missing data (MacGill, 2018). Furthermore, *cohort studies* are not suited to finding clues about rare diseases, as it follows disclosed data and remains on the lookout for any evolving cases of diseases. The latter means that one can also not use *cohort studies* to identify a sudden outbreak of disease, for example, COVID-19. Lastly, *cohort studies* are expensive and take many years—at times even decades—to yield results.

Highlights for Best Practices for Current and Emerging Scholars

With *cohort research*, one is able to track different aspects over time. The studies are larger, with a longer-term focus, and in this way, more data can be obtained, which enables researchers to unpack a vast amount of information on large scales.

Case Study 6: Pragmatic Trials

Intervention trials in healthcare are often described as *pragmatic* or *explanatory*. *Explanatory trials* work with homogenous populations and aim to test whether an intervention works under optimal situations—striving for effectiveness by using carefully defined subjects in a research clinic to ensure treatment benefits under ideal conditions. The focus for this discussion moves now to *pragmatic trials*.

The term *pragmatic trial* is generally used for trials that asses the differences among treatment approaches involving superfluous factors (e.g., the effects of co-medication, nonadherence, and placebo effects) and aim to get the most out of generalizability to a larger setting or patient population. Researchers use *pragmatic trials* to measure the effectiveness of interventions in real-life, routine settings that produce generalizable results. Therefore, Witt (2009) claims that trials aimed to help select between different care options are *pragmatic*, while trials to test fundamental research hypotheses, where an interference causes a particular biological change, are *explanatory*.

Methodology, Instruments, Outcomes, and Results of the Pragmatic Trial Studies

An efficiency "of **dementia-care mapping (DCM)** for institutionalized people with dementia shows in an *explanatory*, **cluster-randomized controlled trial (cRCT)** with two *DCM* researchers carrying out the *DCM* intervention" (van de Ven, Draskovic, Adang, Donders, Zuidema, Koopmans, et al., 2013, p. 1). Patients at the care centers experienced neuropsychiatric symptoms such as dementia, apathy, anxiety, and hallucinations. These symptoms, experienced by the residents at these care homes, affected their quality of life. It also affected the professional caregivers, who encountered serious challenges that resulted in high absenteeism and turnover rates, leading to shortages of staff (van de Ven, et al., 2013).

To gather new knowledge, researchers studied *DCM* efficiency in a *pragmatic cRCT* comprising a variety of care homes with qualified nursing staff executing the intervention. The nurses at the care homes where the intervention took place received *DCM* training and conducted the *DCM* intervention over four months, twice during the study. A primary outcome was agitation, which was measured with the Cohen-Mansfield Agitation Inventory (CMAI). The 29-item questionnaire is used to measure the types and frequencies of agitated behaviors of elderly nursing home residents. The CMAI measures the occurrence on a 7-point scale ranging from "1—never engages in" to "7—establishes the behavior on the average of several times an hour." "Pacing," "cursing or verbal aggression," and "repetitive sentences or questions" are some examples of the items in the inventory (van de Ven, et al., 2013, p. 1).

Two researchers carried out the intervention in the tightly controlled care homes. Tightly controlled refers to surveillance technology to improve social participation, safety, and security of at-risk older people in care homes. Surveillance is implemented to prevent dangerous situations, including falls; to monitor health status; and to track movements of activity. The disadvantages of surveillance are a loss of privacy that contributes to loss of self-confidence, autonomy, and stigmatization.

In this research, dementia special care units were randomly assigned to *DCM* or usual care. While the primary outcome was agitation, measured with the CMAI, the secondary outcomes included "residents' neuropsychiatric symptoms (NPSs) and quality of life, staff stress and job satisfaction" (van de Ven, et al., 2013, p. 1). The nursing staff "made all measurements at baseline and two follow-ups at four-month intervals." The researchers "used linear mixed-effect models to test treatment and time effects" (van de Ven, et al., 2013, p. 1). The study was *pragmatic* in nature, maintaining internal validity by trying to explore the need for research in relation to everyday risks/threats in the real world. By doing this, they could provide information about daily practice.

Wayne, Manor, Novak, Costa, Hausdorff, Goldberger, et al. (2012) researched in another *pragmatic* randomized trial a systems biology approach by using Tai Chi to study physiological complexity (cardiovascular, locomotor, and balance systems) in older adults towards healthy aging. The researchers used a continuing, two-armed, randomized clinical trial where they assessed at three and six months the possibility of Tai Chi mind–body exercise to diminish age-related loss of said physiological complexity.

Wayne, et al. (2012, p. 24) explain that Tai Chi, also referred to as Taiji, Tai Chi Chuan, or Taijiquan, a "mind–body exercise that originated in China, is growing in status in the West. Tai Chi is grounded on slow purposeful movements, often harmonized and coordinated with breathing and images." The main objective of using Tai Chi was to help older adults reinforce and relax the physical body and mind, to grow in personal development, and to improve the natural flow of energy (Wayne, et al., 2012, p. 24). In this article, the authors argue, "aging is typically associated with progressive multi-system impairment that leads to decreased physical and cognitive function and reduced adaptability to stress" (Wayne, et al., 2012, p. 23). The researchers evaluated cardiovascular dynamics, "postural control during quiet standing, gait dynamics, complexity and adaptability," and restoration of complexity (Wayne, et al., 2012, p. 21). The authors concluded their results emphasizing the importance of understanding the biology of aging and appraising interventions that encourage healthy aging. Emerging research supports the idea that aging is associated with loss of complexity in multiple physiology systems.

Pragmatic trials are preferable, as they provide meaningful information on which to base decision-making in healthcare. Furthermore, *pragmatic trials* evaluate effects of treatment in real-world situations. Another positive outcome is that *pragmatic trials* can update practice because they offer proof that the treatment/intervention is effective in usual practice.

However, Ernst and Canter (2005) believe that this not a reasonable claim, and they state that "while pragmatic trials may approximate more closely to the day-to-day clinical situation in which patients are treated, the results they produce are frequently meaningless" (Ernst & Canter, 2005, p. 1). The latter is mainly because one can read the findings as either positive or negative. Therefore, the "spin" in understanding results becomes greatly subject to bias, and the audience may perceive *pragmatic trials* more as propaganda tools than science (Ernst & Canter, 2005). Other disadvantages include first, that *pragmatic trials* offer more design and analytic challenges than *explanatory trials* due to the probable heterogeneity of treatment effect. Second, researchers may need to invest more time and resources to conduct *pragmatic trials* compared to *explanatory trials*. Lastly, a negative result in a *pragmatic trial* cannot offer data on whether the treatment/intervention is effective under prime conditions.

Highlights for Best Practices for Current and Emerging Scholars

In complementary medicine, clinical research studies focus on the efficacy "of a treatment compared to placebo in an experimental setting" (Witt, 2009, p. 293), while other studies access "the effectiveness of additional treatment in a real world setting" (Witt, 2009, p. 293). Current research discussions are focused on the benefits and limitations of efficacy and effectiveness studies in real-world settings.

Conclusion

From this discussion of the six case studies explaining various research methodologies, one realizes the importance of well-being, health, and quality of life as people age. Therefore, research to improve a positive psychological state is core in the aged. *Qualitative research* methodologies are an affordable way to collect data through a variety of methods such as focus groups and in-depth interviewing, among other forms. *Participatory research* is specifically applicable to working with diverse cultural healthcare issues. *EMA* is a good research methodology to track behavior change together with intervention, qualitative, experimental, and *pragmatic trial* methodologies. Although *cohort studies* are expensive and time consuming, they are very important when it comes to longitudinal gender and health outcome research. Continued financial investment in cohort studies is essential.

As males and females age, they become socially dependent, although they want to be more independent. From the discussions earlier, issues of identities arise as people age in relation to the different roles that men and women need to fulfil as they age. Women are usually labeled "caregivers," while men work and excel more in jobs before the retirement phase. Both genders can become more socially segregated due to various reasons, as outlined in this chapter.

References

aan het Rot, M., Hogenelst, K., & Schoevers, R. A. (2012). Mood disorders in everyday life: A systematic review of experience sampling and ecological momentary assessment studies. *Clinical Psychology Review*, *23*(6), 510–523. https://doi.org/10.1016/j.cpr.2012.05.007

Agboka, G. Y. (2014). Decolonial methodologies: Social justice perspectives in intercultural technical communication research. *Journal of Technical Writing and Communication*, *44*(3), 297–327. https://doi.org/10.2190/TW.44.3.e

Andrews, G. R., Sidorenko, A. V., Gutman, G., Gray, J. E., Anisimov, V. N., Bezrukov, V. V., et al. (2006). Research on aging: Priorities for the European region. *Advances in Gerontology*, *18*, 7–14. https://doi.org/10.1016/j.regg.2008.12.007

Arber, S. (1991). Class, paid employment and family roles: Making sense of structural disadvantage, gender and health status. *Social, Science and Medicine*, *32*(4), 425–436.

Bartlett, H., Warburton, J., Lui, C. W., Peach, L., & Carroll, M. (2013). Preventing social isolation in later life: Findings and insights from a pilot Queensland intervention study. *Aging & Society*, *33*(7), 1167–1189. https://doi.org/10.1017/S0144686X12000463

Bryman, A. (2012). *Social research methods* (4th ed.). New York, NY: Oxford University Press.

Cain, A. E., Depp, C. A., & Jeste, D. V. (2009). Ecological momentary assessment in aging research: A critical review. *Journal of Psychiatric Research*, *43*, 987–996. https://doi.org/10.1016/j.jpsychires.2009.01.014

Datta, R. (2018). Decolonizing both researcher and research and its effectiveness in Indigenous research. *Research Ethics*, *14*(2), 1–24. https://doi.org/10.1177/1747016117733296

Dunton, G. F., Atienza, A. A., Castro, C. M., & King, A. C. (2009). Using ecological momentary assessment to examine antecedents and correlates of physical activity bouts in adults age 50+ years: A pilot study. *Annals of Behavioral Medicine*, *38*(3), 249–255. https://doi.org/10.1007/s12160-009-9141-4

Du Plooy, G. M. (2009). *Communication research techniques, methods and applications* (2nd ed.). Cape Town: Juta & Co.

Ernst, E., & Canter, P. H. (2005). Limitations of "pragmatic trials". *Postgraduate Medical Journal*, *81*(954), 203. https://doi.org/10.1016/j.cpr.2012.05.007

Frankel, R. M., & Devers, K. J. (2000). Study design in qualitative research 1: Developing questions and assessing resource needs. *Education for Health*, *13*(2), 251–261. https://doi.org/10.1080/13576280050074534

Gilbert, N., & Stoneman, P. (2016). *Researching social life*. Los Angeles, CA: Sage.

Hamilton, D. F., Lane, J. V., Gaston, P. G., Patton, J. T., MacDonald, D., Simpson, A. H., et al. (2013). What determines patient satisfaction with surgery? A prospective cohort study of 4709 patients following total joint replacement. *BMJ Open*, *3*, 1–7. https://doi.org/10.1136/bmjopen-2012-002525

Hasse, B., Ledergerber, B., Furrer, H., Battlegay, M., Hirschel, B., Cavassini, M., et al. (2011). Mobility and aging in HIV-infected persons: The Swiss HIV-cohort study. *Clinical Infectious Diseases*, *53*(11), 1130–1139. https://doi.org/10.1093/cid/cir626

HelpAge International. (2002). *Gender and aging briefs*. Retrieved April 10, 2020, from www.helpage.org/silo/files/gender-and-ageing-briefs.pdf

Hogan, S., & Warren, L. (2012). Dealing with complexity in research processes and findings: How do older women negotiate and challenge images of aging? *Journal of Women & Aging*, *24*(4), 329–350. https://doi.org/10.1080/08952841.2012.708589

Jankowski, G. S., Diedrichs, P. C., Williamson, H., Harcourt, D., & Christopher, G. (2016). Looking age-appropriate while growing old gracefully: A qualitative study of aging and body image amongst older adults. *Journal of Health Psychology*, *21*(4), 550–561. https://doi.org/10.1177/1359105314531468

Keyton, J. (2011). *Communication research: Asking questions, finding answers*. New York, NY: McGraw-Hill Book Company.

Knodel, J., & Ofstedal, M. B. (2003). Gender and aging in the developing world: Where are the men? *Population and Development Review*, *29*(4), 677–698. https://doi.org/10.1111/j.1728-4457.2003.00677.x

Kumar, R. (2011). *Research methodology: A step-by-step guide for beginners*. Los Angeles, CA: Sage Publications.

MacGill, M. (2018). *What is a cohort study in medical research?* Retrieved February 12, 2019, from www.medicalnewstoday.com/articles/281703.php

Makiwane, M., Ndinda, C., & Botsis, H. (2012). Gender, race and aging in South Africa. *Agenda*, *26*(4), 15–28. https://doi.org/10.1080/10130950.2012.755380

Moola, S. (2015). *Communication dynamics in producing effective patient care: A case study at Stanger Hospital's diabetes clinic in Kwa-Zulu Natal, South Africa* (Unpublished thesis). Retrieved February 5, 2019, from http://hdl.handle.net/10500/20679

Patton, M. Q. (2005). *Qualitative research*. Retrieved February 11, 2019, from https://doi.org/10.1002/0470013192.bsa514

Rodriguez, I., & Inturias, M. L. (2018). Conflict transformation in indigenous peoples' territories: Doing environmental justice with a "decolonial turn". *Development Studies Research*, *5*(1), 90–105. https://doi.org/10.1080/21665095.2018.1486220

Russell, C. (2007). What do older women and men want? Gender differences in the "lived experience" of aging. *Current Sociology, 55*(2), 173–192. https://doi.org/10.1177/0011392107073300

Statistics South Africa. (2012). *South Africa: General household survey 2016.* Retrieved February 6, 2019, from https://datacatalog.worldbank.org/dataset/south-africa-general-household-survey-2016-0

Shiffman, S., Stone, A. A., & Hufford, M. R. (2008). Ecological momentary assessment. *Annual Review of Clinical Psychology, 4,* 1–32. https://doi.org/10.1146/annurev.clinpsy.3.022806.091415

Smyth, J. M., & Stone, A. A. (2003). Ecological momentary assessment research in behavioral medicine. *Journal of Happiness Studies, 4*(1), 35–52. https://doi.org/10.1023/A:1023657221954

van de Ven, G., Draskovic, I., Adang, E. M., Donders, R., Zuidema, S. U., Koopmans, R. T., et al. (2013). Effects of dementia-care mapping on residents and staff of care homes: A pragmatic cluster-randomized controlled trial. *PLPS One, 8*(7), 1–7. https://doi.org/10.1371/journal.pone.0067325

Venn, S., & Arber, S. (2012). Understanding older people's decisions about the use of sleeping medication: Issues of control and autonomy. *Sociology of Health & Illnesses, 34*(8), 1215–1229. https://doi.org/10.1111/j.1467-9566.2012.01468.x

Wayne, P. M., Manor, B., Novak, V., Costa, M. D., Hausdorff, J. M., Goldberger, A. L., et al. (2012). A systems approach to studying tai chi, physiological complexity and health aging: Design and rationale of a pragmatic randomized controlled trial. *Contemporary Clinical Trials, 34*(1), 21–34. https://doi.org/10.1016/j.cct.2012.09.006

Witt, C. M. (2009). Efficacy, effectiveness, pragmatic trials: Guidance on terminology and the advantage of pragmatic trials. *Forsch Komplementmed, 16,* 293–294. https://doi.org/10.1159/000234904

Wray, S. (2003). Women growing older: Agency, ethnicity and culture. *Sociology, 37*(3), 511–527. https://doi.org/10.1177/00380385030373007

Zavala, M. (2013). What do we mean by decolonizing research strategies? Lessons from decolonizing, Indigenous research projects in New Zealand and Latin America. *Decolonization: Indigeneity, Education, and Society, 2*(1), 55–71.

19

SOCIOECONOMIC CONTEXT OF ADOLESCENT HEALTH RISK BEHAVIORS

Life Course Developmental Research Methods

Tae Kyoung Lee, Catherine Walker O'Neal, and Kandauda A. S. Wickrama

Overview

Health studies have documented that contextual adversities can have longitudinal effects on adolescents' development leading to health-risk behaviors and/or health problems in later life stages (Cable, 2014). These findings are consistent with the life course perspective, which posits that developmental processes (or mechanisms) with health consequences stem from one's socioeconomic context (Kuh & Ben-Shlomo, 2004). As such, the life course approach offers substantial insight into the etiology of health disparities in later stages and provides a framework for health researchers seeking to better understand how risk exposure shapes adolescent health behaviors (Jones, Gilman, Cheng, Drury, Hill & Geronimus, 2019). The life course approach, which often involves taking a "long view" (Alwin, 2012, p. 213) to study life trajectories, or histories, is appropriate for health researchers testing developmental models of health behavior based on longitudinal and complex datasets and advanced analytical techniques.

In studies of how early socioeconomic context affects adolescent health or health behavior, five prominent areas of health psychology research with applications to the life course perspective are 1) multiple early risk exposure, 2) health behaviors trajectories, 3) transitions in health behavior trajectories, 4) heterogeneity in health behavior trajectories, and 5) health disparity interventions. Advances in statistical methods, including structural equation modeling (SEM) approaches, allow health researchers to address these five areas of study. More specifically, some of the SEM approaches that are often employed in life course research addressing early socioeconomic context and adolescent health/behavior include confirmatory factor analysis (CFA), latent growth curve modeling (LGCM), piecewise latent growth curve modeling (PLGCM), and growth mixture modeling (GMM). The purpose of this chapter is to illustrate these analytical approaches in research employing a life course perspective to study adolescents' health behaviors. To achieve this purpose, empirical studies are presented, along with a discussion of challenges that health researchers face and possible future directions.

Research in Practice

The Modeling of Multiple Early Risk Exposure

Health risks at the individual and population levels can be attributed to multiple sources across the life course. For instance, some early life course risk factors and adverse exposures that may have implications for health behaviors and health outcomes are family negative life events, low family income, low parental education, and being a single-parent family (Lee, Wickrama, & O'Neal, 2019). This research is consistent with the life course perspective, which emphasizes that multiple contextual exposures additively and multiplicatively influence health and health behaviors (Kuh & Ben-Shlomo, 2004; Jones, et al., 2019). Consequently, this perspective can inform research that sheds light on how multiple risk exposures combine to influence adolescents' health and health behaviors. This section describes the premise of multiple risk exposure, emphasizing the various ways researchers have conceptualized this concept. We introduce two mechanisms that are widely documented in health research: additive effects and multiplicative effects.

Additive effects refer to the relationship between a health risk behavior (e.g., substance use or sedentary behavior) and a set of predictor variables (e.g., maltreatment, family poverty, and community adversity), where the overall effect of the set of predictors is determined by summing their individual unique effects (VandenBos, 2007). That is, the additive effects of these multiple predictor variables (i.e., multiple risk exposures) on the occurrence of a health behavior can be examined by specifying several risk exposures as unique predictors of the health behavior in a multiple regression model. In these models, a coefficient for each risk exposure effect is estimated after adjusting for the effect of the other individual risk exposures. An additive model assumes that each risk exposure uniquely and independently "adds to" the health outcome over and above the other risk exposures captured in the regression model (Kuh, Ben-Shlomo, Lynch, Hallquist, & Power, 2003).

Instead, *multiplicative effects* refer to the synergistic, or interactive, effects of two or more predictors on an outcome (VandenBos, 2007). In a regression model, multiplicative effects can be examined by specifying interaction terms among predictors (e.g., a product term between two risk predictors, such as family economic strain × single-parent family; Aiken & West, 1991). This model allows researchers to examine whether the overall (or combined) effect of multiple risk factors on a health behavior is greater than their separate, or additive, effects (Raviv, Taussig, Culhane, & Garrido, 2010). For example, variables indicating childhood maltreatment and family poverty may combine multiplicatively to influence youth health behaviors such that the health effect of these two risk exposures is substantially greater than simply adding the effect of each risk exposure individually (e.g., Hammen, Henry, & Daley, 2000).

Although incorporating additive and multiplicative effects in the same regression model allows health researchers to investigate how multiple risk exposures affect health behaviors, these models also have several limitations. First, many contextual risk factors in adolescence co-occur (e.g., low-income family, single-parent family, and low parental education) and are confounding, which creates concerns about multicollinearity. *Multicollinearity* is indicated by highly correlated predictors, and, in a regression model, these occurrences can cause biased estimation coefficients. Second, assessing multiplicative effects is appropriate when a researcher is estimating interaction effects for only a few risk exposures (e.g., two or three risk predictors). The standard method for testing the interaction hypothesis is to add each risk into the regression model and then to incorporate the product term(s) between the risk predictors. However, this approach is limited when the research question requires considering a large number (i.e., more than five risk factors) of risk exposures simultaneously. Statistically, the main limitation of this approach is that it requires a large number of parameter estimates. For example, if five risk factors are included in a model, the regression model includes five additive effects and 26 possible interaction effects (including two-way, three-way, four-way, and five-way interaction effects). The large number of interactions makes the results difficult to interpret. Such difficulties can be avoided using *SEM* (Ettekal, Eiden, Nickerson, & Schuetze, 2019), which focuses on the shared variance of closely related, multiple exposure indicators (e.g., low-income family, single-parent family, and low parental education).

The *SEM* approach entails specifying a measurement model using multiple risk predictors as indicators of an unobserved latent factor construct (Bollen & Bauldry, 2011). With the *SEM* approach, the latent factor can be estimated using a *confirmatory factor analysis* (*CFA*; see the circle in Panel *a* of Figure 19.1; Brown, 2006). In a *CFA*, a latent factor is specified, treating each individual contextual risk variable as an indicator. Statistically, indicators with standardized factor loadings larger than .40 are thought to indicate acceptable psychometric properties (see λ_1 to λ_6 in Panel *a* of Figure 19.1; Matsunaga, 2010). Loadings less than .40 suggest that the contextual risk variable does not "load" onto the larger latent factor. After estimating the latent contextual risk factor in a *CFA*, this latent factor is specified as a predictor of the outcome (e.g., health behaviors, such as substance use or sedentary behavior) in the *SEM*, which estimates a regression coefficient, β (see Panel *a* of figure 19.1).

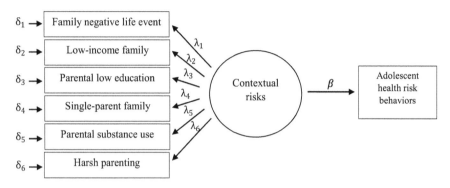

Panel *a*. Latent variable model (LVM)

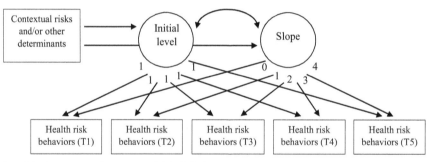

Panel *b*. Latent growth curve model (LGCM)

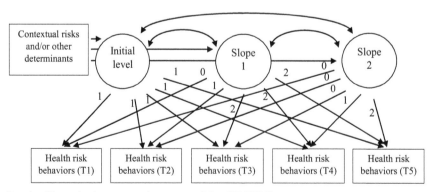

Panel *c*. Piecewise latent growth curve model (PLGCM)

Figure 19.1 Structural equation modeling (SEM) for life course research (Part I).

Note: T = Timepoint.

SEM has several theoretical and statistical advantages. Theoretically, a *SEM* approach is particularly advantageous when researchers seek to aggregate the individual contextual risk indicators into a single underlying general risk factor. Statistically, this latent variable is estimated based on the strength of correlations among individual contextual risk indicators, which avoids collinearity issues experienced in regression models assessing additive and multiplicative effects. In addition, *SEM* explicitly accounts for measurement error (see δ1 to δ6 in Panel *a* of Figure 19.1; Raykov & Marcoulides, 2000) and allows researchers to separate **true variance**, or variance that is common among indicators of a single construct, from **error variance**, or variance due to other factors like measurement error. In standard multiple regression, measurement error within each predictor variable is not accounted for, which may attenuate the regression coefficients from the predictor to the outcomes (Baron & Kenny, 1986). This underestimation reduces a researcher's ability to explain the associations between risk exposures and health behaviors. Because *SEM* uses a latent variable that adjusts for measurement error in each predictor, *SEM* generally provides more accurate estimates of the associations between the latent risk variable and the health behavior outcome. In addition, the *SEM* approach allows researchers to specify non-normal variables (e.g., categorical variables, such as yes/no occurrences of specific contextual risk factors) as indicators when estimating latent factors (e.g., Lee, Wickrama, & O'Neal, 2018).

An Example Study: Modeling Multiple Early Risk Exposure

A recent study by Sharma, Mustanski, Dick, Bolland, and Kertes (2019) utilized *SEM* to examine how multiple risk exposures contribute to adolescents' health behaviors in a sample of African American youth residing in high-poverty neighborhoods. The authors examined the potential negative effects of risk exposures on internalizing problems, externalizing problems, and polydrug use outcomes and the buffering effects of individual- and community-level protective factors. They used a cross-sectional design with 576 adolescents (307 females; M_{age} = 16 years, SD = 1.44 years). Four risk indicators were measured: 1) exposure to stressors (e.g., death, serious illness, and/or loss of employment of a family member), 2) exposure to violence, 3) racial discrimination, and 4) neighborhood problems. The three protective factors evaluated were 1) religiosity, 2) parental monitoring, and 3) neighborhood collective efficacies.

First, a *CFA* examined whether the four multiple risk indicators loaded onto a single latent construct (i.e., "contextual risk"). The results indicated an appropriate fit to the data with standardized loadings above 0.50. Second, the associations between contextual risk and the three health outcomes (internalizing problems, externalizing problems, and polydrug use) were examined using *SEM*. The results revealed that risk exposure significantly predicted adolescents' risk of all three outcomes.

Finally, they examined how individual- and community-level protective factors reduce these negative associations between risk exposure and health behavior using three interaction terms between contextual risk and each protective factor (i.e., adolescents' religiosity, parental monitoring, and neighborhood collective efficacy). They found that the association between risk exposure and internalizing problems was buffered by adolescents' religiosity and neighborhood collective efficacy, such that risk exposure was not associated with adolescents' internalizing symptoms when they reported high levels of religiosity and neighborhood collective efficacy. Similarly, the association between risk exposure and externalizing problems was buffered by parental monitoring and collective efficacy. The findings from Sharma, and colleagues (2019) highlight the usefulness of *SEM* for assessing risk more broadly and identify potential protective factors that can buffer against the effects of cumulative risk for adolescents' health outcomes.

The Modeling of Health Risk Behavior Trajectories

The term trajectory refers to a pattern of health, or health behavior, that a person engages in over time (Wethington, 2005), such as the longitudinal changes in an individual's tobacco use. Health research has generally inferred longitudinal processes of health behaviors across adolescence, implying the existence of trajectories of health behaviors over time. Measuring health behavior trajectories explicitly enables researchers to examine the continuity and change (i.e., increase or decrease) of health behaviors over time, rather than focusing on an outcome at a single occasion or, perhaps, two discrete occasions. A proper analysis of change through the examination of trajectories requires three or more repeated measures of the outcome of interest in order to estimate a continuous developmental process (Wickrama, Lee, O'Neal, & Lorenz, 2016). This section addresses the conceptualization and estimation of trajectories and provides an empirical illustration of how trajectories can be applied to life course research focused on health behaviors.

The research on trajectories mainly focuses on two research interests/hypotheses: 1) sensitive periods and 2) duration of risk exposure. The ***sensitive period hypothesis***, according to the life course perspective, refers to the notion that events, experience, or contexts affect individuals differently depending on their timing in the life course. For example, some research suggests that individuals are more susceptible to contextual events in earlier stages of development, such as childhood and early adolescence. (Hostinar, Lachman, Mroczek, Seeman, & Miller, 2015). Fitting with this research, stronger negative effects of contextual risk exposures (or effects of other predictors such as personality, genetic disposition, or neurological factors) on health and health behaviors are expected in early adolescence compared to later developmental stages. Second, the ***duration hypothesis*** emphasizes the effect of exposure length on outcomes of interests (Wethington, 2005). For example, a previous health study reported long-term, persistent effects of adversities in adolescence on trajectories of health risk behaviors (such as substance use and sedentary behavior) in adolescence and young adulthood (Lee, et al., 2019). Specifically, the effect of early adversity on the change parameter (i.e., slope) of behavior trajectories reflects an increasing influence of adversity over time. The duration hypothesis also can be applied when considering the effect of risk exposure (i.e., time-varying predictor) on outcomes of interest. For example, researchers can examine the effects of trajectories of adverse childhood experiences on adolescents' substance use.

Estimation of Trajectories

A *latent growth curve modeling LGCM* is a type of longitudinal SEM that allows researchers to evaluate an individual's change over time (Meredith & Tisak, 1990; Wickrama, et al., 2016). It can be described as two different processes. First, a latent initial level and a latent slope (i.e., the growth factors) are estimated based on each individual's trajectory (known as intraindividual changes; Wickrama, et al., 2016). Second, growth factors provide an estimate of the *average* trajectory and *variation* among individuals' trajectories (known as interindividual differences). In a *LGCM*, these two processes are modeled as a function of time. They are represented through the specification of latent (i.e., unobserved) variables referred to as 1) initial level and 2) slope (rate of change; see the two circles in Panel *b* of Figure 19.1; Wickrama et al., 2016). The *initial-level* variable reflects the level of health risk behaviors at the first measurement occasion. The *slope* variable reflects the rate of change in health risk behaviors over time. Values of the time metric (e.g., age, day, or wave of measurement) are built into the factor loading matrix to form the hypothesized trajectory. The most common form, or shape, for a trajectory models a linear trend over time (e.g., $t = 0, 1, 2, 3$, and 4; see a latent slope factor in Panel *b* of Figure 19.1). It is noted that nonlinear trajectories, such as quadratic trajectories, can also be specified (e.g., $t = 0, 1, 4, 9$, and 16). Nonlinear trajectory specification for a *LGCM* is detailed in Wickrama et al. (2016). After estimating parameters in a *LGCM*, researchers also can specify predictors (e.g., multiple risk exposures) of the growth factors (i.e., initial level and slope), which estimate regression coefficients between predictors and growth factors. These regression coefficients allow health researchers to examine the long-term effects of early multiple risk exposures on individuals' health risk behavior trajectories over time.

An Example Study: Modeling Health Risk Behavior Trajectories

One study using a *LGCM* in adolescent health behavior research examined the effects of contextual risk factors on adolescents' smoking behavior trajectories. More specifically, Tjora, Hetland, Aarø, and Øverland (2011) examined longitudinal associations between multiple contextual factors (i.e., family socioeconomic status [SES]; smoking behaviors of parents, siblings, and friends) and trajectories of smoking behaviors. They employed data from the Norwegian Longitudinal Health Behaviors Study (NLHB), which followed participants from the ages of 13 to 30 (*n* = 1,053). They analyzed data from the first five waves, covering the age span from 13 to 18. They computed a binary variable of smoking behavior (i.e., smoker/nonsmoker) for each year to use as indicators of the growth factors (i.e., initial level and rate of change). In addition, they measured smoking behaviors from the adolescents' siblings, parents, and peers. The analytical processes consisted of two steps. First, a linear *LGCM* was used to estimate trajectories of smoking behaviors over adolescence (ages 13 to 18). Second, family SES and parent, sibling, and friends' smoking behaviors were then specified as predictors of the growth factors into the *LGCM*.

The results showed that adolescents' smoking rates increased from 3% to 31% from age 13 to age 18. Participants' *initial level* of smoking (age 13) was most strongly associated with their best friends' smoking. However, parental SES, parents' smoking, and older siblings' smoking predicted adolescents' initial level of smoking, as well as the *rate of change* in the adolescents' smoking behaviors from ages 13 to 18. This study indicates that initial levels of adolescents' smoking are much more strongly associated with their peers' smoking habits than with their parents' or siblings' smoking habits. However, from a longitudinal perspective (i.e., considering the rate of change), it seems that parents' SES and parental and older siblings' smoking behaviors are of enduring importance for adolescents' smoking. These findings are consistent with calls for more specific substance use interventions that specifically target at-risk individuals and smokers (Thomas, McLellan, & Perera, 2013). Furthermore, the findings emphasize that driving factors implicated in smoking initiation in early adolescence (i.e., peer smoking in the current study) are distinct from factors that are implicated in the *change* in smoking status across adolescence. These findings can inform prevention and intervention research, as they shed light on multiple points of intervention (e.g., peer smoking, sibling smoking, parent SES) and begin to identify which points of intervention may be most productive during specific developmental periods, such as targeting peer smoking in early adolescence and targeting parent SES as an enduring influence over time.

Modeling Transitions in Health Risk Behavior Trajectories

Consistent with the life course perspective, the period of "transition" from one life stage to another can include changes in various attributes, including health behaviors (Gotlib & Wheaton, 1997). The term "transition" has been defined in various ways within social and behavioral sciences; however, definitions commonly reference "a change in social roles or responsibilities" (Wethington, 2005, p. 116). This definition can apply to the various transitions experienced by young adults (e.g., employment, marriage, and/or parenthood; Lee, Wickrama, O'Neal, & Prado, 2018). The life course perspective assumes that transitions from one life stage to another lead to major changes in life course trajectories (i.e., turning points). For example, the transition period to young adulthood (aged 18 to 25) is thought of as a particularly sensitive period due to the educational, relationship, and socioeconomic changes that may occur (Naicker, Galambos, Zeng, Senthilselvan, & Colman, 2013). That is, young adulthood is often a time with sizeable changes in habits and behaviors (Wethington, 2005), and these turning points may involve nonlinear trajectories in adolescents' health behaviors during the transition period to young adulthood.

During this transition period, contextual exposures (or environment conditions) often change considerably, which can directly influence health behaviors (Ames, Leadbeater, & MacDonald, 2018).

For example, as the primary socializing agent for younger adolescents (before age 18), parents typically have considerable control over their adolescent's health risk behaviors (Mollborn & Lawrence, 2018). However, during the transition to young adulthood (ages 18 to 25), health behavior choices are thought to become more autonomous (Ames et al., 2018). By young adulthood (ages 25 to 30), research suggests that individuals' health behaviors are likely to interact with their own SES (separate from their family's SES; Ames, et al., 2018). Therefore, in order to understand health risk behaviors across the early life course, it is necessary to employ a long-term view that considers trajectories of health risk behaviors across adolescence *and* young adulthood.

Estimation of Trajectories With Transitions

This section addresses the conceptualization and measurement of transitions as they relate to health risk behavior trajectories. Building on the *LGCM* introduced previously, researchers can examine distinct trajectories across multiple life stages by specifying additional latent slope factors (McNeish & Matta, 2018). For example, a *piecewise latent growth curve modeling PLGCM* (also known as a multiphase *LGCM*; Ram & Grimm, 2007) is a common approach to studying individuals' trajectories over multiple developmental phases. In this approach, each individual's trajectory can be estimated separately for each developmental stage (or phase). In Panel *c* of Figure 19.1, two slope factors (see slope 1 and slope 2) estimate two distinct trajectories using five repeated measures. One slope estimates trajectories from time points 1 to 3, and the other estimates trajectories from time points 3 to 5. Similar to time metric specification in a *LGCM*, values of the time metric in a *PLGCM* are built into the factor loading matrix to reflect the form of the hypothesized trajectory. Typically, a linear trajectory for each slope segment is specified, as is shown in Panel *c* of Figure 19.1. More specifically, in this example, to estimate a linear trajectory with two slopes, the factor loadings for the first slope are specified as 0, 1, 2, 2, and 2, and the factor loadings for the second slope are specified as 0, 0, 0, 1, and 2 (see the latent slope factor in Panel *c* of Figure 19.1; Wickrama, et al., 2016). The main advantage of a *PLGCM* is the estimation of unique slope segments, which assess the possibility of distinct trajectories in health risk behaviors across different life course stages (e.g., trajectories in adolescence and young adulthood).

Similar to other *LGCM* approaches, after estimating piecewise trajectories, predictors (e.g., multiple risk exposures) can also be incorporated into the model to estimate regression coefficients between the predictors and growth factors (i.e., initial levels and rates of change). These regression coefficients allow health researchers to examine how risk exposure is associated with health risk behavior trajectories across different life course stages. Although a *PLGCM* can be a useful tool for researchers studying health behaviors, they have not appeared in the literature frequently. In order to provide an example of this approach, we analyzed a *PLGCM* examining health risk behaviors from adolescence to young adulthood.

An Example Study: Modeling Health Risk Behavior Trajectories
With Transitions

To examine the trajectories of health risk behaviors from adolescence and young adulthood (ages 15 to 30), we conducted the research with the data from a nationally representative sample of adolescents participating in the National Longitudinal Study of Adolescent to Adult Health (Add Health). Add Health participants between the ages of 15 and 30 years (n = 9,166; 5,012 females, *M* age = 15.77 years, *SD* = 1.56 years at wave one reported on seven health risk behaviors: 1) smoking, 2) binge drinking, 3) marijuana use, 4) improper sleep duration, 5) unhealthy eating, 6) physical inactivity, and 7) sedentary behaviors. Unless otherwise stated, dichotomous indicators were created from the original continuous measures by adapting the criteria of previous studies (Lee, et al., 2019). Then, all dichotomous indicators were summed to create an index of health risk behaviors at each time point.

A *PLGCM* was used to estimate four unique latent factors of health risk behavior trajectories: 1) initial levels (age 15), 2) a slope during adolescence (ages 15 to 18; slope 1), 3) a slope during emerging adulthood (age 19 to 25; slope 2), and 4) a slope during young adulthood (age 26 to 30; slope 3). After estimating the initial *PLGCM*, multiple risk factors at wave one (i.e., parental low education, family economic hardship, and adolescent depressive symptoms) were specified as predictors of the initial level of health risk behavior and the three slope segments. Additional information regarding the study procedures and measures is available from Lee, and colleagues (2019).

Observed means of health risk behaviors are shown in Panel *a* of Figure 19.2. A *PLGCM* was used to estimate similar trajectories. For example, the estimated growth parameters indicated that the mean of initial level (i.e., health risk behaviors at age 15) was 2.03, $p < .001$. The mean rates of change (i.e. slope of health risk behaviors) during adolescence, emerging adulthood, and young adulthood were

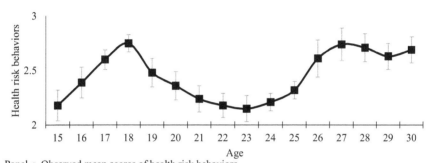

Panel *a*. Observed mean scores of health risk behaviors.
Note. Error bars represent the 95% confidence interval of mean parameters).

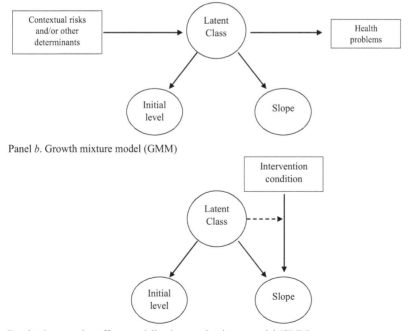

Panel *b*. Growth mixture model (GMM)

Panel *c*. Intervention effects modeling in growth mixture model (GMM).
Note. The dotted line indicates separate estimates of the effect of intervention condition on slope for each of the latent slope classes.

Figure 19.2   Structural equation modeling (SEM) for life course research (Part II).

0.15, −0.08, and 0.14, respectively. All means were significant at $p < .001$. Thus, on average, there was an increase in health risk lifestyle across adolescence (mean slope = 0.15), followed by a decreasing rate of change during emerging adulthood (mean slope = −0.08), and then another increase in health risk behaviors during young adulthood (mean slope = 0.14). In addition, the variances of these growth parameters were statistically significant (0.24, 0.12, 0.06, and 0.08, $p < .001$ for the initial level and rate of change over adolescence, emerging adulthood, and young adulthood, respectively), indicating significant interindividual variation in these trajectories. The findings suggest unique health risk behavior trajectories between adolescence, emerging adulthood, and young adulthood. Moreover, the significant variance statistics suggest there is interindividual variation in these values (i.e., the initial level and rates of changes) that may be explained by predictors such as indicators of socioeconomic context.

Next, predictor variables were added to the *PLGCM* to investigate the possibility that early risk exposures affect health risk behavior trajectories. Early family adversities (i.e., parents with low education, family economic hardship) uniquely predicted health risk behaviors in all three life stages (adolescence, emerging adulthood, and young adulthood), indicating additive and long-term effects of early family adversities on health trajectories. By using *PLGCM*, unique shapes of health risk behavior trajectories were identified from adolescence to young adulthood. Moreover, the findings identified how early family adversity persistently influenced health behaviors over multiple life stages. Findings such as these highlight the need for federal and state policies that focus on eradicating economic hardship, including funding for intervention programs that reduce the likelihood of family socioeconomic hardship, which also includes the truncation of education and lack of resources. The findings also suggest the value of parenting interventions designed to help families cope during times of economic distress.

Modeling Heterogeneity in Health Risk Behavior Trajectories

The life course perspective posits that trajectories of health and, relatedly, health behaviors vary among adolescents depending on their degree of exposure to environmental factors. Thus, these trajectories may vary not only in the rate of change (i.e., slope) but also in their qualitative functional form (Wickrama, et al., 2016). Similarly, epidemiological perspectives have emphasized that early risk exposure may result in unique groupings of developmental trajectories. Accordingly, separate from general trends across the population, some social groups are likely to have overall healthier behaviors than others, whereas other groups (e.g., socioeconomically disadvantaged groups) generally fare worse in most health dimensions, including their poorer health behaviors (Nagin, 2005). These variations are often referred to as heterogeneity in health and health behavior trajectories. Although existing health research has contributed significantly and substantively to our understanding of the overall (homogeneous) trajectories of adolescents' health risk behaviors, less attention has been given to the existence of heterogeneity in these behavior trajectories. Understanding the heterogeneity in patterns of health risk behaviors in adolescence has clear implications for both prevention and intervention science. Such research can identify groups that are at higher risk of poor health behaviors and poor health. This section addresses the conceptualization and measurement of trajectory heterogeneity.

The previously discussed models (i.e., *CFA*, *LGCM*, and *PLGCM*) are variable-centered approaches, meaning that they assume all individuals (or trajectories) are drawn from a single population for which a single set of "averaged" parameters can be estimated. However, this assumption may not be valid when the sample is composed of multiple unknown subpopulations of trajectories (i.e., population heterogeneity) because each subpopulation may be best characterized by a different set of parameters. For example, some youth may show high and decreasing health risk behavior trajectories over adolescence, and another subgroup of individuals may exhibit low and increasing health risk behavior trajectories over adolescence.

As an alternative to variable-centered analyses, person-centered analyses can be utilized to identify unobserved subpopulations of similar individuals using latent class variables in a SEM framework

(Wickrama, et al., 2016). As such, a unique feature of a person-centered approach is that it relaxes the assumption that all individuals in the sample are drawn from a single population for which a single set of "averaged" parameters can be estimated. A *growth mixture model GMM* is one type of longitudinal, person-centered analysis that combines aspects of a *LGCM* and latent class variables to identify discrete trajectories in longitudinal data (see panel *b* of Figure 19.2; Wickrama, et al., 2016). Latent class variables can also be utilized in a nonlinear *LGCM* (e.g., *PLGCM*) or quadratic trajectory models. With this analytical approach, trajectory class membership is not known but inferred from the data based on posterior class membership probability (Muthén, 2004).

To identify the optimal class trajectory model in the *GMM*, an incrementally larger number of classes is estimated and fit indices are compared. For instance, one fit index that can be used to evaluate class classification is the Bayesian Information Criterion (BIC). It is a relatively reliable fit index that can inform the selection of the best model by comparing the BIC between two nested class models (e.g., two-class model vs. three-class model; the class model with lower BIC value is preferred; Muthén, 2004). In addition, predictors and outcomes can be incorporated into a *GMM* (Wickrama, et al., 2016), allowing researchers to address the concurrent and/or predictive validity of the classification (Muthén, 2004).

An Example Study: Modeling Heterogeneity in Health Risk Behavior Trajectories

An example of this approach with health behavior research is a study that examined heterogeneity in substance use trajectories among adolescents (Sittner, 2016). The purpose of the study was to 1) identify heterogeneity in trajectories of substance use (i.e., alcohol, marijuana, and cigarettes) with a sample of indigenous adolescents from the northern Midwest and Canada, and 2) examine the associations between heterogeneity in substance use trajectories and early contextual adversities and health problems in young adulthood. More specifically, the study examined early contextual adversities (e.g., family income, peers who drink/smoke, adolescent's conduct problems, and depressive symptoms) as predictors of the heterogeneous substance use trajectories. Various health outcomes (e.g., substance use disorder) were examined as outcomes of the substance use trajectories during the transition to young adulthood (18 years). For the trajectory analyses, data were utilized from waves one, two, three, five, and seven (spanning ages 10 to 18 years) ($n = 619$, 50.4% female, mean age = 11 years at wave one). At each wave, binary responses of use of all three substances were summed into a count variable indicating substance use over the past year, with a possible range of 0 to 3. Detailed descriptions of the other measures are available in Sittner (2016).

First, class trajectory modeling was used to identify heterogeneity in trajectories of substance use. Based on the BIC value, three distinct shapes of substance use trajectories were evident. For members of the first group (36.3%), termed the early-adolescence onset group, there was a steep increase in substance use during the past year between the ages of 10 and 15. Use peaked at about two substances in the past year and remained stable through age 18. The second trajectory group, with substance use onset in mid-adolescence, was composed of slightly more than a third of the sample (38.3%). This group had virtually no substance use from ages 10 to 11, but they experienced a steep increase in use between ages 12 and 17. By late adolescence, this group had used approximately 1.5 to 2 substances in the past year. The last group, termed the late-onset group (25.3%), used practically no substances until age 15, which was followed by a gradual increase through age 18. By that time, the group averaged using one substance in the past year.

Second, to identify associations between these trajectory classes and early contextual adversities, baseline measures were used to create profiles of trajectory group members. The means and proportions of the profile variables were compared across the trajectory groups using analysis of variance (ANOVA) and chi-square tests. Compared to the other two trajectory groups, a significantly larger proportion of the early-onset group was female (61.3%), met the criteria for conduct disorder (22.1%), and had been expelled from school (24.9%). In addition, compared to adolescents with a late-onset trajectory of substance use, the mid-onset group was composed of a larger percentage of adolescents who met the criteria for conduct disorder (9.7%) and had been expelled from school (18%). The mid-onset and late-onset groups did not differ in their proportion of females, mean per-capita family income, or mean number of friends who drank or smoked.

Third, the trajectory groups were used to predict health outcomes measured in the final wave of the study (wave eight, average age of 18). The results showed that the early-onset group experienced more negative health characteristics (i.e., a higher prevalence of substance use disorder) than did the middle onset group. The late-onset group reported significantly better health outcomes (i.e., lower prevalence of substance use disorder and risky sexual behavior) than the other two groups. These findings suggest early substance use is accompanied by multiple health problems, which have important prevention implications.

Integrating the Life Course Perspective Into Health Disparities Intervention Research

Over the past several decades there has been considerable research focused on uncovering the causes of risk behaviors during childhood and adolescence, with a primary focus on factors involved in the development of health risk behaviors (e.g., Capaldi, Kerr, Eddy, & Tiberio, 2016). There have been calls for more dynamic intervention models bridging strong theoretical models with advanced methodology (e.g., Lerner, 2012). One notable shortcoming of most research on preventive intervention programs targeting adolescents' health risk behaviors is their reliance on the assumption of a homogeneous sample population. That is, existing research on intervention effectiveness has used analysis techniques that treat the sample as a homogeneous group when assessing how interventions affect adolescents' behavioral outcomes (Brincks, Perrino, Howe, Pantin, Prado, Huang, et al., 2018).

As introduced previously, the life course perspective emphasizes the possibility of distinct developmental patterns of health risk behaviors (i.e., *heterogeneity* in health behavior trajectories). Consonant with this perspective, prevention scientists have begun to focus on identifying effective prevention programs for heterogeneous groups of youths (Connell, Stormshak, Dishion, Fosco, & Van Ryzin, 2018). For example, Brincks, and colleagues (2018) reported differential intervention effects among Hispanic youth with different trajectories of health problems (i.e., internalizing problems) using *GMM*. They identified three distinct trajectories of health problems: 1) low internalizing symptoms (60% of the sample), 2) moderate internalizing symptoms (27% of the sample), and 3) high internalizing symptoms (13% of the sample). They found that intervention was most beneficial for the youth with high internalizing symptom levels. That is, within this class, youth receiving the intervention experienced reduced trajectories of internalizing symptoms over time, whereas youth in the control condition experienced increased internalizing symptoms. This type of person-centered approach allows health researchers to identify which adolescents are most likely to benefit from the intervention. Therefore, the results can help direct the intervention to youth who are most likely to gain from it and identify youth who are not likely to benefit, for whom other interventions may be more effective.

In a *GMM*, when a predictor variable is the intervention indicator (i.e., a dichotomous variable indicating whether the individual received the intervention or not), the model specification is slightly different from the previously introduced *GMM*, where predictors are entered as independent variables that are thought to explain the latent class variable (see Panel *a* of Figure 19.2). Class membership should be independent of condition assignment so that the discrete groups (or classes) defined by the trajectory are not influenced by whether the participants are assigned to intervention or control (Brincks, et al., 2018). Instead, the intervention condition may interact with the class membership trajectories to explain the differential effects of the intervention depending on class membership. Therefore, a latent class variable is used to estimate interaction effects between class membership and intervention condition on trajectories of health risk behaviors (see a dotted line in Panel *c* of Figure 19.2; Brincks, et al., 2018).

An Example Study: Integrating the Life Course Perspective Into Health Disparities Intervention Research

A study by Liu, Hedeker, Segawa, and Flay (2010) is an example of this analytic approach. The study employed a *GMM* to identify classes of substance use behavior trajectories with a sample of African American male adolescents, and they identified differential intervention effects among these subgroups of individuals. The study used data from the Aban Aya Youth Project (AAYP), which is a longitudinal preventive intervention trial targeting health-compromising behaviors among adolescents in disadvantaged areas of Chicago. An ordinal scale was used to assess substance use behavior as the outcome of interest. Self-reported data were collected from the participating youth at the beginning of fifth grade and at the end of grades five, six, seven, and eight ($n = 668$ adolescents, $M = 10.8$ years in fifth grade).

First, a *GMM* indicated two classes of adolescent drug use trajectories: Class 1 (44.7% of the sample) reported a relatively higher initial level of drug use (fifth grade) and had a small increase over time; Class 2 had a lower baseline level and a greater increase over time. Next, the intervention condition was entered into the *GMM* to predict the slope factor. The results showed an interaction effect between youth in Class 2 and intervention condition (b = −0.912, $p < .05$). That is, in Class 2 (the group with the lower baseline drug use but greater increase), the adolescents in the intervention group showed a slower increase in drug use trajectories compared to adolescents in the control group, while the drug use trajectory pattern for adolescents in Class 1 did not differ significantly between the intervention and control groups. These findings suggest that interventions are more (or less) effective for certain individuals based on their trajectory pattern. Consequently, these heterogeneous intervention effects indicate the need for varied, targeted interventions based on trajectory patterns. For example, based on this study, the intervention was not helpful for youth who displayed higher levels of drug use at the first measurement occasion (fifth grade). Instead, the intervention was appropriate for youth with lower levels of early drug use. Together, these findings could signal the need for more targeted intervention for youth who exhibit early initiation of drug use behavior.

Strengths and Limitations

The major advantage of the life course perspective for health research is in the area of epidemiology of health and illness. Researchers are applying the life course perspective to understand group differences in health and how health behaviors develop and persist across time. The life course perspective emphasizes the accumulation of threats for individuals exposed to persistent disadvantage over time and how these threats can negatively affect health. This focus provides etiologic insights about the developmental processes that generate health disparities.

However, many existing studies have statistical limitations. Despite their methodological sophistication and public health relevance, many observational (or quasi-experimental) studies have been limited by their inability to make causal conclusions about the associations between contextual risk factors and health behaviors because of possible confounder effects. To address this limitation, many studies incorporate a broad array of possible confounder variables into the statistical models as predictors (i.e., control variables) using traditional regression, which may result in limited statistical power.

Under such circumstances, ***inverse propensity weight*** (IPW) can be used. Conceptually, *IPW* is similar to using survey weights in an analysis. *IPW* is the probability of assignment to, or membership in, a specific group, conditional on a set of observed confounder variables (Rosenbaum & Rubin, 1983). For example, in *IPW*, individuals with a low probability of having a reported level of contextual risk factors, given their levels of confounders, are up-weighted, and individuals with a high probability of having a reported level of contextual risk factors, given their levels of confounders, are down-weighted. Thus, the weighted sample mimics a randomized sample where individuals are randomly assigned to levels of contextual risk factors and confounders are evenly distributed between individuals with different levels of contextual risk factors. *IPW* allows researchers to adjust the data for confounding variables in the absence of randomization, assuming that all possible confounders are measured (Rosenbaum & Rubin, 1983). In addition, *IPW* allows researchers to control for a larger, more diverse array of potential confounders than traditional regression methods, and the ability to more accurately control for these confounders increases the confidence that can be placed in the findings and enhances the ability to draw causal inferences.

Recommendations for Future Research

Several important extensions to the analytical approaches presented earlier are important to emphasize for future research. First, more research should investigate the existence of underlying global risk, such as youth health risk lifestyle (Lawrence, Mollborn, & Hummer, 2017; Wickrama, Conger, Wallace, & Elder, 1999), rather than focusing on specific health behaviors. Such global factors can be captured under latent constructs defined by multiple health risk behaviors as observed indicators. Second, because socioeconomic context can change over time, it is important to investigate the effects of time-varying socioeconomic context on health behavior trajectories. For example, trajectories of family economic hardship may influence adolescent health behavior trajectories. Such investigations can uncover parallel processes between elements of the socioeconomic context and health risk behaviors. Similarly, more research is needed to identify parallel processes between specific health risk behaviors (e.g., substance use and eating a poor diet). Such investigations can identify the extent of longitudinal comorbidity between health risk behaviors. Third, continued research is needed focused on the onset timing of health risk behaviors, such as substance use and risky sex. In order to investigate these event outcomes, categorical regression can be utilized predicting the onset of these risky health behaviors as logistic coefficients or odds ratios. More importantly, the onset timing of health risk behaviors may be influenced by socioeconomic factors, and this possibility can be investigated using survival models.

Conclusion

The life course perspective can lead to etiologic insights about the developmental processes that generate health disparities through adolescence and across life stages, which has clear implications for designing interventions and educational programs. This chapter introduces analytical methods (i.e., *SEM, LGCM, PLGCM,* and *GMM*) that have been utilized to research multiple early risk exposure, health behavior trajectories, and transitions and heterogeneity in health behavior trajectories. Moreover, for each method, we provided an example of how the method can be utilized to identify points of prevention and intervention for minimizing the detrimental effects of socioeconomic contexts. The analytical methods discussed in this chapter can be further strengthened by integrating more cutting-edge techniques, such as second-order constructs, parallel processes, and analyzing the onset timing of health risk behaviors. Research using the analytical methods introduced and rooted in life course studies can further the understanding of the interplay between socioeconomic contexts and youth health risk behaviors and generate findings that positively affect federal, state, and local programs that work to combat the negative contextual effects on youth health risk behaviors.

References

Aiken, L. S., & West, S. G. (1991). *Multiple regression: Testing and interpreting interactions.* Thousand Oaks, CA: Sage Publications.

Alwin, D. F. (2012). Integrating varieties of life course concepts. *The Journals of Gerontology, Series B: Psychological Sciences and Social Sciences*, *67*(2), 206–220. https://doi.org/10.1093/geronb/gbr146

Ames, M. E., Leadbeater, B. J., & MacDonald, S. W. S. (2018). Health behaviors changes in adolescence and young adulthood: Implications for cardiometabolic risk. *Health Psychology*, *37*(2), 103–113. https://psycnet.apa.org/doi/10.1037/hea0000560

Baron, R. M., & Kenny, D. A. (1986). The moderator-mediator variable distinction in social psychological research: Conceptual, strategic, and statistical considerations. *Journal of Personality and Social Psychology*, *51*(6), 1173–1182.

Bollen, K. A., & Bauldry, S. (2011). Three Cs in measurement models: Causal indicators, composite indicators, and covariates. *Psychological Methods*, *16*(3), 265–284. https://psycnet.apa.org/doi/10.1037/a0024448

Brincks, A., Perrino, T., Howe, G., Pantin, H., Prado, G., Huang, S., et al. (2018). Preventing youth internalizing symptoms through the Familias Unidas intervention: Examining variation in response. *Prevention Science*, *19*(Suppl 1), 49–59. https://doi.org/10.1007/s11121-016-0666-z

Brown, T. A. (2006). *Confirmatory factor analysis for applied research*. New York, NY: The Guilford Press.

Cable, N. (2014). Life course approach in social epidemiology: An overview, application and future implications. *Journal of Epidemiology*, *24*(5), 347–352. https://doi.org/10.2188/jea.JE20140045

Capaldi, D. M., Kerr, D. C., Eddy, J. M., & Tiberio, S. S. (2016). Understanding persistence and desistance in crime and risk behaviors in adulthood: Implications for theory and prevention. *Prevention Science*, *17*(7), 785–793. https://doi.org/10.1007/s11121-015-0609-0

Connell, A. M., Stormshak, E., Dishion, T., Fosco, G., & Van Ryzin, M. (2018). The family checkup and adolescent depression: An examination of treatment responders and non-responders. *Prevention Science*, *19*(Suppl 1), 16–26. https://doi.org/10.1007/s11121-015-0586-3

Ettekal, I., Eiden, R. D., Nickerson, A. B., & Schuetze, P. (2019). Comparing alternative methods of measuring cumulative risk based on multiple risk indicators: Are there differential effects on children's externalizing problems? *PLoS One*, *14*(7), e0219134. https://dx.doi.org/10.1371%2Fjournal.pone.0219134

Gotlib, I. H., & Wheaton, B. (1997). *Stress and adversity over the life course: Trajectories and turning points*. New York, NY: Cambridge University Press.

Hammen, C., Henry, R., & Daley, S. E. (2000). Depression and sensitization to stressors among young women as a function of childhood adversity. *Journal of Consulting and Clinical Psychology*, *68*(5), 782–787. https://psycnet.apa.org/doi/10.1037/0022-006X.68.5.782

Hostinar, C. E., Lachman, M. E., Mroczek, D. K., Seeman, T. E., & Miller, G. E. (2015). Additive contributions of childhood adversity and recent stressors to inflammation at midlife: Findings from the MIDUS study. *Developmental Psychology*, *51*(11), 1630–1644. https://psycnet.apa.org/doi/10.1037/dev0000049

Jones, N. L., Gilman, S. E., Cheng, T. L., Drury, S. S., Hill, C. V., & Geronimus, A. T. (2019). Life course approaches to the causes of health disparities. *American Journal of Public Health*, *109*(Suppl 1), S48–S55.

Kuh, D., & Ben-Shlomo, Y. (2004). *A life course approach to chronic disease epidemiology* (2nd ed.). Oxford, England: Oxford University Press.

Kuh, D., Ben-Shlomo, Y., Lynch, J., Hallquvist, J., & Power, C. (2003). Life course epidemiology. *Journal of Epidemiology and Community Health*, *57*(10), 778–783. https://dx.doi.org/10.1136%2Fjech.57.10.778

Lawrence, E. M., Mollborn, S., & Hummer, R. A. (2017). Health lifestyles across the transition to adulthood: Implications for health. *Social Science & Medicine*, *193*, 23–32. https://doi.org/10.1016/j.socscimed.2017.09.041

Lee, T. K., Wickrama, K. A. S., & O'Neal, C. W. (2018). Application of latent growth curve analysis with categorical responses in social behavioral research. *Structural Equation Modeling*, *25*(2), 294–306. https://doi.org/10.1080/10705511.2017.1375858

Lee, T. K., Wickrama, K. A. S., & O'Neal, C. W. (2019). Early socioeconomic adversity and cardiometabolic risk in young adults: Mediating roles of risky health lifestyle and depressive symptoms. *Journal of Behavioral Medicine*, *42*(1), 150–161. https://doi.org/10.1007/s10865-018-9952-5

Lee, T. K., Wickrama, K. A. S., O'Neal, C. W., & Prado, G. (2018). Identifying diverse life transition patterns from adolescence to young adulthood: The influence of early socioeconomic context. *Social Science Research*, *70*, 212–228. https://doi.org/10.1016/j.ssresearch.2017.12.001

Lerner, R. M. (2012). Developmental science: Past, present, and future. *International Journal of Developmental Science*, *6*(1), 29–36. doi:10.3233/DEV-2012-12102

Liu, L. C., Hedeker, D., Segawa, E., & Flay, B. R. (2010). Evaluation of longitudinal intervention effects: An example of latent growth mixture models for ordinal drug use outcomes. *Journal of Drug Issues*, *40*(1), 27–43. https://doi.org/10.1177%2F002204261004000103

Matsunaga, M. (2010). How to factor-analyze your data right: Do's, don'ts, and how-to's. *International Journal of Psychological Research*, *3*(1), 97–110. www.redalyc.org/articulo.oa?id=299023509007

McNeish, D., & Matta, T. (2018). Differentiating between mixed-effects and latent-curve approaches to growth modeling. *Behavior Research Methods*, *50*(4), 1398–1414. https://doi.org/10.3758/s13428-017-0976-5

Meredith, W., & Tisak, J. (1990). Latent curve analysis. *Psychometrika*, *55*(1), 107–122. https://doi.org/10.1007/BF02294746

Mollborn, S., & Lawrence, E. (2018). Family, peer, and school influences on children's developing health lifestyles. *Journal of Health and Social Behavior*, *59*(1), 133–150. https://doi.org/10.1177%2F0022146517750637

Muthén, B. O. (2004). Latent variable analysis: Growth mixture modeling and related techniques for longitudinal data. In D. Kaplan (Ed.), *Handbook of quantitative methodology for the social sciences* (pp. 345–368). Newbury Park, CA: Sage Publications.

Naicker, K., Galambos, N. I., Zeng, Y., Senthilselvan, A., & Colman, I. (2013). Social, demographic, and health outcomes in the 10 years following adolescent depression. *Journal of Adolescent Health*, *52*(2), 533–538. https://doi.org/10.1016/j.jadohealth.2012.12.016

Nagin, D. (2005). *Group-based modeling of development*. Cambridge, MA: Harvard University Press.

Ram, N., & Grimm, K. (2007). Using simple and complex growth models to articulate developmental change: Matching theory to method. *International Journal of Behavioral Development*, *31*(4), 303–316. https://doi.org/10.1177%2F0165025407077751

Raviv, T., Taussig, H. N., Culhane, S. E., & Garrido, E. F. (2010). Cumulative risk exposure and mental health symptoms among maltreated youth placed in out-of-home care. *Child Abuse & Neglect*, *34*, 742–751. https://doi.org/10.1016/j.chiabu.2010.02.011

Raykov, T., & Marcoulides, G. A. (2000). A method for comparing completely standardized solutions in multiple groups. *Structural Equation Modeling*, *7*(2), 292–308. https://doi.org/10.1207/S15328007SEM0702_9

Rosenbaum, P. R., & Rubin, D. B. (1983). The central role of propensity score in observational studies for causal effects. *Biometrika*, *70*, 41–55. https://doi.org/10.1093/biomet/70.1.41

Sharma, S., Mustanski, B., Dick, D., Bolland, J., & Kertes, D. A. (2019). Protective factors buffer life stress and behavioral health outcomes among high-risk youth. *Journal of Abnormal Child Psychology*, *47*(8), 1289–1301. https://doi.org/10.1007/s10802-019-00515-8

Sittner, K. J. (2016). Trajectories of substance use: Onset and adverse outcomes among north American indigenous adolescents. *Journal of Research on Adolescence*, *26*(4), 830–844. https://doi.org/10.1111/jora.12233

Thomas, R. E., McLellan, J., & Perera, R. (2013). School-based programs for preventing smoking. *Cochrane Systematic Review*, *4*. No.:CD001293. https://doi.org/10.1002/ebch.1937

Tjora, T., Hetland, J., Aarø, L. E., & Øverland, S. (2011). Distal and proximal family predictors of adolescent's smoking initiation and development: A longitudinal latent curve model analysis. *BMC Public Health*, *11*(1), 911. https://doi.org/10.1186/1471-2458-11-911

VandenBos, G. R. (2007). *APA dictionary of psychology*. Washington, DC: American Psychological Association.

Wethington, E. (2005). An overview of the life course perspective: Implications for health and nutrition. *Journal of Nutrition Education and Behavior*, *37*(3), 115–120. Retrieved from www.sciencedirect.com/science/article/pii/S1499404606602650

Wickrama, K. A. S., Conger, R. D., Wallace, L. E., & Elder, G. H. (1999). The intergenerational transmission of health-risk behaviors: Adolescent lifestyles and gender moderating effects. *Journal of Health and Social Behavior*, *40*(3), 258–272. doi:10.2307/2676351

Wickrama, K. A. S., Lee, T. K., O'Neal, C. W., & Lorenz, F. O. (2016). *Higher-order growth curves and mixture modeling with Mplus: A practical guide*. New York, NY: Taylor & Francis.

PART V

Environmental Studies

20

UNIQUE ENVIRONMENTAL DETERMINANTS OF HEALTH

Natural, Physical, and Community Factors

Yasmin M. Hussein, Stephanie Spero, Alexander Dean Bracken, and Deborah Fish Ragin

Overview

The effect of the environment on an individual's well-being has been documented and studied throughout the years (e.g., Guite, Clark, & Ackrill, 2006). However, recent events such as dramatic climate change and the environmental release of toxins into the air and water have propelled environmental psychology to the forefront when addressing the health outcomes of communities and nations. While the field initially examined the physical characteristics of the environment people lived in (Proshansky, 1976), it has evolved throughout the years to include much more. Currently, the field of environmental psychology investigates not only how the natural world affects the individual's psyche but also how manmade disasters and social environments influence our development and well-being.

It is common knowledge to many that surviving a natural disaster can be a traumatic event. For instance, some assessments now screen for posttraumatic symptoms as a result of natural disasters (Briere & Hedges, 2010). Others have also studied ways with which clinical interventions can be used in order to treat trauma caused by natural disasters, such as hurricanes (Grainger, Levin, Allen-Byrd, Doctor, & Lee, 1997). However, the full extent to which these disasters affect survivors is still not understood. Research suggests that the prevalence rate of psychological effects, including posttraumatic stress disorder (PTSD) and anxiety, after natural disasters is estimated to be approximately 34% (Felix, Afifi, Kia-Keating, Brown, Afifi & Reyes, 2015; Norris, Friedman, Watson, Byrne, & Kaniasty, 2002; Schneider, Rasul, Liu, Corry, Lieberman-Cribbin, Watson, et al., 2019). In this chapter, we discuss the impact of natural disasters on health outcomes. Specifically, we examine the effects of naturally occurring events like hurricanes, as well as manmade events, specifically air pollution and wildfires. We conclude the chapter by exploring research on the impact of the social environment, and while this is different from the previous three sections—here the determinants are not caused by the physical environment—it is important to recognize that one's social environment is also an essential aspect of the field of environmental psychology.

One important note before proceeding. In many of the studies being addressed, the often-discouraged method of ***convenience sampling*** is used (Felix, et al., 2015; Lowe, Rhodes, & Waters, 2015; Schneider, et al., 2019). While ideally, *convenience sampling* is something that most researchers prefer to avoid, this may be the only option when studying the heath impacts of disasters or epidemics resulting in misplaced persons. The reason for this is simple: If one wishes to study the effects of a natural disaster, the sample may be limited or difficult to find. Potential participants may have relocated to a safer environment, may be hospitalized to address serious health issues and unable to participate, or, frankly, may be, understandably, more concerned with piecing their lives back together than with partaking in a research study. Since, in many such cases, *convenience sampling* cannot be avoided, it is essential to attempt to compensate for this with other study strengths.

Research in Practice

Hurricanes

The National Oceanic and Atmospheric Administration (NOAA) defines a *hurricane* as a tropical cyclone, a type of storm that forms over tropical or subtropical waters. *Tropical cyclones* are referred to as *hurricanes* once the storm reaches a windspeed of 74 mph. *Hurricanes* typically emerge from the Atlantic Ocean, Caribbean Sea, Gulf of Mexico, and the eastern North Pacific Ocean, but they can also originate from the central North Pacific Ocean, though at a less frequent rate. There has been growing concern with the issue of *hurricanes* due to changes in the planet's climate. NOAA projects that these *tropical cyclones* will increase in intensity and potentially lead to more destruction (NOAA, 2018).

Given their increasingly destructive properties, *hurricanes* have become a major environmental concern. We consider two cases: Hurricane Sandy, which hit the United States in 2012, and Hurricane Katrina, which devastated New Orleans in 2005. Hurricane Sandy was a *post tropical cyclone* that caused over 650,000 homes to experience damage or destruction (Blake, Kimberlain, Berg, Cangialosi, & Beven, 2013). While the destruction of these homes alone is a tragedy, Hurricane Sandy also prevented first responders from accessing various locations due to flooding and impassible roadways. This flooding caused a delayed response, which allowed fires to erupt and destroy over 100 homes before they could be contained. As a result, many families lost their homes and, with it, their sense of safety. The destruction caused by the disaster is not typically where the story ends, however. Often, natural disasters continue to inflict negative psychological and physical consequences on those affected for years following the event.

Hurricane Katrina was no less devastating. Much has been written about this category five storm that destroyed the levees of New Orleans, flooding the city and killing more than a thousand poor and minority residents (see Nigg, Barnshaw, & Torres, 2006; Schneider, et al., 2019). Much of the attention, however, focused on the aftermath of the storm: the estimated 200,000 who could not or would not evacuate; the over 1,300 dead due to storm or storm-related ailments; and the hundreds who fled to shelters in neighboring Texas, 48% of whom could not locate family members and another 79% who had neither family nor friends who could provide temporary shelter (Washington Post, Kaiser family Foundation & Harvard University, 2005).

When studying natural disasters such as hurricanes, several constructs must be clearly defined. For example, researchers attempt to measure *exposure severity*, although this concept lacks both an agreed definition and method. *Exposure severity* generally refers to a range of stressors such as loss of resources, personal harm, damage to one's home and goods, extent of concern for significant others, and exposure to grotesque events. In addition, there are various ways in which researchers define and study *disaster-related stressors (DRS)*, including threat to life, injury, fear, witnessing injury/death, financial loss, and loss of social and personal resources, just to name a few (Chan & Rhodes, 2014). But there is no consensus regarding this concept either. Many researchers will use more than one of these *DRS* to measure the psychological impact of such events; however, there is no agreement on either how many should be included or which are most appropriate for specific studies.

In addition to the lack of conceptual consensus in this line of research, a limited number of assessment tools have been developed. Two such measures are used extensively: the Traumatic

Exposure Severity Scale (TESS; Elal & Slade, 2005) and the Hurricane Related Traumatic Experiences (HURTE; Vernberg, Greca, Silverman, & Prinstein, 1996). TESS was originally developed in order to assess exposure severity to earthquakes in adults, but its use has evolved to encompass other natural disasters as well. This is a 24-item scale with five subscales and includes items such as "Did you have to relocate because your house became structurally unsafe to live in?" (Elal & Slade, 2005, p. 219). The subscales were derived from a factor analysis to measure Resource Loss, Damage to Home and Goods, Personal Harm, Concern for Significant Others, and Exposure to the Grotesque. Vernberg, Greca, Silverman, and Prinstein's (1996) HURTE, on the other hand, was developed in order to assess traumatic experiences individuals experience that were related to hurricanes. This scale contains 17 items, with closed-end responses (i.e., yes or no) due to the scale's focus on assessing children and not wanting to burden them with complicated answers. The subscales for this measure—perceived life threat, life-threatening experiences, and loss-disruption experiences—included questions such as "Did you or your family have trouble getting enough food or water after the hurricane?" (Vernberg, et al., 1996, p. 241). While such scales have aided in the conceptual consensus on constructs in this field, the nature of natural disasters has caused researchers to approach studying these events in various ways.

One measure that has become more prominent in natural disaster research is the Posttraumatic Growth (PTG) scale. This scale was originated by Tedeschi and Calhoun (1996) but then later revised into a shorter form by Cann, Calhoun, Tedeschi, Taku, Vishnevsky, Triplett, et al. (2010) and Kaur, Porter, LeardMann, Tobin, Lemus, and Luxton, (2017). PTG is unique in that it assesses an individual's positive development after a traumatic event. The original version from 1996 included 21 items that included the following factors: New Possibilities, Relating to Others, Personal Strength, Spiritual Change, and Appreciation of Life. Based on an analysis of the original scale, Cann, et al. (2010) shortened this scale to 10 items comprised of two items from each of the original five factors. Other variations of this scale have been developed over the years; however, the main goal of these updated versions seems to be shortening the number of questions while maintaining the relevance of the original factors.

The theory behind PTG suggests that people can experience positive transformation despite adversity (Collier, 2016). While this is often confused with **resilience**, there are important distinctions between PTG and resilience that warrant separate examination. Unlike *resilience*, PTG focuses on the processes that one uses to cope with tragedy. *Resiliency*, on the other hand, focuses more on an individual's personal attributes. Although PTG is still a relatively new concept, it has become more popular in research due to its unique approach regarding trauma.

Methodology and Findings

Schneider, et al. (2019) investigated the long-term effects of Hurricane Sandy on New York residents in order to study the association between PTG and mental health difficulties (MHD). Their study used a cross-sectional design with convenience sampling and resulted in 1,356 adult participants from the New York metropolitan area. A noted weakness of the study was the *convenience sampling* procedure, as those not as easily accessible were excluded from the study. Normally, this type of sampling is not ideal. Again, due to the nature of the natural disaster, these concerns do not outweigh other potential strengths of studies such as this one.

Schneider et al.'s study employed several questionnaires, including the Patient Health Questionnaire 4 (PHQ-4), Posttraumatic Stress Disorder Checklist-Specific (PCL-S), Post-Traumatic Growth Inventory (PTGI), and a demographic survey. Schneider, et al. (2019) explain that prior research has shown the PCL-S and PTGI to be validated and widely used tools for the study of stress and trauma; however, only PCL-S is shown to be psychometrically sound. This does not negate PTGI's appropriateness as a tool, although it may suggest that improvements are needed. On the other hand,

PHQ-4 is a validated measure for accessing anxiety and depressive symptoms used by many in the field of health.

In addition to these measures, Schneider, et al. (2019) assessed smoking behavior and alcohol abuse as defined by the National Institute on Alcohol Abuse and Alcoholism (NIAAA). In this study, alcohol abuse was defined as five or more drinks in a day on a monthly basis for males and four or more drinks in a day, again on a monthly basis, for females. Of course, they also evaluated hurricane exposure by using a checklist of 30 items that assessed individuals' experience and consequences from the hurricane. This scale included personal exposure measures such as injury/death (either a friend or family member) and damaged/destroyed home (property exposure). This measure was derived from previous hurricane studies, specifically those studying the effects of Hurricanes Katrina (Harville, Xiong, Smith, Pridjian, Elkind-Hirsch, & Buekens, 2011) and Andrew (Norris, Perilla, Riad, Kaniasty, & Lavizzo, 1999). Schneider, et al. (2019) found that participants who had missing data had a higher proportion of alcohol use and were, on average, younger compared to those who did not have missing data. Fully 70.8% of the missing data pertained to participants' current mental health treatment status. They also found that higher PTG scores were associated with study subjects who were non-White, had completed high school, were current smokers, had a history of mental illness, and currently were receiving mental health treatment. Hurricane exposure and PTSD scores also revealed significant positive correlations with PTG scores. Schneider, and colleagues (2019) argue that this relationship may suggest that being exposed to trauma is a possible foundation from which one can undergo growth. Due to the cross-sectional nature of the study, however, no casual nature can be inferred according to the researchers.

Lowe, et al., (2015) studied Hurricane Katrina and its impact on low-income mothers who survived the event. Briefly, Hurricane Katrina was a category five storm that destroyed the water levees built to protect New Orleans from the surges from the Gulf of Mexico and Lake Pontchartrain. The massive flooding due to the failure of the levees caused damage to the sewer systems and resulted in contaminated waters flowing freely throughout the city. Worst still, thousands of city residents were forced to flee their homes. Those who were unable to flee were stranded on house rooftops, in poorly supplied makeshift shelters, or were abandoned. Lowe, and colleague's (2015) study included females who were participants in a study conducted before Katrina that attempted to increase community college retention for low-income students. The pre-Katrina study included two community colleges; however, following the hurricane, these colleges were closed for the fall 2005 semester. Because of this, these participants were no longer included in the data for the original study, but they were now eligible to participate in the Resilience in Survivors of Katrina (RISK) study by Rhodes, Chan, Paxson, Rouse, Waters, and Fussell (2010). RISK is a longitudinal study that began in 2003 and was originally collecting data on low-income families in New Orleans with the goal of increasing educational attainment among community college students. After Hurricane Katrina in 2005, however, the original purpose of the study was disrupted, which then prompted the researchers to focus on the effects of the hurricane on vulnerable populations, such as low-income families. This study continues to collect data to this day, which allowed Lowe, et al. (2015) the opportunity to use the participants that were newly added. The RISK study currently investigates the effect Katrina had on physical and mental health, social relationships, and educational and employment activities.

Lowe, et al. (2015) utilized both quantitative and qualitative methods collecting three waves of data: the first wave (Wave 1) occurred before Hurricane Katrina in 2004, the second wave (Wave 2) was one year after Hurricane Katrina in 2006, and the third wave (Wave 3) occurred four years after Hurricane Katrina in 2009. Retention throughout the three waves of the study was excellent, which is a rare feat for many studies. Typically, one big drawback of longitudinal studies is the difficulty in maintaining participants throughout the study, but we see this was not an issue here. Of the original

492 participants from Wave 1, the study retained almost all (*n* = 409) by the end of Wave 3. Researchers assessed psychological distress using the K6 scale, a six-item measure used for screening nonspecific psychological distress. That has a reasonable Cronbach alpha estimation of .70 to .81 This scale consists of six item statements, such as "During the past 30 days, about how often did you feel so depressed that nothing could cheer you up?" (Lowe, et al., 2015, p. 3) that are rated on a 4-point scale from "none of the time" to "all of the time." Results from this scale fall into three categories: probable absence of mental illness, mild or moderate mental illness, and probable serious mental illness. During each wave, additional quantitative data were collected. In Wave 1, each participant reported demographic information such as their race/ethnicity, age, and number of children. Next, in Wave 2 participants were asked to complete a module for hurricane-related exposure that addressed issues such as lack of food, water, and access to medical care. In all waves, participants were asked to report any social benefits they had received, such as welfare and food stamps, as well as complete the Social Provisions Scale (Cutrona & Russell, 1987). This scale measure perceived social support by looking at the availability of social support reported by the individuals.

For the qualitative data, in-depth interviews with 63 participants were performed four to seven years post hurricane to assess the participants' experiences and the aftermath of the incident (Lowe, et al., 2015). These interviews were conducted in convenient locations (e.g., the interviewee's home, the interviewer's office, a coffee shop). This lack of location consistency is somewhat questionable, but it should be noted that this did not lessen the usefulness of the information collected. In addition, it may have enhanced participant retention. The interviews were designed to understand, from the participants' perspectives, how the hurricane changed their functioning, relationships, and goals. Questions included in the interview focused on the interviewee's childhood family life, employment and education, post-disaster physical and mental health, friendships since the hurricane, and other topics. Due to their in-depth style, interviews typically lasted between one and two hours, so while they were informative, they were also time consuming,

The interviewees for this qualitative part of the study were selected in three different ways. First, all eligible participants were residents of Orleans or Jefferson Parish before the disaster and suffered damage to their residence due to the storm. Second, for the sake of comparison, an equal number of participants who chose either to stay in New Orleans after the hurricane or move to another location after the hurricane were included. Lastly, the researchers attempted to ensure no significant difference between the participants in the qualitative sample and the quantitative sample with regard to the effects of the hurricane on low-income parents. Lowe, and colleagues (2015) found that reports of mental health from the qualitative data sample aligned with the quantitative trajectories. For example, interviewees with resilience in both groups also reported an absence of psychological symptoms throughout their lives.

Lowe, et al.'s (2015) study is unique in the use of quantitative trajectories mixed with qualitative data in order to understand the aftereffects of natural disasters on mental health. There are, however, limitations to this study (as there would be to any other). One concern is a lack of generalizability. The researchers note that while generalizability was not necessarily a goal of theirs due to the qualitative nature of the study, it is still essential to note that participants were predominantly non-Hispanic, Black mothers and are not necessarily representative of Katrina survivors. The benefit of detailed interviewing is that it allows researchers to glean insight into how environmental and interpersonal factors work together to shape the mental health and outcomes of those enduring such tragedies.

While the studies discussed earlier focus on the effects of hurricanes, the methodologies applied can be used for other natural disasters as well. The application of qualitative methods, such as those used by Lowe, et al. (2015), may aid researchers in understanding the disaster victims' perspectives more clearly than would be typical via quantitative methods. Another consideration is the concept of personal growth that may be precipitated by disaster, as seen by Schneider, et al. (2019). In both cases, participant recruitment was quite difficult; this does not imply they are invalid studies, but the nature of disasters creates hurdles in this branch of research. It is best to try to overcome such challenges through less conventional approaches, creative measures, and, possibly, mixed method designs.

Air Pollution

While natural disasters are known to cause trauma to individuals, manmade environmental issues may be equally as traumatizing. In recent years, air pollution has become a larger concern, with the World Health Organization (WHO, 2018) reporting that 2.4 million people die annually from the effects of air pollution. The concept of air pollution generally is understood, but many do not know what specific pollutants may be included. Included in this general term are substances such as gaseous pollutants, metallic or organic compounds, and ***particulate matter (PM)***, which is arguably the substance most responsible for the physical health consequences (WHO, 2016).

With the increasing attention to air pollution and our limited understanding of the phenomenon, various studies have attempted to investigate if there is an association between air pollution and mental disorders, such as depression and anxiety (Braithwaite, Zhang, Kirkbride, Osborn, & Hayes, 2019; D'Antoni, Smith, Auyeung, & Weinman, 2017). These studies focus primarily on *PM,* which is particle pollution that is composed of small particles and liquid drops, since it is understood to be the most serious component and has been associated with oxidative stress in humans and rodents, changes in brain structure, and increased hormone production (Braithwaite, et al., 2019). Since so little is known about the effects air pollution can have on individuals, there have been attempts to correlate it with other more controversial outcomes such as autism (Kalkbrenner, Windham, Serre, Akita, Wang, Hoffman, et al., 2015). The methods employed in such studies are often unfavorable, providing little support for their arguments. These issues are part of the reason why further investigation is warranted regarding air pollution and its effects on not only the environment but also mental well-being.

Methodology and Findings

Researchers are concerned about air pollution's long-term effect on individuals' mental health. Unfortunately, due to budget and time restrictions inherent in longitudinal studies, many researchers are unable to delve into this question. This is, however, not an issue that Pun, Manjourides, and Suh (2017) encountered when they performed a longitudinal study spanning ten years through the National Social Life, Health, and Aging Project (NSHAP), which yielded three waves of data in 2005, 2011, and 2015. This dataset includes 4,008 participants in the United States, aged 57 to 85 years, without cognitive impairments, oversampling African Americans, Hispanics, men, and individuals 75 to 85 years old (Shega, Sunkara, Kotwal, Kern, Henning, McClintock, et al., 2014). Using this dataset, Pun, et al. (2017) investigated air pollution's association with depression and anxiety.

To measure depression and anxiety, Pun, and colleagues (2017) used several validated, standardized questionnaires and well-established cutoffs for clinically relevant cases. These included the Center of Epidemiological Studies Depression 11-item scale (CESD-11) and the Hospital Anxiety and Depression Scale (HADS). For a measurement of air pollution in the participant's environment, a threshold of ***$PM_{2.5}$***—here meaning the aerodynamic diameter of a pollutant's particle was less than or equal to 2.5 *μm*—was established based on ***spatiotemporal models***. They explain that these *spatiotemporal models* collect data at different points in time as well as from different physical points. They are derived from a set of five ***spatiotemporal generalized additive mixed models (GAMMS)*** used by previous researchers. Information regarding air pollution and $PM_{2.5}$ was obtained from the

Environmental Protection Agency. When analyzing the data, Pun, and colleagues (2017) were careful to adjust for demographic variables such as age, sex, race, and external variables including year, season, and day of the week the questionnaire was completed. Among their representative sample of older adults, they found a positive relationship between $PM_{2.5}$ and moderate-to-severe depression and anxiety. Unlike other studies examining the effect of air pollution on mental health (Braithwaite, et al., 2019), Pun, et al. (2017) controlled for socioeconomic status rather comprehensively by using multivariate models in their analysis. They found that participants with low socioeconomic status may be more susceptible to mental disorders after exposure to *PM*. It should be noted, however, that while this study is representative of the population in the United States, the question of whether these findings can be extended to other parts of the world is not addressed.

While Pun et al.'s study focused primarily on air pollution's effects on adults and older individuals, there has also been research on the effects of early life exposure to air pollution. Rivas, Basagaña, Cirach, López-Vicente, Suades-González, Garcia-Esteban, et al.'s (2019) objective was to assess the role of air pollution during different prenatal and postnatal stages of children's cognitive development. Although previous research has looked into the negative effects of air pollution on cognition, there does not seem to be much research on the effect this has on children, specifically in early childhood. In this study, children aged seven to ten from 39 different schools in Spain were recruited, yielding a total sample of 2,897 participants. Using computerized *n-back tests* and the computerized Attentional Network Test (ANT), Rivas, et al. (2019) assessed participants' working memory and attention. For the *n-back test*, participants were asked to click a button when a number appeared on the screen that matched a number that they had viewed *n* steps ago. For the computerized ANT, participants were first shown a screen that included one of three types of cues (no cue, center cue, spatial cue). They were then shown a screen with a target, that is, an arrow pointing either left or right in the center of the screen. Next to the target are other arrows that are also pointing left or right, and these serve as distractor images. The participants are told to indicate the direction the target (the arrow) is pointing while ignoring distractors. The authors note that both the *n-back tests* and ANT have been validated using brain imaging. Using a repeated measures design, the study was administered to each participant twice with a three-month gap between the first and second administration. In addition, in each session, participants performed four repeated tests, hence a mixed-model within- and between-study design.

Further, to estimate $PM_{2.5}$ for the area, Rivas, et al. (2019) used the **land use regression (LUR)** models developed in the European Study of Cohorts for Air Pollution Effects. *LUR* models take several parameters into consideration to predict the concentration of $PM_{2.5}$ in specific locations and periods of time. These models are based on simultaneous measurements of air pollution throughout long periods of time in various urban areas (Eeftens, Beelen, deHoogh, Bellander, Cesaroni, Cirach, et al., 2012). The researchers used *LUR* to estimate the $PM_{2.5}$ concentrations in the participants' places of residence at specific times in order to create a history of exposure to $PM_{2.5}$ from the prenatal period until seven years of age. Rivas, et al. (2019) had difficulty creating a history of exposure for some participants due to these individuals being adopted or the researchers being unable to locate addresses provided by parents. In order to account for potential selection bias in only using participants with available data, Rivas et al. performed an inverse probability weighting for their analysis. Their finding revealed a negative relationship between exposure to $PM_{2.5}$ and working memory at five, six, seven, and ten years of age.

The negative impact of air pollution on working memory in children holds several adverse implications. As these children progress in school, it is highly likely that this disadvantage will hold them back in terms of achievement and/or performance. From the studies discussed here, it seems that vulnerable populations such as children and those in a low socioeconomic class are more likely to experience negative side effects of air pollution due, in part, to poor living conditions or the impediments to their physical development. Studies such as Rivas et al. illustrate the benefits of using creative methods in order to research air pollution and its connection to cognitive and psychological outcomes. The use of longitudinal data for such studies is uncommon but may be worth further investigation based on the findings from Pun, and colleagues (2017). While some may find themselves unable to conduct a longitudinal study, Rivas, et al. (2019) demonstrate that there are other more creative and less labor-intensive methods available to investigate this topic.

Wildfires

Unlike the previously addressed environmental disasters, wildfires are unique in that they are considered both natural and manmade disasters. Wildfires are uncontrollable blazes that can be caused by weather, dry land, and wind. While many are aware of the dangers of wildfires, it should also be noted that they bring certain benefits to the environment. Controlled wildfires allow dead or decaying matter to burn, distributing nutrients to the soil and removing diseased plants and insects that may harm the ecosystem. Despite such benefits, however, recent events have led to more harmful outcomes (Wolters, 2019).

Around the world, climate change has led to increased weather severity and wildfires (also referred to as bushfires; Intergovernmental Panel on Climate Change, 2016; Kitching, 2014). Wildfires can harm property, the environment, and individuals. The United States has the highest number of fires per capita in the industrial world, though the causes range from natural to manmade (U.S. Fire Administration, 2009). In California, for instance, there have been a total of 7,860 wildfires (both man-made and natural) caused by drought, extreme winds, and other factors in 2019 (California Department of Forestry, 2019). One example of a man-made wildfire is the 2008 Tea Fire caused by young adults having a bonfire (California Department of Forestry and Fire Protection, 2008). It should be noted that man-made wildfires tend to be stronger and more destructive, and this may be something researchers consider when examining such phenomena.

Methodology and Findings

In a study by Felix, et al. (2015), the effects of California's wildfires on family functioning (parents and children) was investigated using a conceptual model of post-disaster functioning. Family functioning here can be understood as the interactions between members of the family, but more specifically, the level of conflict and cohesion, as well as quality of communication that occurs as reported by the family. The sample for this study consisted of families affected by wildfires, 60% of whom suffered damage to their homes, while 30% had their homes destroyed. The authors note that efforts to locate participants were not quite uniform, requiring several different methods, partially due to evacuation and relocation, an issue raised earlier in our discussion of recruitment of participants post hurricanes. In Felix et al.'s study, subject recruitment was performed through local newspapers, social media, researchers' door-to-door solicitations in neighborhoods, or other nontraditional methods. A benefit of this study not found in others is that Felix, and colleagues (2015) used parent–youth dyads to study both parents' and children's perspectives regarding how wildfires affected their lives and family functioning.

Felix, et al. (2015) used several measures for this study. One measure, perceived fire-related stress, developed especially for this study by the researchers, focused on what stressors the participants felt related to the fire. This included nine items rated on a 4-point Likert scale, and some examples of items on this scale are "How stressful was the fire right after it happened?" and "How stressed are you now as a result of this fire?" (Felix, et al., 2015, p. 193). Additionally, life stressors were assessed using a ten-item measure for adults and a six-item measure for youth (Freedy, Kilpatrick, & Resnick, 1993). These items addressed serious illnesses, problems at school or work, and having a close friend or family member die, among others. The researchers also used other reliable measures: the PTG short inventory by Cann, et al. (2010), the Mental Health Inventory (commonly used to screen mental health in the general population), and the Protective Factors Survey (which, for this study, focused on the Emotional Support and Family Functioning/Resiliency subscales).

To test the validity of the perceived fire-related stress measure created by the researchers, Felix, and colleagues (2015) compared the information from parent–youth dyads of intact homes with those whose homes were destroyed. Results indicated that, not surprisingly, the group who lost their home showed significantly higher levels of perceived fire-related stress. The authors also found that PTG in youth was related to younger age, being female, and greater perceived fire stress. For parents, PTG was positively related to family type and perceived fire stress. Contrary to past research, however, they explain that income and parent education were not related to PTG for parents and youth. This is possibly due to four critical limitations of this study, such as their small sample size (50 dyads), which limits statistical power. Furthermore, the lack of information on family functioning prior to the wildfires also limits meaningful comparisons between groups. Several of the measures used were either adapted for this study or were developed by the researchers themselves, raising the question of the validity and reliability of the scales. Finally, the timing of data collection also presents an issue, as the researchers did not collect data until one year after the last wildfire, though Felix, and colleagues (2015) argue that this allowed researchers to examine the long-term outcomes of the disaster.

In many studies of disasters, a common limitation is the lack of information about the participants prior to the disaster, as was the case with Felix, et al. (2015). To address this, Brown, Agyapong, Greenshaw, Cribben, MacLean, Drolet, et al. (2019) utilized a control group in their study on the Fort McMurray wildfires in Alberta, Canada, which focused on the effects of this event on adolescent mental health. This wildfire is believed to be manmade due to the scope and magnitude of the fire (CBS, 2016). Brown, et al. (2019) compared two groups of students in grades seven to 12, those from Alberta and therefore directly affected by the disaster, and those from Red Deer, a community similar to Alberta in size but with no recent major disasters. The data were collected 18 months after the initial 2016 wildfires, and the researchers used six questionnaires looking at mental health as well as substance use. These included surveys such as the PHQ, the HADS, and quality-of-life scales (e.g., substance use, self-esteem).

They found that the Alberta residents affected by the Fort McMurray wildfires displayed higher scores for depression symptoms, lower self-esteem, and lower quality-of-life scores compared to those in the Red Deer group. Similarly, this group also scored higher on measures of PTSD, suicidal ideation, and anxiety when compared to the Red Deer group. It should be noted, however, that alcohol and substance use did not differ significantly between the two groups. This finding contradicts previous research suggesting that mental health trends for depression usually coincide with alcohol and substance use. This finding may be due to the limitations of the study, however. Data collection from Red Deer was performed roughly two years before the Fort McMurray wildfire. What is more, this dataset was not initially collected to compare Red Deer residents with others exposed to wildfires.

While having a comparison group is an added benefit, the time difference between data collection for the two groups could affect the results if other events transpired during this time. Alternatively, it could also be considered a benefit that the data were collected before the fire because of the possible indirect effects from a wildfire in another community. Collecting data at a different point in time allows for all communities to be unaffected by the fire. Another issue Brown, and colleagues (2019) acknowledge is that the mean age of the two groups was significantly different; however, they explain that they conducted additional analyses to mitigate this issue.

As we see, study limitations regarding natural and man-made disasters are familiar. Considering the unique quality of wildfires, both natural and man-made, it could be argued that knowing a disaster is natural versus man-made may alter feelings on the perception of the disaster. It does not appear that this has been investigated. Thus, this may be a topic worthy of more attention.

Social Environment

While the first thought that comes to mind when "environment" is introduced is our physical surroundings, social environment—a person's physical and social setting that includes culture and personal relationships—is a second type of environment. Within the social environment, there are narrow and wide social environments, which will be discussed further in this section. More specifically, how individuals seek support and assistance within a social environment will be looked at. This topic has become more relevant than ever considering the recent COVID pandemic.

Methodology and Findings

Often, with trauma, the first source of support that one relies on is family, which is why Hricova (2018) wanted to examine the coping strategies of those who suffer from sudden hearing loss in relation to their social environment. She recruited 64 participants for this study who had been diagnosed with unilateral hearing loss. While previous research has examined coping strategies with hearing loss, many of them, Hricova (2018) noted, did so many months after the initial diagnosis. In order to truly understand how people cope with hearing loss, participants for this study were approached between one and five days after their initial diagnosis with an average of 2.8 days post findings. The Coping Orientation to Problem Experiences (COPE) scale, developed by Carver, Scheier, and Weintraub (1989), was used to measure participant coping. This scale includes two main components: problem- and emotion-focused coping. Within COPE, five items focus on problem-focused coping, six focus on emotion-focused coping, and four focus on maladaptive coping styles. Some examples of items on these scales include "I concentrate my efforts on doing something about it" for problem-focused coping and "I discuss my feelings with someone" for emotion-focused coping. The participant is asked to answer each of these items on a 4-point Likert scale that ranges from "I usually don't do this at all" to "I usually do this a lot" (Hricova, 2018, p. 218). Hricova (2018) found that the most important source of coping for the participants seemed to be the social support of their family. More specifically, she found that, as supported by previous research, there was a preference to avoid coping styles that involved the wider social environment and a greater preference for the narrow social environment. As Hallberg and Carlsson (1991) found, typically individuals will seek support from those within the narrow social environment over the wider social environment. This is possibly due to individuals having a closer connection to the narrow social environment and therefore finding more comfort in it.

While it seems to be understood that the relationships individuals possess within their narrow and wider social environments are considered different, there are some questions regarding the role that the wider environment can play that are often considered. For instance, consider the following scenario: Someone is experiencing a life-threatening condition that renders them unconscious and unable to consent to an experimental treatment that may save their life. In this scenario, is someone within the wider or narrow environment authorized to consent to the novel and unconfirmed treatment even though the person is unable to give informed consent themselves? This may seem like a strange question, but considering the current COVID pandemic, it seems questions such as this have become highly relevant.

Such questions have been asked in the past, in situations where individuals are unable to provide informed consent. Because of this, in the 1900s, US federal regulations adopted protocols which parallel those accepted by the World Medical Association authorizing emergency medical research on patients with a life-threatening condition as long as certain requirements were met (Federal Regulations, 1996; WMA, 2000). Known as the Final Rule, research without informed consent can be conducted as long as five conditions have been met. The first condition states that the individual is experiencing a life-threatening condition and existing treatments are deemed either unsatisfactory or unproven. The second condition states more research is needed to determine the experimental treatment's efficacy or safety. Next, the individual is unable or incapable of rendering consent because of their medical condition. Then, an intervention is deemed necessary before an authorized representative can be located. The final condition is that researchers have observed a number of special protections, one of which is **community consultation** (Ragin, Ricci, Rhodes, Holohan, Smirnoff, & Richardson, 2008). This concept of *community consultation* is not to be confused with **participatory action research**. Under the Final Rule, the community must be consulted as partners, but this role does not give the community the right to veto or overrule the research or impede its implementation. In other words, researchers are required to consult the community, but the community's views are nonbinding on the researchers (NIH, 2002; Ragin, et al., 2008).

The problem with these regulations lies in the concept of *community consultation*. Researchers in the social sciences, geneticists, and community-based participatory researchers have debated the concept and meaning of *community consultation* for more than 60 years (Ragin, et al., 2008). To date, many researchers agree with sociologists that an individual who considers themselves to be a member of a community also agrees to accept, as a condition of that membership, that the community assumes collective responsibility for decisions made on behalf of the individual (Ragin, 2008, Suliman, 1983), thus ceding authority to the social environment. This suggests a deliberative process that engages a sample of the community, consistent with a democratic process that is widely regarded as fair and representative of the community. There are still several questions that require attention regarding *community consultation*, such as whether this is applicable to medical research and who is the "community". Specifically, for the purposes of research, who would be authorized to speak for the incapacitated individual?

A study by Ragin, and colleagues (2008) sought to answer this question as a follow-up to a study determining whether members of the public (i.e., laypersons) could be trained to use automatic electronic defibrillators (AEDs) following an out-of-hospital cardiac arrest. Cardiac arrests are fatal for 95% of persons experiencing such events outside of hospital environments (Engelstein & Zipes, 1998). Participants for the study by Ragin, and colleagues (2008) were recruited in two phases. In Phase One researchers conducted a two-stage cluster random sampling procedure, first selecting a stratified random sample of 35 of the 59 New York City residential apartment buildings used in the original AED study. Then, using a purposive random sampling procedure, Ragin, and colleagues (2008) recruited volunteers for six focus groups to inform and refine the development of an interview instrument called the Community VOICES Interview Instrument (see Ragin, et al., 2008). The focus group instrument obtained participants' views on informed consent for research, the definition of community, research risks and benefits, and research burdens (Richardson, 2005).

In Phase Two, Ragin, and colleagues (2008) again employed a two-stage random cluster sampling procedure to recruit participants for the in-person interviews. Selecting from the same 35 buildings used in Phase One, the researchers conducted active, on-site recruitment for interviews, which were conducted on-site at the point of contact. All participants were screened for eligibility (i.e., residents or employees of the building at least three months prior to the interview). The Community VOICES instrument designed for this study obtained demographic information (e.g., length of residence/employment; number of household members; descriptive information including age, ethnicity, and gender), definition of community (e.g., how do you define community), self-defined community membership (e.g., which community/ies do you belong to, which community they are most closely affiliated with), and community spokesperson (i.e., who is the community spokesperson and who should be consulted to discuss emergency medical research for incapacitated persons).

Ragin, and colleague's (2008) study identified five core definitions of community: demographic cohorts (people with similar demographic characteristics), experience cohorts (people with similar interests and experiences), geographic cohorts (community as location), intimates (close friends or family), and professional or workplace cohorts (occupation or workplace). More telling, however, few respondents named or identified persons from their respective social communities to be spokespersons for community matters. What is more, the identified spokespersons were rarely the same surrogate to whom responders granted decision-making authority for emergency medical research. Rather, most people identified medical experts or people with the disease (Ragin, et al., 2008).

What do these findings imply with respect to the role of the social environment? In the abstract, they suggest that while respondents understand and define their social community on five distinct dimensions and appear willing to accept a democratic process for community decision-making in general, they are more prescriptive when delegating responsibility for medical care. They default to medical experts or persons suffering from similar health ailments to make decisions for them if they are incapacitated. Many participants declined to name family or close friends as surrogates. Applying these findings to real events, it suggests that when addressing life-threatening pandemics, such as COVID-19, medical experts and/or previous COVID persons may be the preferred decision-makers for incapacitated persons. Limitations of this study, however, include the instruments, which were developed by researchers for the Community VOICES study and are therefore not validated. Additionally, although the study used cluster random sampling procedures, eligibility was restricted to 35 of the 59 New York City buildings participating in an earlier study, hence limiting generalizability.

Conclusion

The studies presented in this chapter show that environmental psychology is a diverse field. Natural limitations are present when conducting research on hurricanes, wildfires, and other natural disasters, requiring unique and creative methods to access the affected populations. Studies investigating relationships in the social environment can also encounter limitations when addressing a unique population. While many of the studies discussed have used convenience sampling, which is typically discouraged in research, this does not take away from their strengths. This method of sampling has been seen to be the most appropriate for environmental studies due to the complications discussed previously that are naturally attached to this field of research. Through the use of creative methodology, such as using preexisting data to create a baseline measure for comparison (Felix, et al., 2015; Lowe, et al., 2015), we can see that this method of sampling does not inherently disqualify a study if it also includes innovative and strong measures to compensate for that limitation.

References

Blake, E. S., Kimberlain, T. B., Berg, R. J., Cangialosi, J., & Beven, J. L. (2013). *Tropical cyclone report: Hurricane sandy.* Retrieved from www.nhc.noaa.gov/data/tcr/AL182012_Sandy.pdf

Braithwaite, I., Zhang, S., Kirkbride, J. B., Osborn, D. P. J., & Hayes, J. F. (2019). Air pollution (particulate matter) exposure and associations with depression, anxiety, bipolar, psychosis and suicide risk: A systematic review and meta-analysis. *Environmental Health Perspectives, 127*(12), 1–23. https://doi.org/10.1289/EHP4595

Briere, J., & Hedges, M. (2010). Trauma symptom inventory. In I. B. Weiner & W. E. Craighead (Eds.), *The Corsini encyclopedia of psychology.* https://doi.org/10.1002/9780470479216.corpsy1010

Brown, M. R. G., Agyapong, V., Greenshaw, A. J., Cribben, I., MacLean, P. B., Drolet, J., et al. (2019). After the Fort McMurray wildfire there are significant increases in mental health symptoms in grade 7–12 students compared to controls. *BMC Psychiatry, 19*(18). https://doi.org/10.1186/s12888-018-2007-1

California Department of Forestry. (2019). *2019 incident archive.* Retrieved from www.fire.ca.gov/incidents/2019/

California Department of Forestry and Fire Protection. (2008). *Tea fire.* Retrieved from http://cdfdata.fire.ca.gov/incidents/incidents_details_info?incident_id307

Cann, A., Calhoun, L. G., Tedeschi, R. G., Taku, K., Vishnevsky, T., Triplett, K. N., et al. (2010). A short form of the posttraumatic growth inventory. *Anxiety, Stress, and Coping, 23*(2), 127–137. http://dx.doi.org/10.1080/10615800903094273

Carver, C. S., Scheier, M. F., & Weintraub, J. F. (1989). Assessing coping strategies: A theoretically based approach. *Journal of Personality and Social Psychology, 56*(2), 267-283. doi:10.1037//0022-3514.56.2.267

CBS. (2016). *Someone likely sparked the Fort McMurray wildfires, but was it a crime? RCMP ask.* Retrieved from www.cbc.ca/news/canada/edmonton/fort-mcmurray-wildfire-cause-investigation-rcmp-1.3635241

Chan, C. S., & Rhodes, J. E. (2014). Measuring exposure in hurricane Katrina: A meta-analysis and an integrative data analysis. *PLoS One, 9*(4), e92899. doi:10.1371/journal.pone.0092899

Collier, L. (2016). Growth after trauma. *American Psychological Association, 47*(10), 48. Retrieved from www.apa.org/monitor/2016/11/growth-trauma

Cutrona, C. E., & Russell, D. W. (1987). The provisions of social relationships and adaptation to stress. In W. H. Jones & D. Perlman (Eds.), *Advances in personal relationships* (Vol. 1, pp. 37–67). Greenwich, CT: JAI Press.

D'Antoni, D., Smith, L., Auyeung, V., & Weinman, J. (2017). Psychosocial and demographic predictors of adherence and non-adherence to health advice accompanying air quality warning systems: A systematic review. *Environmental Health: A Global Access Science Source, 16*(1), 100–118. https://doi:10.1186/s12940-017-0307-4

Eeftens, M., Beelen, R., deHoogh, K., Bellander, T., Cesaroni, G., Cirach, M., et al. (2012). Development of land use regression models for PM(2.5), PM(2.5)absorbance, PM(10) and PM(coarse) in 20 European study areas: Results of the ESCAPE project. *Environmental Science Technology, 46*(20), 11195–11205. https://doi.org/10.1021/es301948k

Elal, G., & Slade, P. (2005). Traumatic Exposure Severity Scale (TESS): A measure of exposure to major disasters. *Journal of Traumatic Stress, 18*(3), 213–220. doi:10.1002/jts.20030

Engelstein, E. D., & Zipes, D. P. (1998). Sudden cardiac death. In R. W. Alexander, R. C. Sclant, & V. Fuster (Eds.), *Hurst's the heart, arteries and veins* (9th ed., Vol. 1, pp. 1081–1112). New York, NY: McGraw-Hill Book Company.

Federal Regulations. (1996). Protection of human subjects informed consent and waiver of Informed consent requirements in certain emergency research: Final rules. *(21c CFR Part 50.24 and 45 Part 46.101), 61*(192), 51497–51531.

Felix, E., Afifi, T., Kia-Keating, M., Brown, L., Afifi, W., & Reyes, G. (2015). Family functioning and posttraumatic growth among parents and youth following wildfire disasters. *American Journal of Orthopsychiatry, 85*(2), 191–200. https://doi.org/10.1037/ort0000054

Freedy, J. R., Kilpatrick, D. G., & Resnick, H. S. (1993). *The psychological impact of the Oakland Hills Fire: Final report.* Charleston, SC: Medical University of South Carolina.

Grainger, R. D., Levin, C., Allen-Byrd, L., Doctor, R. M., & Lee, H. (1997). An empirical evaluation of Eye Movement Desensitization and Reprocessing (EMDR) with survivors of a natural disaster. *Journal of Traumatic Stress, 10*, 665–671. https://doi.org/10.1023/A:1024806105473

Guite, H. F., Clark, C., & Ackrill, G. (2006). The impact of the physical and urban environment on mental wellbeing. *Public Health, 120*(12), 1117–1126. https://doi.org/10.1016/j.puhe.2006.10.005

Hallberg, L. R., & Carlsson, S. G. (1991). A qualitative study of strategies for managing a hearing impairment. *British Journal of Audiology, 25*(3), 201-211. https://doi.org/10.3109/03005369109079853

Harville, E. W., Xiong, X., Smith, B. W., Pridjian, G., Elkind-Hirsch, K., & Buekens, P. (2011). Combined effects of Hurricane Katrina and Hurricane Gustav on the mental health of mothers of small children. *Journal of Psychiatric and Mental Health Nursing, 18*(4), 288–296. http://dx.doi.org/10.1111/j.1365-2850.2010.01658.x

Hricova, M. (2018). Coping strategies and social environment of patients with sudden hearing loss. *Health Psychology Report, 6*(3) 216–221. https://doi.org/10.5114/hpr.2018.75122

Intergovernmental Panel on Climate Change: *Fifth Assessment Report.* (2016). Retrieved January 15, 2020, from www.ipcc.ch/report/ar5/

Kalkbrenner, A. E., Windham, G. C., Serre, M. L., Akita, Y., Wang, X., Hoffman, K., et al. (2015). Particulate matter exposure, prenatal and postnatal windows of susceptibility, and autism spectrum disorders. *Epidemiology, 26*(1), 30–42. https://doi.org/10.1097/EDE.0000000000000173

Kaur, N., Porter, B., LeardMann, C. A., Tobin, L. E., Lemus, H., & Luxton, D. D. (2017). Evaluation of a modified version of the Posttraumatic Growth Inventory-Short Form. *BMC Med Res Methodology, 17*(69). https://doi.org/10.1186/s12874-017-0344-2

Kitching, R. (2014). *IPCC: Australia and New Zealand face greater fire and flood risk, damage to coral reefs.* Retrieved January 15, 2020, from http://theconversation.com/ipcc-australia-andnew-zealand-face-greater-fire-and-flood-risk-damage-to-coral-reefs-24642

Lowe, S. R., Rhodes, J. E., & Waters, M. C. (2015). Understanding resilience and other trajectories of psychological distress: A mixed-methods study of low-income mothers who survived Hurricane Katrina. *Current Psychology*, *34*(3), 537–550. doi:10.1007/s12144-015-9362-6

National Institutes of Health. (2002). *Points to consider when planning a genetic study that Involves members of named populations*. Retrieved from www.nih.gov./sigs/Bioethics/named_populations.html

Nigg, J. M., Barnshaw, J. & Torres, M.R. (2006). Hurricane Katrina & the flooding of New Orleans: Emergent issues in sheltering & temporary housing. The Annals of the American Academy of Political & Social Science, *604*(1), 113–128.

NOAA. (2018). *What is a hurricane?* Retrieved May 20, 2020, from https://oceanservice.noaa.gov/facts/hurricane.html

Norris, F. H., Friedman, M. J., Watson, P. J., Byrne, C. M., & Kaniasty, K. (2002). 60, 000 Disaster victims speak: Part 1. An empirical review of the empirical literature, 1981–2001. *Psychiatry*, *65*(3) 207–239. doi:10.1521/psyc.65.3.207.20173

Norris, F. H., Perilla, J. L., Riad, J. K., Kaniasty, K., & Lavizzo, E. A. (1999). Stability and change in stress, resources, and psychological distress following natural disaster: Findings from Hurricane Andrew. *Anxiety, Stress, and Coping*, *12*(4), 363–396. http://dx.doi.org/10.1080/10615809908249317

Proshansky, H. M. (1976). Environmental psychology and the real world. *American Psychologist*, *31*(4), 303–310. https://doi.org/10.1037/0003-066X.31.4.303

Pun, V. C., Manjourides, J., & Suh, H. (2017). Association of ambient air pollution with depressive anxiety symptoms in older adults: Results from the NSHAP study. *Environmental Health Perspective*, *125*(3), 342–348. doi:10.1289/EHP494

Ragin, D. F., Ricci, E., Rhodes, R., Holohan, J., Smirnoff, M., & Richardson, L. D. (2008). Defining the "community" in community consultation: Findings from the community VOICES study. *Social Science & Medicine*, *66*, 1379–1392.

Rhodes, J. E., Chan, C. S., Paxson, C., Rouse, C. E., Waters, M. C., & Fussell, E. (2010). The impact of Hurricane Katrina on the mental and physical health of low-income parents in New Orleans. *American Journal of Orthopsychiatry*, *80*(2), 237–247. doi:10.1111/j.1939-0025.2010.01027.x

Richardson, L. D. (2005). The ethics of research without consent in emergency situations. *The Mount Sinai Journal of Medicine*, *77*, 242–249.

Rivas, I., Basagaña, X., Cirach, M., López-Vicente, M., Suades-González, E., Garcia-Esteban, R., et al. (2019). Association between early life exposure to air pollution and working memory and attention. *Environmental Health Perspectives*, *127*(5), 1–11. https://doi.org/10.1289/EHP3169

Schneider, S., Rasul, R., Liu, B., Corry, D., Lieberman-Cribbin, W., Watson, A., et al. (2019). Examining posttraumatic growth and mental health difficulties in the aftermath of hurricane sandy. *Psychological Trauma: Theory, Research, Practice, and Policy*, *11*(2), 127–136. http://dx.doi.org/10.1037/tra0000400

Shega, J. W., Sunkara, P. D., Kotwal, A., Kern, D. W., Henning, S. L., McClintock, M. K., et al. (2014). Measuring cognition: The Chicago cognitive function measure in the national social life, health and aging project, Wave 2. *Journal of Gerontology: Series B*, *69*(2), 166–176. doi:10.1093/geronb/gbu106

Suliman, A. (1983). Effective refugee health depends on community participation. *Carnets de L'enfance*, *2*, 2.

Tedeschi, R. G., & Calhoun, L. G. (1996). The posttraumatic growth inventory: Measuring the positive legacy of trauma. *Journal of Traumatic Stress*, *9*(3), 455–471. doi:10.1007/bf02103658

U.S. Fire Administration/National Fire Data Center. (2009). *Fire in the United States 2003–2007*. Emmitsburg, MD: Federal Emergency Management Agency. Retrieved from www.usfa.dhs.gov/applcations/publications

Vernberg, E. M., Greca, A. M., Silverman, W. K., & Prinstein, M. J. (1996). Prediction of posttraumatic stress symptoms in children after Hurricane Andrew. *Journal of Abnormal Psychology*, *105*(2), 237–248. https://doi.org/10.1037/0021-843X.105.2.237

Washington Post, Kaiser Family Foundation & Harvard University. (2005). *Survey of Hurricane Katrina Evacuees*. September, No 7401. Retrieved May 24, 2020, from www.kff.org/newsmedia/upload/7401.pdf

WHO. (2016). *Ambient air pollution: A global assessment of exposure and burden of disease*. Geneva, Switzerland: World Health Organization. Retrieved from https://apps.who.int/iris/bitstream/handle/10665/250141/9789241511353-eng.pdf

WHO (World Health Organization). (2018). *Joint effects of air pollution data by country*. Retrieved from http://apps.who.int/gho/data/node.main.ENVHEALTHJOINTAAPHAP?lang=en

Wolters, C. (2019). *California fires are raging: Get the facts on wildfires*. Retrieved from www.nationalgeographic.com/environment/natural-disasters/wildfires/#close

World Medical Association. (2000). *Declaration of Helsinki: Ethical principles for medical research involving human subjects*. World Medical Association. Adopted by the 18th WMA General Assembly, Kelsinki, Finland, June 1964. Amended by the 52nd WMA General Assembly, Edinburgh, Scotland, October.

21

MULTIPLE WAYS OF UNDERSTANDING VACCINE HESITANCE AND REFUSAL

Jennifer A. Reich

"My daughter is coming up on her second birthday, which is when we decided we'd start selectively vaccinating. I definitely want to keep shots to a minimum . . . but I'm struggling with what I want to move forward with. I was hoping the community could share what alternative schedules they've followed."

"We haven't vaccinated our 4½ year old daughter at all. After we did a ton of research into what vaccines actually do and don't do, we can clearly see that vaccines do nothing good, don't prevent any diseases, all they cause is harm in the body's every system possible."

Overview

This exchange in an online forum where mothers share information about their children's health and family goals illustrates some of the contemporary disagreements about vaccines (see Reich, 2018b). Both of these mothers have rejected the vaccine schedule recommended by federal advisory boards, government agencies, and pediatric associations, yet each has landed on different views about whether vaccines are beneficial, when they might be necessary, and if and how they should be administered. Although they may seem like outliers in the world of healthcare decision-making, their views represent a growing trend.

The Gallup poll in early 2020 released data to show that while most Americans—84 percent—agree that parents should vaccinate their children, this figure is much lower than it was in 2001, when 94 percent of Americans answered that parents should (Reinhart, 2020). Of course, what people say they think is important on a poll may not fully represent what people actually do. However, when it comes to vaccines, we do know that a growing number of parents are opting out of some or all vaccines for their children (Samuel, 2017). Both **vaccine refusal**, meaning parents opting out of all vaccines by choice, and **vaccine hesitance**, in which parents reject select vaccines or delay them beyond when they are recommended by experts, are increasing. The result has been a rise in vaccine-preventable diseases (Phadke, Bednarczyk, Salmon, & Omer, 2016). This trend raises important questions. How has a technology that 20 years ago was overwhelmingly seen as an essential tool in protecting individual and community health come to be increasingly seen as a personal choice and one that is not really necessary or important? Who are the parents rejecting vaccines and expert recommendations for them? What can be done to change their minds?

Part of what is most perplexing about this trend is that those who reject vaccines are not, in fact, uneducated or anti-science, despite how they are often portrayed in the media. In fact, as I detail later in this chapter, parents who reject some or all vaccines for their children are more likely to be white, college-educated, and have economic resources that support access to healthcare (Leask, 2011; McNutt, Desemone, DeNicola, El Chebib, Nadeau, Bednarczyk, et al., 2016). It is important that students and scholars of health understand the complexities of decision-making about vaccines as a way of understanding how parents make decisions for their children in hopes of protecting their health.

This chapter provides an overview of research on *vaccine refusal* and *vaccine hesitance* with particular attention to the different kinds of methods that reveal different information. Identifying how researchers design their studies in varied ways to answer particular questions about *vaccine hesitance* is key. For example, understanding population-level characteristics of families who opt out requires the use of existing datasets with hundreds of thousands of respondents. Some researchers wanting to understand what families do in medical encounters use administrative data that may record billing or health information like state vaccine records to identify patterns. These data were not created for the purposes of research, and thus researchers are limited by the information collected in these systems. However, they can be informative for understanding what is happening more quickly, with more generalizability, and many more participants than if researchers set out to collect that information themselves. When researchers want answers to more targeted questions, many conduct surveys to understand attitudes, decisions, and perceptions or conduct experiments where they control the options available to see how participants respond to controlled situations. To understand more in-depth questions, often with more exploratory goals, others conduct in-depth interviews with a smaller number of people or observe them in their social worlds to understand how interaction, experience, and context shape their decisions. Each of these research designs trades our ability to understand something about the broader population for a deeper understanding of a smaller number of participants. All approaches contribute to our understanding of this important topic.

In this chapter, I begin with an overview of the policies and practices of vaccination in the United States. I then highlight some studies that use quantitative data—from existing datasets and surveys—to provide important measures of patterns among parents of children who are not fully immunized. Next, I describe key ways that qualitative methods—including interviews and ethnographic observations—build on these quantitative studies to identify more subtle processes that inform parental decision-making. Finally, I point to some research that aims to identify ways to persuade parents to choose differently and fully participate in public health campaigns like those for childhood immunization.

Research in Practice

Vaccines in Context

Vaccine policy alongside vaccine decision-making are significant issues for those interested in health. Unlike most other healthcare and medical interventions in which the individual derives all of the benefit, vaccines are most effective when used by approximately 85 to 95 percent of the community (depending on the disease) to create what public health experts call herd immunity (CDC, 2001). These high levels of protection keep infectious disease contained and protect those in the community who are most vulnerable to infection, including those who are immune-compromised, are too young to be vaccinated, have lost immunity with age or illness, or for whom immunizations are not effective (Sobo, 2016).

In pursuit of these broader public health goals, parents in the United States are expected to consent to immunize their children against 13 diseases on a schedule set by a federal advisory panel, approved by the American Academy of Pediatrics, and then administered in doctors' offices as part of routine pediatric care to children. Experts typically recommend use of these vaccines between birth and six years of age, with other vaccines offered later into adolescence and young adulthood.

The expectation that parents will provide consent is communicated culturally through public health messaging, during appointments with healthcare providers, and through institutional requirements in which parents must show evidence of immunization for admission to schools or childcare settings or must file an application for an exemption as allowed in their state. Currently, all states and the District of Columbia (WDC) allow exemption for medical reasons and 45 states and WDC allow exemptions for people who have religious objections to immunizations. Additionally, 15 states allow philosophical exemptions for those who object to immunizations because of personal, philosophical, or conscientiously held beliefs (NCSL, 2020). Exemptions to vaccine requirements allow kids to attend school without evidence of immunization and are used most often by white, affluent families (McNutt, Desemone, DeNicola, El Chebib, Nadeau, Bednarczyk, et al., 2016; Smith, Chu, & Barker, 2004; Yang, Delamater, Leslie, & Mello, 2016). Studies of California, a state that until 2016 had a religious and philosophical belief exemption, suggest that by removing exemptions from law, fewer families are opting out (Buttenheim, Jones, Mckown, Salmon, & Omer, 2018).

These legal requirements for vaccination affect children prior to enrolling in school. However, many vaccines are most beneficial to younger children. As a result, pediatricians and family practitioners who provide medical care to children often must persuade parents to consent to vaccines in the first few years of life, since infants and toddlers are at highest risk of the devastating complications of infection. Whether parents perceive healthcare providers are trustworthy, empathetic, honest about what they perceive to be the possible risks of vaccination, and independent of government or pharmaceutical sources of information matters in these encounters (Leask, 2009; Paulussen, Hoekstra, Lanting, Buijs, & Hirasing, 2006; Ward, Peretti-Watel, Bocquier, Seror, & Verger, 2019). Public health agencies and pharmaceutical companies encourage parents to see the benefits of vaccines for their babies with campaigns and advertisements that promise that "vaccines help strengthen your baby's immune system and keep him safe from vaccine-preventable diseases" and that advise parents "Love them. Protect them. Immunize them" (Reich, 2020). The result is that parents largely see vaccines as technology for personal benefit, rather than part of a community strategy and view their decision as a personal one in which they must weigh the risks and benefits for their own children but not for anyone else's (Reich, 2016; Sobo, 2016). As an increasing number of parents approach vaccines in a cafeteria style of picking and choosing which vaccines, if any, they want for their children, rates of infectious diseases are growing, which increases risk to others (Reich, 2016). How then do we understand who the refusers are, how they come to reject vaccines, and possible solutions to this challenge to public health? It turns out that the solution requires a variety of methods and tools.

Who Are These Parents?

When the polio vaccine was licensed in 1955, it was broadly seen as a miracle that could relieve the sense of fear parents experienced as they worried about their children's well-being (Oshinsky, 2005). Yet upon licensing, there was immediately more demand than supply. Passionate arguments about how the vaccine should be distributed, followed by whether those with private physicians and able to pay full price for the vaccine should have first claim to it, soon followed (Colgrove, 2006). As new vaccines were licensed through the 1960s, these arguments continued, particularly as good evidence showed that low-income children did not access vaccines in equal numbers as higher-income children. Public health researchers became increasingly concerned about these under-vaccinated children who lacked resources or access to medical care. In fact, many of the state-level mandates for vaccines became law through the 1960s and 1970s as a way to increase access by leveraging new federal funding for vaccines (Conis, 2015).

Despite long-standing concern about the under-vaccinated, a new trend emerged that would also concern public health experts. In 2003, county health departments began reporting the problem of children who were unvaccinated because their parents refused vaccines. In one New York county, the county health commissioner identified an outbreak of pertussis (also known as whooping cough) that started with children who were not vaccinated because their parents had decided against it. That outbreak then spread into a neighboring county where up to 25 children also contracted pertussis (Smith, et al., 2004). Understanding which children were unvaccinated by choice was important.

Efforts to understand this outbreak specifically and broad patterns in *vaccine refusal* generally required large-scale epidemiological data that can tell us something about the population. Public health researchers Smith and colleagues from the federal Centers for Disease Control and Prevention (CDC) responded to the aforementioned pertussis outbreak in New York in the article "Children Who Have Received No Vaccines: Who Are They and Where Do They Live?" and provided an important framework for understanding vaccine refusal.

These researchers analyzed the National Immunization Survey (NIS), a survey that since 1994 has sampled parents of children 19 to 35 months of age in 27 metropolitan statistical areas in all 50 states. The CDC conducts the NIS to collect statistical information on health and does not include identifiable information about individuals. At the time (around 2001), the larger NIS was conducted by contacting households with children who are age one year or older by using list-assisted, random-digit dialing to call people. Individuals with children the right age answered a survey about each child in the home as well as demographic and socioeconomic information about the child's mother and household, as well as answering questions about the child's vaccination history. Interviewers then asked for consent to access children's medical records. If parents provided consent, someone from NIS contacted these healthcare providers by mail to get children's vaccination histories, which allowed researchers to verify whether children have received all doses of recommended vaccines and to estimate vaccination coverage rates.

This study found that in 2001, about 62.8 percent of all children 19 to 35 months of age (the age range reported for evaluations of early vaccines) in the United States were fully vaccinated, an estimated 36.9 percent were under-vaccinated, and approximately 0.3 percent were unvaccinated (Smith, et al., 2004). What was perhaps most significant in this study was the differences they uncovered between the families of children who were under-vaccinated and those that were unvaccinated by choice. The researchers found that compared with fully vaccinated children, under-vaccinated children were significantly more likely to be black (than Hispanic or white), younger, and foreign-born. Under-vaccinated children also were significantly more likely to have a mother who was young; widowed, divorced, or separated; and whose highest level of educational attainment was high school or less than a college degree. In addition, under-vaccinated children were significantly more likely to live in a household with an annual income below the poverty level and to have moved across state lines since birth. In contrast, the researchers found that unvaccinated children whose parents did not want vaccines were significantly more likely to be white, to have a mother who had a college degree, to have a mother older than 30 years of age, and to live in a household with an annual income at or exceeding $75,000 (Smith, et al., 2004).

These findings, along with subsequent ones, have provided important information about which families opt out of vaccines. Yet over time, the question of which parents are rejecting some vaccines has become more complex. There is information that parents who would have been classified as the under-vaccinated based on the aforementioned characteristics are also intentionally skipping and spacing vaccines and that the number of parents doing so is increasing (Robison, Groom, & Young, 2012). At times, parents appear to be following an alternative schedule—consenting to some vaccines in a manner inconsistent with expert recommendations. Understanding these patterns has become increasingly important to thinking about herd immunity. Different research teams have set out to understand this trend in different ways. One group used a cross-sectional (data collected at one point in time), internet-based survey of a nationally representative sample of parents of children six months to six years of age to understand patterns in vaccine decision-making and "malleability" (Dempsey,

Schaffer, Singer, Butchart, Davis, & Freed, 2011). Their findings suggest that 13 percent of parents reported following an alternative vaccine schedule. Most delayed certain vaccines or delayed some vaccines until their children were older. They also found that even among parents who fully vaccinated their children, many feel uncertain this was the safest course. Specifically, 28 percent of parents following the recommended vaccination schedule thought that delaying vaccine doses was safer than the schedule they had used, and 22 percent disagreed that the best vaccination schedule to follow was the one recommended by vaccination experts. This study is significant in providing information about parents who delay vaccines, but also about how many parents who fully vaccinate their children lack confidence in that choice.

Another research group aimed to understand the use of alternative vaccine schedules using existing immunization information system data (Nadeau, Bednarczyk, Masawi, Meldrum, Santilli, Zansky, et al., 2014). They evaluated children born in New York State (outside of New York City) between 2009 and 2011 and identified those vaccine patterns are consistent with use of an alternative schedule. They found that of the 222,628 children studied, the proportion of children following an alternative schedule was about 25 percent. These children were significantly less likely to be up-to-date with recommended vaccines at nine months of age (15 percent) compared with those following the routine schedule (90 percent). This study is significant in suggesting that as many as one in four children may not be fully vaccinated consistent with expert-recommended schedules because of parental choice. Using newer data from the aforementioned NIS, a more recent study suggests the number of children not fully vaccinated may be even higher. Hargreaves, Nowak, Frew, Hinman, Orenstein, Mendel, et al. (2020) estimate that only 63 percent of children ages 19 to 35 months were classified as following recommended vaccine schedules and only 58 percent were up-to-date on those recommendations. This study suggests that as many as one-third of children are receiving vaccines on an alternate or delayed schedule.

How Do We Understand Parental Decision-Making?

How parents come to delay or refuse vaccines is not only a complex question but important for public health goals. Some survey data identify reasons parents space or skip vaccines, including fear of a complication or reaction (Dempsey, et al., 2011; Salmon, Sotir, Pan, Berg, Omer, Stokley, et al., 2009). Survey methods are good for understanding patterns in preferences, particularly in well-powered and randomly selected samples. However, they require a limited number of options from which respondents can choose. Those options must be known to those who design and deploy the survey and thus potentially eliminate other possibilities. Although these quantitative health data are essential for understanding broader patterns among parents in communities, they cannot necessarily elucidate the myriad reasons parents may opt to space or skip vaccines and the reasons for those decisions. They also miss the cultural contexts in which parents make these choices. A deeper exploration of how parents view vaccines requires more fine-grained measurements. How do parents decide? What values and goals do these decisions represent? How do social networks and communities shape these outcomes? Which sources of information do they trust?

In a broader effort to measure vaccine concerns in different countries, researchers from the Social Science and Immunization Project (SSIM) drew on ethnographic data along with interviews, focus groups, and surveys from Bangladesh, Ethiopia, India, Malawi, The Netherlands, and The Philippines. The SSIM was a transnational multi-institutional research project that used mixed methods to understand vaccine acceptance. With these data, the SSIM researchers were able to identify "local vaccine cultures" that reflect how parents understand health systems, share information with neighbors and families, view disease, and perceive the potency of modern medicine—including preventative measures (Streefland, 1999). This is a significant reminder of how cultural context shapes perceptions, even as the specific contexts may be different.

To understand the cultural contexts that lead to *vaccine refusal*, researchers must study vaccines and families in contexts. Returning to the United States, anthropologist Elisa Sobo, for example, used focus groups and in-depth interviews to examine the views of vaccines held by parents in a Waldorf school, a private school with low rates of immunization. Sobo found that parents were not ignorant about vaccines and infection, but rather saw vaccines as unnecessary, toxic, developmentally inappropriate, and profit driven. Most notable, Sobo found that vaccine concerns grew after school enrollment, suggesting that refusal is cultivated in social contexts and through networks—including in a school that encourages questioning health and vaccines. Quantitative studies have shown that *vaccine refusal* clusters in networks (Lieu, Ray, Klein, Chung, & Kulldorff, 2015; May & Silverman, 2003; Omer, Enger, Moulton, Halsey, Stokley, & Salmon, 2008; Salathé & Bonhoeffer, 2008)—that knowing others who do not vaccinate increases the odds that someone also will not vaccinate. Qualitative findings like these help provide explanation of these processes (Poltorak, Leach, Fairhead, & Cassell, 2005; Reich, 2018a, 2018b; Sobo, 2015). Sobo also showed that even when parents understood the scientific goals of herd immunity, they were not necessarily inclined to believe those goals were important or to perceive their role in contributing to it.

My own sociological research explored patterns of vaccine refusal and vaccine hesitance, including how parents make decisions in the context of law, health policy, cultural information, and pediatric encounters (Reich, 2016). To do so, I drew on a range of data. First, I analyzed in-depth interviews with parents, pediatricians, other healthcare providers, and key informants, which included vaccine researchers and policy makers. Second, I collected data during ethnographic observations in spaces where vaccines are discussed, including at meetings of organizations opposed to vaccine mandates, parent education events about vaccines, hearings in the vaccine injury compensation program, meetings of parenting groups discussing vaccines, and pediatric trainings at a local children's hospital. Unlike interview data, where participants respond to questions the researcher poses, ethnographic observation allowed me to analyze conversations as they occur without my prompting and to observe different social worlds that contribute to shaping the social meanings that in turn shape vaccine encounters. Additionally, I analyzed popular cultural media, online parenting blogs in which parents talk to each other about vaccines, like the ones at the beginning of the chapter, and policies relating to vaccines. Together, this research aimed to understand parent decision-making in context and to identify how broader cultural definitions of good parenting and of good health inform vaccine decisions. Rather than focusing solely on vaccines, my research identified how parents in general, and mothers specifically, see themselves as experts on their own children and able to make the best healthcare decisions for their family. Given the aforementioned patterns that White women with higher incomes are most likely to deliberately reject vaccines, this study allowed me to understand how women with privilege view both definitions of good parenting and health as a series of individual informed consumption choices (Reich, 2014).

What Changes Perceptions of Vaccines?

These different lines of research—both quantitative and qualitative—have allowed for a more nuanced understanding of how parents make decisions, what the outcomes of those decisions are, and how they are based on individually held values and views. The question then is what to do about this? Newer research has aimed to find empirically tested ways to design and implement interventions that might change parents' minds. This has led to innovative experimental designs to test how communication about vaccines affects views, which in turn has yielded some mixed results.

A group of political scientists and public health researchers set out to test how vaccine messaging affected parental views (Nyhan, et al., 2014). To do so, they conducted a two-wave online survey. In the first wave, before the intervention, participants answered questions about health and vaccine attitudes, including questions about the health status of their children and eight "agree/disagree" questions about attitudes toward vaccines. Participants were also asked if they had ever delayed or refused a recommended vaccine, how important vaccines were to them personally, and how much trust they placed in various health professions and institutions. Then the researchers randomly assigned participants from that first survey to receive one of four pro-vaccine messages or to a control message. The messages provided information about the safety of the vaccine against measles, mumps, and rubella (MMR) or the danger of contracting MMR. The four strategies, the authors explained, were adopted from messages distributed by public health agencies and included text from the CDC. One test condition aimed specifically to correct misinformation (like debunking false claims that the MMR vaccine can cause autism). A second presented information on disease risks (including symptoms and risks of MMR infection). A third condition used dramatic narratives (including stories of parents whose children were hospitalized for MMR). The fourth test condition displayed visuals to make disease risks more salient or accessible (including images of children who are infected). After viewing the assigned message, the participants were asked a series of questions designed to assess misperceptions about the MMR vaccine, concerns about side effects, and intent to give MMR to future children.

This study found that none of the interventions increased parental intent to vaccinate a future child. They also found that "refuting claims of an MMR/autism link successfully reduced misperceptions that vaccines cause autism but nonetheless decreased intent to vaccinate among parents who had the least favorable vaccine attitudes" (Nyhan, et al., 2014: e835). Images of sick children surprisingly increased expressed belief in a link between vaccine and autism. A dramatic narrative about an infant in danger actually increased participant-reported beliefs in serious vaccine side effects. In this study and a related one of efforts to correct misinformation about the flu vaccine (Nyhan & Reifler, 2015), the authors conclude that "public health messaging might not be successful in increasing vaccination and might in fact unintentionally increase misperceptions about vaccines, thereby lowering usage. Notably, efforts to correct false information "may be especially likely to be counterproductive" (Nyhan, et al., 2014, p. e835).

Experimental studies have been important in revealing how public education efforts can have unintended consequences. However, follow-up experiments have suggested that not all messaging is unsuccessful. For example, in an effort to increase confidence in vaccines in adults (who were not necessarily parents), one study tested the effects of consensus statements like, "90 percent of medical scientists agree that vaccines are safe" or "90 percent of medical scientists agree that all parents should be required to vaccinate their children" or a combination of both. The authors found that these consensus statements appear to be positive in increasing support for vaccines (van der Linden, et al., 2015, p. 2). Information criticizing vaccines may also be influential in changing minds. Other research suggests that accessing vaccine-critical websites for as little as five to ten minutes increased the perception that vaccination carries risks, decreased fear of skipping vaccines, and possibly decreased intent to vaccinate (Betsch, et al., 2010).

Rather than focusing solely on parents, some research has focused on pediatricians and family practitioners who see children in their offices and recommend vaccines to see how they advise parents. For example, one survey of pediatricians found that 87 percent of providers in 2013 encounter *vaccine refusal*, an increase of about 12.5 percent since 2006. Exploring the outcomes of these encounters, the researchers found that 11.7 percent of pediatricians report that they always dismiss families from their practice for continued *vaccine refusal*, an increase from 6.1 percent in 2006 (Hough-Telford, et al., 2016).

How tolerant physicians should be of *vaccine refusal* is controversial, with some advocates suggesting pediatricians should no longer treat families who distrust or reject their judgment about vaccines presenting a risk to other patients, and others suggesting that partnerships with families can provide opportunities for ongoing discussions (Reich, 2016). How pediatricians emerge from their residency training programs and the experience they have with supervisors appear to shape their approaches.

One study examined how pediatric residents felt about advising parents about vaccines. The authors surveyed 87 residents at two institutions in a region with relatively high *vaccine hesitancy* and found that most residents (68 [79.1 percent]) reported feeling confident in their ability to discuss vaccines. They found, though, that residents who had observed their pediatric faculty agreeing to alternative or delayed vaccinations were more likely to believe this to be acceptable vaccine practice, which they suggest raises questions about how pediatricians are trained (Arora, Lehman, Charlu, Ross, Ardy, Gordon, et al., 2019). Others have evaluated physician views on the importance of particular vaccines (Daley, Crane, Markowitz, Black, Beaty, Barrow, et al., 2010) and to what degree parents trust physicians as a source of information (Freed, Clark, Butchart, Singer, & Davis, 2011).

Other research more directly tested provider communication to identify approaches that are comfortable for providers and more effective (Leask, 2009). One of the more interesting studies tested whether vaccine uptake was higher when a provider announced a child would be vaccinated that day or when they invited an open-ended conversation about vaccination with parents. To test this, the researchers randomized 30 pediatricians to receive no training (which served as a control), training in the "announcement" of vaccines approach, or training in the "conversation" approach. Announcements are described as brief statements that assume parents are ready to vaccinate, whereas conversations engage parents in open-ended discussions. Each approach focused specifically on encouraging use of the vaccine against the human papilloma virus (HPV), which is recommended for boys and girls between 11 and 12 years of age and older. The researchers then monitored vaccines according to a state vaccine registry and found that there was no difference in HPV vaccine rates between the control group who had not received any training and the test group that participated in open-ended discussion. However, they did find that the announcement approach led to increases in HPV uptake by about 5 to 6 percent (Brewer, Hall, Malo, Gilkey, Quinn, & Lathren, 2017). However, this approach did not lead to an increase in other vaccines recommended for teens.

One study asked four stakeholder groups to advise them on which kinds of communication and outcomes are important and to advise them on a survey. These stakeholders included parents or community members, healthcare providers, researchers, and government or non-governmental organization representatives. This method, known as a *Delphi survey*, works to find consensus on particular measures. Participants were asked to rate the importance of eight outcome domains for each of the three communication types, which included efforts to inform and educate, to communicate reminders, and to encourage community engagement. All three communication types were rated as important, but the communication styles that prioritized the "attitudes or beliefs" domain and included "trust" scored the highest and was rated most important. The authors concluded from this process that although some domains were rated higher, communication about vaccination cannot be a "single homogenous intervention," but "has a range of purposes." They suggest that researchers evaluating vaccination communication should select outcomes accordingly (Kaufman, Ryan, Lewin, Bosch-Capblanch, Glenton, Cliff, et al., 2018, 6520). This study reminds us that as researchers continue to evaluate which communication styles are most promising, it is clear that how information is communicated is as important as what is communicated and to whom (Thomson, Vallee-Tourangeau, & Suggs, 2018).

Conclusion

Different research designs answer different questions, and thus yield different results. Quantitative data from surveys and analysis of administrative data are important for providing descriptions of trends about who rejects vaccines, where they live, and how providers respond. Qualitative data have been used to advance contextual meanings of *vaccine hesitance* and *vaccine refusal* by examining the perspectives of those who make vaccine decisions as they perceive meanings and values. At times, findings from qualitative studies inform quantitative studies and at other times, they help to explain patterns. Together, we can see fairly consistent patterns in qualitative and quantitative data about who rejects vaccines and some indications of why. The mechanisms by which individuals come to reject vaccines and the interventions that might change their minds are multifaceted. As a result, research cannot provide easy answers or simple solutions to affect healthcare decision-making. One research method is unlikely to yield the information researchers, practitioners, and policy makers need to advance this issue. Instead, the body of research that draws on multiple methods offers the best path forward to finding the multiple tools that may affect decision-making.

It is tempting to dismiss *vaccine refusal* as simply a personal choice and one that does not require as much attention or tests of intervention as it has received. Unlike other personal health choices, infectious disease does not reside with the individual. The outcomes can be far-reaching for everyone in a community, particularly those that are most vulnerable to the worst outcomes of infection. Looking at infectious disease historically reveals that vaccines have been seen at times as a miraculous solution to life-threatening conditions and also as a source of misgivings (Colgrove, 2006). Yet as parents increasingly voice distrust of vaccines and delay or reject them, they undermine the power vaccines have to potentially save lives. As Australian vaccine researcher Julie Leask cautions, "The safest and most effective vaccines are of little use if too few people take them" (Leask, 2011, p. 445). Thus, it is up to researchers to represent parents' concerns authentically and accurately, and also to find ways to alleviate their concerns.

References

Arora, G., Lehman, D., Charlu, S., Ross, N., Ardy, A., Gordon, B., et al. (2019). Vaccine health beliefs and educational influences among pediatric residents. *Vaccine*, *37*(6), 857–862. https://doi.org/10.1016/j.vaccine.2018.12.038

Betsch, C., Renkewitz, F., Betsch, T., & Ulshöfer, C. (2010). The influence of vaccine-critical websites on perceiving vaccination risks. *Journal of Health Psychology*, *15*(3), 446–455. https://doi.org/10.1177%2F1359105309353647

Brewer, N. T., Hall, M. E., Malo, T. L., Gilkey, M. G., Quinn, B., & Lathren, C. (2017). Announcements versus conversations to improve HPV vaccination coverage: A randomized trial. *Pediatrics*, *139*(1), e20161764. doi:https://doi.org/10.1542/peds.2016-1764

Buttenheim, A. M., Jones, M., Mckown, C., Salmon, S., & Omer, S. B. (2018). Conditional admission, religious exemption type, and nonmedical vaccine exemptions in California before and after a state policy change. *Vaccine*, *36*(26), 3789–3793. https://doi.org/10.1016/j.vaccine.2018.05.050

CDC. (2001). *History and epidemiology of global smallpox eradication*. Atlanta, GA: Centers for Disease, Control Prevention and World Health, Organization.

Colgrove, J. (2006). *State of immunity: The politics of vaccination in twentieth-century America*. Berkeley: University of California.

Conis, E. (2015). *Vaccine nation: America's changing relationship with immunization*. Chicago, IL: University of Chicago Press.

Daley, M. F., Crane, L. A., Markowitz, L. E., Black, S. R., Beaty, B. L., Barrow, J., et al. (2010). Human papillomavirus vaccination practices: A survey of US physicians 18 months after licensure. *Pediatrics*, *126*(3), 425–433. doi:10.1542/peds.2009-3500

Dempsey, A. F., Schaffer, S., Singer, S., Butchart, A., Davis, M., & Freed, G. L.(2011). Alternative vaccination schedule preferences among parents of young children. *Pediatrics*, *128*(5). doi:10.1542/peds.2011-0400

Freed, G. L., Clark, S. J., Butchart, A. T., Singer, D. C., & Davis, M. M. (2011). Sources and perceived credibility of vaccine-safety information for parents. *Pediatrics*, *127*(Supplement 1), S107–S112. https://doi.org/10.1542/peds.2010-1722P

Hargreaves, A. L., Nowak, G., Frew, P., Hinman, A. R., Orenstein, W. A., Mendel, J., et al. (2020). Adherence to timely vaccinations in the United States. *Pediatrics*, *145*(3), e20190783. doi:10.1542/peds.2019-0783

Hough-Telford, C., Kimberlin, D. W., Aban, I., Hitchcock, W. P., Almquist, J., Kratz, R., et al. (2016). Vaccine delays, refusals, and patient dismissals: A survey of pediatricians. *Pediatrics*, *138*(3), e20162127. https://doi.org/10.1542/peds.2016-2127

Kaufman, J., Ryan, R., Lewin, S., Bosch-Capblanch, S., Glenton, C., Cliff, J., et al. (2018). Identification of preliminary core outcome domains for communication about childhood vaccination: An online delphi survey. *Vaccine*, *36*(44), 6520–6528. https://doi.org/10.1016/j.vaccine.2017.08.027

Leask, J. (2009). How do general practitioners persuade parents to vaccinate their children? A study using standardised scenarios. *NSW Public Health Bull*, 20. https://doi.org/10.1071/NB08064

Leask, J. (2011). Target the fence-sitters. *Nature*, 473. https://doi.org/10.1038/473443a

Lieu, T. A., Ray, G. T., Klein, N. P., Chung, C., & Kulldorff, M. (2015). Geographic clusters in underimmunization and vaccine refusal. *Pediatrics*, *135*(2), 280–289. https://doi.org/10.1542/peds.2014-2715

May, T., & Silverman, R. D. (2003). Clustering of exemptions' as a collective action threat to herd immunity. *Vaccine*, *21*(11–12), 1048–1051. https://doi.org/10.1016/S0264-410X(02)00627-8

McNutt, L.-A., Desemone, C., DeNicola, E., El Chebib, H., Nadeau, J. A., Bednarczyk, R. A., et al. (2016). Affluence as a predictor of vaccine refusal and underimmunization in California private kindergartens. *Vaccine*, *34*(14), 1733–1738. https://doi.org/10.1016/j.vaccine.2015.11.063

Nadeau, J. A., Bednarczyk, R. A., Masawi, M. R., Meldrum, M. D., Santilli, L., Zansky, S. M., et al. (2014). Vaccinating my way: Use of alternative vaccination schedules in New York State. *The Journal of Pediatrics*, *166*(1), 151–156. https://doi.org/10.1016/j.jpeds.2014.09.013

NCSL. (2020). States with religious and philosophical exemptions from school immunization requirements. *National Conference of State Legislatures*. Retrieved from www.ncsl.org/research/health/school-immunization-exemption-state-laws.aspx

Nyhan, B., & Reifler, J. (2015). Does correcting myths about the flu vaccine work? An experimental evaluation of the effects of corrective information. *Vaccine*, *33*(3), 459–464. https://doi.org/10.1016/j.vaccine.2014.11.017

Nyhan, B., Reifler, J., Richey, S., & Freed, G. L. (2014). Effective messages in vaccine promotion: A randomized trial. *Pediatrics*, *133*(4), e835–e842. doi:10.1542/peds.2013-2365

Omer, S. B., Enger, K. S., Moulton, L. H., Halsey, N. A., Stokley, S., & Salmon, D. A. (2008). Geographic clustering of nonmedical exemptions to school immunization requirements and associations with geographic clustering of pertussis. *American Journal of Epidemiology*, *168*(15), 1389–1396. https://doi.org/10.1093/aje/kwn263

Oshinsky, D. M. (2005). *Polio: An American story*. Oxford: Oxford University Press.

Paulussen, T. G. W., Hoekstra, F., Lanting, C. I., Buijs, G. B., & Hirasing, R. A. (2006). Determinants of Dutch parents' decisions to vaccinate their child. *Vaccine*, *24*(5), 644–651. https://doi.org/10.1016/j.vaccine.2005.08.053

Phadke, V. K., Bednarczyk, R. A., Salmon, D. A., & Omer, S. B. (2016). Association between vaccine refusal and vaccine-preventable diseases in the United States: A review of measles and pertussis. *JAMA: Journal of the American Medical Association*, *315*(11), 1149–1158. doi:10.1001/jama.2016.1353

Poltorak, M., Leach, M., Fairhead, J., & Cassell, J. (2005). "Mmr talk" and vaccination choices: An ethnographic study in Brighton. *Social Science & Medicine*, *61*(3), 709–719. https://doi.org/10.1016/j.socscimed.2004.12.014

Reich, J. A. (2014). Neoliberal mothering and vaccine refusal: Imagined gated communities and the privilege of choice. *Gender & Society*, *28*(5), https://doi.org/10.1177%2F0891243214532711

Reich, J. A. (2016). *Calling the shots: Why parents reject vaccines*. New York, NY: NYU Press.

Reich, J. A. (2018a). We are fierce, independent thinkers and intelligent: Social capital and stigma management among mothers who refuse vaccines. *Social Science & Medicine*, 112015. https://doi.org/10.1016/j.socscimed.2018.10.027

Reich, J. A. (2018b). I have to write a statement of moral conviction: Can anyone help?: Parents' strategies for managing compulsory vaccination laws. *Sociological Perspectives*, *61*(2), 222–239. https://doi.org/10.1177%2F0731121418755113

Reich, J. A. (2020). Vaccine refusal and pharmaceutical acquiescence: Parental control and ambivalence in managing children's health. *American Sociological Review*, *85*(1), 106–127. doi:10.1177/0003122419899604

Reinhart, R. J. (2020). Fewer in U.S. continue to see vaccines as important. *Gallup*. Retrieved from https://news.gallup.com/poll/276929/fewer-continue-vaccines-important.aspx

Robison, S. G., Groom, H., & Young, C. (2012). Frequency of alternative immunization schedule use in a metropolitan area. *Pediatrics*, *130*(1), 32–38. doi:10.1542/peds.2011-3154

Salathé, M., & Bonhoeffer, S. (2008). The effect of opinion clustering on disease outbreaks. *Journal of the Royal Society Interface*, *5*(29), 1505–1508. https://doi.org/10.1098/rsif.2008.0271

Salmon, D. A., Sotir, M. J., Pan, W. K., Berg, J. L., Omer, S. B., Stokley, S., et al. (2009). Parental vaccine refusal in Wisconsin: A case-control study. *WMJ*, *108*(1), 17–23. PMID: 19326630

Samuel, L. (2017, January 20). Vaccine exemptions are on the rise in a number of Us States. *Stat News*.

Smith, P. J., Chu, S. Y., & Barker, L. E. (2004). Children who have received no vaccines: Who are they and where do they live? *Pediatrics*, *114*(1), 187–195. https://doi.org/10.1542/peds.114.1.187

Sobo, E. J. (2015). Social cultivation of vaccine refusal and delay among Walldorf (steiner) school parents. *Medical Anthropology Quarterly*, 381–399. https://doi.org/10.1111/maq.12214

Sobo, E. J. (2016). What is herd immunity, and how does it relate to pediatric vaccination uptake? Us parent perspectives. *Social Science & Medicine*, *165*, 187–195. https://doi.org/10.1016/j.socscimed.2016.06.015

Streefland, P., Chowdhury, A. M. R., & Ramos-Jimenez, P. (1999). Patterns of vaccination acceptance. *Social Science and Medicine*, *49*(12), 1705–1716. https://doi.org/10.1016/S0277-9536(99)00239-7

Thomson, A., Vallee-Tourangeau, G., & Suggs, L. S. (2018). Strategies to increase vaccine acceptance and uptake: From behavioral insights to context-specific, culturally-appropriate, evidence-based communications and interventions. *Vaccine*, *36*(44), 6457–6458. https://doi.org/10.1016/j.vaccine.2018.08.031

van der Linden, S. L., Clarke, C. E., & Maibach, E. W. (2015). Highlighting consensus among medical scientists increases public support for vaccines: Evidence from a randomized experiment. *BMC Public Health*, *15*(1), 1207. https://doi.org/10.1186/s12889-015-2541-4

Ward, J. K., Peretti-Watel, P., Bocquier, A., Seror, V., & Verger, P. (2019). Vaccine hesitancy and coercion: All eyes on France. *Nature Immunology*. doi:10.1038/s41590-019-0488-9. https://doi.org/10.1038/s41590-019-0488-9

Yang, Y. T., Delamater, P. L., Leslie, T. F., & Mello, M. M. (2016). Sociodemographic predictors of vaccination exemptions on the basis of personal belief in California. *American Journal of Public Health*, *106*(1), 172–177. Retrieved from https://ajph.aphapublications.org/doi/abs/10.2105/AJPH.2015.302926

22

VIOLENCE AND HEALTH THROUGH THE LIFESPAN

The Critical Role of Childhood Exposures
and Developmental Context

Kathy Sanders-Phillips

Overview

Violence is one of the leading and most costly causes of death worldwide. ***Violence*** is the "intentional use of physical force or power, threatened or actual, against oneself, another person, or against a group or community that either results in or has a high likelihood of resulting in injury, death, psychological harm, maldevelopment or deprivation" (World Health Organization, 2002, p. 5). It includes public and private acts; victimization and perpetration; and acts resulting from an imbalance of power that significantly burdens individuals, families, and communities worldwide (e.g., threats, intimidation, acts of neglect, omission, and commission). There are three subcategories of violence (World Health Organization, 2002). ***Interpersonal violence*** occurs between family members, intimate partners, friends, acquaintances, and strangers and includes child maltreatment, youth violence, violence against women, and elder abuse. ***Self-directed violence*** is inflicted against oneself such as suicide. In ***collective violence***, larger groups such as nation-states, militia groups, and terrorist organizations inflict violence in order to achieve political, economic, or social objectives.

This chapter focuses on ***childhood violence exposure***, child physical and psychological impacts, and their implications for adult health. We also explore the impact of interpersonal violence, as well as collective violence in the form of racial discrimination on health outcomes in youth and adults.

Research in Practice

Adverse Childhood Experiences: A Retrospective Study of Health Impacts Over the Life Cycle

Exposure to violence in childhood affects adult health outcomes, although the impact may not emerge until years after the initial event (World Health Organization, 2002). *Childhood violence exposure* predicts chronic diseases in adulthood related to biological, physiological and genetic changes that may be due to ***allostasis***—a measure of the "wear and tear" on the body related to chronic responses to environmental stress, as well as its subsequent return to a resting state (Danese, Moffitt, Pariante, Ambler, Poulton, & Caspi, 2008; Danese, Moffitt, Harrington, Milne, Polanczyk, Pariante, et al., 2009; Danese & McEwan, 2012; Danese, Caspi, Williams, Ambler, Sugden, Mika, et al., 2011).

The constant physiological adjustments are associated with elevated heart rate variability, changes in sweat gland activity, and body mass index. Child abuse and neglect are also related to sleep disturbances and risks such as smoking and alcohol use (Burt, Simons, & Gibbons, 2012; Chapman, Liu, Presley-Cantrell, Edwards, Wheaton, Perry, et al., 2013; Chamberlain, 2011). Some researchers (e.g., Logan, Hasler, Forbes, Franzen, Torregrossa, Huang, et al., 2017) suggest that these risky substance use behaviors may be efforts to self-medicate in response to chronic states of physiological reactivity, anxiety, or depression.

Bellis, Lowey, Leckenby, Hughes, and Harrison's (2013) study focuses on relationships between **adverse childhood experiences (ACEs)** and adult health and social outcomes. *ACE*s include exposure to domestic violence and child abuse. The study was designed to examine associations between *ACE*s and poor health and social outcomes in adulthood. The study sample was drawn from outside of the United States—an approach that helps to identify commonalities in prevalence and outcomes that may be universal (Priest, Perry, Ferdinand, Paradies, & Kelaher, 2014).

To ensure that specific measures were appropriate for their sample and culture, the study employed a variety of instruments (Charmaraman & Grossman, 2010). Ethnicity was self-identified—an important approach, since self-identity is a significant predictor of outcomes (American Psychological Association, 2012). A multilanguage questionnaire was administered by trained researchers through face-to-face interviews or self-reported.

The methods to recruit a sample that approximated the characteristics of a larger population included establishing criteria for participants, as well as using a composite score and random sampling to stratify the sample by poverty. The inclusion criteria were resident in the study area, aged 18 to 70 years, and cognitively able to participate in a face-to-face interview. Neighborhoods were classified based on a national deprivation composite measure that included 38 economic and social indicators and yielded five categories of poverty, ranging from one (least deprived) to five (most deprived). Postal addresses were used to identify houses in areas representing each of the five poverty categories.

To identify variables that best predicted health (Freedman, 2009), the first step was to examine correlations between all study variables. Regression analyses were used to identify the best predictive variables.

Reports of higher numbers of childhood adversity (*ACE*s) were associated with poor outcomes and behaviors in adulthood that included having been hit and hitting someone else in the last 12 months, having spent one night in prison or in a police station in the last 12 months, and substance use, including heroin or crack cocaine. Morbid obesity, having a sexually transmitted infection, having spent nights in the hospital, ever broken a bone, and having respiratory disease or digestive/liver disease were significantly higher in those with more *ACE*s. Thus, adults who reported more *ACE*s were more likely to report violent behaviors, drug use, and health problems during adulthood.

These findings indicated that cumulative *ACE* counts were strongly related to adverse outcomes throughout life, independent of poverty. The authors suggest that these effects may result in a cycle of poor health by promoting risk behaviors such as drug use and early pregnancy that increase the likelihood of poor adult outcomes. In turn, the authors speculate that if these adults become parents, their *ACE*s may predispose them to behaviors that affect the health of the next generation. Significant associations were not found between *ACE* counts and cancer, type 2 diabetes, and cardiovascular disease. The authors explain this finding by suggesting that people with higher *ACE* counts may have died prematurely before the study was even initiated.

Recommendations for Future Research

Information was not collected on the 30% who chose not to participate. Therefore, bias introduced through selective participation cannot be excluded. The use of face-to face interviews also increases the possibility of a social desirability bias where individuals may deliberately or inadvertently (e.g., poor recall, blocking certain memories) provide incorrect answers or answers that they think are more "desirable" (Gove & Geerken, 1977).

Longitudinal studies have empirically documented the findings of Bellis, and colleagues (2013) and identified the biological mechanisms by which poor child and adult health outcomes may occur in children exposed to adverse events (Danese & McEwan, 2012, Sumner, Colich, Uddin, Armstrong, & McLaughlin, 2018). For example, adults who experience childhood violence may show genetic and physiological changes that begin in childhood but are not fully apparent until adulthood and maturity of the brain. However, there are pros and cons to Bellis, and colleague's (2013) suggestion that prospective longitudinal studies on *ACEs* would avoid problems of potential sampling bias and provide data to map and quantify the full impact of childhood adversity. The strength of a prospective longitudinal design is that repeated observations of the same variables over time help determine whether one variable actually causes another (Manolio, Bailey-Wilson, & Collins, 2006; Shadish, Cook, & Campbell, 2002).

However, longitudinal studies can also raise potential ethical issues (see Danese, et al., 2008; Herrenkohl, Hong, Klika, Herrenkohl, & Russo, 2013). In some studies, data on child maltreatment may have been recorded without intervention—a possibility that raises troubling ethical questions about the role of researchers and their obligations to study participants. Similar ethical questions may be raised when collecting data on child and family functioning during times of war and collective upheaval in a country. Reports of child abuse and maltreatment are now mandated in the United States and in some, but not all, countries (European Union Agency for Fundamental Rights, 2014; Mathews, 2014), though this may not solve the problem. A critical overall question any researcher should always ask is "do the benefits of participation in a study outweigh the potential harms and/or trauma to participants?" This is necessary in order to *do no harm* in our research on youth violence exposure and health.

The findings of Bellis, and colleagues (2013) also strongly suggest that effective public health and social policies to address *ACEs* will require greater attention to upstream and downstream factors. *Upstream factors* include social inequality and its markers, such as economic variables and policies regarding education, health workforce training, and child welfare, as well as laws governing children's rights. *Downstream factors* include individual risks like smoking and depression. Limiting our focus to the *downstream factors* related to health fails to acknowledge critical *upstream factors*, like racial discrimination, that are often seen as fundamental contributors to health.

Exposure to Collective Violence, Children's Health, and Perceived Safety in Society: A Community Participation Perspective and Approach

As noted, collective violence occurs when larger groups such as nation-states, militia groups and terrorist organizations inflict violence in order to achieve political, economic, or social objectives. It is based on power differences that exist between groups in a society and is seen both in poor urban communities with high incidences of violence, as well as during times of war, refugee relocation, mass violence, and terrorism.

For example, African American adolescents and other youth of color are disproportionately exposed to community and other types of violence. Homicide is the leading cause of death for African Americans ages 10 to 19 (Sheats, Irving, Mercy, Simon, Crosby, Ford, et al., 2018), the second leading cause of death for Hispanics, and the third leading cause of death for Native Americans and Alaska Natives (Centers for Disease Control, 2010). African Americans are also more likely than Whites to be involved in violence perpetration and the juvenile justice system (Elsaesser & Voisin, 2015; Sheats, et al., 2018). Native American children report high rates of child abuse and neglect and are twice as likely as any other group to die before the age of 24 (Indian Law & Order Commission, 2013). Finally, gang members are more likely to be Hispanic/Latino and African American/Black than other races/ethnicities (National Gang Center, 2012), and rates of physical and sexual dating violence are also higher in Latino youth (Reyes, Vangie, & Foshee, 2017).

Alcohol and other drug use is often reported by children who are victims or perpetrators of violence and is related to higher rates of assaultive crime, more serious youth crime, and becoming a crime victim (Daane, 2003; Margolin & Gordis, 2000; Sanders-Phillips, Settles-Reaves, Walker, & Brownlow, 2009). Some children may try to control their environments through repeated encounters with life-threatening situations and involvement in gang activity or with violent peers (Garbarino, 2001; Stewart, Simons, & Conger, 2002).

Children may have similar reactions to collective violence witnessed in the media that includes mass shootings in schools, terrorist activity such as 9/11, and war-related events (Garbarino, 2001; Leiner, Peinado, Villanos, Lopez, Uribe, & Pathak, 2016). For example, girls and children in grades four and five may be the most affected by school shootings (Hoven, Duarte, Lucas, Wu, Mandell, Goodwin, et al., 2005), although conduct disorders as well as drug use are reported by many youth who have witnessed such events (Crum, Cornacchio, Coxe, Green, & Comer, 2018). The degree of proximity and age of exposure may exacerbate these effects in children (Drury & Williams, 2012; Garbarino, 2001). In addition, since some children may have difficulty distinguishing between events they have seen in the media versus events that occur in proximity to them, they may experience heightened feelings of being unsafe, hopelessness, helplessness, or aggression (Garbarino, 2001; Williams, 2007).

Youth responses to collective violence and the authority figures they associate with such violence are significantly influenced by direct interactions with these individuals and by witnessing the encounters of others (Sheats, et al., 2018). These experiences affect attitudes toward authority, the way that youth are socialized in their community environment, and their association with antisocial peers (Leiber, Nalla, & Farnworth, 1998; Skogan, 2009). In turn, these outcomes may affect health directly or indirectly by influencing psychological functioning and increasing the likelihood of exposure to violent situations. Fine, Freudenberg, Payne, Perkins, Smith, and Wanzer (2003) were among the first to examine these relationships in a US urban sample. Their study examines the experiences of urban youth in New York City (NYC) with adults in positions of authority, including police officers, educators, social workers, security guards, teachers, and store and restaurant workers. The findings provide an overview of responses to police surveillance that expands our knowledge of the sources, extents, and impacts of violence exposure for youth in this country as well as the fact that, in some communities, interactions with authority figures such as the police may cause stress, violence, and trauma that significantly influence health and development.

Fine et al.'s study utilized data collection methods that directly involved the target community. The methodology is known as ***participatory action research (PAR)*** and represents a partnership that equitably involves community members, organizational representatives, researchers, and others in all aspects of the research process. The aim of *PAR* is to increase knowledge and understanding of a phenomenon and integrate the knowledge gained into interventions for policy or social change (Israel, Schulz, Parker, & Becker, 1998).

Participants in Fine et al.'s study were recruited from "the street," that is public spaces in NYC, using quantitative (e.g., a structured survey) and qualitative (e.g., in-depth interviews with a subsample) methods that resulted in four research questions: a) To what extent do urban youth experience adult surveillance as evidence of mistrust and harassment versus comfort and safety? b) To what extent do race/ethnicity and gender differentiate youth experiences of adult surveillance, particularly by teachers, police, and security guards? c) Can we begin to identify the consequences of surveillance on urban youth? d) To what extent does the perception of adult surveillance affect youths' trust in adult society, civic institutions, and democratic engagement?

NYC youth and young adults (*n* = 24) were hired as co-investigators; trained in *PAR*; and provided wisdom, cautions, and language for instrument design. This process resulted in a 112-item survey entitled *Young Adults and Public Spaces*, a multidimensional measure that included indicators of trust, alienation, harassment, and help-seeking across four scales: Attitudes toward Police, Comfort in School, Trust toward Adults, and Safe Places.

Recruitment was conducted at multiple public sites to attract different types of youth in different types of settings based on a sampling framework that was calculated using the 1990 Census and the race/ethnic distribution by borough. The survey was completed by participants or read to participants when necessary.

Findings from the Attitudes toward Police Scale indicated that youth of African descent (i.e., African American or African Caribbean) had more negative attitudes toward the police than other ethnic groups. Males also had more negative attitudes toward police than females. Many reported that they did not feel psychologically or physically safe in schools: 21% felt unsafe (or very unsafe), 45% saw fights often or all the time, 50% believed police/security officers did not make school safer, and only 11% felt comfortable talking to a teacher if they witnessed a fight.

This study by Fine, and colleagues (2003) is notable for its use of quantitative and qualitative methods in a community-focused design that acknowledges the fact that community residents often have knowledge of a problem that investigators may lack if they have not grown up in similar communities. Training community residents as members of the study team also creates a cadre of community members who understand the basic principles of research and serve as advocates and gatekeepers in evaluating community participation in research projects.

Since young people who spend time on the streets may be at higher risk for interacting with police, the findings may not be generalizable to other populations. Reading the survey to some participants may have also introduced biases (Furnham, 1986). If this happens, study results may be due to a systematic response bias rather than to the hypothesized effect. Face-to-face interviews, where a respondent has to reveal his or her answer to another person, may also increase the likelihood of social desirability biases (Gove & Geerken, 1977).

Recommendations for Future Research

Future violence research should examine interactions between youth and authority figures such as the police in urban communities of color (Butler, 2011). We also need to examine the impact of youth exposure to violence under conditions of state-sanctioned violence—especially in countries with large populations of refugees (Garbarino, 2001). In addition, few studies have evaluated whether violence in childhood may contribute to youth affiliation with terrorist groups (Schilis & Verhage, 2017).

Finally, critical questions remain: What does it mean to feel unsafe as a child? How does feeling unsafe change a child's developmental trajectory? What are the consequences of distrusting the societal institutions (e.g., schools) in which children develop? Studies based on these questions help us understand children's responses to one form of violence in the context of exposures to other types of violence (Garbarino, 2001).

In order to shift the theoretical lens of how we view violence and how best to design research to address the effects on youth, we need multilevel interventions as well as multidisciplinary teams to examine the broad range of variables (e.g., education, economic, housing, poverty) related to children's exposure to violence.

Collective Violence in the Form of Racial Discrimination: An Empirical Study of the Effects on Health and Perceived Safety in a School Setting

Defining violence outcomes solely in terms of injury or death limits our understanding of the full impact of violence. Violence is best understood in the context of social and interpersonal variables and experiences, such as those described by Fine, and colleagues (2003), that often exist in countries like the United States where there are social hierarchies and stratification (Blume, 1996). **Social strat-ification** is the categorization of people into social and economic groups based on their occupation, income, social status, castes, kinship, physical characteristics, gender, beliefs, or other characteristics. *Social stratification* creates dominant and secondary groups, with lower status ascribed to members of secondary social groups. Secondary social status influences health and psychological well-being by increasing the likelihood of social inequalities, exposure to discrimination, exposure to environmental hazards, and access to health resources (Brown, 1995; Grusky, 2014).

Direct exposure to racial discrimination is related to feelings of powerlessness, alienation, low life satisfaction, low self-esteem, a sense of invisibility, and greater substance use (Sanders-Phillips, 1997, 2009; Sanders-Phillips, Settles-Reaves, Walker, & Brownlow, 2009). Immigrant children and families from impoverished and violence-torn countries are often victims of racial discrimination (Listenbee, Torre, Boyle, Sharon, Cooper, et al., 2012). Additionally, structural racism (i.e., at policy and other institutional levels of society) is most likely to influence health risks by fostering anxiety, depression, and hopelessness (Gee & Ford, 2011).

Priest, and colleagues (2014) identified associations between depressive symptoms, loneliness, and **motivated fairness** (i.e., the extent to which children and adolescents feel motivated to respond without prejudice because they view the world as fair and safe) in Australian students who had directly experienced racism, as well as those who had experienced racism vicariously. The researchers also documented feelings of alienation and marginalization in these two groups. The findings are important because feelings of alienation, isolation, and marginalization are related to depression and other symptoms of psychological distress that foster high levels of aggression in youth as well as criminal activity (Burt, et al., 2012; Simons, Murry, McLoyd, Lin, Cutrona, & Conger, 2002; Simons, Chen, Stewart, & Brody, 2003). This study also examined whether children attribute their discrimination experiences to an identity or to specific personal characteristics, such as their race or ethnicity. This is an interesting and novel study question that has not been widely studied.

Priest, et al., (2014) also assessed **vicarious racial discrimination** as a moderator that may intensify the effects of direct experiences of racial discrimination on negative outcomes (i.e., depressive symptoms and loneliness) because it leads youth to conclude that racism is pervasive. Priest, and colleagues (2014) and Stroebe, Dovido, Barreto, Ellmers, and John (2011) have concluded that the belief that discrimination is pervasive can be especially damaging to youth outcomes, since it threatens a basic need to perceive the world as just and fair. The second study hypothesis was that individual differences in racial/ethnic attitudes might also moderate responses to racism.

The findings of Priest, et al., (2014) are potentially important to the development of effective school-based programs to prevent racial discrimination (Paradies, 2006). Schools also provide a critical developmental context for children in which peer relationships evolve (Mansouri & Jenkins, 2010). Negative experiences in school "distance youth from important and necessary structures of support rather than engage them" (Schiff, 2013, p. 4), resulting in feelings of injustice, risky or illegal behaviors, and encouraging dropout rates, creating a school-to-prison pipeline (Raffaele-Mendez, Knoff, & Ferron, 2002).

Issues of fairness and social justice significantly affect child and adult health behaviors and are critically influenced by both the social environment and individual personality (Farrington, Loeber, & Stouthamer-Loeber, 2003; Sanders-Phillips, 2009). Priest, and colleagues' (2014) findings expand these findings (Duckitt, 2001; Mischel & Shoda, 1995) and help to refine or modify existing models and theories (Brittian, 2012).

Finally, since Priest el al.'s (2014) study was conducted in Australia, the findings help identify the "universal" aspects of exposure to racial discrimination, while reinforcing that racism and marginalization exist across the globe and operate as vectors affecting the health of people worldwide. Like the United States, Australia has a history of racial discrimination. Although antidiscrimination laws were enacted in Australia in the 1970s after decades of legal and illegal racial discrimination targeting Aboriginal and other indigenous peoples (Australian Human Rights Commission, 2007), problems with racism and racial discrimination persist.

Data for the Priest et al. study were collected via self-report surveys. Items were read to primary school students, while secondary school students completed it independently. The final sample consisted of 263 (82.4% primary and 17.6% secondary) students who were divided into four groups based on student and parent(s) place of birth/birth categories: a) reference group (student and parents both born in English-speaking countries), b) minority English group (student born in English-speaking country and parents born in non-English-speaking countries), c) minority non-English group (student and parents born in non-English-speaking countries), and d) unknown parental country of birth group. Country of birth was chosen as a proximal indicator of majority versus minority ethnic group status.

Results of the study revealed that at least one form of racism was experienced directly by 32.2% of the overall sample, and 22.1% experienced at least one form of direct racism every day. A majority of students (71.7%) reported at least one form of vicarious racism, and 26.3% reported all three forms of vicarious racism. Almost half of the overall sample (47.3%) reported at least one form of vicarious racism every day. Exposure to direct racism was most likely to come from other students who felt that some groups did not "belong" in Australia. Vicarious racism usually took the form of seeing others being called names or teased because of their cultural group. A total of 65.7% of the overall sample experienced this, at a minimum, on a monthly basis.

Reporting both loneliness and depressive symptoms was associated with a greater likelihood of experiencing direct racism. Depressive symptoms were related to a lower likelihood of having positive racial/ethnic attitudes and, as expected, students from all three minority birth-country categories reported higher levels of loneliness relative to the majority ethnic group students.

Only majority-birth students who reported having more friends from other cultures also reported higher levels of loneliness and depressive symptoms. According to Priest, and colleagues (2014), this may have occurred because majority-group students with friends from other cultures may have witnessed their friends experiencing racism and may have been more sensitive to the negative emotional consequences of these experiences. Or majority-birth students may have experienced exclusion due to having friends from other cultures or made friends with students from other cultures after being excluded by those from their own culture.

The results also suggested that the level of *motivated fairness* modified the relationship between exposure to direct racism and depressive symptoms. The investigators suggest that this may be due to a cumulative effect, since youth who view the world as unfair or unjust, who experience racial discrimination, *and* who perceive racial discrimination as common are more likely to have depressive symptoms (Stroebe, et al., 2011). Therefore, a child's perceptions of the world as "fair" and "safe" may be critical determinants of how youth respond to racial discrimination.

Priest et al.'s study is limited by its small sample size, nonrandom selection of schools, and possible bias related to the use of inconsistent data collection methods when administering the surveys to students. More extensive measures of loneliness and depression would have been helpful. Furthermore, the decision to label the largely English-speaking and Australian-born students as the "reference" group is conceptually problematic, since it implies that this group is the standard by which all other groups are judged.

Recommendations for Future Research

Future studies should assess larger groups of students in the United States and other countries to identify how experiences of racial discrimination influence developmental milestones such as peer group affiliations, school achievement, and health. Since the association between racial discrimination and poor mental health is considerably weaker among youth with strong national and ethnic identifications who also respect other groups (Huynh, Devos, & Goldberg, 2014; Phinney, Jacoby, & Silva, 2007; Umaña-Taylor, Quintana, Lee, Cross, Rivas-Drake, Schwartz, et al., 2014), these variables should be explored in future studies. Finally, how do we help children who are living in circumstances where racial discrimination and other forms of violence actually are, in fact, historically and currently pervasive? Future studies are needed.

Racial Discrimination and Health: Prevention at the Individual Level

Repeated exposure to violence may be cumulative, leading to anger, despair, and emotional numbing (Burt, et al., 2012; Garbarino, 2001; Simons, Simons, Burt, et al., 2006). To address these realities, parents of color often use **racial socialization approaches**, which can be defined as messages that parents send to their children regarding racial identity and status (Brittian, 2012; Rodriguez, McKay, & Bannon, 2008).

As documented in the Bellis, et al., (2013) and Priest, and colleagues (2014) studies, psychological distress, related to *ACEs* such as racial discrimination, is associated with higher youth aggression and crime. In turn, greater involvement in crime is associated with violence-related morbidity and mortality (Elsaesser & Voisin, 2015; Sheats, et al., 2018). Simons, et al.'s (2006) study examined the extent to which supportive parenting may mitigate the impact of racial discrimination on youth and thereby reduce youth crime. The authors concluded that children who experienced violence related to racial discrimination may require both tailored interventions and/or treatment, as well as supportive parenting. The investigators warn against "the dangers of adopting a 'one model fits all' approach when studying children . . . and . . . the importance of considering factors common to the everyday lives of a cultural group" (Simons, et al., 2006, p. 374).

The Simons, et al. (2006) study is one of the few longitudinal studies to examine the effects of racial discrimination on family and youth outcomes. The sample for the 2006 study was drawn from the Family and Community Health Study (FACHS)—a longitudinal, multisite investigation of neighborhood and family effects on health and development in African American families living in Georgia and Iowa. Thus, the study recruited both urban and rural African American families. Using census data, block groups were identified in both Iowa and Georgia in which the percentage of African American families was 10% or higher and the percentage of families with children living below the poverty line ranged from 10% to 100%. Using these criterion, 259 block groups were identified and the study families were recruited from these block groups. Each family included a child who was in fifth grade (aged 10 to 12) at the time of recruitment. Interviews were conducted with the target child and his or her primary caregiver. Child reports were used to construct measures of discrimination, violence, anger, and hostile view of relationships. Caregiver and child reports were used for assessments of supportive parenting and parental control. Supportive parenting was based on the cumulative parent responses to three measures that assessed warmth/affection, providing children with reasons for their parenting actions and helping children to problem-solve, and avoidance of harsh parenting.

Using two waves of data collected two years apart from 332 African American boys, the investigators found that parental support moderates the association between discrimination and violent delinquency in two ways: by decreasing the chances that discrimination will lead to either anger or a hostile view of relationships or by providing a model of relationships that may counter the cynical view fostered by acts of discrimination. However, discrimination continued to have a main effect on youth anger and aggression even after taking supportive parenting into account (see Brown & Tylka, 2010). These findings underscore the lack of attention in the extant literature that is given to racial discrimination and its impact on youth and health outcomes.

The results of this longitudinal study suggest causality by indicating that the relationship between discrimination and aggression flows from discrimination to violent adolescent behavior, rather than the reverse (Simons, et al., 2003). High levels of discrimination or experiencing an increase in discrimination predicted an escalation in violent delinquency (Simon, et al., 2003; Simons, et al., 2006). As Priest, and colleagues (2014) found, feelings of anger and development of a hostile view of relationships mediated much of the association between discrimination and violence in the Simons, et al. (2006) study, but depression and anxiety did not.

Recommendations for Future Research

The discrimination measure in the Simons, et al. (2006) study only assessed perceptions of discrimination, and these perceptions may not represent reality. However, both Priest, and colleagues' (2014) findings and other reports of high levels of racial discrimination for African American youth suggest that this is not the case (Martin, McCarthy, Conger, Gibbons, Simons, Cutrona, et al., 2011). In addition, the composite parenting score utilized in the Simons, et al. (2006) study assessed supportive parenting but did not identify whether parents used a specific approach such as a ***preparation for bias*** approach to racial socialization or a ***cultural adaptation*** to racial socialization. According to Burt, and colleagues (2012), *preparation for bias* approaches include talking to youth about the potential for experiencing discrimination and discussing ways to cope with such experiences so that children learn to place experiences of racial discrimination in a context of race relations and develop strategies to address them. *Cultural adaptation* practices emphasize racial heritage and promote cultural customs and traditions in order to foster children's racial pride and sense of belonging, as well as negate racial stereotypes that they may encounter in the broader society (Winkler & Bouncken, 2011). In subsequent studies, Burt, and colleagues (2012) found that the specific parenting technique of *preparation for bias* significantly reduced the effects of discrimination on youth criminal behavior. Lastly, in light of the potential biological impacts of violence exposure, future research on violence and health might also focus on relationships between adult physiological responses to violence and parenting behaviors (Mills-Koonce, Propper, Jean-Louis, Barnett, Moore, Calkins, et al., 2009).

The Continuum of Exposure and Cumulative Effects of Violence Exposure: Youth at High Risk for Poor Health Outcomes

In countries like the United States and South Africa that are racially or ethnically stratified and have high levels of collective violence, health outcomes are generally poor for those in socially devalued groups, yet factors like racial discrimination are generally not examined in health and violence research (Sanders-Phillips & Kliewer, 2019). Nonetheless, researchers have argued for a developmentally based understanding of children's health outcomes that requires greater knowledge of the cumulative effects of experiences that disrupt behavioral, cognitive, and/or emotional development (Conti & Heckman, 2013; Garbarino, 2001; Gregorowski & Seedat, 2013). Childhood is a critical period for developing healthy behaviors that are based on positive self-perceptions and for achieving a sense of mastery over life outcomes that affect healthy behaviors over the life cycle (Farrington, Loeber, Stouthamer-Loeber, 2003). These perceptions, attitudes, and behaviors develop in the context of home, schools, and communities (Daiute & Fine, 2003). Unfortunately, chronic and cumulative exposure to many types of violence, including the collective violence of ethnic or racial discrimination, may significantly influence risk behaviors and health outcomes (e.g., Bellis, et al., 2013; Dubow, Huesmann, & Boxer, 2009; Gregorowski & Seedat, 2013; Sanders-Phillips, 2009; Sanders-Phillips, et al., 2009).

The study by Sanders-Phillips and Kliewer (2019) identified groups of youth in South Africa who were most vulnerable to risk-taking behaviors and poor health outcomes based on multiple indicators of violence exposure. It builds on the findings of the Bellis, and colleagues (2013), Fine, and colleagues (2003), Priest et al. (2013), and Simons, et al. (2006) studies by examining the role of racial discrimination as a form of violence that occurs in the context of exposure to other forms of violence, exacerbates the effects of exposure to other types of violence, and increases risk-taking in South African youth (Brondolo, Halen, Pencille, Beatty, & Contrada, 2009; Goff, Jackson, Allison, Di Leone, Culotta, & DiTomasso, 2014; Sanders-Phillips, et al., 2009).

Apartheid, a legal form of racial discrimination from 1948 to 1994 in South Africa, remains a central contributing factor to the country's endemic violence (Seedat, Van Niekerk, Jewkes, Suffla, & Ratele, 2009). Perceptions and reports of personal racial discrimination also heighten the negative effects of exposure to other types of violence among South African youth (Duncan, 2012; Eagle, 2015).

In the Sanders-Phillips and Kliewer (2019) study, surveys were administered to a representative sample of 1,317 high school students (Black, Colored/Mixed Race, White) in Cape Town, South Africa. Measures of violence exposure reflected lifetime exposure and included the frequency of both witnessing and victimization due to interpersonal violence. Outcomes included indicators of substance use and sexual risks.

We identified five profiles of violence exposure: a) a low-violence exposure class; b) an average violence exposure class; c) a high-exposure to violence at home class; d) a high-community victimization class; and e) a very high-violence exposure group that included youth who reported high community violence as a victim and witnessing violence in the home, school, and community in addition to experiencing high levels of racial discrimination. Whites were overrepresented in the low-exposure class and were underrepresented in all other classes. Overall, as compared to females, males were overrepresented in high community victimization and very high exposure profiles. Youth in the very high-violence exposure profile were older than youth in the low-violence exposure and high family violence exposure profiles.

Violence exposures were highest among the youth of color. Youth with very high exposures to violence, including the exposure to personal racial discrimination, were at greater risk on every measure of substance use risk except frequency of alcohol use; had the earliest onset of marijuana use; and were more likely to use glue, prescription medication, or hard drugs to get high. Consistent with Priest, and colleagues (2014) findings, youth with very high levels of exposure to violence in multiple forms who also reported personal racial discrimination were at the highest risk for substance use and sexual risk behaviors.

The youth in this sample were born after 1994 when apartheid was dismantled. Therefore, they were not directly exposed to the political violence and marginalization of apartheid. Yet as Bellis, and colleagues (2013) suggested, the effects of marginalization can be enduring and may persist from one generation to the next. This cycle can sustain unfavorable social conditions that often include greater violence exposure as victims and perpetrators (Yahyavi, Zarghami, & Marwah, 2014). Poor outcomes associated with historical group trauma have been reported in the second generation of youth born after significant violence and conflict in a society (Bowers & Yehuda, 2016; Kellerman, 2013; Yahyavi, et al., 2014).

Strengths of this study include the assessment of individual perceptions of experiences of racial discrimination, documentation of violence exposure across multiple contexts, use of analytic techniques to model profiles of exposure, inclusion of a large sample of South African youth, and linkages to both substance use and sexual risk behavior as outcomes, using well-validated measures.

The data are limited, since they are based on self-report, are cross-sectional, and are assessed at one point in time. Further, the study sample was drawn from the Western Cape of South Africa, which may or may not be representative of the entire country.

Recommendations for Future Research

To prevent future violence and promote youth resiliency in racially stratified countries such as the United States and South Africa, effective programs will need to address the legacies of racial segregation, the continuing interface between youth health outcomes and social justice, and ongoing structural inequalities. In order to accomplish this goal, considerably more studies of racial discrimination and health are needed and strategies to ameliorate the effects identified and tested.

Conclusion

As we witness the separation and detainment of children at the US/Mexico border, the marginalization of children in the Middle East, and children facing war in Syria and other countries, the cumulative effects of exposure to multiple types of violence must be evaluated, particularly for youth whose experiences of inequality place them at a higher risk of being victimized or encountering other types of violence. For many of these children, exposure to violence and/or war may be just one event in a series of adverse events in their lives

A sense of safety, stability, and trust in the future are preconditions for healthy lives, since they reinforce perceptions of control, health, and life outcomes (Weinstein, 1993). In other words, without a sense of future, being healthy means little. For children, successful integration into social institutions, such as the family, school, and neighborhood, is also a prerequisite for healthy behaviors (Raffaele-Mendez, et al., 2002; Schiff, 2013). Life under conditions of violence may severely limit the degree to which these preconditions can be met.

The findings in this chapter strongly support Garbarino's (2001) *Accumulation of Risk Model*, which predicts that the children at highest risk for negative consequences associated with violence already live in the context of accumulated risk. When experiences of violence are internalized into painful feelings of anger, detachment, rejection, failure, and being unsafe, as Fine, and colleagues (2003) and Simons, et al. (2006) found, youth are vulnerable to psychological and biological effects that can be lifelong. A child's exposure to multiple forms of violence is more than simply additive. When the violence exposure includes the collective violence of racial discrimination, there may be interacting and confounding effects on health outcomes (Sanders-Phillips & Kliewer, 2019). A child's emotional responses to such realities will always reflect the cumulative load of these stressful events (Leiner, et al., 2016). Thus, our ability to accurately describe how violence exposure affects child and adult health is significantly improved by considering a broader spectrum of violence exposure. And as Garbarino (2001) notes, whether a child faces the discrimination and collective violence of urban streets or warfare, there must be a major concentration of opportunities (e.g., education, community resources) available to children to avoid youth adversity (Garbarino, 2001).

These findings also document that high levels of violence exposure co-vary with the violence of discrimination and may become part of a lifetime burden of adversities that serve as latent factors predicting psychological distress and poor health (Brondolo, et al., 2009). Therefore, a limited focus on poverty as the primary "driver" of violence may obscure the critical impact of social inequalities on youth. The poorest outcomes are likely to occur in children when exposure to violence is chronic and require alterations in perceptions of safety and major changes in behavior that allow for interpretation and accommodation of the danger. Youth with access to resources, social support, and adults who model social competence might better accept and deal with the developmental challenges posed by violence, even if they show short-term disturbances (Garbarino, 2001). However, interventions based primarily on changing individual health behaviors rather than the underlying social inequalities that give rise to poor health outcomes in children and adults will not suffice (Braveman, Egerter, & Williams, 2011; Sanders-Phillips, 2009). To improve child and adult health outcomes, we must acknowledge the full range of children's exposure to multiple concurrent forms of violence and conduct research that recognizes violence exposure as it is maintained in the context of children's and families' social conditions.

References

American Psychological Association. (2012). *Cultural adaptations: Tools for evidence-based practice with diverse populations* (G. Bernal, D. Rodríguez, & M. Melanie, Eds.). https://doi.org/10.1037/13752-000

Australian Human Rights Commission. (2007). *A guide to Australia's anti-discrimination laws.* Retrieved April 29, 2020, from www.humanrights.gov.au

Bellis, M. A., Lowey, H., Leckenby, N., Hughes, K., & Harrison, D. (2013). Adverse childhood experiences: Retrospective study to determine their impact on adult health behaviours and health outcomes in a UK population. *Journal of Public Health.* doi:10.1093/pubmed/fdt038

Blume, T. W. (1996). Social perspectives on violence. *Michigan Family Review, 2,* 9–23. https://doi.org/10.3998/mfr.4919087.0002.102

Bowers, M. E., & Yehuda, R. (2016). Intergenerational transmission of stress in humans. *Neuropsychopharmacology Reviews, 41,* 232–244. https://doi.org/10.1038/npp.2015.247

Braveman, P., Egerter, S., & Williams, D. R. (2011). The social determinants of health: Coming of age. *Annual Review of Public Health, 32,* 381–398. doi:10.1146/annurev-publhealth-031210-101218

Brittian, A. S. (2012). Understanding African American adolescents' Identity development: A relational developmental systems perspective. *Journal of Black Psychology, 38*(2), 172–200. doi:10.1177/0095798411414570

Brondolo, E., Halen, N. B., Pencille, M., Beatty, D., & Contrada, R. J. (2009). Coping with racism: A selective review of the literature and a theoretical and methodological critique. *Journal of Behavioral Medicine, 32,* 64–88. https://doi.org/10.1007/s10865-008-9193-0

Brown, D. L., & Tylka, T. L. (2010). Racial discrimination and resilience in African American young adults: Examining racial socialization as a moderator. *Journal of Black Psychology, 37*(3), 259–285. https://doi.org/10.1177/0095798410390689

Brown, P. (1995). Race, class, and environmental health: A review and systematization of the literature. *Environmental Research, 69*(1), 15–30. doi:10.1006/enrs.1995.1021

Burt, C. H., Simons, R. L., & Gibbons, F. X. (2012). Racial discrimination, ethnic-racial socialization, and crime: A micro-sociological-model of risk and resilience. *American Sociological Review, 77,* 648–677. https://doi.org/10.1177/0003122412448648

Butler, F. (2011). Rush to judgment: Prisoners' views of juvenile justice. *Western Criminology Review, 12*(3), 106–119. Retrieved from http://wcr.sonoma.edu/v12n3/Butler.pdf

Chamberlain, L. (2011). *Assessment for lifetime exposure to violence as a pathway to prevention.* National Resource Center on Domestic Violence. Retrieved April 29, 2020, from https://vawnet.org/material/assessment-lifetime-exposure-violence-pathway-prevention

Chapman, D., Liu, Y., Presley-Cantrell, L. R., Edwards, V. J., Wheaton, A. G., Perry, G. S., et al. (2013). Adverse childhood experiences and frequent insufficient sleep in 5 U.S. States, 2009: A retrospective cohort study. *BMC Public Health, 13*(3). doi:10.1186/1471-2458-13-3

Charmaraman, L., & Grossman, J. M. (2010). Importance of race-ethnicity: An exploration of Asian, Black, Latino, and multiracial adolescent identity. *Cultural Diversity and Ethnic Minority Psychology, 16*(2), 144–151. doi:10.1037/a0018668

Conti, G., & Heckman, J. J. (2013). The developmental approach to child and adult health. *American Academy of Pediatrics,* (Supplement 2), S133–S141. https://doi.org/10.1542/peds.2013-0252d

Crum, K. I., Cornacchio, D., Coxe, S., Green, J. G., & Comer, J. S. (2018). A latent profile analysis of co-occurring youth posttraumatic stress and conduct problems following community trauma. *Journal of Child and Family Studies, 27,* 3638–3649. https://doi.org/10.1111/j.1468-2850.2007.00078.x

Daane, D. (2003). Child and adolescent violence. *Orthopedic Nursing, 22,* 23–31. doi:10.1097/00006416-200310000-00008

Daiute, C., & Fine, M. (2003). Youth perspectives on violence and injustice. *Journal of Social Issues, 59,* 1–14. https://doi.org/10.1111/1540-4560.00001

Danese, A., Caspi, A., Williams, B., Ambler, A., Sugden, K., Mika, J., et al. (2011). Biological embedding of stress through inflammation processes in childhood. *Molecular Psychiatry, 16*(3), 244–246. doi:10.1038/mp.2010.5

Danese, A., & McEwan, B. (2012). Adverse childhood experiences, allostasis, allostatic load, and age-related disease. *Physiology & Behavior, 106*(1), 29–39. https://doi.org/10.1016/j.physbeh.2011.08.019

Danese, A., Moffitt, T. E., Harrington, H., Milne, B. J., Polanczyk, G., Pariante, et al. (2009). Adverse childhood experiences and adult risk factors for age-related disease: Depression, inflammation, and clustering of metabolic risk markers. *Archives of Pediatrics & Adolescent Medicine*, *163*(12), 1135–1143. doi:10.1001/archpediatrics.2009.214

Danese, A., Moffitt, T. E., Pariante, C. M., Ambler, A., Poulton, R., & Caspi, A. (2008). Elevated inflammation levels in depressed adults with a history of childhood maltreatment. *Archives of General Psychiatry*, *65*(4), 409–415. doi:10.1001/archpsyc.65.4.409

Drury, J., & Williams, R. (2012). Children and young people who are refugees, internally displaced persons or survivors or perpetrators of war, mass violence and terrorism. *Current Opinion in Psychiatry*, *25*(4), 277–284. doi:10.1097/YCO.0b013e328353eea6

Dubow, E. F., Huesmann, L. R., & Boxer, P. (2009). A social-cognitive-ecological framework for understanding the impact of exposure to persistent ethnic-political violence on children's psychosocial adjustment. *Clinical Child and Family Psychology Review*, *12*, 113–126. https://doi.org/10.1007/s10567-009-0050-7

Duckitt, J. (2001). A dual-process cognitive-motivational theory of ideology and prejudice. *Advances in Experimental Psychology*, *33*, 41–113. https://doi.org/10.1016/S0065-2601(01)80004-6

Duncan, N. (2012). Reaping the whirlwind: Xenophobic violence in South Africa. *Global Journal of Community Psychology Practice*, *3*, 104–112. Retrieved from www.gjcpp.org/pdfs/V3i1-0011%20Duncan.pdf

Eagle, G. (2015). Crime, fear and continuous traumatic stress in South Africa: What place social cohesion? *Psychology in Society*, *49*, 83–98. https://doi.org/10.17159/2309-8708/2015/n49a7

Elsaesser, C. M., & Voisin, D. R. (2015). Correlates of polyvictimization among African American youth: An exploratory study. *Journal of Interpersonal Violence*, *30*(17), 3022–3042. doi:10.1177/0886260514 554424

European Union Agency for Fundamental Rights. (2014). *Specific legal obligations for civilians to report cases of child abuse, neglect and violence*. Retrieved August 15, 2015, from https://fra.europa.eu/en/publication/2015/mapping-child-protection-systems-eu/reporting2

Farrington, D., Loeber, R., & Stouthamer-Loeber, M. (2003). How can the relationship between race and violence be explained? In D. Hawkins (Ed.), *Violent crime: Assessing race and ethnic differences* (pp. 213–237). Cambridge, UK: Cambridge University Press. doi:10.1017/CBO9780511499456.014

Fine, M., Freudenberg, N., Payne, Y., Perkins, T., Smith, K., & Wanzer, K. (2003). "Anything can happen with police around": Urban youth evaluate strategies of surveillance in public places. *Journal of Social Issues*, *59*(1), 141–158. https://doi.org/10.1111/1540-4560.t01-1-00009

Freedman, D. A. (2009). *Statistical models: Theory and practice*. Cambridge: Cambridge University Press. https://doi.org/10.1017/CBO9780511815867

Furnham, A. (1986). Response bias, social desirability and dissimulation. *Personality and Individual Differences*, *7*(3), 385–400. doi:10.1016/0191-8869(86)90014-0

Garbarino, J. (2001). An ecological perspective on the effects of violence on children. *Journal of Community Psychology*, *29*(3), 361–378. https://doi.org/10.1002/jcop.1022

Gee, G. C., & Ford, C. L. (2011). Old issues, new directions. *Du Bois Review*, *8*(1), 115–132. doi:10.1017/S1742058X11000130

Goff, P. A., Jackson, M. C., Allison, B., Di Leone, L., Culotta, C. M., & DiTomasso, N. A. (2014). The essence of innocence: Consequences of dehumanizing black children. *Journal of Personality and Social Psychology*, *106*, 526–545. https://doi.org/10.1037/a0035663

Gove, W. R., & Geerken, M. R. (1977). Response bias in surveys of mental health: An empirical investigation. *American Journal of Sociology*, *82*(6), 1289–1317. doi:10.1086/226466.JSTOR 2777936. PMID 889001

Gregorowski, C., & Seedat, S. (2013). Addressing childhood trauma in a developmental context. *Journal of Child and Adolescent Mental Health*, *25*, 105–118. https://doi.org/10.2989/17280583.2013.795154

Grusky, D. B. (2014). Theories of Stratification and Inequality. In *International encyclopedia of social and behavioral sciences* (2nd ed.). Oxford: Elsevier. Retrieved from www.elsevier.com/books/international-encyclopedia-of-the-social-andampamp-behavioral-sciences/wright/978-0-08-097086-8

Herrenkohl, T. I., Hong, S., Klika, J. B., Herrenkohl, R. C., & Russo, M. J. (2013). Developmental impacts of child abuse and neglect related to adult mental health, substance use, and physical health. *Journal of Family Violence*, *28*, 191–199. doi:10.1007/s10896-012-9474-9

Hoven, C. W., Duarte, C. S., Lucas, C. P., Wu, P., Mandell, J., Goodwin, R. D., et al. (2005). Psychopathology among New York City public school children 6 months after September. *Archives of General Psychiatry*, *62*(5), 545–551. Retrieved from www.ncbi.nlm.nih.gov/pubmed/15867108

Huynh, Q. L., Devos, T., & Goldberg, R. (2014). The role of ethnic and national identifications in perceived discrimination for Asian Americans: Toward a better understanding of the buffering effect of group identifications on psychological distress. *Asian American Journal of Psychology*, *5*(3), 161–171. doi:10.1037/a0031601

Indian Law & Order Commission. (2013). *Report to the President & Congress of the United States: A road map for making Native Americans safer*. Retrieved April 29, 2020, from https://dps.mn.gov/divisions/ojp/forms-documents/Documents/MMIWTaskForce/IndianLawandOrder CommissionReport.pdf

Israel, B. A., Schulz, A. J., Parker, E. A., & Becker, A. B. (1998). Review of community-based research: Assessing partnership approaches to improve public health. *Annual Review of Public Health, 19*, 173–202. doi:10.1146/annurev.publhealth.19.1.173

Kellerman, N. P. F. (2013). Epigenetic transmission of holocaust trauma: Can nightmares be inherited? *The Israel Journal of Psychiatry and Related Sciences, 50*, 33–39. Retrieved from www.ncbi.nlm.nih.gov/pubmed/24029109

Leiber, M. J., Nalla, M. K., & Farnworth, M. (1998). Explaining juveniles' attitudes toward the police. *Justice Quarterly, 15*(1), 151–174. doi:10.1080/07418829800093671

Leiner, M. J., Peinado, J., Villanos. M. T. M., Lopez, I., Uribe, R., & Pathak, I. (2016). Mental and emotional health of children exposed to news media of threats and acts of terrorism: The cumulative and pervasive effects. *Frontiers in Pediatrics, 4*, 26. doi:10.3389/fped.2016.00026. PMCID: PMC4803729. PMID: 27047909

Listenbee, R. L., Torre, J. J., Boyle, G., Sharon, S. J., Cooper, W., et al. (2012). *Report of the Attorney General's national task force on children exposed to violence.* doi:10.1017/S1742058X11000130. Retrieved April 20, 2020.

Logan, R. W., Hasler, B. P., Forbes, E. E., Franzen, P. L., Torregrossa, M. M., Huang, Y. H., et al. (2017). Impact of sleep and circadian rhythms on addiction vulnerability in adolescents. *Biological Psychiatry, 83*(12), 987–996. https://doi.org/10.1016/j.biopsych.2017.11.035

Manolio, T. A., Bailey-Wilson, J. E., & Collins, F. S. (October 2006). Genes, environment and the value of prospective cohort studies. *Nature Reviews Genetics, 7*(10), 812–820. doi:10.1038/nrg1919

Mansouri, F., & Jenkins, L. (2010). Schools as sites of race relations and intercultural tension. *Australian Journal of Teacher Education, 35*(7), 93–108. http://dx.doi.org/10.14221/ajte.2010v35n7.8

Margolin, G., & Gordis, E. (2000). The effects of family and community violence on children. *Annual Review of Psychology, 51*, 445–479. https://doi.org/10.1146/annurev.psych.51.1.445

Martin, M. J., McCarthy, B., Conger, R. D., Gibbons, F. X., Simons, R. L., Cutrona, C. E., et al. (2011). The enduring significance of racism: Discrimination and delinquency among Black American youth. *Journal of Research on Adolescence, 21*(3), 662–676. doi:10.1111/j.1532-7795.2010.0069

Mathews, B. (2014). Mandatory reporting laws and identification of child abuse and neglect: Consideration of differential maltreatment types, and a cross-jurisdictional analysis of child sexual abuse reports. *Social Sciences, 3*(3), 460–482. doi:10.3390/socsci3030460

Mills-Koonce, W. R., Propper, C., Jean-Louis, G., Barnett, M., Moore, G. A., Calkins, S., et al. (2009). Psychophysiological correlates of parenting behavior in mothers of young children. *Developmental Psychobiology, 51*(8), 650–661. https://doi.org/10.1002/dev.20400

Mischel, W., & Shoda, Y. (1995). A cognitive-affective system theory of personality: Reconceptualizing situations, dispositions, dynamics, and invariance in personality structure. *Psychological Review, 102*(2), 246. https://doi.org/10.1037/0033-295X.102.2.246

National Gang Center. (2012). *National youth gang survey analysis.* Office of Juvenile Justice and Delinquency Prevention, Bureau of Justice Assistance. Retrieved May 20, 2020, from www.nationalgangcenter.gov/Survey-Analysis

Paradies, Y. (2006). A systematic review of empirical research on self-reported racism and health. *International Journal of Epidemiology, 35*, 888–901. doi:10.1093/ije/dyl056

Phinney, J. S., Jacoby, B., & Silva, C. (2007). Positive intergroup attitudes: The role of ethnic identity. *International Journal of Behavioral Development, 31*(5), 478–490. https://doi.org/10.1177/0165025407081466

Priest, N., Perry, R., Ferdinand, A., Paradies, Y., & Kelaher, M. (2014). Experiences of racism, racial/ethnic attitudes, motivated fairness and mental health outcomes among primary and secondary school students. *Journal of Youth and Adolescence, 43*, 1672–1687. doi:10.1007/s10964-014-0140-9

Raffaele-Mendez, L. M., Knoff, H. M., & Ferron, J. M. (2002). School demographic variables and out-of-school suspension rates: A quantitative and qualitative analysis of a large, ethnically diverse school district. *Psychology in the Schools, 39*, 259–277. https://doi.org/10.1002/pits.10020

Reyes, H. L. M., Vangie, A., Foshee, V. A., et al. (2017). Patterns of dating violence victimization and perpetration among Latino youth. *Journal of Youth and Adolescence, 46*(8), 1727–1742. doi:10.1007/s10964-016-0621-0

Rodriguez, J., McKay, M. M., & Bannon, W. M. (2008). The role of racial socialization in relation to parenting practices and youth behavior: An exploratory analysis. *Social Work in Mental Health, 6*(4), 30–54. doi.org/10.1080/15332980802032409

Sanders-Phillips, K. (1997). Assaultive violence in the community: Psychological responses of adolescents and their parents. *Journal of Adolescent Health, 21*, 356–365. https://doi.org/10.1016/S1054-139X(97)00165-1

Sanders-Phillips, K. (2009). Racial discrimination: A continuum of violence exposure for children of color. *Clinical Child and Family Psychology Review, 12*(2), 174–195. https://doi.org/10.1007/s10567-009-0053-4

Sanders-Phillips, K., & Kliewer, W. (2019). Violence and racial discrimination in South African youth: Profiles of a continuum of exposure. *Journal of Child and Family Studies, 29*, 1336–1349. https://doi.org/10.1007/s10826-019-01559-6

Sanders-Phillips, K., Settles-Reaves, B., Walker, D., & Brownlow, J. (2009). Social inequality and racial discrimination: Risk factors for health disparities in children of color. *Pediatrics, 124*(Supplement 3), S176–S186. doi:10.1542/peds.2009-1100E

Schiff, M. (2013). *Dignity, disparity and desistance: Effective restorative justice strategies to plug the "school to prison pipeline".* Retrieved May 20, 2020, from http://civilrightsproject.ucla.edu/resources/projects/center-for-civil-rights-remedies/school-to-prison

Schilis, N., & Verhage, A. (2017). Understanding how and why young people enter radical or violent extremist groups. *International Journal of Conflict and Violence, 11.* doi:10.4119/UNIBI/ijcv.473

Seedat, M., Van Niekerk, A., Jewkes, R., Suffla, S., & Ratele, K. (2009). Violence and injuries in South Africa: Prioritising an agenda for prevention. *Lancet Special Issue: Health in South Africa, 374*(9694), 1011–1022. https://doi.org/10.1016/S0140-6736(09)60948-X

Shadish, W. R., Cook, T. D., & Campbell, D. T. (2002). *Experimental and quasi-experimental designs for generalized causal inference* (2nd ed.). Boston, MA: Houghton Mifflin. Retrieved from https://pdfs.semanticscholar.org/9453/f229a8f51f6a95232e42acfae9b3ae5345df. pdf

Sheats, K. J., Irving, S. M., Mercy, J. A., Simon, T. R., Crosby, A. E., Ford, D. C., et al. (2018). Violence-related disparities experienced by Black youth and young adults: Opportunities for prevention. *American Journal of Preventive Medicine, 55*(4), 462–469. doi:10.1016/j.amepre.2018.05.017

Simons, R. L., Chen, Y., Stewart, E. A., & Brody, G. H. (2003). Incidents of discrimination and risk for delinquency: A longitudinal test of strain theory with an African American sample. *Justice Quarterly, 20*, 82. Retrieved from www.tandfonline.com/doi/abs/10.1080/07418820300095711

Simons, R. L., Murry, V., McLoyd, V., Lin, K. H., Cutrona., C., & Conger, R. D.(2002). Discrimination, crime, ethnic identity, and parenting as correlates of depressive symptoms among African American children: A multilevel analysis. *Development and Psychopathology, 14*, 371–393. Retrieved from www.ncbi.nlm.nih.gov/pubmed/12030697

Simons, R. L., Simons, L. G., Burt, C. H., et al. (2006). Supportive parenting moderates the effect of discrimination upon anger, hostile view of relationships, and violence among African American boys. *Journal of Health and Social Behavior, 47*(4), 373–389. Retrieved from www.ncbi.nlm.nih.gov/pubmed/?term=simons+et+al.+2006+supportive+parenting

Skogan, W. G. (2009). Concern about crime and confidence in the police reassurance or accountability? *Police Quarterly, 12*(3), 301–318. https://doi.org/10.1177/1098611109339893

Stewart, E., Simons, R., & Conger, R. (2002). Assessing neighborhood and social psychological influences on childhood violence in an African American sample. *Criminology, 40*, 801–829. https://doi.org/10.1177/1043986216660009

Stroebe, K., Dovido, J. F., Barreto, M., Ellmers, N., & John, M. S. (2011). Is the world a just place? Countering the negative consequences of pervasive discrimination by affirming the world as just. *British Journal of Social Psychology, 50*, 484–500. doi:10.1348/014466610X523057

Sumner, J. A., Colich, N. L., Uddin, M., Armstrong, D., & McLaughlin, K. A. (2018). Early experiences of threat, but not deprivation, are associated with accelerated biological aging in children and adolescents. *Biological Psychiatry, 85*(3), 268–278. doi:10.1016/j.biopsych.2018.09.008

Umaña-Taylor, A. J., Quintana, S. M., Lee, R. M., Cross, W. E., Rivas-Drake, D., Schwartz, S. J., et al. (2014). Ethnic and racial identity during adolescence and into young adulthood: Am integrated conceptualization. *Child Development, 85*(1), 21–39. doi:10.1111/cdev.12196

Weinstein, N. D. (1993). Testing four competing theories of health-protective behavior. *Health Psychology, 12*, 324–333. https://doi.org/10.1037/0278-6133.12.4.324

Williams, R. (2007). The psychosocial consequences for children of mass violence, terrorism and disasters. *International Review of Psychiatry, 19*(3), 263–277. https://doi.org/10.1080/09540260701349480

Winkler, V. A., & Bouncken, R. B. (2011). How does cultural diversity in global innovation teams affect the innovation process? *Engineering Management Journal, 23*(4), 24–35.

World Health Organization. (2002). *World report on violence and health* (E. Krug, L. Dahlberg, J. Mercy, A. Zwi, & R. R. Lozano, Eds.). Retrieved May 20, 2020, from https://apps.who.int/iris/bitstream/handle/10665/42495/9241545615_eng.pdf;sequence=1

Yahyavi, S. T., Zarghami, M., & Marwah, U. (2014). A review on the evidence of transgenerational transmission of posttraumatic stress disorder vulnerability. *Revista Brasilieria de Psiquiatria, 36*, 89–94. https://doi.org/10.1590/1516-4446-2012-0995

23

ENVIRONMENTAL EXPOSURES
Lead Studies

Bryce Hruska and Brooks B. Gump

Overview

Health psychology is an interdisciplinary field that aims to promote human health and prevent illness. Guided by the biopsychosocial model, it places emphasis on the role played by cognitions, behaviors, and physiological processes as determinants of health. In contrast, the field of environmental health focuses on the role of environmental exposures in human health and disease. Environmental exposures consist of all of the chemicals and compounds that come into human contact, including residual pesticides from fruit and vegetables, **phthalates** (chemicals used to increase the flexibility and permanence of plastics), **parabens** (chemicals used to preserve personal care products), and **bisphenol A** (a chemical used to manufacture plastics; National Biomonitoring Program, 2017c, 2017b, 2017a).

Lead exposure represents a well-researched environmental exposure with established human health effects. Although naturally occurring in the environment, human exposure to lead was less common before the industrial revolution. While government regulations in the United States have resulted in a continuing decline in lead exposure, it remains a threat due to its presence in deteriorating residential paint and aging infrastructure. Since 1976, the Centers for Disease Control and Prevention (CDC) has monitored **blood lead levels (BLLs)** in the general US population using the National Health and Nutrition Examination Survey (NHANES), a program of studies assessing the health and nutrition of both children and adults in the United States. Given that the developing nervous system is particularly sensitive to the effects of lead (Sanders, Liu, Buchner, & Tchounwou, 2010), public health attention has focused on identifying and preventing lead exposure in children. In 1991, the CDC defined a *BLL* of 10 μg/dL as its "level of concern" for children aged one to five years (CDC, 1991). However, given research showing that there is no safe level of lead exposure, the CDC abandoned this terminology in 2012 and instead calculated an upper reference value of lead exposure based upon the 97.5th percentile of the *BLL* distribution in the two most recent NHANES datasets. This upper reference value is updated every four years. The current *BLL* reference value is 5 μg/dL (CDC, 2020); children whose *BLL* meets or exceeds this reference value should be monitored to ensure no further exposure occurs (CDC, 2012).

Considerations that should be made when designing a study in which lead exposure is a key measure of interest include the selection of an appropriate lead biomarker, assessment of other toxicants and nonessential metals that may accompany lead exposure, exposure routes, selection of an appropriate health outcome, and exposure cohort effects that may be present in the sample. In the following chapter, we provide a discussion of each of these topics, as well as key studies that either represent important exemplars or classic studies in the field of lead exposure.

Research in Practice

Biomarker Selection

A key decision in the design of a study in which lead exposure is a measure of interest is the selection of a lead biomarker that is consistent with the purpose and aims of the project. Two of the most common lead biomarkers are in blood and bone. Lead in blood is typically assessed using blood from either ***capillary*** (via a finger stick) or ***venous*** (via venipuncture) samples. With a 35-day half-life, it provides a measure of the circulating levels of lead present in the body (Rabinowitz, Wetherill, & Kopple, 1976); thus, it offers an indication of acute exposure and ongoing effects, as well as the fraction of lead present in the body that may be actively contributing to adverse health outcomes. As such, it may be most appropriately employed in studies interested in the active, ongoing effects of lead exposure on health outcomes. For example, current *BLL* may affect vascular responses to acute stress (Gump, Reihman, Bendinskas, Morgan, Dumas, Palmer, et al., 2005, p. 2005) via interference with ion channels that alter ***intracellular Ca2+ homeostasis***, which refers to the tendency for the body to maintain balanced amounts of calcium inside and outside of its cells (Ferreira de Mattos, Costa, Savio, Alonso, & Nicolson, 2017; Webb, Winquist, Victery, & Vander, 1981).

In contrast, bone lead is typically measured *in vivo* from the dense cortical bone present in the tibia using x-ray fluorescence (Hu, Rabinowitz, & Smith, 1998); it has a variable five- to 19-year half-life that is influenced by age, health, pregnancy and lactation, and pubertal and menopausal status (Hu, Rabinowitz, & Smith, 1998; Rabinowitz, 1991). Bone lead provides a measure of absorbed levels of lead present in the body and can be used as an indication of cumulative exposure. Notably, bone lead may be re-released into circulation in response to physiological processes (e.g., pregnancy, menopause) or disease states (e.g., osteoporosis; Nash, Magder, Sherwin, Rubin, & Silbergeld, 2004; Tellez-Rojo, Hernández-Avila, Lamadrid-Figueroa, Smith, Hernández-Cadena, Mercado, et al., 2004). Thus, in addition to providing a measure of cumulative exposure that may be related to current health status, it provides an indication of future health risks that may be incurred from bone lead stores that are released back into circulation in the body.

Given the complementary viewpoints provided by *BLL* and bone lead levels, inclusion of both in a study protocol has the potential to yield greater insight into the relationship between lead exposure and the selected health outcome of interest. An observational case-control study performed by Hu, Aro, Payton, Korrick, Sparrow, Weiss, et al. (1996) provides a representative example of this approach. Utilizing data from the National Aging Study (Bell, Rose, & Damon, 1972), Hu, et al. (1996) examined the relationship between lead exposure and hypertension. Participants consisted of 590 male veterans who were, on average, 66.6 years old. Cases were defined as individuals with hypertension, as defined by taking daily blood pressure medication or by having a blood pressure reading that met or exceeded 160/96 mmHg at the time of the study's physical examination. Blood lead was assessed via venipuncture, and bone lead was assessed using K-shell x-ray fluorescence measured at the tibia and patella.

On average, participants had a *BLL* equal to 6.3 μg/dL. While considered elevated by today's standards, this *BLL* was below the 10 μg/dL level of concern in place at the time (CDC, 1991). Tibia and patella bone lead levels were 21.6 μg/g and 32.1 μg/g, respectively. While the CDC does not offer bone lead level guidelines, these levels were reported as comparable to those levels typically observed at the time that the study was performed. In unadjusted models, both *BLL* and bone lead levels were found to be greater for participants classified as hypertensive compared to participants classified as nonhypertensive. After controlling for body mass index and family history of hypertension, only bone lead levels in the tibia remained a statistically significant predictor of hypertensive status.

This study is notable because it included both blood lead and bone lead biomarkers. Lead exposure has a documented association with blood pressure (Navas-Acien, Guallar, Silbergeld, & Rothenberg, 2007). Without the inclusion of both types of biomarkers, this association would not have been evident. Furthermore, while *BLLs* were not statistically significantly related to hypertension after controlling for covariates, it is notable that all of the participants were older adult males. Had the study been conducted with menopausal females or if osteoporosis disease status had been assessed, a relationship may have been detected. Including both lead biomarkers in such a hypothetical study would further highlight the different sources of information afforded by each of these measures, as well as the potential value in including both in a study protocol. Similarly, ongoing and repeated cardiovascular perturbations due to circulating lead (as outlined earlier) might, in the context of chronic and repeated exposure, lead to vascular remodeling, elevated blood pressure, and ***cardiovascular disease (CVD)***. As such, bone lead levels might be a stronger predictor of disease endpoints, while *BLL* might predict the functional precursors (i.e., mediators) for these effects. Nevertheless, despite the advantages of measuring both blood and bone lead, measuring bone lead does require a small degree of radiation exposure, and the equipment cost and availability of radiation source can be significant hurdles depending upon the desired sample size and study design. Therefore, it may be unrealistic for many projects.

Other Important Methodological Issues Related to the Measurement of Lead

When making plans for the measurement of lead (or any toxicant, for that matter), one must consider the ***method detection limit (MDL)*** for the proposed sample analysis. The *MDL* refers to the level of precision for a particular laboratory's analytic method—and these levels can vary greatly. For example, analysis of postnatal lead in the Oswego Children's Study (Gump, Reihman, Bendinskas, Morgan, Dumas, Palmer, et al., 2005) relied on abstracting lead levels from primary care charts in New York State (NYS) as a consequence of the state's mandated lead testing for one- to two-year-old children. However, for this sort of routine testing, finger/toe sticks are frequently used, and the subsequent lead analytic methods are designed for low-cost/high-throughput analyses with relatively high *MDLs* (typically 4.0 or 5.0 µg/dL). The high *MDLs* offered by these methods may be adequate if the investigator is considering the effects of high lead exposure; however, recent research has identified variables that are significantly associated with lead in cohorts in which nearly the entire sample has *BLLs* below 4 µg/dL. For example, our recent work documenting an association between lead and vascular responses to acute psychological stress (Gump, MacKenzie, Bendinskas, Morgan, Dumas, Palmer, et al., 2011) required a venous blood draw coupled with an analytic method having an *MDL* of 0.34 µg/dL.

Presence of Other Toxicants and Nonessential Metals

Exposure to nonessential metals rarely occurs as a single metal exposure, particularly when considering low-level exposures. Similarly, exposure to nonessential metals frequently occurs in the context of exposure to other toxicants (e.g., pesticides). In addition to simply using these exposures and potential confounds as covariates, a number of investigators have suggested a need to consider the effect of "metal mixtures" (Agay-Shay, Martinez, Valvi, Garcia-Esteban, Basagaña, Robinson, et al., 2015; Dorea, 2014), as well as specific interactions between different toxicants (Stewart, Reihman, Lonky, Darvill, & Pagano, 2003). However, there are a number of methodological and analytic issues to consider when addressing these more complex models. First, it is necessary to consider sample collection issues. There are legal and ethical limitations with respect to the quantity of biological samples (e.g., blood draw limits) as well as potential budgetary limits to analysis of multiple toxicants (e.g., measurement of multiple organic compounds—such as perfluorochemicals—could quickly exceed $1000 per participant). With these considerations in mind, investigators should carefully consider the relevant literature and study hypotheses when selecting the appropriate toxicants to monitor.

Second, an analysis of multiple toxicants requires a large enough sample size to provide the power to test an interaction. Third, and related to the prior consideration of power, testing interactions between three or more toxicants ("mixtures") within a general linear model requires a sample size that is unrealistic in many situations. New analytic methods are currently being developed to specifically test these higher-order interactions as well as potential nonlinear associations without requiring excessively large samples (Carlin, Rider, Woychik, & Birnbaum, 2013; Forns, Mandal, Iszatt, Polder, Thomsen, Lyche, et al., 2016; Kelley, Banker, Goodrich, Dolinoy, Burant, Domino, et al., 2019). Such interactions among toxicants are important to understand, as toxicant associations may vary across studies (producing inconsistencies) as a result of differences in levels of other toxicants across these study populations.

Exposure Routes

When designing a study considering the effects of lead on human health, it is important to consider potential routes of exposure that may contribute to any lead levels detected. This consideration is important both for the purposes of designing interventions intended to limit exposure and for providing information on potential confounding variables (e.g., socioeconomic status). While lead exposure is declining in the United States, it remains present in the modern environment, creating potential exposure risks that carry significant health effects. Historically, lead exposure in the United States and in most developed countries originated from lead-based gasoline in automobiles and lead-based paint in home residences. Growing recognition of the health effects of lead in the 1970s ushered in governmental regulation. In 1973, the Environmental Protection Agency initiated regulations requiring reductions in the amount of lead content in gasoline (Lewis, 1985), while in 1990, revisions to the Clean Air Act resulted in a complete ban on lead-based gasoline. In addition, in 1978 a ban was issued on lead-based residential paint, followed in 1986 by a ban on lead products used in plumbing (Brown & Margolis, 2012). Collectively, these regulations—particularly the restrictions on lead-based gasoline—have produced a dramatic decline in *BLLs* in both children and adults (Pirkle, 1994).

While these regulations have been effective, they have not curbed occupational exposure, which remains the leading cause of lead exposure in adults. According to the most recent estimates from the Adult Blood Lead Epidemiology and Surveillance Program, 20.4 per 100,000 employed adults in the United States have a *BLL* of 10 μg/dL or higher (Alarcon, 2016). Elevated lead exposure is prevalent for individuals employed in manufacturing (e.g., storage battery manufacturing), construction (e.g., highway, street, and bridge construction), remediation services, or mining industries (e.g., copper, nickel, lead, zinc; reviewed in Shaffer & Gilbert, 2018), as well as for workers in developing countries where regulations limiting worker lead exposure are absent (e.g., Gottesfeld & Pokhrel, 2011).

In contrast to adults, ingestion of lead present in soil, dust, and paint chips is the primary cause of exposure in children (Council on Environmental Health, 2016). Lead may be present in the soil surrounding a home due to its proximity to the street, deteriorating exterior paint, or renovations performed on the home's exterior (e.g., Mielke, Powell, Shah, Gonzales, & Mielke, 2001; Zahran, Laidlaw, McElmurry, Filippelli, & Taylor, 2013). Indoor household dust may contain lead particles from contaminated soil brought into the home from footwear worn outside (Clark, Menrath, Chen, Succop, Bornschein, Galke, et al., 2004). Aside from external sources of lead brought into the home, interior sources of lead may also be ingested. Most notably, paint chips from deteriorating indoor lead-based paint (Su, Barrueto, & Hoffman, 2002) and lead present in water from aging pipes can contribute to children's lead exposure, most recently demonstrated by the Flint water crisis (Hanna-Attisha, LaChance, Sadler, & Champney Schnepp, 2016; Ngueta, Abdous, Tardif, St-Laurent, & Levalloi, 2016). The risk for exposure conveyed by these different routes varies depending upon a child's age. Lead ingested from soil or household dust is the major lead exposure route in children from birth to six months, while lead ingested from water is the major route of exposure in children between one and two years old (Zartarian, Xue, Tornero-Velez, & Brown, 2017).

Well-designed research exploring lead exposure routes is essential, given the established effects of lead on various health outcomes (see "Health Outcome Selection" later for a review). A natural experiment conducted by Mielke, Gonzales, Powell, and Mielke (2017) provides an example of a creative research design that demonstrates the impact of lead-contaminated soil on children's *BLLs*. In the study, soil lead concentrations and *BLLs* in children under six years were compared before and after Hurricane Katrina. Following Katrina, the city of New Orleans razed and replaced all public housing using lead-free paint and amended landscapes on both public and private properties with fresh soil. These actions provided an unplanned opportunity for lead abatement. Soil samples were collected as part of an ongoing series of soil surveys performed in New Orleans (Mielke, Gonzales, Powell, & Mielke, 2005, 2016).

In total, 3314 pre-Katrina soil samples were collected from 1998 to 2001 and 3320 post-Katrina soil samples were collected from 2013 to 2015. Blood samples were obtained from the Louisiana Childhood Blood Lead Surveillance System, a local program conducted by the Louisiana State Department of Health to monitor the *BLLs* of children residing within the state. In total, 13,379 pre-Katrina and 4,820 post-Katrina blood samples were collected. Soil and blood samples were divided into four groups according to their geographical location within the city of New Orleans (i.e., public vs. private properties located within the core vs. outer regions of the city). Results demonstrated large reductions in the soil lead content and corresponding decreases in the *BLLs* of children residing in New Orleans in all groups. In particular, soil lead concentrations decreased 59% to 81% in the private and public *core* areas of the city—regions in which congested traffic patterns, deteriorating housing, and aging lead smelting plants are located. Likewise, in these regions of the city, the percentage of children with *BLLs* exceeding 5 μg/dL decreased by 70% to 88%. Collectively, these results highlight the profound impact that soil replacement can have on child *BLLs* and provide a compelling argument for the implementation of polices and soil replacement practices in the city of New Orleans.

Although relatively high *BLLs* are likely a consequence of these important exposure routes, low-level *BLLs* might occur as a result of more pervasive and repeated low-level exposure to sources such as airborne dust from contaminated soil (Laidlaw, Mielke, Filippelli, Johnson, & Gonzales, 2005) and food (Leroux, Ferreira, Silva, Bezerra, da Silva, Salles, et al., 2018). For example, in the Environmental Exposures and Child Health Outcomes (EECHO) cohort, we have found that African American (AA) children have significantly higher *BLLs* than European American (EA) children, and, furthermore, this difference in *BLL* is a result of AAs consuming more total fruit (based on total dietary records) than EAs (Gump, Hruska, Parsons, Palmer, MacKenzie, Bendinskas, et al., 2020). From a public health standpoint, these prevalent, low-level, persistent sources of lead exposure may be more important than isolated, high-level, acute sources of lead exposure (e.g., water pipes in Flint, Michigan; Ruckart, Ettinger, Hanna-Attisha, Jones, Davis, & Breysse, 2019). Moreover, such chronic low-level exposures might be particularly important in the etiology of slow-developing diseases such as *CVD* and hypertension.

Health Outcome Selection

The selection of an appropriate health outcome is another important choice when designing a study examining lead exposure effects. Lead has pervasive health consequences due to its impact on a variety of target organs in the cardiovascular, nervous, skeletal, and renal systems of the body. Its effects on cardiovascular and neurocognitive function are some of the more well-documented associations.

The cardiovascular effects of lead exposure have been the primary health outcome of interest in adults. Both experimental and observational studies have demonstrated that lead exposure can cause cardiac and vascular damage (Kopp, Barron, & Tow, 1988). For example, while *CVD* rates in the United States have decreased in tandem with decreasing lead levels (Ruiz-Hernandez, Navas-Acien, Pastor-Barriuso, Crainiceanu, Redon, Guallar, et al., 2017), recent estimates suggest that nearly a third of *CVD* cases in the United States may be attributable to lead exposure, and an increase in *BLLs* from 1.0 to 6.7 µg/dL is associated with a 1.7 times increased risk for *CVD* mortality (Lanphear, Rauch, Auinger, Allen, & Hornung, 2018). In an effort to better understand the mechanism for lead-induced *CVD* later in life, some recent research has focused on *CVD* risk factors in children that are associated with lead exposure (Gump, Stewart, Reihman, Lonky, Darvill, Parsons, et al., 2008; Gump, et al., 2011; Pawlas, Płachetka, Kozłowska, Broberg, & Kasperczyk, 2015).

In contrast to adults, the neurocognitive effects of lead exposure have been the primary health outcome examined in children. The nervous system absorbs a greater proportion of circulating lead relative to other organs in the body. Due to its ability to mimic calcium ions and calcium-mediated cell processes, lead readily crosses the blood–brain barrier, where it creates a state of excitotoxicity, oxidative stress, and abnormal neurotransmitter functioning that ultimately results in neuronal dysfunction and death throughout the central nervous system (for a review see Lidsky & Schneider, 2003). Collectively, these effects contribute to a number of neurocognitive problems in children, with intellectual deficits being one of the most studied (Bellinger, 2004).

Meta-analyses examining the relationship between lead exposure and IQ suggest that a doubling of *BLL* concentration (e.g., 5 to 10 µg/dL or 10 to 20 µg/dL) results in a childhood IQ decrement between one and 2.6 points (Pocock, Smith, & Baghurst, 1994; Schwartz, 1994). While these effects may appear small, it is estimated that, at the population level, a one-point IQ decrement attributable to lead exposure translates into earnings reductions totaling over $15 billion (Salkever, 2014). Notably, given the decreasing *BLLs* present in the general US population, research also suggests that the IQ decrement resulting from lead exposure may be greater at lower *BLLs* than at higher levels (e.g., <7 µg/dL vs. ≤7.5 µg/dL; Lanphear, Hornung, Khoury, Yolton, Baghurst, Bellinger, et al., 2005). Thus, the effect of lead on IQ continues to be a highly relevant health outcome despite decreasing BLLs.

Aside from its effect on intelligence, lead exposure is also associated with socioemotional and behavioral problems in children. Increasing *BLLs* at age two have been shown to be associated with emotion regulation deficits, while increasing levels of bone lead at age 10 have been shown to predict both externalizing and internalizing symptoms (via teacher report) at age 11 (Mendelsohn, Dreyer, Fierman, Rosen, Legano, Kruger, et al., 1998; Needleman, Riess, Tobin, Biesecker, & Greenhouse, 1996). In adolescence, increasing *BLLs* have been shown to predict subsequent aggressive behaviors and physical violence (Nkomo, Mathee, Naicker, Galpin, Richter, & Norris, 2017;, Nkomo, Naicker, Mathee, Galpin, Richter, & Norris, 2018). These latter findings have also been observed at the population level: census tracts in the United States that consist of a higher percentage of children with BLLs ≥5 µg/dL have been shown to have a higher level of both violent and nonviolent crime even after controlling for neighborhood disadvantage (defined by a composite measure reflecting household income, poverty, unemployment, and housing conditions; Boutwell, Nelson, Emo, Vaughn, Schootman, Rosenfeld, et al., 2016).

Only a handful of prospective longitudinal studies examining the effects of lead exposure from birth through early childhood on health outcomes in childhood and adulthood have been conducted. Such studies are crucial contributors to our understanding of effects of lead across the lifespan. The Port Pirie Cohort study is one such study. Initiated in 1979 in the smelting town of Port Pirie, Australia, the study is ongoing, with the most recent follow-up assessment performed in 2008–2009 when participants were 25 to 29 years old. A variety of key insights into the effects of lead exposure on childhood development have been documented (for review see Searle, Baghurst, van Hooff, Sawyer, Sim, Galletly, et al., 2014), and the findings pertaining to intellectual functioning are particularly notable. In an early report from the study, Tong, Baghurst, McMichael, Sawyer, and Mudge (1996) examined the relationship between prenatal (via venous blood samples from the mother), perinatal (via umbilical cord blood samples assessed at birth), and postnatal (via venous blood from the children assessed roughly yearly) *BLLs* and intelligence in 375 members (79.4% of eligible cohort members) of the Port Pirie Cohort. The average prenatal *BLL* was 9.52 µg/dL; the average perinatal *BLL* was 8.49 µg/dL; the average *BLL* at age 11 to 13 was 7.87 µg/dL; and the lifetime average at age 11 to 13 (i.e., *BLLs* averaged over all assessments through age 11 to 13) was 14.08 µg/dL. Intelligence was assessed using the Wechsler Intelligence Scale for Children (WISC). Total IQ, verbal comprehension IQ, and performance IQ subscale scores were considered. Results indicated that after controlling for socioeconomic status, maternal IQ, and enrichment in the home environment, an inverse relationship between *BLLs* and total scores and all subscales on the WISC was observed for all *BLLs* except perinatal. Notably, the relationship with lifetime average was particularly strong. At the time of publication, this study was one of the few to consider the effects of lead exposure on intelligence in early childhood. Collectively, these results demonstrated the persistent effects of lead exposure on intelligence. Furthermore, given that *BLLs* declined across time in the sample, the demonstration that lifetime average levels were particularly associated with intelligence decrements was a key finding because it signaled the importance of primary over secondary prevention.

Cohort Effects

BLLs have been declining in the United States for decades, and because of this trend it is important to consider the age of the target population to be included in a study examining lead exposure. The average *BLL* of adults in the general US population today is approximately half of what it was a decade ago (Tsoi, Cheung, Cheung, & Cheung, 2016). At the time of this writing, the CDC's blood lead reference value is 5 µg/dL (based upon the 2007–2008 and 2009–2010 NHANES datasets); however, more recent data (from the 2011–2012 and 2013–2014 NHANES datasets) suggest that a lower reference value of 3.48 µg/dL may be warranted (Caldwell, Cheng, Jarrett, Makhmudov, Vance, Ward, et al., 2017).

While these decreasing levels are encouraging, it is important to remember that no level of lead exposure is safe (CDC, 2012). In addition, the average *BLL* in children one to five years old in the most recent NHANES datasets (NHANES 2011–2014) is still estimated to be 50 times greater than the average *BLL* extrapolated from bone lead levels present in the remains of preindustrial humans (0.82 µg/dL vs. 0.016 µg/dL; Caldwell, Cheng, Jarrett, Makhmudov, Vance, Ward, et al., 2017; Flagel & Smith, 1992). Thus, even today's low *BLLs* greatly exceed what was typical prior to the industrial revolution, necessitating further examination in order to better understand their health implications. Understanding associations at the low exposure range might be particularly important, as it is possible that physiological changes associated with *BLLs* occur at very low levels of lead and "saturate" quickly. In other words, perhaps risk factors increase as *BLL* rises from no exposure to low levels (e.g., 1.0 mg/dL), but exposures beyond 1.0 accrue no greater risk. Further investigation is required to determine if and when such nonlinear associations operate. On a related note about toxicant levels and human health, toxicants with high body burdens are not necessarily more important to human health and functioning than lower-level exposures. The critical question is the level at which a particular toxicant begins to have a significant and large effect and whether this effect increases with increasing exposures (as opposed to a nonlinear association suggesting saturation, followed by a plateau, cf. [Lanphear, et al., 2005]). For example, some toxicants are highly impactful on the body, even at very low levels, and quickly become lethal (e.g., dimethylmercury).

As lead exposure continues to decline in the general population, it is becoming concentrated in historically disenfranchised populations through residential segregation and a corresponding racial divide in exposure to older housing stock that may have lead paint and pipes (Gee & Payne-Sturges,

2004). An estimated 37.1 million homes in the United States contain lead-based paint, affecting 40% of poorer households (i.e., household income <$30,000/year) compared to 32.3% of more affluent households (i.e., household income ≥$30,000/year). Furthermore, 45.3% of households headed by African Americans live in a home with lead-based paint compared to 31.6% of households headed by Caucasians (Dewalt, Cox, O'Haver, Salatino, Holmes, Ashley, et al., 2015). Consequently, when designing a research study that includes lead exposure, it is important to consider whether the study should oversample individuals based upon demographic characteristics such as socioeconomic status or race/ethnicity. This may be particularly important if the study is concerned with examining the main effects of lead exposure on the selected health outcome. On the other hand, if the goal of the study is to consider how demographic factors, including socioeconomic status and race, modify the relationship between lead exposure and a selected health outcome, it is important to design a study to recruit an adequate number of participants with qualifying characteristics to detect hypothesized moderating effects (Bellinger, 2000).

A prospective observation study performed by Bellinger, Leviton, and Sloman (1990) represents one of the initial studies highlighting the importance of this consideration. Using a sample of 249 children, the researchers examined the relationship between *perinatal BLLs* (via umbilical cord); *post-natal BLLs* (via capillary blood samples at six, 12, 18, 24, and 57 months); and cognitive functioning at six, 24, and 57 months. Participants were divided into three groups based upon their *BLL* at birth: a low group (<3 μg/dL), a medium group (3 to 10 μg/dL), and a high group (≥10 μg/dL). Results indicated that cognitive deficits observed at six months tended to improve through 57 months of age for all groups. However, these effects were dependent upon the socioeconomic status of the children's families. More specifically, cognitive deficits observed at 24 months persisted through 57 months for children belonging to low-income families; however, a marked improvement was observed during this same time frame for children whose *BLL* was elevated at birth but who belonged to high-income families. These findings highlight the influential role that socioeconomic status potentially plays in buffering the adverse health effects of lead exposure on child development.

Strengths and Limitations

The impact of lead on human health has been well-established by existing research. Indeed, the studies reviewed in this chapter have played an important role in informing public health policy surrounding lead exposure. Collectively, their strengths lie in their careful attention to design regarding the topics reviewed in this chapter. As a result, the consistent decline in *BLLs* in the United States is regarded by many as one of the best examples of public health research translated into regulatory actions that have led to tangible results.

Even so, there are a number of limitations facing all lead exposure research conducted today. First, the limitations associated with assay sensitivity remain an outstanding challenge for contemporary lead exposure research. As discussed earlier, decreasing *BLLs* necessitate ever more sensitive assays in order to reliability and accurately investigate the significance of low levels of lead exposure. Second, most existing lead exposure research has not adequately accounted for the potential effect of other toxicant and nonessential metals that may co-occur with lead exposure. As noted earlier, new analytic methods are being developed to account for these interactions and are needed in order to fully understand the significance of environmental exposures on human health.

Conclusion

Recommendations for Future Research

This review suggests a number of important directions for future research. First, public health policy research will need to address the issue of how best to respond to low-level exposures. If, as the CDC now asserts, there are no known safe levels of lead, are public health efforts best directed at acute exposure events as in Flint, Michigan or are we best served by primary prevention efforts such as lead abatement in homes, identification and elimination of contaminated foods, and soil removal/replacement? Perhaps the answer to this question also depends upon the particular health outcome that is prioritized: IQ might be most strongly affected by high exposures at critical developmental periods for the child (suggesting a need to address emergent high-level exposures), whereas *CVD* risk might be most strongly associated with low-level chronic exposures (suggesting a need to identify and eliminate low-level exposure sources).

Second, although there are relatively well-established associations between *BLLs* and IQ as well as hypertension/*CVD*, establishing a mechanism to explain these associations remains an area in need of study. This is a particularly important line of work, as it can help establish whether prior associations found with lead are a result of poorly controlled confounds (i.e., whether the associations are spurious) or if lead actually causes the changes in these outcomes.

Finally, low-level lead exposures may be unavoidable at this point (i.e., the industrial revolution and consequent widespread mining of lead may have created exposure routes that will exist indefinitely). If so, are there methods to safely remove lead from the body? Currently, exposure to chelating agents can convert metal ions into chemically and biochemically inert forms that can then be excreted; however, there are a number of side effects to these treatments (Andersen, 2004), and therefore, most chelation is only recommended for high-exposure situations. Perhaps additional research on "natural" chelators will identify approaches that are safer and can be implemented even for low-level lead exposure (Amadi, Offor, Frazzoli, & Orisakwe, 2019). For example, the CDC recommends greater consumption of iron, vitamin C, and calcium as a means to lower *BLL*; however, there is research suggesting that such nutrient intake may be ineffective in mitigating exposure to nonessential metals (Kordas, 2017).

References

Agay-Shay, K., Martinez, D., Valvi, D., Garcia-Esteban, R., Basagaña, X., Robinson, O., et al. (2015). Exposure to endocrine-disrupting chemicals during pregnancy and weight at 7 years of age: A multi-pollutant approach. *Environmental Health Perspectives*, *123*(10), 1030–1037. https://doi.org/10.1289/ehp.1409049

Alarcon, W. A. (2016). Elevated blood lead levels among employed adults: United States, 1994–2013. *Morbidity and Mortality Weekly Report*, *63*, 59–65.

Amadi, C. N., Offor, S. J., Frazzoli, C., & Orisakwe, O. E. (2019). Natural antidotes and management of metal toxicity. *Environmental Science and Pollution Research*, *26*(18), 18032–18052. https://doi.org/10.1007/s11356-019-05104-2

Andersen, O. (2004). Chemical and biological considerations in the treatment of metal intoxications by chelating agents. *Mini Reviews in Medicinal Chemistry*, *4*(1), 11–21. https://doi.org/10.2174/1389557043487583

Bell, B., Rose, C. L., & Damon, A. (1972). The normative aging study: An interdisciplinary and longitudinal study of health and aging. *Aging and Human Development*, *3*(1), 5–17. https://doi.org/10.2190/GGVP-XLB5-PC3N-EF0G

Bellinger, D. C. (2000). Effect modification in epidemiologic studies of low-level neurotoxicant exposures and health outcomes. *Neurotoxicology and Teratology*, *22*(1), 133–140. https://doi.org/10.1016/S0892-0362(99)00053-7

Bellinger, D. C. (2004). Lead. *Pediatrics*, *113*(Supplement 3), 1016–1022.

Bellinger, D. C., Leviton, A., & Sloman, J. (1990). Antecedents and correlates of improved cognitive performance in children exposed in utero to low levels of lead. *Environmental Health Perspectives*, *89*, 5–11. https://doi.org/10.1289/ehp.90895

Boutwell, B. B., Nelson, E. J., Emo, B., Vaughn, M. G., Schootman, M., Rosenfeld, R., et al. (2016). The intersection of aggregate-level lead exposure and crime. *Environmental Research*, *148*, 79–85. https://doi.org/10.1016/j.envres.2016.03.023

Brown, M. J., & Margolis, S. (2012). Lead in drinking water and human blood lead levels in the United States. *Morbidity and Mortality Weekly Report*, *61*, 1–9.

Caldwell, K. L., Cheng, P.-Y., Jarrett, J. M., Makhmudov, A., Vance, K., Ward, C. D., et al. (2017). Measurement challenges at low blood lead levels. *Pediatrics*, *140*(2), e20170272. https://doi.org/10.1542/peds.2017-0272

Carlin, D. J., Rider, C. V., Woychik, R., & Birnbaum, L. S. (2013). Unraveling the health effects of environmental mixtures: An NIEHS priority. *Environmental Health Perspectives*, *121*, 1. https://doi.org/10.1289/ehp.1206182

CDC. (1991). *Preventing lead poisoning in young children*. Washington, DC: Centers for Disease Control and Prevention.

CDC. (2012). *Low level lead exposure harms children: A renewed call for primary prevention*. Washington, DC: Centers for Disease Control and Prevention.

CDC. (2020). *CDC: Lead: Blood lead reference value*. Retrieved from www.cdc.gov/nceh/lead/data/blood-lead-reference-value.htm

Clark, S., Menrath, W., Chen, M., Succop, P., Bornschein, R., Galke, W., et al. (2004). The influence of exterior dust and soil lead on interior dust lead levels in housing that had undergone lead-based paint hazard control. *Journal of Occupational and Environmental Hygiene*, *1*(5), 273–282. https://doi.org/10.1080/15459620490439036

Council on Environmental Health. (2016). Prevention of childhood lead toxicity. *Pediatrics*, *138*(1), e20161493–e20161493. https://doi.org/10.1542/peds.2016-1493

Dewalt, F. G., Cox, D. C., O'Haver, R., Salatino, B., Holmes, D., Ashley, P. J., et al. (2015). Prevalence of Lead Hazards and Soil Arsenic in U.S. Housing. *Journal of Environmental Health*, *78*(5), 22–29. JSTOR.

Dorea, J. G. (2014). Chemical mixtures, maternal exposure and infant neurodevelopment: Did we miss positive (breastfeeding) and negative (mercury) confounders? *Neurotoxicology and Teratology*, *45*, 93. https://doi.org/10.1016/j.ntt.2014.06.006

Ferreira de Mattos, G., Costa, C., Savio, F., Alonso, M., & Nicolson, G. L. (2017). Lead poisoning: Acute exposure of the heart to lead ions promotes changes in cardiac function and Cav1.2 ion channels. *Biophysical Reviews*, *9*(5), 807–825. https://doi.org/10.1007/s12551-017-0303-5

Flagel, A. R., & Smith, D. R. (1992). Lead levels in preindustrial humans. *New England Journal of Medicine*, *326*(19), 1293–1294. https://doi.org/10.1056/NEJM199205073261916

Forns, J., Mandal, S., Iszatt, N., Polder, A., Thomsen, C., Lyche, J. L., et al. (2016). Novel application of statistical methods for analysis of multiple toxicants identifies DDT as a risk factor for early child behavioral problems. *Environmental Research*, *151*, 91–100. https://doi.org/10.1016/j.envres.2016.07.014

Gee, G. C., & Payne-Sturges, D. C. (2004). Environmental health disparities: A framework integrating psychosocial and environmental concepts. *Environmental Health Perspectives*, *112*(17), 1645–1653. https://doi.org/10.1289/ehp.7074

Gottesfeld, P., & Pokhrel, A. K. (2011). Review: Lead exposure in battery manufacturing and recycling in developing countries and among children in nearby communities. *Journal of Occupational and Environmental Hygiene*, *8*(9), 520–532. https://doi.org/10.1080/15459624.2011.601710

Gump, B. B., Hruska, B., Parsons, P. J., Palmer, C. D., MacKenzie, J. A., Bendinskas, K., & Brann, L. (2020). Dietary contributions to increased background lead, mercury, and cadmium in 9–11 year old children: Accounting for racial differences. *Environmental Research*, *185*, 109308. https://doi.org/10.1016/j.envres.2020.109308

Gump, B. B., MacKenzie, J. A., Bendinskas, K., Morgan, R., Dumas, A. K., Palmer, C. D., et al. (2011). Low-level Pb and cardiovascular responses to acute stress in children: The role of cardiac autonomic regulation. *Neurotoxicology and Teratology*, *33*(2), 212–219. https://doi.org/10.1016/j.ntt.2010.10.001

Gump, B. B., Reihman, J., Bendinskas, K., Morgan, R., Dumas, A. K., Palmer, C. D., et al. (2005). Prenatal and early childhood blood lead levels and cardiovascular functioning in 9.5 year-old children. *Neurotoxicology and Teratology*, *27*(4), 655–665. https://doi.org/10.1016/j.ntt.2005.04.002

Gump, B. B., Stewart, P., Reihman, J., Lonky, E., Darvill, T., Parsons, P. J., et al. (2008). Low-level prenatal and postnatal blood lead exposure and adrenocortical responses to acute stress in children. *Environmental Health Perspectives*, *116*(2), 249–255. https://doi.org/10.1289/ehp.10391

Hanna-Attisha, M., LaChance, J., Sadler, R. C., & Champney Schnepp, A. (2016). Elevated blood lead levels in children associated with the flint drinking water crisis: A spatial analysis of risk and public health response. *American Journal of Public Health*, *106*(2), 283–290. https://doi.org/10.2105/AJPH.2015.303003

Hu, H., Aro, A., Payton, M., Korrick, S., Sparrow, D., Weiss, S. T., et al. (1996). The relationship of bone and blood lead to hypertension: The normative aging study. *JAMA: Journal of the American Medical Association*, *275*(15), 1171. https://doi.org/10.1001/jama.1996.03530390037031

Hu, H., Rabinowitz, M., & Smith, D. (1998). Bone led as a biological marker in epidemiological studies of chronic toxicity: Conceptual paradigms. *Environmental Health Perspectives*, *106*(1), 1–8.

Kelley, A. S., Banker, M., Goodrich, J. M., Dolinoy, D. C., Burant, C., Domino, S. E., et al. (2019). Early pregnancy exposure to endocrine disrupting chemical mixtures are associated with inflammatory changes in maternal and neonatal circulation. *Scientific Reports*, *9*(1), 1–14. https://doi.org/10.1038/s41598-019-41134-z

Kopp, S. J., Barron, J. T., & Tow, J. P. (1988). Cardiovascular actions of lead and relationship to hypertension: A review. *Environmental Health Perspectives*, *78*, 91–99. https://doi.org/10.1289/ehp.887891

Kordas, K. (2017). The "lead diet": Can dietary approaches prevent or treat lead exposure? *The Journal of Pediatrics*, *185*, 224–231, e1. https://doi.org/10.1016/j.jpeds.2017.01.069

Laidlaw, M. A. S., Mielke, H. W., Filippelli, G. M., Johnson, D. L., & Gonzales, C. R. (2005). Seasonality and children's blood lead levels: Developing a predictive model using climatic variables and blood lead data from Indianapolis, Indiana, Syracuse, New York, and New Orleans, Louisiana (USA). *Environmental Health Perspectives*, *113*(6), 793–800. https://doi.org/10.1289/ehp.7759

Lanphear, B. P., Hornung, R., Khoury, J., Yolton, K., Baghurst, P., Bellinger, D. C., et al. (2005). Low-level environmental lead exposure and children's intellectual function: An international pooled analysis. *Environmental Health Perspectives*, *113*(7), 894–899. https://doi.org/10.1289/ehp.7688

Lanphear, B. P., Rauch, S., Auinger, P., Allen, R. W., & Hornung, R. W. (2018). Low-level lead exposure and mortality in US adults: A population-based cohort study. *The Lancet Public Health*, *3*(4), e177–e184. https://doi.org/10.1016/S2468-2667(18)30025-2

Leroux, I. N., Ferreira, A. P. S. da S., Silva, J. P. da R., Bezerra, F. F., da Silva, F. F., Salles, F. J., et al (2018). Lead exposure from households and school settings: Influence of diet on blood lead levels. *Environmental Science and Pollution Research*, *25*(31), 31535–31542. https://doi.org/10.1007/s11356-018-3114-8

Lewis, J. (1985). Lead poisoning: A historical perspective. *EPA Journal*, *15*, 15–18.

Lidsky, T. I., & Schneider, J. S. (2003). Lead neurotoxicity in children: Basic mechanisms and clinical correlates. *Brain*, *126*(1), 5–19. https://doi.org/10.1093/brain/awg014

Mendelsohn, A. L., Dreyer, B. P., Fierman, A. H., Rosen, C. M., Legano, L. A., Kruger, H. A., et al. (1998). Low-level lead exposure and behavior in early childhood. *Pediatrics*, *101*(3), e10–e10. https://doi.org/10.1542/peds.101.3.e10

Mielke, H. W., Gonzales, C. R., Powell, E. T., & Mielke, P. W. (2005). Changes of Multiple Metal Accumulation (MMA) in New Orleans soil: Preliminary evaluation of differences between survey I (1992) and survey II (2000). *International Journal of Environmental Research and Public Health*, *2*(2), 308–313. https://doi.org/10.3390/ijerph2005020016

Mielke, H. W., Gonzales, C. R., Powell, E. T., & Mielke, P. W. (2016). Spatiotemporal dynamic transformations of soil lead and children's blood lead ten years after Hurricane Katrina: New grounds for primary prevention. *Environment International*, *94*, 567–575. https://doi.org/10.1016/j.envint.2016.06.017

Mielke, H. W., Gonzales, C. R., Powell, E. T., & Mielke, P. W. (2017). Spatiotemporal exposome dynamics of soil lead and children's blood lead pre- and ten years post-Hurricane Katrina: Lead and other metals on public and private properties in the city of New Orleans, Louisiana, U.S.A. *Environmental Research*, *155*, 208–218. https://doi.org/10.1016/j.envres.2017.01.036

Mielke, H. W., Powell, E. T., Shah, A., Gonzales, C. R., & Mielke, P. W. (2001). Multiple metal contamination from house paints: Consequences of power sanding and paint scraping in New Orleans. *Environmental Health Perspectives*, *109*(9), 973–978. https://doi.org/10.1289/ehp.01109973

Nash, D., Magder, L. S., Sherwin, R., Rubin, R. J., & Silbergeld, E. K. (2004). Bone density-related predictors of blood lead level among peri- and postmenopausal women in the United States the third national health and nutrition examination survey, 1988–1994. *American Journal of Epidemiology*, *160*(9), 901–911. https://doi.org/10.1093/aje/kwh296

National Biomonitoring Program. (2017a). *Bisphenol a (BPA) factsheet|National Biomonitoring Program|CDC*. Retrieved from www.cdc.gov/biomonitoring/BisphenolA_FactSheet.html

National Biomonitoring Program. (2017b). *Parabens factsheet|National Biomonitoring Program|CDC*. Retrieved from www.cdc.gov/biomonitoring/Parabens_FactSheet.html

National Biomonitoring Program. (2017c). *Phthalates factsheet|National Biomonitoring Program|CDC*. Retrieved from www.cdc.gov/biomonitoring/Phthalates_FactSheet.html

Navas-Acien, A., Guallar, E., Silbergeld, E. K., & Rothenberg, S. J. (2007). Lead exposure and cardiovascular disease: A systematic review. *Environmental Health Perspectives*, *115*(3), 472–482. https://doi.org/10.1289/ehp.9785

Needleman, H. L., Riess, J. A., Tobin, M. J., Biesecker, G. E., & Greenhouse, J. B. (1996). Bone lead levels and delinquent behavior. *JAMA: Journal of the American Medical Association*, *275*(5), 363–369. https://doi.org/10.1001/jama.275.5.363

Ngueta, G., Abdous, B., Tardif, R., St-Laurent, J., & Levallois, P. (2016). Use of a cumulative exposure index to estimate the impact of tap water lead concentration on blood lead levels in 1- to 5-year-old children (Montréal, Canada). *Environmental Health Perspectives*, *124*(3), 388–395. https://doi.org/10.1289/ehp.1409144

Nkomo, P., Mathee, A., Naicker, N., Galpin, J., Richter, L. M., & Norris, S. A. (2017). The association between elevated blood lead levels and violent behavior during late adolescence: The South African birth to twenty plus cohort. *Environment International*, *109*, 136–145. https://doi.org/10.1016/j.envint.2017.09.004

Nkomo, P., Naicker, N., Mathee, A., Galpin, J., Richter, L. M., & Norris, S. A. (2018). The association between environmental lead exposure with aggressive behavior, and dimensionality of direct and indirect aggression during mid-adolescence: Birth to twenty plus cohort. *Science of the Total Environment, 612*, 472–479. https://doi.org/10.1016/j.scitotenv.2017.08.138

Pawlas, N., Płachetka, A., Kozłowska, A., Broberg, K., & Kasperczyk, S. (2015). Telomere length in children environmentally exposed to low-to-moderate levels of lead. *Toxicology and Applied Pharmacology, 287*(2), 111–118. https://doi.org/10.1016/j.taap.2015.05.005

Pirkle, J. L. (1994). The decline in blood lead levels in the United States: The National Health and Nutrition Examination Surveys (NHANES). *JAMA: Journal of the American Medical Association, 272*(4), 284. https://doi.org/10.1001/jama.1994.03520040046039

Pocock, S. J., Smith, M., & Baghurst, P. (1994). Environmental lead and children's intelligence: A systematic review of the epidemiological evidence. *BMJ, 309*(6963), 1189–1197. https://doi.org/10.1136/bmj.309.6963.1189

Rabinowitz, M. B. (1991). Toxicokinetics of bone lead. *Environmental Health Perspectives, 91*, 33–37. https://doi.org/10.1289/ehp.919133

Rabinowitz, M. B., Wetherill, G. W., & Kopple, J. D. (1976). Kinetic analysis of lead metabolism in healthy humans. *Journal of Clinical Investigation, 58*(2), 260–270. https://doi.org/10.1172/JCI108467

Ruckart, P. Z., Ettinger, A. S., Hanna-Attisha, M., Jones, N., Davis, S. I., & Breysse, P. N. (2019). The flint water crisis: A coordinated public health emergency response and recovery initiative. *Journal of Public Health Management and Practice, 25*, S84–S90. https://doi.org/10.1097/PHH.0000000000000871

Ruiz-Hernandez, A., Navas-Acien, A., Pastor-Barriuso, R., Crainiceanu, C. M., Redon, J., Guallar, E., et al. (2017). Declining exposures to lead and cadmium contribute to explaining the reduction of cardiovascular mortality in the US population, 1988–2004. *International Journal of Epidemiology, 46*(6), 1903–1912. https://doi.org/10.1093/ije/dyx176

Salkever, D. S. (2014). Assessing the IQ-earnings link in environmental lead impacts on children: Have hazard effects been overstated? *Environmental Research, 131*, 219–230. https://doi.org/10.1016/j.envres.2014.03.018

Sanders, T., Liu, Y., Buchner, V., & Tchounwou, P. B. (2010). *Nihms190515, 24*(1), 15–45.

Schwartz, J. (1994). Low-level lead exposure and children's IQ: A metaanalysis and search for a threshold. *Environmental Research, 65*(1), 42–55. https://doi.org/10.1006/enrs.1994.1020

Searle, A. K., Baghurst, P. A., van Hooff, M., Sawyer, M. G., Sim, M. R., Galletly, C., et al. (2014). Tracing the long-term legacy of childhood lead exposure: A review of three decades of the port pirie cohort study. *NeuroToxicology, 43*, 46–56. https://doi.org/10.1016/j.neuro.2014.04.004

Shaffer, R. M., & Gilbert, S. G. (2018). Reducing occupational lead exposures: Strengthened standards for a healthy workforce. *NeuroToxicology, 69*, 181–186. https://doi.org/10.1016/j.neuro.2017.10.009

Stewart, P. W., Reihman, J., Lonky, E. I., Darvill, T. J., & Pagano, J. (2003). Cognitive development in preschool children prenatally exposed to PCBs and MeHg. *Neurotoxicology and Teratology, 25*(1), 11–22. https://doi.org/10.1016/S0892-0362(02)00320-3

Su, M., Barrueto, F., & Hoffman, R. S. (2002). Childhood lead poisoning from paint chips: A continuing problem. *Journal of Urban Health, 79*(4), 491–501. https://doi.org/10.1093/jurban/79.4.491

Tellez-Rojo, M. M., Hernández-Avila, M., Lamadrid-Figueroa, H., Smith, D., Hernández-Cadena, L., Mercado, A., et al. (2004). Impact of bone lead and bone resorption on plasma and whole blood lead levels during pregnancy. *American Journal of Epidemiology, 160*(7), 668–678. https://doi.org/10.1093/aje/kwh271

Tong, S., Baghurst, P., McMichael, A., Sawyer, M., & Mudge, J. (1996). Lifetime exposure to environmental lead and children's intelligence at 11–13 years: The Port Pirie cohort study. *BMJ, 312*(7046), 1569–1575. https://doi.org/10.1136/bmj.312.7046.1569

Tsoi, M.-F., Cheung, C.-L., Cheung, T. T., & Cheung, B. M. Y. (2016). Continual decrease in blood lead level in Americans: United States national health nutrition and examination survey 1999–2014. *The American Journal of Medicine, 129*(11), 1213–1218. https://doi.org/10.1016/j.amjmed.2016.05.042

Webb, R. C., Winquist, R. J., Victery, W., & Vander, A. J. (1981). In vivo and in vitro effects of lead on vascular reactivity in rats. *American Journal of Physiology-Heart and Circulatory Physiology, 241*(2), H211–H216. https://doi.org/10.1152/ajpheart.1981.241.2.H211

Zahran, S., Laidlaw, M. A. S., McElmurry, S. P., Filippelli, G. M., & Taylor, M. (2013). Linking source and effect: Resuspended soil lead, air lead, and children's blood lead levels in Detroit, Michigan. *Environmental Science & Technology, 47*(6), 2839–2845. https://doi.org/10.1021/es303854c

Zartarian, V., Xue, J., Tornero-Velez, R., & Brown, J. (2017). Children's lead exposure: A multimedia modeling analysis to guide public health decision-making. *Environmental Health Perspectives, 125*(9), 097009. https://doi.org/10.1289/EHP1605

24

GEOGRAPHIC DETERMINANTS

Joy E. Obayemi and Roy H. Hamilton

Overview

Our lived experiences are inextricably linked to our environments. From the quality of the air that we breathe to our perceived sense of safety when walking throughout our neighborhood, much of our physical and psychological health can be affected by the physical, social, and even political realities of our surroundings. This concept has long been studied in the field of environmental psychology, which focuses on "relating the physical environment to human behavior" (Devlin, 2018, p. xvi). For approximately 50 years, experts in this field have attempted to study how and in what ways the environment can affect an individual's health, employing a variety of biological and psychological methodologies. One must also recognize that an individual's mental or physical illness is rife with external influences. The aim of this chapter is to discuss how geographic influences affect the psychosocial health of an individual and to present and critique methodologies used to study this impact.

Family structure and housing conditions are two proximal and profoundly influential environmental factors that affect child development. Familial and emotional stability can prevent the perpetually elevated cortisol levels seen in children who are subject to volatility, which can predispose them to conduct disorders, anxiety, and depression (Bucci, Marques, Oh, & Harris, 2016; Oh, Jerman, Silvério Marques, Koita, Purewal Boparai, Burke Harris, et al., 2018). This can occur when children do not have steady, consistent sources of emotional support, whether due to absent or transient caregivers or neglect. Children who are forced to relocate frequently within the foster care system are particularly vulnerable to the effects of home instability. In addition to a person's interpersonal and emotional environment, evidence demonstrates that the physical environment affects their physical and mental health (Devlin, 2018). In one British study, living in poor housing conditions within the past five years—defined as "not enough light, lack of adequate heating, condensation, leaky roof, damp walls or roof, and/or rot in the walls or floor"—was associated with poorer mental health (Pevalin, Reeves, Baker, & Bentley, 2017, p. 305). Research has also shown that those who live in high-rise apartments have higher rates of psychological distress, perhaps due to "concerns about housing, feeling trapped in deprived social environments, fears of falling from windows or balconies, being trapped by fire, earthquake, or terror attacks" (Larcombe, van Etten, Logan, Prescott, & Horwitz, 2019, p. 3). Public housing high-rise apartments built in the mid-20th century in American cities were often poorly constructed and overcrowded. For example, the Robert Taylor homes in Chicago at one time housed over 27,000 people when it was only built to hold 11,000 (Larcombe, et al., 2019). Such housing conditions affect the day-to-day experiences of the inhabitants and can lead to behavior changes that affect health.

Apart from one's immediate living environment, a lack of resources in local communities can negatively or positively affect residents' well-being in a variety of ways. The lack of markets in poorly resourced areas makes it difficult to purchase nutrient-rich foods, such as vegetables, and to establish healthy eating habits. In these *food deserts*, nutritious food is simply not available for purchase, even for residents with economic means. Other community resources also vary dramatically along economic lines. As highlighted in the literature, "resources such as leisure and park facilities, day-care centers, social activities, and other institutional resources are usually more scarce in poor neighborhoods" (Amaddeo, Salazzari, & Salinas-Perez, 2015, p. 39). The absence of these resources can have an enormous impact on the development of young children in these neighborhoods, potentially contributing to poor mental and physical health (Larcombe, et al., 2019). In addition, unsafe communities contribute to differences in physical and mental well-being. If there is violence plaguing the streets of an inner-city neighborhood, children may elect to spend less time exercising or playing outdoors and more time worrying about their physical safety and that of those around them. Of course, these problems with community resources and dynamics are not limited to urban environments. Access to facilities such as mental health clinics, doctors' offices, and other institutions is also limited in rural areas of the country, demonstrating that low-income urban and rural neighborhoods experience similar barriers to optimizing health.

Structural characteristics of a geographic area, such as high levels of pollution, also contribute to poor mental health. Studies from around the world have shown that air pollution is strongly correlated with a variety of psychiatric pathologies, including depression and anxiety (Lim, Kim, Kim, Bae, Park, & Hong, 2012; Power, Kioumourtzoglou, Hart, Okereke, Laden, & Weisskopf, 2015). Researchers have hypothesized that the *oxidative stress* (i.e., the cellular damage caused by exposure to free radicals) and the systemic inflammation associated with prolonged exposure to pollution may be responsible for these findings and for generalized neurobehavioral dysfunction (Power, et al., 2015; Salvi & Salim, 2019). Furthermore, environmental toxins—such as lead in the water of Flint, Michigan—can have chronic effects on health. Studies have found that lead exposure is associated with decreased cognitive functioning and psychiatric conditions such as depression and anxiety (Mason, Harp, & Han, 2014). Exposure to other heavy metal toxins, such as mercury, can also lead to significant neuropathology.

From what has been stated, one could surmise that the working definition of environment being cultivated here is simply a proxy for socioeconomic status. Unfortunately, given the worsening structural and economic inequality in the United States, socioeconomic status greatly dictates one's geography. Poverty is often concentrated in neighborhoods, where a lack of funding for public schools or for local infrastructure frequently leads to decreased access to important resources. It has been shown that one's ZIP code is a powerful predictor of all-cause mortality, more than genetics and medical risk factors (Arias, Escobedo, Kennedy, Fu, & Cisewki, 2018; Goodwin, Nadig, McElligott, Simpson, & Ford, 2016; Murphy, Xu, Kochanek, & Arias, 2018). Similarly, the oppression, racism, and discrimination that are often present in the lived experiences of those who live in these neighborhoods of low socioeconomic status negatively affects their psychosocial well-being. Some American cities are more racially segregated than South Africa under apartheid (Massey & Denton, 1998), showing that race and class undoubtedly affect one's geographical surroundings.

Given the abundant evidence that geography affects an individual's mental and physical health, how can we appropriately and effectively study these interactions? How do we gather the data necessary to elucidate the ways in which the environment can affect the nuances of the human experience? A variety of methodologies propose their own answers to these questions, each with powerful strengths and weaknesses worthy of consideration. In their struggle to balance generalizability with validity, voyeurism with collaboration, and control settings with studying subjects *in situ*, each moves us towards a more complete and inclusive understanding of the world around us.

Research in Practice

Ecological Momentary Assessments

Theory

The work of Barker, Wicker, and Gump in the 1950s and 1960s—at the origins of environmental psychology as a discipline—posits that "behavior is to be understood as part of a larger context or setting that occurs within boundaries" (Devlin, 2018, p. xvii). This begs the question: How do we study this behavior within its geographical boundaries? Presumably, the moment we take our subjects out of their environment into a controlled research setting for an interview or focus group, we have lost the chance to really observe the environmental influences at work. Even if we joined our subjects in their environments, walking the streets alongside them, our data run the risk of being corrupted by our mere presence via the Hawthorne effect or changes to an individual's behavior in response to being observed (O' Sullivan, Orbell, Rakow, & Parker, 2004).

Ecological momentary assessment (EMA) is a methodology that attempts to address these concerns by prompting subjects to report on their behaviors, feelings, and general states of being in real time. By doing so, *EMA* hopes to bring ecological validity to studies of human behavior and interactions. This methodology was initially created in the clinical context based on the premise that humans have tremendous difficulty remembering our own experiences. Our ability to recall past events is plagued with biases that can affect our memory in both unpredictable and systematic ways.

Although the term *EMA* was not established until 1994, one could say that the first versions of *EMA*s took the form of diaries (Shiffman, Stone, & Hufford, 2008). Over the years, this methodology has grown and developed, especially in the realm of psychology, in an attempt to understand more about the nuances of human behavior. Currently, *EMA* often involves a handheld electronic device that study subjects carry around with them. There are two ways that the device can collect data. It can use a *time-based* approach, in which the subject is alerted ("pinged") to respond to a set of questions on the device at predetermined intervals throughout the day. It can also take an *event-based* approach, in which subjects are directed to respond to questions on the device whenever they are having particular experiences, such as cravings or interpersonal conflicts.

It is also possible to combine these approaches and gather even more data points for analysis. More recent studies have also used global positioning system (GPS) data at the time of response as yet another focal point for analysis (Shaughnessy, Reyes, Shankardass, Sykora, Feick, Lawrence, et al., 2018). An *EMA* study that utilizes GPS data is often referred to as a *geographic ecologic momentary assessment (GEMA)* or *geographic momentary assessment (GMA)*; this methodological subgroup is particularly pertinent for studying how environmental factors such as access to green space, pollution, and the financial wealth of the surrounding community can affect subject responses (Epstein, Tyburski, Craig, Phillips, Jobes, Vahabzadeh, et al., 2014; Kirchner & Shiffman, 2016; Mennis, Mason, & Ambrus, 2018; Shaughnessy, et al., 2018) With all of the information that can be gathered, researchers are able to piece together a detailed story of a subject's lived experience over the course of a day as his or her environment and conditions shift. One could say, "Data provided by *EMA* studies may be likened to a movie, in which dynamic relationships emerge over time, whereas global or recall measures are analogous to a still photograph, a single static snapshot of time" (Shiffman, et al., 2008, p. 10). *EMA* has been used to study a variety of behavioral and psychological phenomena, including smoking cessation, toddler exercise habits, and self-esteem (Campbell, Babiarz, Wang, Tilton, Black, & Hager, 2018; Hager, Tilton, Wang, Kapur, Arbaiza, Merry, et al., 2017; Shiffman, et al., 2008).

There are a number of advantages to using *EMA*, including the ability to characterize the changes in an individual's experience (e.g., different levels of pain a patient experiences throughout the day while recovering from surgery), the natural history of a phenomenon (e.g., the pattern of cigarette cravings when trying to quit), the relevant contextual associations (e.g., what type of events can trigger sadness or anger throughout one's day), and the impact of temporality on experience (e.g., how does the impact of an event change over time; Shiffman, et al., 2008). In relation to the environment's impact on the human experience, the geospatial and social contextualization allotted by EMA is paramount.

Like any other methodology, *EMA* has weaknesses. While these assessments are not being performed in a room filled with researchers, one must consider that the mere act of being evaluated and knowing that your responses will be closely analyzed may affect how you respond. This reactivity is often present when a subject is asked to actively participate in the research in some way. Another related challenge of *EMA* as a methodology is both conscious and subconscious deception. Many of these studies aim to understand complex psychological conditions, such as addiction and depression. However, subjects may not be eager to share their struggles with drug use or suicidal ideation due to powerful social stigma surrounding these topics. Due to this social desirability bias, they may alter their responses in order to provide answers that they perceive as being more socially acceptable or pleasing to the researchers. It may also be that some subjects have a difficult time being honest with themselves about their true feelings.

Lastly, compliance is another common challenge associated with *EMA*s. Depending on the intervals chosen by the research team, subjects may be prompted to respond to questions a number of times throughout the day. Some studies have required assessments more than 20 times per day (Shiffman, et al., 2008). These assessments can be very intrusive over the course of one's day and could easily lead to survey fatigue. Reports of compliance in *EMA*-type studies range from 11% to over 80% or 90% (Ram, Brinberg, Pincus, & Conroy, 2017). These strengths and weaknesses of *EMA* are best illustrated in the context of a specific study, as seen in the next section.

Case Study

A 2016 study by Mennis, Mason, Light, Rusby, Westling, Way, et al., provides a clear example for how *EMA*, and more specifically *GMA*, can be utilized to understand how one's environment influences behavior. The study aimed to answer the following question: Does substance use moderate the association of neighborhood disadvantage with perceived stress and safety in the activity spaces of urban youth? (Mennis, et al., 2016). The researchers hypothesized that the psychological stress of spending time in impoverished, low-resource neighborhoods might lead adolescents to rely heavily on coping mechanisms, such as substance use. They wanted to see how the geographical location of the adolescents and feelings of safety and stress corresponded to patterns of drug use.

They studied this by utilizing the one-year follow-up data from the Social Spatial Adolescent Study based out of Richmond, Virginia, from 2012 to 2014. As a part of this study, adolescents 13 to 14 years old were enrolled from outpatient clinics in the Richmond area. They were all given a mobile phone on which they received text messages with uniform resource locator (URL) links to the web-based *EMA* survey. Participants were prompted to complete these surveys three to six times per day over a four-day period every other month during the two-year study period (Mennis, et al., 2016). In these surveys, participants were asked about their substance use, feelings of safety, and feelings of stress. Substance use was measured using the validated Adolescent Alcohol and Drug Involvement Scale (AADIS), which asks about the frequency of drug use, time since last use, and type of substance consumed (Moberg & Hahn, 1991). To evaluate feelings of safety, the adolescents were asked "How safe are you right now?" and instructed to give a number between 1 ("Not at all safe") and 9 ("Very safe"). They were also asked "How stressed out are you right now?" with responses ranging from 1 ("Not at all stressed out") to 9 ("Very stressed out"; Mennis, et al., 2016, p. 289). As study participants submitted their responses, GPS data were also being sent from the mobile phones they were given. These data were used to create a variable called **relative neighborhood disadvantage** (Mennis, et al., 2016, p. 289). Neighborhood disadvantage was determined using an established index that factors in percentage of households with income below the poverty level, percentage of female-headed households with children, percentage of adults with at least a bachelor's degree, and percentage of owner-occupied housing obtained from the US census (Ross & Mirowsky, 2001). These variables were used to determine a disadvantage score for a particular location. The *relative neighborhood disadvantage* could then be calculated by subtracting the score of the location associated with the *EMA* response from the score associated with the participant's home. The researchers then performed **general estimating equations (GEE)** to create models correlating momentary stress and safety with the calculated *relative neighborhood disadvantage*. Substance use information from the AADIS was used to create three distinct subpopulations: those with a score indicating abstinence (AADIS = 2), those with a score indicating substance use (AADIS between 3 and 36), and those with a score indicating likely substance use disorder (AADIS >36; Moberg & Hahn, 1991). Models were created and analyzed for each of these populations.

The results show that for the 139 participants in the study, *relative neighborhood disadvantage* was associated with substance use after controlling for race, age, and sex (Mennis, et al., 2016). It was also significantly associated with momentary feelings of stress, an effect that was stronger among those with a history of more substance use. However, this result had a Cohen's *d* value of 0.3, indicating a small-to-medium effect size. Interestingly, there was no correlation between momentary feelings of safety and *relative neighborhood disadvantage*. The data presented did show that those with higher reported substance use also had higher perceptions of stress and felt less safe in their surroundings (Mennis, et al., 2016).

This study concludes by stating, "This research highlights the value of capturing integrated activity space-based neighborhood characteristics and momentary measures of perceived stress and safety for investigating neighborhood associations with substance use and demonstrates the efficacy of *GMA* for this purpose" (Mennis, et al., 2016, p. 291). This paper exemplifies the power of *EMA* and *GMA* as a methodological tool. By using momentary assessments, GPS, and census data, the authors were able to connect perceptions of stress and safety to both substance use and neighborhood conditions. As highlighted in the prior section, this environmental contextualization of human behavior is a powerful advantage of *EMA* and a strength of this particular study. Another strength in this work is how the data points were collected. By assessing participants for several days over the course of years, the authors likely avoided the survey fatigue that would have come with daily assessments, especially in the adolescent population they chose to study. They could also feel confident that the data did not simply reflect the effects of a particular event or a "bad week" because such a long time period was represented.

However, as the authors also highlight, the study had several weaknesses worthy of consideration. The size of the cohort was fairly limited, with data from only 139 adolescents being analyzed in the end. While it is inherently difficult to get continued participation from 13- to 14-year-olds, the incompleteness of the data reflects how compliance can be a huge barrier with this study design. The authors report that they had a 50% response rate among all the adolescents in the study and only 41% of the *EMA* responses submitted from outside of the participants' homes had GPS coordinates (Mennis, et al., 2016). All of the incomplete data collected were therefore excluded from the final analysis. It is possible that systematic bias influenced which adolescents completed all of the *EMA*s as instructed. Social desirability bias could have affected the validity of the AADIS responses, especially given how sensitive adolescents can be to social pressures. Lastly, we should consider that even validated indexes and tools can invigorate prejudicial notions unless they are subject to appropriately rigorous scrutiny. The scoring system described in this study by Mennis, Mason, and Ambrus, which has been used for years in a variety of studies in environmental psychology, utilizes "female-headed households with children" as a marker of a disadvantaged neighborhood (2018, p. 289). We would argue that the choice to highlight "female-headed" households rather than "single-guardian" households is reflective of patriarchal notions that women serving as the head of a household automatically puts those in that household and even the surrounding community at a disadvantage. Such a bias in the calculations used to determine "neighborhood disadvantage" could have pervasive effects on the conclusions drawn from this work. Other studies have chosen to measure social disorder, environmental hazards, and neighborhood disorder—in other words, neighborhood disadvantage—by using a metric such as the Neighborhood Inventory for Environment Typology (Epstein, et al., 2014). This metric utilizes direct observation of the physical layout of the space (such as the layout of the city block, type of structures, adult activity, youth activity, physical disorder, and social order) performed by multiple raters to objectively characterize a neighborhood (Furr-Holden, Campbell, Milam, Smart, Ialongo, & Leaf, 2010, 2008). However, such a nuanced understanding of a neighborhood takes time and means that are not always available.

In the next section, we will introduce genetics as another key factor that can influence behavior and explore how to best study the intersection of one's genetics and environment to further our understanding of human experience.

Twin Studies

Theory

Our consideration of environmental effects would be incomplete without reference to the debate of nurture versus nature. This fiery debate has raged and simmered its way throughout a variety of disciplines, from psychology to biology to medicine. Academics and lay people alike have been intrigued by this question because it demands that we reflect on how our essential traits came to be and forces a philosophical choice between determinism and the unpredictability of life experience. Are we who we are because of our genetics? Or does our environment shape the personalities and beliefs that define us?

While the answer probably lies somewhere between these two extremes, twin studies are a helpful research methodology to answer these questions. Studying the experiences of twins allows researchers to keep genetics constant in order to isolate the impact of the environment on the human experience. However, limiting a study population to twins vastly changes the range of populations and subgroups that can be studied. Often these studies require long and tedious enrollment periods as researchers search for as many identical and fraternal twins to be involved as possible. To facilitate recruitment, there are many twin registries around the world available for research purposes (Hur, Bogl, Ordoñana, Taylor, Hart, Tuvblad, et al., 2020). However, unless these registries make an effort to recruit diverse populations, they run the risk of producing relatively homogenous cohorts with limited generalizability (Younan, Tuvblad, Li, Wu, Lurmann, Franklin, et al., 2016).

In medicine, twin studies are often used to explore the influence of genetic factors on the development of specific pathology, such as schizophrenia or alcoholism. They determine a concordance rate for both **monozygotic** (**MZ**, 100% genetic similarity) and **dizygotic** (**DZ**, average of 50% genetic similarity) twins developing the same medical condition. However, in these types of studies, the premise is that the twins were reared together and therefore shared a common environment, a concept known as the "*equal environment assumption*" (Joseph, 2002, p. 71). With this assumption, researchers can conclude that if the concordance rate is higher among *MZ* twins than *DZ* twins, there is a significant contribution of genetics to the development of that pathology. However, the utility of this methodology in environmental psychology is in denying this assumption of environmental sameness. Much like studies of twins that are reared apart, these psychologists are more interested in how environmental differences affect the lives of the twins. They can do this by choosing adults who were reared together as children and then exposed to separate environments as adults, therefore eliminating confounders associated with vastly different childhoods. Alternatively, they could choose adults reared apart as children to appreciate the impact of a lifetime of environmental differences. Thus, twin studies can take many forms and lead to a wide range of inferences.

It is often said that proximity to plants and greenery can improve one's mood. In the following study, we will see how infrared light calculations and twins as genetic controls can be studied to determine if there is any truth to such a statement.

Case Study

One study that captures the potential for twin studies as a methodology in this field comes out of the University of Washington and their study on the impact of green space on depression, stress, and anxiety (Cohen-Cline, Turkheimer, & Duncan, 2015). The authors utilized the University of Washington Twin Registry, which was described as "a community-based sample of twins reared together identified by the Washington State Department of Licensing" that was recruited between 2008 and 2014 (Cohen-Cline, et al., 2015, p. 523). Psychology literature has suggested for some time that access to green space can have an important impact on an individual's mental health (Lee & Maheswaran, 2011). However, as the authors of this study point out, most of those studies were cross-sectional in nature, which leaves the possibility of reverse causality up for debate. Other studies also have an "inability to control for non-random selection of residents into neighborhoods," meaning that neighborhoods with less green space may be populated by people who have vastly different life experiences and economic means, which could affect their overall mental health (Cohen-Cline, et al., 2015, p. 523). Therefore, the authors posit that a twin study comparing adult twins who were reared together and have a relatively similar life experience would limit potential confounders and highlight the true influence of green space on mental health.

The study recruited 4,338 twins. While 73.5% of the twins had once lived in Washington State, the addresses of the participants at the time of the study spanned almost all 50 states. Green space exposure was measured using the **Normalized Difference Vegetation Index (NDVI)**. This well-established tool uses remote satellite sensors to estimate the light reflected by vegetation within a specified distance around an address; in this study the radius used was 1 km (Cohen-Cline, et al., 2015). Specifically, "Healthy vegetation reflects **near-infrared (NIR) light** while absorbing **visible (VIS) light**.. . . The *NDVI* is calculated by dividing the difference of *NIR* and visible radiation by the sum of *NIR* and visible radiation: $NDVI=(NIR-VIS)/(NIR+VIS)$" (Cohen-Cline, et al., 2015, p. 524). The *NDVI* ranges from a score of -1 to 1, with lower values indicating less vegetation. A score of -1 represents water, while a score of 0.1 or below indicates barren areas of rock, sand, or snow. A score of 0.2 to 0.3 is considered moderate vegetation, and scores of 0.6 to 0.8 indicate environments similar to tropical rainforests. Participants living within 1 km of water were excluded from the analysis.

Depression as an outcome was measured using the Patient Health Questionnaire (PHQ2). Stress and anxiety were also measured using Perceived Stress Scale (PSS) and the Brief Symptom Inventory (BSI), respectively. All three of these validated questionnaires utilize a 4-point Likert scale to evaluate symptoms of depression, life-event scores, social anxiety, and other aspects of their lived experience. The authors also recognize that household income and physical activity were potential confounders, so they gathered these data from participants to include in their analysis. Population density and neighborhood deprivation were two additional measures of the environment that were considered. Statistical analyses were performed using multilevel random intercept models. The first model correlated *NDVI* with mental health, treating each twin as a singleton in order to establish baseline effects of green space on depression, anxiety, and stress (Cohen-Cline, et al., 2015). The subsequent models then explored the within-pair effect of both *MZ* and *DZ* twins. As the authors state, "A significantly different within-pair effect for *MZ* and *DZ* twins suggests genetic confounding in the relationship between green space and mental health" (Cohen-Cline, et al., 2015, p. 525).

The study found that there was a significant inverse association between exposure to green space and depression, anxiety, and stress when all participants were analyzed individually. In the genetically informed models, there was found to be a significant within-pair inverse association between *NDVI* score and markers of depression. As stated,

> the twin with the higher *NDVI* had a lower risk of depression. . . . The *MZ* within-pair effect in the unadjusted model for depression suggests that, on average, people who live in or around dense vegetation have a 0.44 (on a scale of 0–9) lower depression score than those who live in a location without any access to green space.
>
> *(Cohen-Cline, et al., 2015, p. 526)*

This significant association persisted in the models that adjusted for income, physical activity, population density, and the other possible confounders established *a priori*. In the models that adjusted for income and physical activity, there was also found to be a significant difference in this association between *MZ* and *DZ* twins. The within-pair effect of limited green space exposure was more negative for *MZ* twins than *DZ* twins, indicating that genetics could possibly attenuate the impact of green space on an individual's mental health (Cohen-Cline, et al., 2015). There was also a significant inverse association between green space exposure and stress and anxiety. However, these differences were not present in the adjusted models, indicating that those measured confounders likely explained the association between green space and stress and anxiety in the participant population.

These results bolster the notion that the amount of green in our environments can influence our mood and psychiatric health. The authors offer a thought-provoking discussion surrounding the mechanism for lack of green space contributing to depression, hypothesizing that green space indicates increased access to outdoor physical activity, and perhaps those who value physical activity choose to live in greener neighborhoods. But they agree that more work is needed to identify the exact mechanism behind this association. The use of twins in this study strengthens the authors' arguments because it allowed them to control for many known and unknown confounders, such as childhood exposures and family history. The large population accessed also improved the power of their analysis.

However, the study struggles to achieve generalizability for a couple of key reasons. First, the study population was 90% white, which does not reflect the ethnic and cultural diversity of the American society. It would have been useful to see if access to green space affected mental health in the same way among different demographic groups. Since comfort and solidarity can be derived from people of similar ethnic backgrounds living in close proximity, it would be interesting and relevant to study how green space exposure and exposure to people of similar backgrounds could both affect mental health and perhaps counteract each other (Hogg & Abrams, 2001). The choice to remove all individuals who lived near water from the analysis may have also biased the data by excluding wealthier twins who can afford waterfront property. There has also been work describing the benefits of living near water that the authors could have contributed to if they had used alternative exclusion criteria.

In the following section, we will discuss work in environmental and health psychology that attempts to bring members of the community onto the research team, recognizing that they have a deep knowledge of their own communities that researchers can never truly access. What happens when this local grassroots knowledge is utilized in both the design and implementation of community health initiatives?

Participatory Action Research

Theory

There is always an element of voyeurism in psychological research. The act of carefully studying the ins and outs of a community, attempting to dissect behavior and interaction, requires focusing a pair of binoculars on a study population. However, the same binoculars used to view these communities creates an inherent separation between "us" and "them," dividing the world into researchers and their subjects. Not all methodologies require this degree of separation between the two groups. Acknowledging that the goal of the work is to eventually affect the study population positively, one can choose to lower the binoculars and pass them to the subject, asking them what they see and how they might go about improving their own community.

This is the premise of what is known as ***participatory action research (PAR)***. In this paradigm, members of the community being studied are included in the design and execution of the study, offering their feedback on everything from subject selection to intervention to further directions for the research. This work has been described as a "practice that attempts to put the less powerful at the center of the knowledge creation process, to move people and their daily lived experiences of struggle and survival from the margins of epistemology to the center" (Hall, 1992, p. 16). With these marginalized groups placed at the center of this work, researchers are able to appreciate how knowledge is intricately linked to one's vantage point and to see how individuals with different lived experiences can add depth to that knowledge. This realization is also transformative for the community participants, as they are given the means to meaningfully contributing to new knowledge.

The theory behind participatory action work is founded upon the work of Paolo Freire, who spoke boldly about the impact of social participation on creating social change (Khan, Bawani, & Aziz, 2013). In *Pedagogy of the Oppressed*, Freire speaks of how community members, particularly the youth, should be called upon to be co-creators of knowledge rather than empty vessels into which knowledge is placed (Freire, 1993). Through this co-creation, individuals can feel empowered to change their own surroundings. Given its origins, *PAR* is a research methodology born out of community organizing and activism work with a clear intention of dismantling oppressive social systems. Many would argue that this foundation in the principles of social justice allows *PAR* to reduce the wide and oppressive gap between the sources of social knowledge and its disseminators.

There can be many benefits to adopting *PAR* as one's primary methodology. If we accept that there is a truth about human experience to be understood and that knowledge of that truth is often obscured by geopolitical narratives and social constructs, one could argue that incorporating the vantage points of those from wildly different walks of life is the only way to access that truth. Therefore, the validity of the work done in social sciences could potentially improve if diverse voices were given a seat at the table. As researchers employing this methodology have stated, "Some posit that *PAR* is the best methodology that allows us to get closer to the truth . . . and while it cannot claim to always get it right, *PAR* is one tool in the struggle for liberation" (Etowa, Bernard, Oyinsan, & Clow, 2007, p. 352). Participation from the subject's community can also help researchers determine if the questions they are asking will, in fact, capture the ideas or social phenomena they wish to study. In a Canadian *PAR* study of Black women's health in rural Nova Scotia, the authors conducted in-depth interviews with the study subjects and had community participants review the interview questions, reporting back on how best to ask questions about certain topics (Etowa, et al., 2007). As they stated, "the likelihood of the research instruments' alienating the researched is reduced and the questions posed are more likely to be meaningful, enabling the participants to describe their experiences more effectively" (Etowa, et al., 2007, p. 353).

Another important strength of this methodology is that it effectively brings in groups of people who have historically been excluded from the research process. ***Youth-oriented PAR***, or ***YPAR***, has been a robust area of research that has worked specifically to get adolescents and young adults to contribute their ideas to the research process. *YPAR* is used to understand how teenagers can become actively involved in their communities, to provide a grassroots perspective on barriers to maternal and child health, to help build safe social spaces for youth, and to promote health (Foster-Fishman, Law, Lichty, & Aoun, 2010; Khan, et al., 2013; Vaughan, 2014; Wang & Pies, 2004). This participation can take many different forms, from using a ***photovoice*** method that requires participants to take photographs and record their spoken commentary, to using Internet platforms for discussion in what can be called ***e-PAR*** (Flicker, Maley, Ridgley, Biscope, Lombardo, Skinner, et al., 2008; Wang & Pies, 2004).

Lastly, *PAR* has a key element that is often missing from research in the social sciences: action. As a methodology, *PAR* is poised not only to adequately identify psychosocial phenomenon but also to determine how real changes can be made. Some have stated that *PAR* is "a method of social investigation of problems, involving the participation of oppressed and ordinary people in problem posing and problem solving" (Maguire, 1987, p. 29). It can be seen as a way to "empower people to analyze their experience as a means of effecting change" (Etowa, et al., 2007, p. 351).

However, some in academia have pushed back on the utility of *PAR*. Many have wondered: Does mere participation truly equal empowerment? Does participation do enough work to subvert the power that wealthy institutions have over struggling communities? Etowa, and colleagues argue that "[*PAR*] should not be construed as empowerment if it does not result in capacity building to effect change" (2007, p. 351). Therefore, it is important that involving participants is not simply a symbolic gesture but also a launching point for a transfer of true power and agency.

Critics of *PAR* also state that researchers should not take their expertise for granted. Given that the purest *PAR* model allows community participation in the design and analysis of the studies, some would argue that participants do not have the knowledge or analytical skills needed for quality research. Some have even questioned whether or not members of the community wish to be involved in social science research (Etowa, et al., 2007). Much like a Black person being asked to explain racism or a woman educating others about sexism, participating in the social education of others can be tiring and is often an undue burden placed on already marginalized communities. Perhaps members of these key populations worthy of study would rather not entangle themselves in the world of academic research. Lastly, discussions of *PAR* often involve a debate concerning the ownership of the data and the research itself. If the community is the entity being studied, should they have ownership of the research results? Furthermore, if community members are providing their time and energy to improve the quality and applicability of a study, how exactly should they be recognized for their efforts in the dissemination of that work? These are all questions that those choosing to employ *PAR* as a methodology need to explore.

In order to illustrate the power of this methodology, in the following section we will discuss a specific study in which *e-PAR* was used to partner with youth and community organizations to promote healthy living.

Case Study

Researchers based in Toronto, Canada, have thoughtfully been trying to engage youth for many years. Since its inception in 1995, the TeenNet Research Program out of the University of Toronto has been investigating how best to promote health among the city's youth (Norman & Skinner, 2007). Over the years, researchers from this group realized that they could make a larger impact on the community if they focused their efforts on collaborative intervention rather than individual health behaviors. They also saw the value of involving the youth in their research efforts, stating "young people must be viewed as community assets that are capable of partnering in both the identification of community health issues and the development of possible solutions" (Flicker, et al., 2008, p. 286). The authors also recognize the practical benefits of having the perspectives of the population they were trying to engage at the decision table. They stated,

> Some of the benefits of involving youth as co-researchers include valuable youth input in research design to ensure that processes are 'youth friendly' and accessible, assistance in the recruitment of hard-to-reach youth through peer models, increased accessibility and community credibility, improved analysis and the development of creative peer dissemination strategies.
>
> *(Flicker, et al., 2008, p. 286)*

As a result of this reflection, a technology-based e-*PAR* project was determined to be the most effective methodology.

The authors developed a model for youth participation that involved the use of "youth media" (i.e., Internet, photography, video and music production software) to critically research the world around them and propose potential improvements (Flicker, et al., 2008). Instead of recruiting participants individually, the TeenNet Research Group chose to form partnerships with local organizations that already worked with adolescents and teenagers, such as a drop-in center for young adults in the city, a support group for LGBTQ immigrant youth, and others (Flicker, et al., 2008). Through working within established community groups, the researchers were able to integrate seamlessly into the social network of the study participants. Once a team of young people was established, the project they developed was either overseen by TeenNet members or members of the youth center who became co-facilitators of the study. This highlights another strength of the study in that the authors were willing to step back and minimize direct supervision over the work. The research was managed from a distance whenever possible, which gave the youth the flexibility to direct these projects freely.

Fifty-seven young people were involved in seven different projects between 2000 and 2004. Each project had a set number of group members who gathered weekly for anywhere from four to 12 months. Some groups were told to design a project around a specific health concern, such as tobacco use, while others were allowed to choose their own health initiative to address. The youth were able to brainstorm and design an initiative that would best address the topic at hand. The researchers state, "In all cases, the scope of the youths' participation was negotiated transparently by the facilitators at the time of recruitment," indicating that clear expectations were set from the beginning (Flicker, et al., 2008, p. 291). A key strength of how this group employed *PAR* is that they provided the participants with clear tangible benefits in addition to the communal benefits of the overall study. For instance, several participants joined the work due to the promise that they could work with various types of music production software. While they used these skills to create uplifting songs for their community, they also left the project with music production skills that could help them in non-research settings (Flicker, et al., 2008).

This research resulted in a variety of youth-led interventions; however, the focus here is on one project: Rock the Boat. This project was designed by youth participants recruited at Support Our Youth (SOY), a Toronto-based group created to support LGBTQ youth who had recently immigrated to the country. The team consisted of seven people aged 18 to 24 who recently relocated to Canada. In order to determine the topic of their intervention, the group utilized the *photovoice* methodology. As briefly discussed previously, *photovoice* is an established, community-based mechanism for self-reflection that involves taking photographs of your surroundings. Participants are then encouraged to use the ***SHOWED*** acronym to analyze the photo: What do you **S**ee here? What is really **H**appening here? How does this relate to **O**ur lives? **W**hy does this problem/situation exist? How can we become **E**mpowered? What can we **D**o about it? (Flicker, et al., 2008). Using this framework as a launching point for discussion, the group at SOY decided that they wanted to "create a website (www.RocktheBoat.ca) that would educate LGBTQ youth about the social, fun and entertaining side to living in Toronto, Canada, as well as give support and provide resources to legal and social services" (Flicker, et al., 2008, p. 291). The group carefully crafted this resource, even entitling the project *Rock the Boat* to reclaim the "fresh off the boat" epithet applied to recent immigrants and transform it into a source of pride. The authors state that long after the project was formally over, a group at SOY was created to continue the website's mission. This highlights another strength of this work, which is that it has the potential to outlast the presence of a formal research team and have a long-standing impact on a community. Lastly, throughout the creative process, the authors encouraged active self-reflection about the work being done and the impact that it could have.

This study also demonstrates some of the weakness of *PAR*. While the authors had magnanimous intentions, it can often be challenging to engage youth in these types of research efforts. Therefore, the authors chose to provide the participants with payment in the form of an "honorarium" for their participation. Though the study does not list the amount that these participants received, these payments could have added a transactional nature to this work, an important consideration. Many study participants are compensated for their time. However, those participants are often offering their experiences or their opinions in exchange, rather than the design and implementation of community initiatives. What, then, separates paid participants in an action research study from university-sponsored community organizers? One could also argue that *PAR* is still in search of the scientific rigor needed to make its results truly respected by academicians who remain attached to traditional research methodologies.

In the following section, we will remove the subject from the research team and instead explore how longitudinal analysis of a specific cohort can reveal information about the environment's impact on an individual.

Cohort Studies

Theory

Cohort studies are a common observational methodology used in both biomedical and psychological research. In these studies, a subject population is carefully chosen based on an identified risk factor or characteristic. Researchers then follow this group longitudinally, performing evaluations at defined intervals to measure the outcome of interest. These studies can be **retrospective**, with both the risk factor and outcome of interest occurring in the past; **prospective**, with risk factors in the present affecting future outcomes; or a mixture of both, with risk factors from the past affecting future outcomes. In psychological research, prospective cohorts are particularly common.

Cohort studies can be particularly useful when assessing the impact of the environment on an individual or a community. Since study subjects are evaluated over long periods of time, researchers can observe how certain environmental factors can have a persistent or even compounded impact over time. This methodology can be used to study a wide variety of topics in health psychology, including risk factors for suicide, the impact of sunlight and rain frequency on mood, and how a parent's or guardian's stress can affect a child's development (Aktar & Bögels, 2017; Henríquez-Sánchez, Doreste-Alonso, Martínez-González, Bes-Rastrollo, Gea Sánchez-Villegas, 2014; Park, Lee, Lee, Moon, Jeon, Shim, et al., 2019). Developmental psychologists in particular see the benefit of cohort studies, as it allows them to track children as they progress into adulthood. Many studies are designed to explore the impact of local environmental factors or familial stressors on a child's psychological health. For instance, work has shown that children of Mexican immigrants who experience discrimination in their communities are more likely to have lower self-esteem (Espinoza, Gonzales, & Fuligni, 2016). Other cohort studies highlight that experiencing frequent racism as a pregnant mother can result in low birth weight for her child (Dominguez, Dunkel-Schetter, Glynn, Hobel, & Sandman, 2008). *Cohort studies* allow academics to study the intersection of environment and psychology with the added dimension of time, which can often lead to powerful and far-reaching conclusions. Another key strength of this study design is that the researchers are able to study multiple outcomes within the same cohort. By administering multiple surveys on a range of topics, the designers of the study may be able to draw multiple conclusions from work with the same population (Mann, 2003).

Cohort studies are not without their limitations, however. Attrition is arguably one of the biggest limitations for this type of study. While it may be possible to enroll thousands of participants initially, over time participants may drop out of the study for a variety of reasons ranging from disinterest to relocation or even death. Often there is an attrition bias to consider, given the possibility that those who leave the study share certain characteristics that could influence the results. The longer the study continues, the higher the likely attrition rates. However, the statistical power of these studies can be improved by having very large cohort sizes. Some large cohorts, such as the one created by the Framingham study, have greatly affected our understanding of the natural history of medical conditions such as heart disease (Mann, 2003).

Despite its limitations, a cohort study is arguably one of the few effective ways to examine generational phenomena and intergenerational influences because it can span several years, if not decades. In the following section, we will consider the investigative value that this approach provides by examining the work of the UK Millennium Cohort Study.

Case Study

Through research funded by the Economic and Social Research Council, children born in the UK between September 2000 and January 2002 were heavily recruited into the Millennium Cohort Study (MCS; Dex & Joshi, 2005). This longitudinal study was created with the hope of studying various aspects of childhood development, ranging from obesity and physical health to cognitive abilities. Infants and their families were approached for the study based on residential location, with immigrants and ethnic minorities purposefully overrepresented (Kelly, Becares, & Nazroo, 2013) The children and the responding guardians—often their mothers—responded to a number of surveys and assessments when each child was nine months (MCS1), three years (MCS2), and five years old (MCS3; Kelly, et al., 2013). At MCS1, the study had 18,552 families involved, which increased to 19,244 at MCS2 as more families enrolled. While there was some natural attrition and general loss to follow-up, there remained over 15,000 families enrolled at MCS3 when the authors of the study gathered their data.

When the children in the cohort were five years old, Kelly, and colleagues (2013) performed home visits to question parents about their experiences with racism and discrimination. Specifically, the mothers were first asked about their neighborhoods, "how common are insults or attacks to do with someone's race or colour?" and instructed to respond on a scale of 0 (not at all common) to 3 (very common; Kelly, et al., 2013, p. 36). Mothers who identified as ethnic minorities were then asked the following four additional questions about interpersonal racism:

> How often has someone said something insulting to you because of your race or ethnicity? How often have you been treated unfairly just because of your race or ethnicity? How often has a shopkeeper or salesperson treated you in a disrespectful way just because of your race or ethnicity? How often have members of your family been treated unfairly just because of their race or ethnicity?
>
> *(Kelly, et al., 2013, p. 36)*

They were asked to select "never, once or twice, several times, many times, and can't say" in response to each question (p. 36). The five questions that were asked of these mothers formed the five "measures of racism" and were dichotomized from 0 (not at all common) to 1 (fairly common). In dichotomizing these data about experiences of racism, one could argue that the authors lose important granularity in the variation of these experiences. Reducing racism to a binary scale ignores the nuances of how racism affects day-to-day life, taking different forms with different frequencies. Although this likely simplified the data analysis, one could argue that the authors oversimplified the dynamic and complicated nature of experiences of racism, the very exposure that they hoped to study.

After speaking with the mothers, the researchers turned their attention to the children. Toddlers' height and weight were measured to assess obesity. Mothers were also asked to complete a Strength and Difficulties Questionnaire (SDQ), a validated tool used to evaluate social and emotional behavior of children four to 15 years of age. The mothers were asked to score their child on the following categories: conduct problems, hyperactivity, emotional symptoms, peer problems, and pro-social behavior (Kelly, et al., 2013). Data from the first four categories were used to create a "total difficulties score," which was then analyzed as a continuous variable. The children also underwent three cognitive ability assessments. The Naming Vocabulary Test evaluated expressive language and vocabulary by asking children to name pictures in a booklet. The Pictures Similarities Test evaluated the participant's ability to reason and identify items that are conceptually similar. Lastly, the Pattern Construction Test assessed children's spatial ability with small timed tasks (Kelly, et al., 2013).

The authors also considered the possibility of confounders in their work. They collected information about ethnicity, languages spoken at home, economic status (income), education, and area-level deprivation using the Index of Multiple Deprivation 2004. They also collected critical information about the mothers, such as the mother's age at time of birth and current mental health status.

Analysis of these data was a multistep process involving multilevel logistic and linear regression models. The authors used likelihood ratios to determine if markers of racism and child health varied by ethnic group. Finding no statistically significant differences between ethnic groups, ethnicity was used to adjust rather than stratify the data (Kelly, et al., 2013). They then performed three models. The first model, or Step 1, examined how the five measures of racism independently affected child health outcomes, adjusting for ethnicity, age at time of birth, and gender. The Step 2 model additionally adjusted for socioeconomic markers (i.e., education, income, and neighborhood deprivation). Lastly, the Step 3 model considered all five markers of racism simultaneously, rather than individually.

Upon analyzing the data for demographic-based differences, they found that there was some nuance in how different ethnic groups perceived the world around them. They state, "For example, Bangladeshi mothers were most likely to perceive problems to do with racism in their residential areas, while Black Caribbean and African mothers were most likely to report unfair treatment, disrespectful treatment in shops and unfair treatment of family members" (Kelly, et al., 2013, p. 37). They also found a statistically significant association between mothers who reported acts of racism or discrimination in their neighborhood and the socioemotional difficulties of their children. Spatial ability was also found to be affected by racism reports in the neighborhood and perceptions of the family being treated unfairly. The nonverbal ability of the children in the cohort was also significantly associated with their mothers receiving racially motivated insults.

It is challenging to know the best way to interpret these results, as the authors admit in their discussion. Child development is a complicated process, influenced by a myriad of internal and external factors. Such factors may include the effects of parents who regularly face racism, the systemic policies that relegate people of color to disadvantaged neighborhoods, and the lack of opportunities for upward economic mobility given to black and brown job applicants. What exactly is affected these kids: the poor housing, the poverty, or the racism? The authors hypothesize that cognitive ability could be affected by racism in the family's neighborhood by suggesting living in an area where racist attacks are perceived to be common may lead to children spending less time outside the home environment than might otherwise be the case, thus limiting the breadth of interactions and experiences with others outside the home setting.

(Kelly, et al., 2013, p. 39)

They also propose that the impacts of racism on a parent's mental health, which are well documented, could lead to "non-favorable parent-child interactions and parenting behaviors" (Kelly, et al., 2013, p. 39; Williams, Lawrence, Davis, & Vu, 2019).

The limitations of this study largely pertain to the narrow scope of experiences of racism that were considered. Given that a mere five questions were used to summarize these experiences, the authors themselves argue that they were unable to assess the "full range of chronic and acute experienced racism" (Kelly, et al., 2013, p. 40). Though they worked with an established cohort, they performed a single, cross-sectional survey of the participants. The results may have been richer had they harnessed the temporal power of *cohort studies* and surveyed the participants at multiple time points. That being said, this study was an ambitious attempt to understand how aspects of our social environment can affect our offspring, recognizing the intergenerational effects of our lived experiences and interactions with others. As knowledge of adverse childhood events deepens, an important body of work is developing around the many ways (e.g., through epigenetics) that trauma and systemic oppression can be passed from parent to child (Espinoza, et al., 2016; Ford, Hurd, Jagers, & Sellers, 2013; Heard-Garris, Cale, Camaj, Hamati, & Dominguez, 2018).

By virtue of its reductive nature, quantitative data analysis is inherently limited in its ability to capture the dynamic and multifaceted qualities of many lived experiences. It is, for instance, impossible to summarize the deep and pervasive effects of racism with a series of numbers. As we will see in the next section, qualitative data can be an effective way to fill these gaps and to enrich our understanding of complex social phenomena.

Qualitative Studies

Theory

It is always challenging to capture human experiences with a *p*-value or a logistical regression. Certain aspects of life can be captured more appropriately with in-depth interviews, ethnographic observation, and other powerful qualitative methods. One could argue that, "many health psychology topics are particularly suited to the rich, detailed, in-depth inquiries that are able to be achieved with many qualitative research approaches" (Lyons, 2011, p. 1). As Lyons states in her review, health psychology research has lagged behind other disciplines of the field, such as community psychology and cultural psychology, in the use of qualitative methods. She argues that this resistance stems from the field's alignment with the biomedical paradigm, which places value in quantitative work and often treats qualitative research as "soft" science (Morse, 2010). However, understanding how patients experience health-related phenomena is crucial to improving the healthcare system. An in-depth, 45-minute interview is more likely to capture the essence of an individual's thought process or emotions surrounding an illness than a five-question survey. This is because a patient's complete narrative can be more powerful than a momentary experience. With the realization that the personal touch of medicine is being threatened by the increasingly electronic aspects of clinical care, there are some who are now turning to qualitative work to deepen our understanding of the patient perspective (Lyons, 2011; Morse, 2010).

One major challenge to qualitative work is how it is perceived. Many see the methodology as lacking rigor and subject to the bias of the researchers performing the analysis. One could argue that these critiques stem from a very rigid view of scientific principles such as reliability, validity, and generalizability. In the biomedical framework, results are seen as reliable if two scientists can independently run the same test and obtain the exact same results. However, if two researchers have in-depth interviews with the same individuals, it is possible that they will have slightly different conversations and arrive at different conclusions. This stems simply from the reality that both researchers could have captured different but equally legitimate aspects of the same psychosocial phenomenon. As Collingridge and Gantt (2019) state, "Slight differences in findings should not immediately be construed as the result of employing a flawed method of investigation or analysis. Differences often reflect a multifaceted understanding of complex social phenomena" (p. 390). The same flexibility should be afforded to concerns about validity and generalizability, which can be optimized if researchers "build on existing theoretical concepts through comprehensive literature reviews, employ theory-based sampling procedures, follow well-defined data analysis procedures, clearly define how the findings apply to other contexts, and integrate results into existing research in a coherent fashion" (Collingridge & Gantt, 2019, p. 392).

Qualitative research methods can be conducted with a high degree of rigor, a notion many in the biomedical paradigm are just beginning to accept. This rigor is often the result of months, if not years, of painstaking research conducted in field sites or time spent by multiple researchers to code hours of interview transcripts. The work can therefore be limited by manpower, time, and funding, which may result in the use of a fairly small study population. However, the richness of the interactions with each participant can be seen as an acceptable trade-off.

Qualitative studies can help us understand a wide variety of topics in health psychology. In the following example, we will see how in-depth interviews can bring to life the challenges of having limited access to healthy food in one's environment.

Case Study

The African American community has high rates of obesity, hypertension, and heart disease—all chronic conditions that can be modified with dietary changes. As a result, access to healthy food options has become a prominent area of research. Once individuals have knowledge about healthy dietary choices, they must also have the means to apply that knowledge in their grocery selections. However, there are many intertwining factors that influence how individuals shop for groceries and choose which stores to frequent, especially in urban and under-resourced settings.

In order to understand this decision-making process and identify changes that could promote health, a team at the University of Illinois conducted a qualitative study in which they interviewed 30 African American women about this topic. The authors state:

> Research has shown that low-income and African-American neighborhoods have fewer supermarkets and more liquor stores and convenience stores than higher income and White neighborhoods, respectively. . . . Understanding perceived environmental influences on food acquisition in neighborhoods with few food resources is critical to inform environmental and policy interventions to expand access to healthy food and promote healthy eating.
>
> *(Zenk, Odoms-Young, Dallas, Hardy, Watkins, Hoskins-Wroten, et al., 2011, p. 282)*

The study recruited African American women living in Greater Englewood, a predominantly African American neighborhood in Chicago, Illinois, with 32% to 44% of people living below the poverty line. Women between ages 21 and 45, with at least one child younger than 18 years old, were recruited from the Englewood Neighborhood Health Center, a city-sponsored community health clinic. Semi-structured interviews were performed by an interviewer who was matched on race at the location of the participant's choosing. Interview questions covered perceptions of the neighborhood food environment, barriers to healthy food choices, the selection process, and general store and location preferences (Zenk, et al., 2011). These interviews, which ranged from 45 to 120 minutes long, were transcribed and then coded for thematic patterns by three separate coders in an iterative process involving frequent checks for intercoder discrepancies. Overarching themes were then pulled from the data by grouping the initial codes, and the research team refined the themes to identify actionable conclusions (Zenk, et al., 2011). All participants were given a $25 gift certificate for their participation.

The study found that numerous material, economic, and social-interactional factors influence the grocery selection process for these women. In discussing the material factors, many of the women reported that store availability was limited in their neighborhoods, indicating that they would need to walk long distances or drive to other communities for a good grocery selection. The women also cited poor upkeep of the stores in their community as a material barrier. They described how a "lack of cleanliness, disorganized shelves and aisles, and poorly maintained shopping carts" would push them to choose another grocery store (Zenk, et al., 2011, p. 285). Some women mentioned seeing cockroaches and rodents in the stores, which would force them to search for higher-quality stores that may be farther from their homes. Many women also spoke of items such as baby food and vegetables being out of stock in local stores or even simply difficult to find. Per one participant, "[When you first walk in] it's the cake, it's the chips, it's the soda . . . then you have to hunt for the fruits, the vegetables, the bottled water, and things like that" (Zenk, et al., 2011, p. 285). From an economic perspective, many of the women claimed that there were higher prices at both small local stores and supermarkets. They often spoke of how other ethnic groups, such as Arabs and Asians, were inflating the prices of groceries in their communities. One woman spoke of how many people in the neighborhood use food assistance programs, which means that the store owners cannot charge taxes. "So, they jack-up the regular price of the food so that they can make their money that way," she concluded (Zenk, et al., 2011, p. 285). Lastly, the social-interactional factors that the women described were in reference to negative experiences they had with store employees, whom they perceived as providing little customer service and following them closely "like you're going to steal something" (p. 286). They also spoke of feeling unsafe in the spaces around the local stores, where people are often found panhandling, soliciting drugs, or sexually harassing shoppers as they approached (Zenk, et al., 2011).

The researchers also discussed the adaptive strategies that these women employed in order to provide food for their families despite these obstacles. The first strategy involved optimizing their situation, which included traveling long distances for better options or shopping at multiple retailers for different items. The women interviewed shopped at an average of 4.3 different food retailers and on average traveled 2.3 miles from their home to food shop (Zenk, et al., 2011). As the authors describe, "A typical pattern was purchasing lower priced canned and packaged goods at discount grocers and buying fresh meat and produce at supermarkets or specialty stores, which were perceived as having better selection and quality" (p. 286). Another identified strategy was termed ***settling*** and consisted of shopping at local stores, paying the higher prices, and purchasing junk food when healthy food was desired. In the stores that were perceived as unclean, mothers spoke of how they would only purchase canned or packaged items. Another strategy involved ***being proactive***. This meant the mothers employed methods such as shopping during the day when they felt safer, avoiding shopping at times of the month when people receive food assistance benefits, or carrying themselves in such a way that the store employees would be less likely to disrespect them (Zenk, et al., 2011). Lastly, some women used ***advocacy*** as a strategy, contacting the local health department and regulatory bodies about the conditions seen within the local stores.

One important strength of this study is that it was able to paint a clear picture of the obstacles to healthy living in this Chicago neighborhood. The rich quotes and examples highlight the nuanced choices these women make every day about how to provide food for their families. The women interviewed also highlighted aspects of this topic that often go undiscussed. While the lack of grocery stores in low-income neighborhoods is well-documented, there has been less discussion of the physical environment within those stores and the low standards of cleanliness. These mothers also spoke of the stress of being harassed by men who congregate outside the stores and how that influences their choice of where to shop, pointing to an insidious link between gender relations and dietary health. The authors provide a framework for understanding how these women combat these obstacles, which is instrumental to understanding the behaviors that may or may not promote health. They also emphasize clear, actionable changes that could be made to improve food shopping in the community, such as promoting local ownership and investing in urban agriculture.

Regarding the study's weaknesses, the authors were only able to speak with 30 African American women in one neighborhood of Chicago. While one can readily imagine that the challenges the authors describe could be found in similar urban, inner-city settings, the small sample size may call into question the overall generalizability of the work. The authors also failed to report a measure of intercoder reliability, which often takes the form of a Cohen's *kappa* calculation. This metric allows the reader to evaluate the consistency of the thematic coding between researchers, which speaks to the individual bias that may be present in the analysis.

Conclusion

In this chapter, we have discussed the many ways in which one can study the impact of the environment on an individual's health. *EMA, twin studies, PAR, cohort studies*, and *qualitative research* represent five very different methodologies that can be used to learn more about the human health experience in a variety of settings. From engaging youth in health promotion in their communities to analyzing precisely how vegetation exposure affects mental health, we have seen that our interactions with the surrounding social, economic, and geographic environments are extremely complex. The methodologies discussed here are certainly not exhaustive, nor is our discussion of them comprehensive. However, this chapter aimed to present a snapshot of the range of study types and designs that can be utilized in health psychology as it pertains to geographic influences.

Looking toward the future, advances in science and technology will make it possible to study the environment's impact on the individual in even more sophisticated ways. For example, wearable sensors could be used to provide a steady stream of biophysical data such as heart rate or respiratory rate. At the same time, sensitive monitoring tools and networks of highly interconnected computing devices are capable of providing massive amounts of data about the physical environment. Technology is also being used increasingly to connect our location in space and time to our social interactions, thoughts, and feelings. For instance, time and location stamps on social media have already been used to track moods and screen for psychopathologies such as depression. As our technology and access to data continue to grow, the key to future research in environmental and health psychology will be to creatively incorporate these advances into the deeply personal and often community-oriented nature of this field.

References

Aktar, E., & Bögels, S. M. (2017, December 1). Exposure to parents' negative emotions as a developmental pathway to the family aggregation of depression and anxiety in the first year of life. *Clinical Child and Family Psychology Review, 20*, 369–390. https://doi.org/10.1007/s10567-017-0240-7

Amaddeo, F., Salazzari, D., & Salinas-Perez, J. A. (2015, February 26). Is a geographical approach worthwhile for epidemiological research in mental health? *Epidemiology and Psychiatric Sciences, 24*, 38–41. https://doi.org/10.1017/S2045796014000705

Arias, E., Escobedo, L. A., Kennedy, J., Fu, C., & Cisewki, J. (2018). U.S. small-area life expectancy estimates project: Methodology and results summary. *Vital and Health Statistics: Series 2, Data Evaluation and Methods Research*, (181), 1–40. Retrieved from www.ncbi.nlm.nih.gov/pubmed/30312153

Bucci, M., Marques, S. S., Oh, D., & Harris, N. B. (2016, August 1). Toxic stress in children and adolescents. *Advances in Pediatrics*, *63*, 403–428. https://doi.org/10.1016/j.yapd.2016.04.002

Campbell, K. L., Babiarz, A., Wang, Y., Tilton, N. A., Black, M. M., & Hager, E. R. (2018). Factors in the home environment associated with toddler diet: An ecological momentary assessment study. *Public Health Nutrition*, *21*(10), 1855–1864. https://doi.org/10.1017/S1368980018000186

Cohen-Cline, H., Turkheimer, E., & Duncan, G. E. (2015). Access to green space, physical activity and mental health: A twin study. *Journal of Epidemiology and Community Health*, *69*(6), 523–529. https://doi.org/10.1136/jech-2014-204667

Collingridge, D. S., & Gantt, E. E. (2019). The quality of qualitative research★. *American Journal of Medical Quality*, *34*(5), 439–445. https://doi.org/10.1177/1062860619873187

Devlin, A. S. (2018). *Environmental psychology and human well-being: Effects of built and natural settings*. San Diego, CA, US: Elsevier Academic Press.

Dex, S., & Joshi, H. (2005). *Children of the 21st century: From birth to nine months*. Bristol, UK: Policy Press.

Dominguez, T. P., Dunkel-Schetter, C., Glynn, L. M., Hobel, C., & Sandman, C. A. (2008). Racial differences in birth outcomes: The role of general, pregnancy, and racism stress. *Health Psychology*, *27*(2), 194–203. https://doi.org/10.1037/0278-6133.27.2.194

Epstein, D. H., Tyburski, M., Craig, I. M., Phillips, K. A., Jobes, M. L., Vahabzadeh, M., et al. (2014). Real-time tracking of neighborhood surroundings and mood in urban drug misusers: Application of a new method to study behavior in its geographical context. *Drug and Alcohol Dependence*, *134*(1), 22–29. https://doi.org/10.1016/j.drugalcdep.2013.09.007

Espinoza, G., Gonzales, N. A., & Fuligni, A. J. (2016). Parent discrimination predicts Mexican-American adolescent psychological adjustment 1 year later. *Child Development*, *87*(4), 1079–1089. https://doi.org/10.1111/cdev.12521

Etowa, J. B., Bernard, W. T., Oyinsan, B., & Clow, B. (2007). Participatory Action Research (PAR): An approach for improving black women's health in rural and remote communities. *Journal of Transcultural Nursing : Official Journal of the Transcultural Nursing Society*, *18*(4), 349–357. https://doi.org/10.1177/1043659607305195

Flicker, S., Maley, O., Ridgley, A., Biscope, S., Lombardo, C., Skinner, H. A., et al. (2008). e-PAR using technology and participatory action research to engage youth in health promotion A R T I C L E. *Action Research*, *6*(3), 285–303. https://doi.org/10.1177/1476750307083711

Ford, K. R., Hurd, N. M., Jagers, R. J., & Sellers, R. M. (2013). Caregiver experiences of discrimination and African American adolescents' psychological health over time. *Child Development*, *84*(2), 485–499. https://doi.org/10.1111/j.1467-8624.2012.01864.x

Foster-Fishman, P. G., Law, K. M., Lichty, L. F., & Aoun, C. (2010). Youth React for social change: A method for youth participatory action research. *American Journal of Community Psychology*, *46*(1), 67–83. https://doi.org/10.1007/s10464-010-9316-y

Freire, P. (1993). Pedagogy of the oppressed, 1970. Reprint, New York: Continuum (Vol. 68). Retrieved from www.ncbi.nlm.nih.gov/pubmed/4527926%5Cnhttp://scholar.google.com/scholar?hl=en&btnG=Search&q=intitle:Pedagogy+of+the+oppressed#3

Furr-Holden, C. D. M., Campbell, K. D. M., Milam, A. J., Smart, M. J., Ialongo, N. A., & Leaf, P. J. (2010). Metric properties of the neighborhood inventory for environmental typology (NIfETy): An environmental assessment tool for measuring indicators of violence, alcohol, tobacco, and other drug exposures. *Evaluation Review*, *34*(3), 159–184. https://doi.org/10.1177/0193841X10368493

Furr-Holden, C. D. M., Smart, M. J., Pokorni, J. L., Ialongo, N. S., Leaf, P. J., Holder, H. D., & Anthony, J. C. (2008). The NIfETy method for environmental assessment of neighborhood-level indicators of violence, alcohol, and other drug exposure. *Prevention Science*, *9*(4), 245–255. https://doi.org/10.1007/s11121-008-0107-8

Goodwin, A. J., Nadig, N. R., McElligott, J. T., Simpson, K. N., & Ford, D. W. (2016). Where you live matters: The impact of place of residence on severe sepsis incidence and mortality. *Chest*, *150*(4), 829–836. https://doi.org/10.1016/j.chest.2016.07.004

Hager, E. R., Tilton, N. A., Wang, Y., Kapur, N. C., Arbaiza, R., Merry, B. C., et al. (2017). The home environment and toddler physical activity: An ecological momentary assessment study. *Pediatric Obesity*, *12*(1), 1–9. https://doi.org/10.1111/ijpo.12098

Hall, B. L. (1992). From margins to center? The development and purpose of participatory research. *The American Sociologist*, *23*(4), 15–28. https://doi.org/10.1007/BF02691928

Heard-Garris, N. J., Cale, M., Camaj, L., Hamati, M. C., & Dominguez, T. P. (2018). Transmitting trauma: A systematic review of vicarious racism and child health. *Social Science and Medicine*, *199*, 230–240. https://doi.org/10.1016/j.socscimed.2017.04.018

Henríquez-Sánchez, P., Doreste-Alonso, J., Martínez-González, M. A., Bes-Rastrollo, M., Gea, A., & Sánchez-Villegas, A. (2014). Geographical and climatic factors and depression risk in the SUN project. *European Journal of Public Health*, *24*(4), 626–631. https://doi.org/10.1093/eurpub/cku008

Hogg, M. A., & Abrams, D. (2001). *Intergroup relations: Essential readings*. Philadelphia, PA: Psychology Press.

Hur, Y.-M., Bogl, L. H., Ordoñana, J. R., Taylor, J., Hart, S. A., Tuvblad, C., et al. (2020). Twin family registries worldwide: An important resource for scientific research. *Twin Research and Human Genetics*, 1–11. https://doi.org/10.1017/thg.2019.121

Joseph, J. (2002). Twin studies in psychiatry and psychology: Science or pseudoscience? *The Psychiatric Quarterly*, *73*(1), 71–82. https://doi.org/10.1023/a:1012896802713

Kelly, Y., Becares, L., & Nazroo, J. (2013). Associations between maternal experiences of racism and early child health and development: Findings from the UK millennium cohort study. *Journal of Epidemiology and Community Health*, *67*(1), 35–41. https://doi.org/10.1136/jech-2011-200814

Khan, K. S., Bawani, S. A. A., & Aziz, A. (2013). Bridging the gap of knowledge and action: A case for Participatory Action Research (PAR). *Action Research*, *11*(2), 157–175. https://doi.org/10.1177/1476750313477158

Kirchner, T. R., & Shiffman, S. (2016). Spatio-temporal determinants of mental health and well-being: Advances in geographically-explicit ecological momentary assessment (GEMA). *Social Psychiatry and Psychiatric Epidemiology*, *51*, 1211–1223. https://doi.org/10.1007/s00127-016-1277-5

Larcombe, D.-L., van Etten, E., Logan, A., Prescott, S. L., & Horwitz, P. (2019). High-rise apartments and urban mental health: Historical and contemporary views. *Challenges*, *10*(2), 34. https://doi.org/10.3390/challe10020034

Lee, A. C. K., & Maheswaran, R. (2011, June). The health benefits of urban green spaces: A review of the evidence. *Journal of Public Health*, *33*, 212–222. https://doi.org/10.1093/pubmed/fdq068

Lim, Y. H., Kim, H., Kim, J. H., Bae, S., Park, H. Y., & Hong, Y. C. (2012). Air pollution and symptoms of depression in elderly adults. *Environmental Health Perspectives*, *120*(7), 1023–1028. https://doi.org/10.1289/ehp.1104100

Lyons, A. C. (2011, March). Advancing and extending qualitative research in health psychology. *Health Psychology Review*, *5*, 1–8. https://doi.org/10.1080/17437199.2010.544638

Maguire, P. (1987). Doing participatory research: A feminist approach. *Participatory Research & Practice*. Retrieved from https://scholarworks.umass.edu/cie_participatoryresearchpractice/6

Mann, C. J. (2003, January). Observational research methods: Research design II: Cohort, cross sectional, and case-control studies. *Emergency Medicine Journal*, *20*, 54–60. https://doi.org/10.1136/emj.20.1.54

Mason, L. H., Harp, J. P., & Han, D. Y. (2014). Pb neurotoxicity: Neuropsychological effects of lead toxicity. *BioMed Research International*, *2014*. https://doi.org/10.1155/2014/840547

Massey, D. S., & Denton, N. A. (1998). *American apartheid: Segregation and the making of the underclass*. Retrieved April 30, 2020, from www.hup.harvard.edu/catalog.php?isbn=9780674018211

Mennis, J., Mason, M., & Ambrus, A. (2018). Urban greenspace is associated with reduced psychological stress among adolescents: A Geographic Ecological Momentary Assessment (GEMA) analysis of activity space. *Landscape and Urban Planning*, *174*, 1–9. https://doi.org/10.1016/j.landurbplan.2018.02.008

Mennis, J., Mason, M., Light, J., Rusby, J., Westling, E., Way, T., et al. (2016). Does substance use moderate the association of neighborhood disadvantage with perceived stress and safety in the activity spaces of urban youth? *Drug and Alcohol Dependence*, *165*, 288–292. https://doi.org/10.1016/j.drugalcdep.2016.06.019

Moberg, D. P., & Hahn, L. (1991). The adolescent drug involvement scale Wisconsin obesity prevention initiative view project Wisconsin SBIRT project view project. *Article in Journal of Child & Adolescent Substance Abuse*. https://doi.org/10.1300/J272v02n01_05

Morse, J. M. (2010). How different is qualitative health research from qualitative research? Do we have a subdiscipline? *Qualitative Health Research*, *20*(11), 1459–1464. https://doi.org/10.1177/1049732310379116

Murphy, S. L., Xu, J., Kochanek, K. D., & Arias, E. (2018). Mortality in the United States, 2017. *NCHS Data Brief*, (328), 1–8.

Norman, C. D., & Skinner, H. A. (2007). Engaging youth in e-health promotion: Lessons learned from a decade of TeenNet research. *Adolescent Medicine: State of the Art Reviews*, *18*(2), 357–369, xii. Retrieved from www.ncbi.nlm.nih.gov/pubmed/18605651

Oh, D. L., Jerman, P., Silvério Marques, S., Koita, K., Purewal Boparai, S. K., Burke Harris, N., et al. (2018). Systematic review of pediatric health outcomes associated with childhood adversity. *BMC Pediatrics*, *18*(1). https://doi.org/10.1186/s12887-018-1037-7

O' Sullivan, I., Orbell, S., Rakow, T., & Parker, R. (2004). Prospective research in health service settings: Health psychology, science and the Hawthorne' effect. *Journal of Health Psychology*, *9*(3), 355–359. https://doi.org/10.1177/1359105304042345

Park, C. H. K., Lee, J. W., Lee, S. Y., Moon, J. J., Jeon, D. W., Shim, S. H., et al. (2019). The Korean cohort for the model predicting a suicide and suicide-related behavior: Study rationale, methodology, and baseline sample characteristics of a long-term, large-scale, multi-center, prospective, naturalistic, observational cohort study. *Comprehensive Psychiatry*, *88*, 29–38. https://doi.org/10.1016/j.comppsych.2018.11.003

Pevalin, D. J., Reeves, A., Baker, E., & Bentley, R. (2017). The impact of persistent poor housing conditions on mental health: A longitudinal population-based study. *Preventive Medicine*, *105*, 304–310. https://doi.org/10.1016/j.ypmed.2017.09.020

Power, M. C., Kioumourtzoglou, M. A., Hart, J. E., Okereke, O. I., Laden, F., & Weisskopf, M. G. (2015). The relation between past exposure to fine particulate air pollution and prevalent anxiety: Observational cohort study. *BMJ (Online)*, *350*. https://doi.org/10.1136/bmj.h1111

Ram, N., Brinberg, M., Pincus, A. L., & Conroy, D. E. (2017). The questionable ecological validity of ecological momentary assessment: Considerations for design and analysis. *Research in Human Development*, *14*(3), 253–270. https://doi.org/10.1080/15427609.2017.1340052

Ross, C. E., & Mirowsky, J. (2001). Neighborhood disadvantage, disorder, and health. *Journal of Health and Social Behavior*, *42*(3), 258. https://doi.org/10.2307/3090214

Salvi, A., & Salim, S. (2019). Neurobehavioral consequences of traffic-related air pollution. *Frontiers in Neuroscience*, *13*. https://doi.org/10.3389/fnins.2019.01232

Shaughnessy, K., Reyes, R., Shankardass, K., Sykora, M., Feick, R., Lawrence, H., et al. (2018). Using geolocated social media for ecological momentary assessments of emotion: Innovative opportunities in psychology science and practice. *Canadian Psychology*, *59*(1), 47–53. https://doi.org/10.1037/cap0000099

Shiffman, S., Stone, A. A., & Hufford, M. R. (2008). Ecological momentary assessment. *Annual Review of Clinical Psychology*, *4*, 1–32. Retrieved from www.ncbi.nlm.nih.gov/pubmed/18509902

Vaughan, C. (2014). Participatory research with youth: Idealising safe social spaces or building transformative links in difficult environments? *Journal of Health Psychology*, *19*(1), 184–192. https://doi.org/10.1177/1359105313500258

Wang, C. C., & Pies, C. A. (2004). Family, maternal, and child health through photovoice. *Maternal and Child Health Journal*, *8*(2), 95–102. https://doi.org/10.1023/B:MACI.0000025732.32293.4f

Williams, D. R., Lawrence, J. A., Davis, B. A., & Vu, C. (2019). Understanding how discrimination can affect health. *Health Services Research*. https://doi.org/10.1111/1475-6773.13222

Younan, D., Tuvblad, C., Li, L., Wu, J., Lurmann, F., Franklin, M., et al. (2016). Environmental determinants of aggression in adolescents: Role of urban neighborhood greenspace. *Journal of the American Academy of Child and Adolescent Psychiatry*, *55*(7), 591–601. https://doi.org/10.1016/j.jaac.2016.05.002

Zenk, S. N., Odoms-Young, A. M., Dallas, C., Hardy, E., Watkins, A., Hoskins-Wroten, J., et al. (2011). "You have to hunt for the fruits, the vegetables": Environmental barriers and adaptive strategies to acquire food in a low-income African American neighborhood. *Health Education and Behavior*, *38*(3), 282–292. https://doi.org/10.1177/1090198110372877

25

CLIMATE CHANGE

Melinda R. Weathers and Marceleen M. Mosher

Overview

Climate change has created a global public health crisis. With a myriad of serious health harms occurring worldwide, it is nearly certain that, if left unaddressed, these harms will become dramatically worse and more pervasive. These harms include illness, injuries, and deaths from increasingly dangerous weather, worsening air pollution, the spread of infectious diseases, increases in food- and water-borne illnesses, reduced nutrition, and mental health harms. Averting a sustained global public health catastrophe will require rapid mitigation efforts as well as local and regional adaptation actions to protect human health. If taken, these actions offer profound public health and economic benefits, both short- and long-term. Effective public communication has played a vital role in improving and managing a wide range of public health problems, including tobacco and substance abuse, HIV/AIDS, and vaccine-preventable diseases (Hornik, 2002; Maibach, Abroms, & Marosits, 2007). These lessons can be harnessed to alert and engage the American public and policy makers in understanding and responding to climate change today.

As the climate crisis unfolds and the human health harms rise, there is a rapidly growing need for the public health community to employ effective public communication and engagement strategies. Three main factors drive the need. First, the health of Americans is already being harmed by climate change, and the magnitude of this harm is likely to get much worse if effective actions are not taken soon to limit climate change and help communities successfully adapt to inevitable changes. Second, historically, climate change public engagement efforts have focused primarily on the environmental dimensions of the threat. These efforts have mobilized an important, but still relatively narrow, range of Americans. Third, many of the actions that slow or prevent climate change and that protect human health from the harms associated with climate change also benefit health and well-being in ways unrelated to climate change. From a public health perspective, actions taken to address climate change are a "win-win" in that—in addition to responsibly addressing climate change—they can help us make progress on other important public health goals as well (e.g., increased physical activity, reduced air and water pollution, and increased social capital in and connections across communities).

For nearly a decade, US-based researchers have been investigating the factors that shape public views about the health risks associated with climate change, the communication strategies that motivate support for actions to reduce these risks, and the practical implications for public health organizations and professionals who seek to engage individuals and their communities effectively. Their work serves as a model for similar work that can be conducted across the country and internationally to understand the public's response to climate change framed as a public health harm. Until only recently, the voices of public health experts have been largely absent from the public dialogue on climate change, a dialogue that is often inaccurately framed as an "economy versus the environment" debate. Expanding the conversation to include the public health harms of climate change may make the threat immediate, tangible, and relatable to the American public. Introducing the public health voice into the public dialogue can help communities see the issue in a new light, motivating and promoting more thoughtful decision-making and a more positive vision for a healthier, low-carbon future (i.e., reduce greenhouse gases and save nonrenewable resources).

This chapter outlines how communication research can be used to support these important goals. Specifically, this chapter examines American audiences through investigations of textual analysis (e.g., content analysis), survey research (e.g., audience segmentation, interviews, and questionnaires), and experimental research (e.g., selective exposure and quasi-experimental design). These communication efforts work to better understand the American public's response to the critical issue of climate change through a public health messaging perspective.

Research in Practice

Textual Analysis

Content Analysis

News media is of vital importance in the delivery of information about issues that affect the public. Weathers (2013), and later Weathers and Kendall (2015), used content analysis and framing theory to examine the news coverage of climate change as a public health issue. Both studies analyzed two national and three regional newspapers across two 2-year time periods. In the original work, Weathers (2013) set a baseline for the rate of coverage of climate change and public health in newspapers from 2007 to 2008. The research questions asked how much attention was given to the public health impacts of climate change, what dimensions of the health impacts of climate change were covered, and how different frames were used. In the follow-up study, Weathers and Kendall (2015) asked how the media coverage of climate change from 2011 to 2012 has changed and considered a new dimension of media framing levels (i.e., local and national levels).

For each study, the author(s) examined five newspapers: two leading national newspapers (i.e., *The New York Times* and *The Washington Post*) and three regional newspapers that serve communities currently affected by extreme climate-related events (i.e., *Atlanta Journal Constitution*, *Houston Chronicle*, and *The Tampa Tribune*). For both studies, each paper was queried through the Lexis-Nexis online database for keywords that appeared in the headline or lead paragraph. The four search terms were "global warming," "climate change," "greenhouse gas," or "greenhouse effect." In both studies, the author(s) reviewed each article resulting from the searches to ensure it focused substantially on climate change, discarding those that did not. For each newspaper, final totals for climate change–focused articles were recorded by year and entered into an Excel database.

The author(s) established six distinct categories of public health–related impacts and keywords through the examination of key public health texts. The categories of public health–related issues included "general public health–related impacts," "heat-related health impacts," "weather-related health impacts," "respiratory-related health impacts," "water and foodborne disease–related health impacts," and "vector and rodent-borne disease–related health impacts." Each public health–related climate change article was then coded according to the aforementioned six categories. Articles with more than one health impact frame were placed into the frame that was thought to exemplify the most dominant theme or message. The author(s) also examined the articles for their generic framing convention: an ***episodic frame***, an illustration of an issue through a specific example, case study, or event-oriented report; a ***thematic frame***, a broader contextual report of a topic; a ***dramatic frame***, a report focused on conflict or crisis; or a **substantive frame**, a report focused on describing and prescribing issues beyond single events. The second study also coded for media framing at the local and national levels.

The unit of analysis used in these studies was the article. Data were entered into a coding instrument using an Excel spreadsheet and were later transferred to the Program for Reliability Assessment with Multiple Coders (PRAM) database for analysis. Categories were coded using a coding manual that explicitly defined each category and variables within each category. Coding was conducted by the first author and an additional trained coder. About 10% of the news articles were randomly selected and coded separately to ensure intercoder reliability using Scott's *Pi* coefficient in the original study and Cohen's *kappa* coefficient in the follow-up study, both with acceptable levels of agreement. Specifically, Scott's *Pi* coefficient was reported at a level of .90 and Cohen's *kappa* coefficient was reported at a level of .87 for the public health frame variable, .90 for the issue-specific frame variable, and .80 for the dramatic/substantive frame variable. Descriptives and frequencies were run on all variables and were analyzed to provide an overall picture of climate change as a public health issue in the news.

The results of the first study indicate that the human health implications of climate change are dramatically underreported. Of the 2,544 climate change–focused articles analyzed by the author, only 13.9% mentioned health-related impacts, leaving 2,190 articles missing a vital dimension of the climate change story. In the follow-up study, the results showed that while there was a decrease in climate change–focused articles overall, the proportion of articles that mentioned a public health–related issue doubled from 13.9% in 2007–2008 to 27.2% in 2011–2012. There was also more mention of the general public health concerns related to climate change, which aids in building the salience of the idea that climate change affects human health. The follow-up study also included an increase in the number of substantively framed articles across categories. As such, "the increased frequency with which public health frames are used in the news is a testament to the progressive standardization and legitimization of public health as a framing device for climate change discourse" (Weathers & Kendall, 2015, p. 13).

Summary

The problem of framing climate change in a compelling way for mass audiences is already a matter of significant interest and popular discussion. Findings from these studies show that public health–related climate change news continues to be dominated by stories employing *substantive frames*, those most akin to the conventions of scientific discourse. This may be worrisome, as news reporting that takes on a detached tone may skew media consumers' understanding of climate change risks (Smith, 2005). While some may applaud this as an important part of public science education, others recognize the need for varying modes of news writing in order to capture the attention of a wide variety of audiences—some not familiar with the dangers of climate change for public health. The content analysis presented in these studies is a starting point for examining, tracking, and critically assessing the story of climate change in public health terms—a project that deserves further attention from communication, environment, and public health scholars.

Survey Research

Audience Segmentation Design

Central to effective communication and communication research is a basic understanding of any given audience's values, beliefs, desires, and motivations (Gamson, Croteau, Hoynes, & Sasson, 1992). These characteristics inform how people conceptualize information, what captures their attention, and what prompts action. ***Audience segmentation*** allows communicators to know their audience so that they can tailor the message content, message context, and channel that will best reach their audience. Maibach, Leiserowitz, Roser-Renouf, and Mertz's (2011) groundbreaking research defined distinct multidimensional audience segments of the American public based on their existing perceptions of climate change (see also Leiserowitz, Maibach, E., & Roser-Renouf, 2009; Leiserowitz, Maibach, Roser-Renouf, Rosenthal, Cutler, & Kotcher, 2018; Maibach, Roser-Renouf, & Leiserowitz, 2009). The researchers analyzed and categorized the results of a large-scale, nationally representative survey of American adults in order to develop the six audience segments, now known as "Global Warming's Six Americas."

Using an in-depth questionnaire, the authors conducted a representative survey of US adults (*n* = 2,164) that contained three major categories of variables as inputs into a segmentation analysis: ***global warming motivations***, ***behaviors***, and ***policy preferences***. The *global warming motivations* category included two distinct subcategories: "beliefs about global warming and degree of involvement in the issue" (Maibach, et al., 2011, p. 2). The authors then analyzed the responses with 36 variables in four categories—***global warming beliefs***, ***issue involvement***, *policy preferences*, and *behaviors*. In order to "maximize the practical value of the segmentation findings, the researchers limited the analysis to five-, six-, and seven-segment solutions"; they determined that the six-segment solution (i.e., the six audience segments) was ideal (Maibach, et al., 2011, p. 2). The authors expanded on their analysis of the survey data by creating extensive profiles for each of the six audience segments. The profiles both described each segment's characteristics and contrasted their differences and can be used by anyone seeking to communicate about climate change with the American public.

The results of the audience segmentation analysis identified six distinct groups within the American public—"Global Warming's Six Americas"—the alarmed, concerned, cautious, disengaged, doubtful, and dismissive. Each group responds differently to the issue of global warming based on varied experiences, values, beliefs, and motivations. The identification of each audience segment serves as a guide for communicators across America to craft messages tailored to each segment's individual needs and to meaningfully engage the public with the issue of climate change through a diversity of messages, messengers, and methods. The national survey of the public's perception of climate change that the authors analyzed to define "Global Warming's Six Americas" is routinely readministered to provide up-to-date audience segment data. The most recent analysis was published in 2018 and shows that the alarmed segment has nearly doubled, with the other segments seeing reductions in their percentages; the dismissive segment gained a modest 2% of the population (Leiserowitz, et al., 2018).

Summary

Climate change communication and engagement efforts must start with the fundamental recognition that people are different and have different psychological, cultural, and political reasons for acting—or not acting—to reduce greenhouse gas emissions. This study identifies "Global Warming's Six Americas"—six unique audiences within the American public that each responds to the issue of climate change in their own distinct way. ***Audience segmentation*** research provides essential knowledge grounded in social science that can be leveraged by climate educators and communicators throughout the United States to facilitate the changes required to achieve a transition to a low-carbon future.

Questionnaire Survey Research

Survey research allows researchers to gather specific data from groups of people with relative ease. In large enough numbers, survey research uncovers trends about the way people think and act, their understanding and perceptions of a given issue, and their values and beliefs (Blair, Czaja, & Blair, 2014). Maibach, Kreslake, Roser-Renouf, Rosenthal, Feinberg, and Leiserowitz (2015) performed an online national survey using both open- and closed-ended questions to assess respondents' perceptions of the risk of climate change and its public health–related impacts. The questionnaires were self-administered online and included measures related to general attitudes and beliefs about climate change, affective assessment of health effects, vulnerable populations and specific health conditions (open- and closed-ended), perceived risk, trust in sources, and support for government response.

Data were obtained from a nationally representative survey of US adults. Participants (*n* = 1,275) were recruited using both random digit dialing and address-based sampling techniques. Participants were asked open-ended questions about the health problems they saw related to global warming (e.g., "In your view, what health problems related to global warming are Americans currently experiencing, if any?"; Maibach, et al., 2015, p. 399). A coding scheme was developed for the responses using an iterative grounded-theory approach. Codes and examples of responses in each coding category are provided in the original article (see Maibach, et al., 2015).

The authors asked a series of closed-ended questions to measure the dimensions of perceived risk for health harm associated with global warming. These items measured participants' perceptions of the severity of harm global warming is currently causing and will cause in the future; perceptions of harm to the respondent, the respondent's family, and other Americans; and perceptions of near-future local effects (e.g., "Do you think each of the following will become more or less common in your community over the next 10 years as a result of global warming, if nothing is done to address it?"; Maibach et al., 2015, p. 400). Fifteen health-related conditions were listed. Response scales ranged from 1 (much less common) to 7 (much more common). Perceived current and distant-future global health harm was also assessed. Participants

> were asked to estimate the number of people worldwide who, due to global warming, are currently injured or become ill each year; are currently killed each year; will be injured or become ill each year 50 years from now; and will die each year 50 years from now. Response categories were: none, hundreds, thousands, millions, or don't know.
>
> *(Maibach, et al., 2015, p. 400)*

The authors asked participants to consider the role of governmental response to climate change's health effects: what branches of government should respond and if they support funding health agencies. Scales ranging from one (much less) to seven (much more) assessed the desired level of response from President Obama, the US Congress, federal agencies (e.g., the Centers for Disease Control and Prevention [CDC], the National Institutes of Health [NIH], and the Federal Emergency Management Agency), and participant's state and local governments (Maibach, et al., 2015). Participants were also asked to rate the credibility of specific sources for information on the health effects of global warming. Finally, participants were asked two questions to assess their prior cognitive and affective investment in the health aspects of global warming:

> Before taking this survey, how much if at all . . . a) had you thought about how global warming might affect people's health? and b) did you worry about how global warming might affect people's health? Response categories were: not at all, a little, a moderate amount, a great deal, and not sure.
>
> *(Maibach, et al., 2015, p. 400)*

Analyses were conducted using SPSS 19.0 and Stata 13.1.

Most participants "(61%) reported that, before taking the survey, they had given little or no thought to how global warming might affect people's health" (Maibach, et al., 2015, p. 400). In response to a closed-ended question, many participants (64%) indicated global warming is harmful to health, yet in response to an open-ended question, few (27%) accurately named one or more specific type of harm. In response to a closed-ended question, 33% indicated some groups are more affected than others, yet on an open-ended question, only 25% were able to identify any disproportionately affected populations. Perhaps not surprising given these findings, respondents demonstrated only limited support for a government response: Less than 50% of respondents said the government should be doing more to protect against health harms from global warming, and about 33% supported increased funding to public health agencies for this purpose. Respondents said their primary care physician is their most trusted source of information on this topic, followed by the CDC, the World Health Organization (WHO), and their local public health department.

Summary

Findings from this questionnaire survey indicate that the American public is only vaguely aware of the human health consequences of climate change and this lack of awareness manifests in relatively weak support for protective action by public health agencies. Central to the research design, the researchers suggest that people's unprompted responses to their open-ended questions are likely a more accurate reflection of their actual understanding of the effects of global warming on human health than are their responses to close-ended questions. As such, there is a clear need to better inform the public of the health threats associated with climate change. Primary care physicians and public health officials appear well positioned to educate the public about the health relevance of climate change.

Interview Survey Research

Interviews are qualitative methods that allow researchers to examine an issue in a meaningful and in-depth way through individual participants. The stories participants tell are used as a way to "explore a particular research phenomenon and may help in clarifying a less-well-understood problem, situation, or context" (Sutton & Austin, 2015, p. 226). Maibach, Nisbet, Baldwin, Akerlof, and Diao (2010) used an innovative exploratory research method by combining an interactive activity and in-depth interviews to measure the efficacy of climate change messaging. Specifically, the study sought to explore how American adults respond to an essay about climate change framed as a public health issue.

Participants (*n* = 70) were "recruited to participate in semi-structured, in-depth elicitation interviews that lasted an average of 43 minutes (ranging from 16 to 124 minutes) and included the presentation of a public health framed essay on climate change" (Maibach, et al., 2010, p. 3). The recruitment process was designed to yield completed interviews with a demographically and geographically diverse group of at least 10 people from each of the previously identified "Global Warming's Six Americas" (Maibach, et al., 2011). Audience segment status (i.e., which one of the "Six Americas" a person belonged to) was assessed with a previously developed 15-item screening questionnaire that identifies segment status with 80% accuracy (see Maibach, et al., 2010).

The interview was composed mostly of open-ended questions that asked "how and for whom global warming was a problem, how global warming is caused, if and how global warming can be stopped or limited, and what, if anything, an individual could do to help limit global warming" (Maibach, et al., 2010, p. 3). At the end of the interview, participants read a brief essay that framed climate change as a human health issue. Respondents were also given a green and a pink highlighter pen and asked to "use the green highlighter pen to mark any portions of the essay that you feel are especially clear or helpful, and use the pink highlighter pen to mark any portions of the essay that are particularly confusing or unhelpful" (Maibach, et al., 2010, pp. 3–4).

After reading the essay, participants were asked to describe their reaction. For each portion of the essay they marked in green/pink, they were then asked: "What about each of these sentences was especially clear/confusing or helpful/unhelpful to you?" (Maibach, et al., p. 4). To evaluate the participant's general reactions to the essay the authors reviewed their individual statements ($n =$ 193). Based on this review, the authors developed eight thematic categories (see Maibach, et al., 2010) that captured the range of statements made by participants. The statements were then coded into one of the thematic categories. To assess reliability, the authors used Krippendorff's alpha, "a conservative measure that corrects for chance agreement among coders" (Maibach, et al., 2010, p. 5). For seven of the eight thematic categories, a reliability of .80 or higher was achieved; "Lack of Evidence or Stylistically Confusing" was the exception, with an intercoder reliability of .70 (Maibach, et al., 2010, p. 5). After establishing reliability, the authors categorized the rest of the remaining statements.

To code the respondent's sentence-specific reactions made with the highlighter pens, sentences deemed helpful or clear by the participants (highlighted in green) were scored positively (+1), while confusing or unhelpful sentences (highlighted in pink) were scored negatively (−1). Sentences without highlights or with both green and pink were given a neutral score (0). The researchers then calculated a composite score for the overall essay per respondent. Using the nonparametric Kruskal-Wallis test, the authors assessed "the between-segment differences in the dependent measures (i.e., respondents' overall reaction to the essay and composite sentence-specific reactions to the entire essay" Maibach, et al., 2010, p. 6). The Wilcoxon signed rank test was used to see "if the median response to the essay on each dependent measure was greater than zero (i.e., a positive reaction)" and "to test the hypothesis that five of the six audience segments (the Dismissive being the one exception) would respond positively to the essay" (Maibach, et al., 2010, p. 6). Post-hoc analyses were conducted to test for two possible main effects: to examine the possibility that the essay's later focus on the public health benefits of mitigation-related policy actions (compared to the essay's earlier focus on the public health–related threats) and concluding framing section (as opposed to the opening framing section) were seen by the respondents as clearer and more useful (Maibach, et al., 2010).

There was clear evidence that reading the public health framed essay was positive for most groups, but its effect was tied to participants' existing ideology as defined by "Global Warming's Six Americas" audience segments. Participants who were already concerned about climate change (e.g., alarmed and concerned segments) demonstrated consistent positive responses, while people without clear concern (e.g., cautious, disengaged, and doubtful segments) were less consistent in their responses to the essay. Post-hoc analyses revealed that five of the six audience segments responded more positively to information about the health benefits associated with mitigation-related policy actions (e.g., making communities easier to navigate on foot or bike) than to information about the health risks of climate change. Therefore, the authors suggest a focus not on the problems, but the solutions, "a perspective that makes the problem more personally relevant, significant, and understandable to members of the public" (Maibach, et al., 2010, p. 1).

Summary

Presentations about climate change that encourage people to consider its human health relevance appear likely to provide many Americans with a useful and engaging new frame of reference. In-depth interviews revealed that information about the potential health benefits of specific mitigation-related policy actions appears to be particularly compelling. As a point of strategy, however, the findings from this study may suggest that continuing to communicate about the *problem of climate change* is not likely to generate wider public engagement. Instead, public health voices may be wise to focus their communication on the *solutions and the many co-benefits* that matter most to people.

Experimental Research

Selective Exposure Design

Selective exposure theory draws on cognitive dissonance theory to examine how an individual's personal preferences and biases affect their selection of information based on how it aligns with their existing values and beliefs and any tendency to avoid information counter to their beliefs (Festinger, 1957). Selective exposure theory also intersects with the concepts of confirmation bias and partisan selective exposure and is a useful tool when investigating the role that message frames have across audience segments (Stroud, 2011).

Feldman and Hart (2018) tested the effects of climate change frames through "two online news-browsing experiments assessing selective exposure to climate change news stories" (Feldman & Hart, 2018, p. 510). The researchers asked how multiple climate change frames affect individuals' exposure to news stories about climate change and how those effects vary according to political orientation. The studies were designed to approximate real-world news browsing experiences similar to that of results from a Google News search. Participants (*n* = 2,174) were asked to browse through and select six stories based on their headline and lead. In the first study, all of the articles were about climate change, each with a different frame—conflict, economic, environmental, morality, national security, and public health—and the headlines and lead paragraphs included the keyword from the frame. In the second study, the six articles included a collection of topics—national politics, business, fitness and health, sports, foreign affairs, and climate change. The single climate change article had to compete against other topics. In each case, it was one of the six aforementioned articles from the first study assigned at random. After six article selections, or if the participant indicated they were not interested in reading any more articles, they were redirected to a questionnaire that identified their party identification and political ideology (e.g., liberal-Democrats, moderate-Independents, and conservative-Republicans).

The public health frame showed increased exposure to climate change news articles, albeit mainly with liberal-Democrats. In the first study, participants were more likely to choose the news article with the public health frame in the headline and lead paragraph than the other climate change stories. However, in the second study, where the climate change article had to compete for the readers' attention, the framing did not affect selective exposure. These findings support prior research (e.g., Maibach, et al., 2010; Myers, Nisbet, Maibach, & Leiserowitz, 2012) that shows the importance of utilizing a public health emphasis in climate change communication due to its ability to connect readers to the tangible and immediate impacts of climate change, making it more personal and relevant to the segments of the American public, notably liberal-Democrats.

Summary

Results from this study offer some support for the idea that framing climate change as a human health risk "can stimulate exposure to climate change news relative to news framed in other ways" (Feldman & Hart, 2018, p. 520). From a practical perspective, this suggests that using a health frame may help encourage public engagement with climate change, particularly given evidence for this frame's positive effects on public opinion and perceptions related to climate change (Myers, et al., 2012).

However, the small observed effects and the fact that conservative-Republicans were unaffected by the frame suggest limits to these influences, particularly as a way to overcome confirmation bias in information exposure.

Quasi-Experimental Design

Quasi-experimental design is a practical way to examine general trends found in evaluating frame efficacy, especially in social science disciplines like communication studies (Lewis-Beck, Bryman, & Liao, 2004). Ranking, one such tool, is used to evaluate subjects against one another; in this case, to uncover the most compelling climate change message frames. Kotcher, Maibach, and Choi (2019) sought to assess how people respond to information about the neurological health harms of air pollution from fossil fuels, which are intricately linked to climate change. Specifically, they sought to identify the specific messages about the health implications of air pollution from fossil fuels that are most and least concerning to people and whether rankings of concern vary among different audiences. The authors also hypothesized that reading the messages "would influence people's attitudes and behavioral intentions in a manner supportive of a transition to cleaner sources of energy" (Kotcher, et al., 2019, p. 1).

Participants were recruited via Qualtrics to obtain a diverse sample that approximates the general American population (n = 1,025) along with an oversampling of six target groups (n = 619). The target groups included various subgroups of women, minorities, and caretakers and were used to contrast the way these groups ranked each statement in comparison to the general population. Participants were first asked a series of questions to identify demographic details and measure their attitudes toward air pollution, fossil fuels, and clean energy and their behavioral intentions regarding consumer and political advocacy. Next, participants engaged in a maximum difference scaling (i.e., MaxDiff) exercise to elicit their ranking of 10 different statements about fossil fuels and health from most to least concerning, each designed to represent a broad range of factual information about the health consequences of air pollution caused by burning fossil fuels. The statements included

> well-established health harms such as asthma, cancer, and heart disease; emerging neurological health harms to children; emerging neurological health harms to older adults; mechanisms by which air pollution causes harm to health; and statements about who is most likely to be harmed by air pollution from fossil fuels.
>
> *(Kotcher, et al., 2019, p. 4)*

All of the statements were evidence-based and reviewed before use by experts on the health impacts of air pollution caused by fossil fuel use (e.g., WHO, Environmental Health Perspectives).

The 10 statements were shown to each participant multiple times across eight screens, with each screen displaying a different combination of four statements. Respondents were asked to select the statement that "causes them the most concern" and the one that "causes them the least concern" (Kotcher, et al., 2019, p. 4). These selections

> provide five data points per screen on a respondent's preferences about the four statements displayed: if a respondent selects A as the greatest concern and D as the least concern, we learn that: A > B; A > C; A > D; B > D; C > D.
>
> *(Kotcher, et al., 2019, p. 4)*

Through a hierarchical Bayes estimation method, "these data points—40 per respondent from the eight screens—allow for the calculation of individual respondent-level utility scores for each of the items tested" (Kotcher, et al., 2019, p. 4). As a result, there were a total of 65,760 data points for the MaxDiff exercise (1,644 survey interviews × 40 data points). In addition to calculating the individual utility scores for each message, the authors conducted a reach analysis to identify the combination of messages that pertain to the largest portion of respondents. While the utility scores demonstrate the relative ranking of the messages for all respondents, a statement's "reach" equals the percentage of respondents ranking that item as their greatest or second greatest concern (Kotcher, et al., 2019, p. 4). This study examined the "total reach for every possible combination of statements and determined the package that causes participants the most concern" (Kotcher, et al., 2019, p. 4). After completing the MaxDiff exercise, participants were again asked the same attitude and behavioral intention questions (e.g., perceived health risk of air pollution and fossil fuels, support for fossil fuel and clean energy use, and consumer and political advocacy intentions). Finally, participants were asked questions about their political orientation.

The cumulative effect of reading and ranking the statements on participants' attitudes and behavioral intentions were measured using a "series of mixed-design ANOVAs with time (T1- pre-test vs. T2- post-test) as a within-subjects factor and party affiliation as a between-subjects factor" (Kotcher, et al., 2019, pp. 4–6) . A ***Bonferroni adjustment***, a statistical technique that minimizes the risk of false-positives, was used for all pairwise comparisons. Effect size estimates for specific contrasts were provided in terms of Cohen's *d*. The effect size descriptors—small, medium, and large—specific to communication research were derived from a quantitative review of meta-analyses (Weber & Popova, 2012).

Across all subgroups examined, participants were most concerned by a message about the neurological impacts of air pollution on infants and children, including all three statements that referenced neurological impacts on infants and children. In addition to high agreement in the three most concerning statements, there was agreement across all subgroups about the three least concerning statements: a statement that called attention to and explained why low-income populations are particularly vulnerable to air pollution, a statement about general health problems, and a statement about the impacts on the elderly. Additionally, the reach analysis showed 84% of participants ranked one of four statements as first or second most concerning: specific neurological health impacts on children, well-established health effects, lasting effects on children and the elderly, and toxic chemicals released when burning fossil fuels.

Summary

To our knowledge, this is the first study to investigate how people respond to information about the neurological risks associated with air pollution from fossil fuels. Findings from this quasi-experimental study build on the body of literature illuminating the value of climate change messages framed as a public health issue. It draws attention to participants' concern for the health impacts of burning fossil fuels and the resulting well-established forms of human health harms. Specifically, these findings suggest that efforts should now be organized to communicate the health impacts of climate change on infants and children, especially the neurodevelopmental effects of air pollution from fossil fuels on infants and children.

Strengths and Limitations

The impacts of climate change on public health are compelling, novel, and tangible. The research presented here suggests that Americans rank health issues as highly important. In fact, Maibach, and colleagues (2010) found that all groups surveyed agreed on the importance of good health— that is, "human health and wellbeing is a widely-shared value" (p. 11). Research also suggests that the health-centered frame of climate change may better resonate with the American public and that healthcare professionals (e.g., primary care physicians) are uniquely positioned to deliver this message to the public. Additionally, framing climate change impacts through the positive outcomes and opportunities for mitigation may motivate public engagement because the "co-benefits" are not only empowering but also good for individual health; "the public health perspective offers a vision of a better, healthier future—not just a vision of environmental disaster averted, and it focuses on a range of possible policy actions that offer local as well as global benefits" (Maibach, et al., 2010, pp. 10–11). While the findings presented in this chapter are promising, climate change communication researchers are just beginning to uncover the value of a public health frame, and, as such, further research is needed to understand its impact more fully.

Research communicating human health implications of climate change faces many limitations. Given the limited research that has been conducted, much being exploratory, findings cannot be generalized without further study. In addition, multiple analyses presented here employ modest research designs in order to conduct initial investigations of the phenomena and call for more rigorous and realistic study designs as next steps in the investigation of their findings (Feldman & Hart, 2018; Levine & Kline, 2017; Maibach, et al., 2010; Maibach, et al., 2015). Further, without replication, the research methods themselves have not been tested to uncover how they may have affected the findings. For example, in one study, the authors expressed a need to examine the impact that the order in which questions are presented in surveys has on responses (Maibach, et al., 2015). Researchers also note the need to consider the role that extensive exposure to issues may have on participants. For instance, does exposure engage them in "effortful processing," which may trigger the phenomena of priming—reflecting a more significant concern about the public health impacts of climate change (Feldman & Hart, 2018)?

Most of the studies examining communicating about climate change as a public health issue are focused on Americans. It will be essential for future research to include populations outside of the United States and, as such, consider the varied audiences of those countries as well. In addition, many studies use the terms "global warming" and "climate change" nearly interchangeably without concern for the negative connotations associated with the term "global warming" among Americans. Researchers may fail to consider the differences in meaning across cultural and social variations in the United States, weakening the connections between findings using contrasting terms (Akerlof et al., 2010).

Subsequent research will require a deeper understanding of the relevance of people's socioeconomic status, health, age, and other factors of audience segmentation in the respondent's assessment of the health issues associated with climate change. For example, respondents with low levels of risk due to their fiscal and physical health may not accurately assess the risk their families and communities face (Maibach, et al., 2015). It is also likely that messages that highlight risks to vulnerable populations, most notably people in poverty, may not resonate with more affluent populations who do not relate with those groups or see themselves as vulnerable (Lane, 2001; Maibach, et al., 2015).

Using closed-ended questions, like the ones used in survey research, may give a false perception of the salience of an issue (Akerlof, et al., 2010). For example, Maibach, et al. (2015) discovered that participants recognize the public health impacts of climate change through close-ended questioning, but were largely unable to replicate familiarity with the issue in an open-ended format. Conducting more research using open-ended questions will help to more accurately reflect the public's understanding of climate change as a public health issue.

Scholars in the field of climate change communication know it is vital that studies be designed to investigate the behavioral aspects of interfacing with climate change messaging. Further research must be done to determine framing effects' overall impact on public engagement with the issue of climate change—it is critical to balance the efficacy of a frame against how it affects public engagement. A message that receives a positive value judgment by a participant may not foster engagement with the issue, or worse, may depress engagement (Levine & Kline, 2017). If engagement is the ultimate goal of effective climate change communication, framing effects must be fully understood.

The findings presented in this chapter offer a rich base from which to grow a meaningful field of research across disciplines, agencies, and into the community. While there are limitations to the studies presented in this chapter, scholars agree that "using a public health frame helps encourage public engagement with climate change" (Feldman & Hart, 2018, p. 520). Therefore, it is essential that researchers fully examine and leverage the power that the public health frame may have to engage the public in society's transition toward a low-carbon future.

Recommended Future Research

Given the public's lack of understanding surrounding climate change and public health and its strong association with global warming as a heat-related issue, climate change lacks salience as a health issue. Therefore, it is critical to build public awareness surrounding the issue using consistent messaging. "Re-defining climate change in public health terms should help people make connections to already familiar problems . . . shifting the visualization of the issue away from remote Arctic regions, and distant peoples and animals" (Maibach, et al., 2010, p. 9).

Efforts should be made to ensure the risks and effects outlined in research instruments are localized and relevant to study participants (Akerlof, et al., 2010). Maibach, and colleagues (2015) call researchers to examine how the "actual risk status of respondents and their family (e.g., age and health status), and their community (e.g., high poverty rates and environmental exposures) influences people's assessments of the health risks associated with climate change" (p. 407). For example, Kotcher, Maibach, Montoro, and Hassol (2018) note that respondents "may see themselves as relatively less vulnerable to mental health and food-related impacts from global warming" (p. 272), while others found that affluent audiences underestimated the risk to their food supply (Maibach, et al., 2015).

The threats associated with the human health impacts of climate change are not the only important aspect of a health-centered frame. There are positive and personally relevant health benefits to reducing personal carbon emissions, such as those associated with exercise, which may further engage the public in the issue of climate change. "The problem of climate change is not likely to generate wider public engagement. Instead, public health voices may be wise to focus their communication on the solution and the many co-benefits that matter most to people" (Maibach, et al., 2010, pp. 10–11). A choice to commute to work on foot or bike rather than driving a vehicle is good for the planet and good for the individual—empowering them to tackle climate change and their health.

It is also critical to recognize, however, that people are different, with widely diverse backgrounds, experiences, knowledge, and values. There is a spectrum from those Americans who know a lot about climate change, to those who have never heard of it. Likewise, some Americans have taken personal action to reduce their own carbon footprint, while others have not. At a deeper level, different groups within American society emphasize different values, which strongly shape their interpretations and preferred solutions to climate change. Thus, the American public does not respond to climate change with a single voice—there are many different groups that each respond to this issue in different ways. Constructively engaging each of these groups in climate change solutions will therefore require tailored approaches. One of the first rules of effective communication is to "know thy audience"—what they currently understand and misunderstand about the issue; how they perceive the threat; their current and intended behaviors; their values, beliefs, and policy preferences; and the barriers to change and underlying motivations that either constrain or can inspire their further engagement with the solutions (Maibach, et al., 2009). Only with this knowledge can effective strategies be designed to help individuals and organizations make more informed decisions, empower them to make and enact better choices, and build public support for policies that institute systemic and structural change.

It is imperative for future studies to analyze the impact of messages about climate change framed as a human health issue on both attitude and behavior (Levine & Kline, 2017). Maibach, and colleagues (2010) call for researchers to "look carefully for examples of associations that trigger counter and negative reactions" and to "identify the conditions under which message about the health implications of global warming can motivate protective actions to mitigate and adapt to the problem" and how messages can reduce advocacy (pp. 10–11). Similarly, Kotcher, Maibach, Montoro, and Hassol (2018) call for further research to "ascertain how presenting this information in more dynamic engaging, and realistic formats in field settings may affect responses to the messages" (p. 273).

Finally, public health officials, most notably primary care doctors, have been ranked as the most trusted messengers to deliver vital information about the human health implications of climate change. Americans value health and they trust their doctors (Maibach, et al., 2015). Agencies like the CDC and public health departments are considered trusted sources as well. Coupled with the efficacy of positively framed mitigation practices, such as those associated with health benefits and reinforcement by members of the public (e.g., friends and family), there is no doubt about the potential value of the healthcare community educating its constituency and the public at large about the issue of climate change. However, further research is needed to reconcile America's high ranking of health issues and corresponding low investment interest in climate change–related health priorities and programs (Maibach, et al., 2015).

Conclusion

The ultimate goal of the climate change communication research summarized in this chapter goes well beyond an effort to understand the implications of communicating about climate change through a public health frame, aiming to foster engagement with the issue of climate change through effective communication. The findings presented here support the premise that efforts should be made to start a large-scale, public health professionals–led communication campaign to educate the public about the human health implications of climate change—both the risks and the positive "health benefits associated with taking actions to address climate change" (Maibach, et al., 2015, p. 407). With further research, communication scholars can work with healthcare professionals to equip agencies (e.g., CDC) and professionals (e.g., primary care physicians) with the information and tools they need to communicate with their patients and the public about the looming threats to human health brought on by climate change and the positive benefits of health-focused mitigation practices.

References

Akerlof, K., DeBono, R., Berry, P., Leiserowitz, A., Roser-Renouf, C., Clarke, K., et al. (2010). Public perceptions of climate change as a human health risk: Surveys of the United States, Canada and Malta. *International Journal of Environmental Research and Public Health, 7*(6), 2559–2606. https://doi.org/10.3390/ijerph7062559

Blair, J., Czaja, R., & Blair, E. (2014). *Designing surveys: A guide to decisions and procedures.* Thousand Oaks, CA: Sage Publications.

Feldman, L., & Hart, P. S. (2018). Broadening exposure to climate change news? How framing and political orientation interact to influence selective exposure. *Journal of Communication, 68*(3), 503–524. https://doi.org/10.1093/joc/jqy011

Festinger, L. (1957). *A theory of cognitive dissonance.* Evanston, IL: Row, Peterson, & Co.

Gamson, W. A., Croteau, D., Hoynes, W., & Sasson, T. (1992). Media images and the social construction of reality. *Annual Review of Sociology, 18*, 373–393. https://doi.org/10.1146/annurev.so.18.080192.002105

Hornik, R. (2002). *Public health communication: Evidence for behavior change.* Mahwah, NJ: Lawrence Erlbaum Associates.

Kotcher, J., Maibach, E., & Choi, W. T. (2019). Fossil fuels are harming our brains: Identifying key messages about the health effects of air pollution from fossil fuels. *BMC Public Health*, *19*(1), 1–12. https://doi.org/10.1186/s12889-019-7373-1

Kotcher, J., Maibach, E., Montoro, M., & Hassol, S. J. (2018). How Americans respond to information about global warming's health impacts: Evidence from a national survey experiment. *GeoHealth*, *2*(9), 262–275. https://doi.org/10.1029/2018GH000154

Lane, R. E. (2001). Self-reliance and empathy: The enemies of poverty: And of the poor. *Political Psychology*, *22*(3), 473–492. https://doi.org/10.1111/0162-895X.00250

Leiserowitz, A., Maibach, E., & Roser-Renouf, C. (2009). *Climate change in the American mind: Americans' climate change beliefs, attitudes, policy preferences, and actions*. Retrieved February 10, 2019, from http://climatecommunication.yale.edu/publications/climate-change-american-mind-2009/

Leiserowitz, A., Maibach, E., Roser-Renouf, C., Rosenthal, S., Cutler, M., & Kotcher, J. (2018). *Climate change in the American mind: March 2018*. Retrieved February 10, 2019, from http://climatecommunication.yale.edu/publications/climate-change-american-mind-march-2018/

Levine, A. S., & Kline, R. (2017). A new approach for evaluating climate change communication. *Climatic Change*, *142*(1–2), 301–309. https://doi.org/10.1007/s10584-017-1952-x

Lewis-Beck, M. S., Bryman, A., & Liao, T. F. (2004). *The Sage encyclopedia of social science research methods*. Thousand Oaks, CA: Sage Publications.

Maibach, E. W., Abroms, L., & Marosits, M. (2007). Communication and marketing as tools to cultivate the public's health: A proposed "people and places" framework. *BMC Public Health*, *7*(88), 1–15. Retrieved from https://bmcpublichealth.biomedcentral.com/articles/10.1186/1471-2458-7-88#citeas

Maibach, E. W., Kreslake, J. M., Roser-Renouf, C., Rosenthal, S., Feinberg, G., & Leiserowitz, A. A. (2015). Do Americans understand that global warming is harmful to human health? Evidence from a national survey. *Annals of Global Health*, *81*(3), 396–409. https://doi.org/10.1016/j.aogh.2015.08.010

Maibach, E. W., Leiserowitz, A., Roser-Renouf, C., & Mertz, C. K. (2011). Identifying like-minded audiences for global warming public engagement campaigns: An audience segmentation analysis and tool development. *PLoS One*, *6*(3), e17571. doi:10.1371/journal.pone.0017571

Maibach, E. W., Nisbet, M., Baldwin, P., Akerlof, K., & Diao, G. (2010). Reframing climate change as a public health issue: An exploratory study of public reactions. *BMC Public Health*, *10*(1), 1–11. Retrieved from https://link.springer.com/article/10.1186/1471-2458-10-299#citeas

Maibach, E. W., Roser-Renouf, C., & Leiserowitz, A. (2009). *Climate change in the American mind: Global Warming's Six Americas*. Retrieved February 10, 2019, from www.climatechangecommunication.org/climate-change-in-the-american-mind/

Myers, T. A., Nisbet, M. C., Maibach, E. W., & Leiserowitz, A. A. (2012). A public health frame arouses hopeful emotions about climate change. *Climatic Change*, *113*(3–4), 1105–1112. https://doi.org/10.1007/s10584-012-0513-6

Smith, J. (2005). Dangerous news: Media decision making about climate change risk. *Risk Analysis*, *25*, 1471–1482. https://doi.org/10.1111/j.1539-6924.2005.00693.x

Stroud, N. J. (2011). *Niche news*. New York: Oxford University Press.

Sutton, J., & Austin, Z. (2015). Qualitative research: Data collection, analysis, and management. *The Canadian Journal of Hospital Pharmacy*, *68*(3), 226–231. doi:10.4212/cjhp.v68i3.1456

Weathers, M. R. (2013). Newspaper coverage of Global Warming and Climate Change (GWCC) as a public health issue. *Applied Environmental Education & Communication*, *12*(1), 19–28. https://doi.org/10.1080/1533015X.2013.795829

Weathers, M. R., & Kendall, B. E. (2015). Developments in the framing of climate change as a public health issue in U.S. newspapers. *Environmental Communication*, *10*(5), 593–611. Retrieved from www.tandfonline.com/doi/abs/10.1080/17524032.2015.1050436

Weber, R., & Popova, L. (2012). Testing equivalence in communication research: Theory and application. *Communication Methods & Measures*, *6*(3), 190–213. https://doi.org/10.1080/19312458.2012.703834

PART VI

Health Policy and Future Directions in Research

26

IMPACT OF NUTRITION HEALTH POLICY ON OUTCOMES

Jessica Devine, Krystal Lynch, Dennis A. Savaiano, and Heather A. Eicher-Miller

Overview

Nutrition health policy is designed to improve diet quality, thereby preventing nutrient deficiencies and reducing the risk of certain chronic diseases. While health policies may be implemented in various environments or through different interventions, individual behavior change is ultimately a primary goal. Social ecological and other health behavior models have been used to describe the relationship between individual, organizational, social, environmental, and policy-related factors and health. A variety of methods may be used to evaluate the relationship between policy and health in each of these social ecological contexts. In this chapter, we overview select methods that may be used to evaluate health policy, with a specific focus on nutrition as a modifiable risk factor for health outcomes. Dietary intake and quality contribute to the development of obesity, type 2 diabetes, cardiovascular disease, and many cancers. Nutrition research has been important in providing science-based information aimed at regulating the safety of the food supply, the prevention of nutrient deficiencies, and more recently, the promotion of healthy food intake for the reduction of chronic disease (Kessler, 1995). Nutrition research methodology has been developed to evaluate interventions directed through the various levels of the social ecological model, including large populations, communities, and individuals. The impact of these interventions on health may vary depending on the target population or individuals. For example, methods that focus on individual nutrition knowledge or perceptions provide a basis for understanding individual choice. Other methods focus on determining how restricting or regulating certain foods may influence population-level dietary intake. Thus, diverse nutrition methodologies are powerful tools in successfully transcending the link between nutrition interventions, policies, and resulting health outcomes.

This chapter describes five nutrition policies or systems that are influential factors in promoting public health nutrition: 1) national school lunch programs, 2) nutrition education (the example being the US Supplemental Nutrition Assistance Program Education [SNAP-Ed]), 3) menu labeling policies, 4) taxation of low-nutrient dietary components (e.g., sweetened beverages), and 5) the social networks that influence nutrition policy. Each of the studies reviewed uses a unique method, including the specific exposure and outcome, to evaluate the program, policy, or system related to the authors' hypothesis. The studies are arranged according to the social ecological model. Presented first are studies aimed at changing individual dietary intake through direct changes to school lunch and nutrition education to the household. Next, studies focusing on environmental-level changes through menu labeling and taxation are presented. Finally, we present an example that examines policy influence through social networks. Through the course of this chapter, strengths and weaknesses of each method to evaluate health policy are discussed in order to promote best practices for future research.

Research in Practice

Impact of National School Lunch Program on Fruit and Vegetable Selection in Northeastern Elementary Schoolchildren, 2012-2013

The US National School Lunch Program was a result of a federal policy created in 1946 in recognition of the effect the school food environment has on a child's diet, with some children consuming up to two meals at school every weekday. The National School Lunch Program feeds almost 31 million children, directly affecting the school food environment of children throughout the United States. Therefore, changes to the federal policy guiding the National School Lunch Program have the potential to significantly affect dietary intake and the health of US children. In 2012, the US Department of Agriculture added a requirement to the National School Lunch Program that all children eating a school lunch must choose a fruit or vegetable for the lunch meal that is subsidized as part of the National School Lunch Program.

Such widespread changes in policies provide an opportunity for natural observational study designs that should not be missed by researchers, as they are very difficult to replicate in experimental conditions. Further, evaluation of such potentially consequential changes are critical to ensure the intended results. Methods to quantify the impact of policy and program changes may be tailored to the environment and outcome, but the use of a pre-post or before-after study design capitalizes on such opportunities. Amin, Yon, Taylor, and Johnson (2015) used this approach to evaluate the outcomes of the 2012 change in school lunch policy on food choice, food consumption, and food waste among schoolchildren. Inadequate consumption of fruits and vegetables among schoolchildren during lunch prior to 2012 was the basis for creating new requirements that children select fruits and vegetables as part of the reimbursable school meal (Amin, et al., 2015). The changes were met with much support as well as some skepticism, as many expected increased food waste or unaffected consumption. Subjective reports indicated increased waste. Thus, Amin and colleagues evaluated changes in food waste as well as fruit and vegetable selection and consumption before and after the implementation of the requirements (Amin, et al., 2015).

This study used an observational study design evaluating food selection, consumption, and waste prior to the changes in the National School Lunch Policy and after the changes. Two cross-sectional assessments were completed, and the estimated dietary intake and food waste of third- through fifth-grade children from two schools were quantified. The study was a secondary analysis of data collected to validate digital imaging methods to measure fruit and vegetable consumption and waste. Both schools were considered low-income, with 40% to 60% of students qualifying for free or reduced-priced lunches; schools were also 84% to 90% white.

Digital imaging is an emerging tool that is used to estimate the amount of food wasted and the assumed amount of food consumed. Images of lunch trays were taken before and after students ate their lunches. The fruit and vegetable portions discarded were estimated as fruit and vegetable waste and then subtracted from the food portions selected to determine the fruit and vegetable portion assumed to be consumed. In addition, the amount of waste returned on the tray after lunch was weighed and compared with initial serving weight to determine the estimated cups consumed and wasted. Before the policy changed, 10 data collection visits were completed, with a total of 498 tray observations. After the 2012 policy change, 11 data collection visits were completed, with a total of 944 tray observations. Data analysis included chi-squared tests and independent sample t-tests. All were two-tailed tests comparing fruit and vegetable selection, consumption, and waste before and after the regulation change.

Researchers found that students took more fruits and vegetables after the policy change, but consumption of fruit and vegetables decreased while waste of fruits and vegetables increased in the school year following implementation of the new fruit and vegetable requirement. Approximately one tablespoon less was consumed and two tablespoons more were wasted on average. Such changes in intake, held consistent over time, may be meaningful with regard to nutrient and energy intake but are limited by the context of only quantifying one eating occasion in a day. These results may not reflect long-term adaptation or intake following the new requirement.

Strengths/Limitations

Before and after study designs allow researchers to observe and quantify changes before and after policy implementations in natural settings. Researchers, unaware of impending policy changes, may not have the ability to plan for these experiments and, as in this study, may need to use secondary data intended to test other hypotheses. Several limitations exist in these conditions, but the value of well-done studies is critical to determining effectiveness. Amin, et al. (2015) collected data from two schools before and after the change in National School Lunch Policy, allowing researchers to evaluate how the policy change affected student's behaviors. The study compared averages for the desired outcomes but not individual-level changes; thus, the mean changes describe the group but may not describe the behavior of individual students. The actual school menus were not shown and may not be a representative sample of typical school meals before or after implementation of the policy. The fruits and vegetables provided during data collection may be more or less well liked by students and could bias results. This study design is similar to other studies that evaluated changes in student dietary behaviors as a result of the National School Lunch Policy. The study would have been strengthened by the inclusion of a control group, but this would have been practically impossible in this setting, as the policy change affected all US schools. Further, Amin, et al.'s pre-/post-test study does not allow for conclusions regarding any period of adaptation, as only one post-intervention time point was evaluated.

The novel methods of visualizing and weighing plate waste also have some limitations. Although plate waste was an objective measure that was not dependent on self-report, dietary intake was assumed and not directly quantified. Children's selection and consumption of fruits and vegetables could have been affected by the presence of the researchers. In addition, the results have limited generalizability due to geographic location, cafeteria dynamics, and sociodemographic factors that may affect social norms and behaviors.

Recommendations for Future Research

Unpredictability in the implementation of policy may limit the attainment of perfect study conditions; however, recommendations to improve on the methods described in Amin, et al.'s study (2015) include the introduction of a longitudinal cohort component to the study design that would allow researchers to match individual intake and plate waste before and after the policy to determine long-term, individual-level changes. Extension of dietary measures to quantify children's intake at other meals during the day would allow inferences of whether intake changes at lunch have the desired impact of improving overall dietary intake. Assessments should also quantify barriers such as insufficient time to eat during lunch or fruit and vegetable preferences that could discourage children from consuming these items during school lunches. The representativeness of the schools and children sampled may be improved and further consideration given to the extent to which fruit and vegetable offerings are tailored to regional and cultural preferences, the overall diet of the children, and fruit and vegetable consumption at other meals, as these factors may also affect fruit and vegetable consumption and food waste at lunch. Finally, follow-up studies should be conducted to see how children adapt to the changes in policy, whether the changes captured here are maintained, or if fruit and vegetable intake improves once children are accustomed to the new guidelines.

Summary

Before and after public health policy studies are necessary to quantify whether the intended changes in behavior actually occur after public health policy changes are made. Methods to quantify and visualize plate waste were an objective measure that was practical and matched to the school lunch setting.

SNAP-Ed Increases Long-Term Food Security Among Indiana Households With Children in a Randomized Controlled Study

SNAP-Ed, a federally funded grant program, is the nutrition education component of the Supplemental Nutrition Assistance Program (formerly the food stamp program). SNAP-Ed provides direct nutrition education to SNAP-eligible populations to further improve food security by increasing knowledge of nutrition, healthy food preparation, and food resource management to promote healthy food consumption. More recently, SNAP-Ed has also focused on community public health initiatives and multilevel interventions to increase access to healthy foods in resource-limited populations. A significant budget supports SNAP-Ed, yet few evaluations of effectiveness have been completed. Rivera, Maulding, Abbott, Craig, and Eicher-Miller (2016) evaluated changes in long-term food security due to SNAP-Ed programming.

Use of a randomized, controlled experimental trial is well known as a "gold-standard" method of study design in clinical trials research and other areas of health research. The additional methods of randomization and use of a control group strengthen experimental study designs by removing bias that may otherwise be present in the allotment or assignment of participants to treatment groups. Such methods may also be applied in a public health setting depending on the nature of the intervention to be evaluated.

Direct nutrition education has been included as a public health intervention to promote nutrition knowledge, positive attitudes toward healthy food-related behaviors, and intake of fruits and vegetables (Beydoun & Wang, 2008; Carbone & Zoellner, 2012; Devine, Farrell, & Hartman, 2005; Eyles & Mhurchu, 2009). Education as an intervention indirectly addresses disparities in knowledge of how to access resources and to use health and nutrition information. Those receiving a direct nutrition education intervention may gain health literacy and resource management skills that may aid ability to make healthier choices, engage in health promotion, and improve overall lifestyle health.

Nutritional education, as a public health intervention, is conducive to evaluation using an experimental trial, with an experimental group receiving education and a control group with no educational intervention, or a placebo intervention. Such a study design is not always possible. For example, experimental designs for a food assistance intervention where the investigator assigns treatment, such as the resources provided through SNAP, is unlawful, as SNAP is an entitlement program available to anyone who is eligible for it. Other designs may not be possible due to ethical or practical constraints. However, nutrition education provided through SNAP-Ed is conducive to a more rigorous experimental design. This nonentitlement program serves as a complementary educational program to SNAP and aims to support SNAP, promote food security, and improve healthy behaviors and dietary intake among the SNAP-eligible population.

Rivera, Maulding, Abbott, Craig, and Eicher-Miller (2016) applied a randomized, controlled experimental design to evaluate the SNAP-Ed program in a sample of 575 participants who were eligible in Indiana. In this study design, a parallel-arm nutrition education intervention with two treatment groups, an intervention and control, was used. The intent of the evaluation was to determine if SNAP-Ed improved food security among households with children, consistent with SNAP-Ed's goals.

At the direction of Purdue University Health and Human Sciences Cooperative Extension, 41 county-level, Indiana SNAP-Ed paraprofessionals in 38 counties recruited participants following SNAP-Ed protocol. Only SNAP-Ed–eligible households with children were included and were identified through screening via a questionnaire. As part of the recruitment and screening process, all participants were asked if they were willing to wait at least one year to receive SNAP-Ed. Those who agreed were eligible. Participants were randomized to the experimental or control groups with an allocation ratio of approximately 1:1 and then completed a baseline assessment. A 10-week intervention period followed. Participants in the intervention group 1) completed four or more SNAP-Ed lessons, 2) had a child still living in the household at least a year after the assessment period, and 3) followed all protocols of the study, while participants in the control group fulfilled components 2 and 3 and were asked to wait one year to fulfill component 1. The intervention consisted of four SNAP-Ed lessons that fulfilled federal guidelines and were taught by paraprofessionals either in participants' homes or to groups of participants in other settings. All participants completed the post-intervention assessment after the intervention period and again one year later. Food security was quantified by using the US Household Food Security Survey Module (Bickel, Nord, Price, Hamilton, & Cook, 2000). Analysis evaluated the effect of the treatment group (SNAP-Ed intervention or control) on the change in food security from baseline to one year later, using a linear mixed model. Several covariates, including sex, age, marital status, race, household education, household poverty status, household employment, number of people in household, participation in food assistance programs, frequency of food pantry use, and number of SNAP-Ed lessons, were considered in the selection of the model. Household food security in the intervention group significantly improved by about 25% from baseline over the one-year study period compared with the control group.

Strengths/Limitations

The longitudinal design of the study was a strength. Improvement over the long term may not have been captured in a limited short-term trial. The use of a randomized, controlled trial methodology was a strength, as the assignment of the intervention was the only variable manipulated by researchers. Thus, the change in the outcome, food security in this case, can be attributed to the intervention of SNAP-Ed. Caution must be taken, however, in interpreting these findings, as factors that made the control participants different from the intervention participants may also be inherent to the results. For example, some of the SNAP-Ed paraprofessionals may not have strictly adhered to the randomization protocol and may have assigned intervention participants as those that they felt could not wait for the education. True randomization mitigates this flaw and provides the strongest evidence for causality, as participants are not assigned based on any characteristic or situation, and thus, these qualities are removed as potential causes for the behavior change.

Attrition also may have played a role in the findings. The 43% attrition may have affected the representativeness of the sample. There may be characteristics or situations that made certain participants less likely to complete the study that may be related to the effectiveness of the intervention. The authors quantified the differences in characteristics of those who completed the study compared with those who did not, potentially describing biasing factors. Representativeness is also a factor in the selection of the sample. Participants were not chosen randomly from the Indiana SNAP-eligible population, but had to agree to participate in both SNAP-Ed and the study. As a result, the study sample may not truly reflect the population who qualify for SNAP-Ed and thus limit the applicability of the results to the SNAP-Ed–eligible population.

The paraprofessional contact with study participants was both a benefit and a limitation. Paraprofessional involvement replicates the normal administration of the program by health educators, but may also bias the outcome toward a better or stronger intervention. For example, paraprofessionals were encouraged to stay in contact with participants to prevent attrition. This may have biased participants to form a stronger relationship with the paraprofessional and potentially receive further advice or direction to resources.

The "gold-standard" measure of food security used in this study was a strength. Alignment of assessment to study design was also a strength. For example, at the final assessment participants reported on their food security over the last year, a period of time matching the follow-up period after the intervention. Finally, statewide and nationwide economic trends, unemployment, and other environmental factors may have influenced food security over the one-year study period, potentially affecting the results.

Recommendations for Future Research

Rivera, et al.'s (2016) study population was primarily non-Hispanic white and evaluated only one statewide program; thus, future research should replicate this study with populations that represent the race/ethnic and geographic diversity of other SNAP-Ed programs and curriculums. Questions remain about how SNAP benefits, or other financial assistance programs, affect food security and how SNAP may interact with SNAP-Ed to influence household food security. Further research may build evidence for SNAP-Ed's contribution to improving food security and dietary quality for SNAP recipients.

Summary

Use of randomized, controlled experimental trial study methodology may be very effective for mitigating bias and determining the effectiveness of public health interventions such as nutrition education where investigator assignment of the intervention is possible.

Meta-Analysis to Determine Impact of Restaurant Menu Labeling on Calories and Nutrients (Ordered or Consumed) by US Adults

Menu labeling is a population-based public health policy designed to provide nutrition information to consumers at the point of purchase. Chain restaurants and other retail food establishments with 20 or more sites are required to post calorie information for menu items regarding food prepared away from home as per the Patient Protection and Affordability Care Act (PPACA) passed in 2010 (U.S. Food & Drug Administration, 2004; Office of the Legislative Counsel for the U.S. House of Representatives, 2010). The intent of such policy is to empower consumers to make "healthier" choices, or choices adherent to the Dietary Guidelines for Americans, when eating away from home. Improved dietary intake away from home includes reducing intake of saturated fat and sodium and increasing the intake of fiber, fruit, and vegetables, ultimately reducing energy intake and the prevalence of obesity in the US population.

Evaluation of the effectiveness of menu labeling as an intervention is important to determine whether such a policy should be expanded or be used to inform similar public health interventions to educate consumers. The introduction of menu labeling in some locations prior to the passing of the PPACA generated much public interest and was evaluated by numerous investigators using a variety of study designs. Energy and nutrients purchased or consumed were the main outcomes of such studies, with results varying from no change to moderate increases or decreases. The diversity of findings and availability of many published investigations presents an opportunity for meta-analysis, an inclusive way of evaluating the effectiveness of menu labeling at the point of purchase across various times, locations, and samples.

Meta-analysis is appropriate when there are numerous published high-quality studies evaluating a policy or intervention. The studies may focus on diverse times, places, and populations. The methodology used in meta-analyses combines data from various studies to provide an overall evaluation of the effect of the policy on dietary intake or health. Meta-analysis may be particularly helpful when the findings of such studies vary, as meta-analysis allows for comprehensive results. This combination of data from many types of study designs and from diverse populations enhances representativeness compared to any single study.

Cantu-Jungles, McCormack, Slaven, Slebodnik, and Eicher-Miller (2017) conducted a meta-analysis with the specific goal of evaluating how exposure to calorie labeling on menus affected consumers and to determine if menu labeling as an intervention is effective to promote health behavior change. Guidance published by Crockett, Hollands, Jebb, and Marteau (2011) and *Cochrane* (Ryan, Hill, Broclain, Horey, Oliver, & Prictor, 2013) was followed by Cantu-Jungles, et al. (2017) in conducting a meta-analysis that aimed to determine if restaurant menu labeling would affect caloric choice or intake or alter carbohydrate, total fat, saturated fat, and sodium choice or intake compared with before menu labeling or compared with a control group in an away-from-home US setting. A systematic search for key words was completed using several databases. The Preferred Reporting Items for Systematic Reviews and Meta-Analysis were also followed (Moher, Liberati, Tetzlaff, & Altman, 2009). Criteria included participants older than 18 years; studies published in English from 1950 to 2014; and comparisons of nutrition labeling at the point of purchase in full-service restaurants, fast-food restaurants, or simulated settings. Two reviewers independently and sequentially assessed titles, abstracts, and then papers according to the inclusion and exclusion protocol. Reviewers compared results and discussed disagreements, and a third party was consulted when disagreements were presented. Data from the studies were systematically collected through use of abstraction forms.

All studies were rated as to the quality of their study designs. Primary analysis included randomized controlled trials (RCTs), quasi-RCTs, controlled before and after studies, and interrupted time series. An additional analysis included cross-sectional studies and uncontrolled before and after studies. Risk of bias was determined, and studies with a high risk of bias were excluded. Fourteen studies ultimately were included in the meta-analysis from the original 42,282 papers gathered. Meta-analysis was performed on means and standard deviations from each study. The change in calories as a result of menu labeling was calculated, as was the standard deviation of the differences. Study-level–weighted mean differences were calculated to determine overall meta-analysis–weighted mean differences using a random effects model. Heterogeneity was also quantified. Menu labeling lowered the number of calories ordered by consumers by a minimal amount when studies were conducted in a laboratory setting. However, no significant difference in calories consumed were observed in away-from-home settings. High heterogeneity was present in the study designs and continued to exist even after adjustment. Further, there was no impact of menu labeling on the amount of carbohydrate, fat, saturated fat, or sodium in foods ordered.

Strengths/Limitations

Meta-analysis to combine various study designs and evaluations, including diverse populations, locations, and times, can be a strength if a sufficient number of high-quality studies are available. Data may be combined to find a single answer to the question of how effective an intervention may be. However, the answer may be more nuanced than a summary result based on the limited number of studies allowed. For example, interventions such as menu labeling may be more effective in certain populations and under certain conditions. Such detailed information is lost using a single integrated meta-analysis and may be best understood by reading the individual studies. Similarly, different study designs may more effectively eliminate different types of bias, but when data from these studies are combined, the bias inherent to the results may be less well understood. Certain uncharacterized or unquantified aspects of the menu-labeling intervention, including where the information is located or the format, may be very important to consumers and thus may not be properly accounted for in the meta-analysis. The finding that menu labeling resulted in fewer calories ordered or purchased only in studies in lab settings lacks the external validity that real-world applications of menu-labeling present, yet real-world studies are difficult to control. Finally, other factors that are specific to the participant's characteristics or to the outcomes may have affected the results. Including nutrients in the outcomes was a strength.

Recommendations for Future Research

Future research on menu labeling may need to include additional investigations into the nutrients or dietary components ordered and consumed. Only a few studies with these outcomes were available in this analysis, but future research may allow more robust findings for these outcomes. Consumers' knowledge and improved estimates of the calories and nutrients contained in away-from-home foods may also improve as a result of menu labeling. Future research may investigate the effects of hunger and the interaction of hunger with menu-labeling. Research could expand on options for how and where menus are labeled and the information included (such as calorie counts or more detailed nutrition information). Finally, a more comprehensive evaluation of dietary intake, not only for the meal where menu labeling was available but in the context of other dietary intake, may reveal additional information about the effectiveness of menu-labeling interventions.

Summary

Meta-analyses are useful to evaluate public health policies and interventions over time, space, and various populations to better quantify their impact. However, meta-analyses are only as strong as the studies they evaluate. Meta-analyses conducted prematurely may lead to erroneous conclusions about the impact of nutrition health policy on diet quality and disease risk.

Modeling the Potential of Taxes on Sugar-Sweetened Beverages to Reduce Consumption and Generate Revenue

Diet is a key health behavior that has a strong health promotion opportunity, as Americans eat a diet that diverges from national recommendations (US Dietary Guidelines, 2015). Recent attention has been given to reducing the consumption of **sugar-sweetened beverages (SSBs)**. Sweetened beverages are associated with an increased risk of negative health outcomes. As a result, several governing agencies have either considered or attempted taxing the sale of these beverages in the hopes of decreasing consumption. To assist public health professionals and policy makers in developing and implementing policies, systems, and environmental changes that improve health, researchers model changes in health behaviors on environmental influences. Andreyeva, Chaloupka, and Brownell (2011) modeled the expected impact of a tax on sweetened beverages and evaluated the changes that may result with regard to revenue and health. The model they present is a useful method for estimating the change in the consumption of *SSB*, based on **price elasticity** (Andreyeva, et al., 2011). Using price to influence health behavior is not new to public health. Similar taxes were enacted on tobacco products. In order to develop a *SSB* and **price elasticity** model, researchers first reviewed existing *SSB* taxes. The authors summarized this literature, citing that increased prices usually decrease consumption (Powell & Chaloupka, 2009; Sturm, Powell, Chriqui, & Chaloupka, 2010). The authors make a case for an excise tax, typically assessed per ounce, based on preliminary evidence of elasticity of demand from their own research and that of others. Finally, the authors predicted the impact of the model on the consumption of *SSBs*.

The development of any model requires numerous assumptions. For this model, the authors developed estimates of consumption, tax rate, and penetration (including SNAP participants); assumed no regional price variation; utilized a sample population defined by the US Census population projections from 2007 to 2015 (United States Census Bureau, 2009); and set the consumption of carbonated soft drinks (CSDs) as a 0.5% increase from the 2008 value (Beverage Marketing Corporation, 2009a). The consumption of CSD was set at a 0.5% increase from the 2008 value after considering patterns for consumption of beverages. Change in consumption, the target health behavior, was also estimated. Using 2008 industry records, the authors estimated consumption of *SSB* for specific regions by the gallon, including CSDs, fruit drinks (excluding 100% fruit juice usually labeled as fruit consumption), and prepared teas (Beverage Marketing Corporation, 2009b, 2009c). The consumption of sports drinks, energy drinks, flavored or enhanced waters, and prepared coffees were estimated using total US sales from 2008. A fixed time point was chosen "because of the perceived stability of the trends," noting that "the initial dramatic growth for a new product is unlikely to continue more than several years" (Andreyeva, et al., 2011, p. 414). Some of the predictions used for the model were derived from known price effects of taxation on alcohol consumption. Data on alcohol taxation indicate that taxes result in decreased consumption and decreased tax revenue (Young & Bielinska-Kwapisz, 2002). While taxing *SSBs* has some analogy to taxing alcohol, the researchers chose to assume that consumption of *SSBs* would remain unchanged after taxation based on elasticity information. The resulting model indicated that an excise tax on *SSB* consumption will be especially significant for children, low-income populations, and other populations at increased risk for developing obesity.

Strengths/Limitations

Results inherent to the final model had significant limitations. First, estimations of price elasticity of demand are limited; that is, the influence of price on demand under all conditions is not known. Second, the authors assumed that the cost of diet beverages would remain constant, but acknowledged that producers and sellers could modify the price of diet beverages in reaction to a tax on sugary beverages. The numerous market ripples that could result were not accounted for in the model and analysis. However, the authors did account for inflation, but not for a shift in beverage preference based on cost. Their simple model focuses on one diet component and only accounted for price and the determinant of consumption. More complex models that consider additional elasticity parameters such as transportation barriers, distance to activity, work and family responsibilities, etc., could be developed to better predict or evaluate *SSB* consumption or other health behaviors.

Recommendations for Future Research

Future research to develop a more complex and accurate model should account for multiple factors that influence diet quality and *SSB* consumption. These include the resulting changes in elasticity of other beverages and foods as a result of a beverage tax. Further, interventions that specifically focus on how a beverage tax would affect children and low-income populations are most relevant to the potential health benefits of a *SSB* tax because of their higher rates of consumption and the risks of obesity.

Summary

Predictive models may provide useful estimates for changes in consumption of a dietary component to inform future policy changes despite the limitations of being only as accurate and comprehensive as the data used in their development.

Exploring Power and Influence in Nutrition Policy in Australia

The final study included in this chapter looked at the broader perspective of societal influencers on food policy. Cullerton, Donnet, Lee, and Gallegos (2016) evaluated the social networks behind Australia's nutrition policy decisions in order to investigate the influence that members of the food industry, nutrition professionals, scientists, and other practitioners have on nutrition policy making. The results may inform those invested in health policy research and implementation to better understand the organizational and individual relationships that can influence outcomes in the legislative arena. Researching relationships can be difficult due to the intangible nature of influence, but the social network study design offers an opportunity to trace these relationships (Swinburn, Kraak, Rutter, Vandevijvere, Lobstein, Sacks, et al., 2015). *Social network analysis (SNA)* offers a way to systematically evaluate the links between individuals and to quantify the closeness of the relationships. Cullerton, et al. (2016) analyzed the closeness of several influencers on nutrition policy in Australia. They chose Australia to build on previous studies that attempted to analyze relationships among policy makers for public health and, in part, because of the lack of movement in nutrition policy since Eat Well Australia concluded in 2010. Since 2010, the only changes in policy were voluntary policies, such as including front-of-package labeling, and a Healthy Food Partnership, in which the food industry collaborated with the health sector to change the formulations of processed foods (Australian Department of Health, 2016). But few additional policy efforts were instituted. Prior *SNA* studies were limited to a few professions that were thought to influence nutrition policy. The study described here expanded the social network to include politicians, academic interest groups, food and agricultural industry, journalists and other media, bureaucrats, and professional organizations. Study participants were chosen based on their perceived ability to influence policy ideas, make policy proposals, influence other policy proposals, and influence the implementation of policies. Cullerton, et al. (2016) adapted this method from Scott (1991). Nine participants were selected after researchers determined their considerable ability to influence nutrition policy, based on the advocacy coalition theory (Kingdon, 1995; Sabatier & Weible, 2007; True, Jones, & Baumgartner, 2007). Influencers were selected from four rounds of data collection through phone interviews and follow-up phone calls querying interpersonal connections. The researchers used NodeXL (Smith, Milic-Frayling, Schneiderman, Medes Rodrigues, Leskovec, Dunne, et al., 2010) and algorithms (Chaturvedi, Dunne, Ashktorab, Zachariah, & Schneiderman, 2014) to produce a cluster network map. Individuals were characterized by their distance from a decision maker on the map. The results support the view that the food industry exerts the most influence on nutrition policy. The authors suggest that nutrition professionals might be limiting their influence by primarily being in contact with peers and not reaching out to those in other sectors that influence policy. Nutrition professionals and other experts on the periphery of policy making could increase their influence by investing in relationships with professionals in other sectors.

Strengths/Limitations

The authors suggest that this case study could be generalized to other policy making relationships, assuming that characteristics of networks apply outside of this specific food environment. However, diverse factors unique to each policy environment such as resource availability and lobbying effort could affect the relevance of the model to policy outcomes. Thus, the nature of environments will affect generalizability. For example, well-capitalized industries such as energy might be very different from less well-capitalized industries. Further, academic/industry networks likely vary by segment (e.g., engineering versus public health). This *SNA* method assumed that one influential person would know another or know their name and function (Scott, 1991). The researchers identified the most powerful nutrition policy influencer in Australia who could be contacted for the sectors of influence. Subjective determinations are always subject to bias. Another limitation was the method of participant responses. Subjective interpersonal ties were investigated, and responses could have been modulated due to expectancy effect. Further, the response rate was only 49%. Those who responded may have different social networks than those who did not, missing critical information regarding network involvement in policy determination. Finally, a limitation of this design relates to the comprehensiveness of the social ecological model. A focused individual *SNA* risks missing consideration of other aspects of social structure, especially as they relate to organizations and the environment.

Recommendations for Future Research

There are opportunities to build on the information learned from this *SNA*. This study used a particular type of analysis: interpreting the distance between individuals to visualize how closely they were in influence to each other and to policy outcomes. This model is a unique analysis of social networks because it evaluates an intangible structure. Additional research could investigate approaches that nutrition professionals and other health professionals can use to network with those who have the greatest influence on national nutrition policy.

Summary

Social network analysis may uncover important relationships that influence health and nutrition policy making. They are limited by the representativeness of the individuals or sectors included, and therefore, they may miss important relationships.

Conclusion

Nutrition policy aims to improve health across populations by utilizing rigorous study designs that critically and accurately evaluate outcomes. The studies featured in this chapter were selected based on their effective use of an array of methods currently used in nutrition health policy, which aim to understand the links between nutritional outcomes for overall health in specific populations. Outcomes such as fruit and vegetable selection, food security, intake and purchasing of nutrients and calories, reductions in consumption of *SSBs*, and individual influences on policy making were evaluated. Specific populations were also chosen based on the goals of the nutrition policy. Children are often the focus of policy, as with the National School Lunch Policy. Lifelong eating patterns can be formed during childhood, making it especially important to introduce children to healthy diets. Another population of interest is those with historically high rates of disease. An example of this was seen with the modeling of the effect of *SSB* taxes on consumption rates in low socioeconomic groups, who often have higher rates of *SSB* consumption, as well as a higher prevalence of diseases that can be influenced by nutrition.

Evaluating policy can be difficult due to the diverse and numerous factors involved in consumer decision-making, as well as the hard-to-define actions and attitudes that influence policy makers. In addition to the challenge presented by the breadth of factors to evaluate, the ethics of a rigorous evaluation with the population at risk are important considerations. For example, the SNAP program cannot be tested against a control group due to ethical concerns that could negatively influence the control group. Additionally, interventions effective for diet quality are not necessarily effective for more distal outcomes such as the prevention of weight gain. Education is typically assumed to be important and effective at increasing public awareness and changing health behavior. Education not only requires evaluation but also an understanding and evaluation of the context in which the education is provided. Policies, systems, and environmental issues likely interact significantly with educational efforts aimed at a healthier diet.

Despite the significant challenges to conducting research on health policy, the studies presented in this chapter demonstrate five methods that can be used to accomplish effective evaluations. Studies that evaluate interventions and outcomes vary by design and scope, as demonstrated by the selections in this chapter. Choice of the most appropriate study design possible, given the natural limitations of public health research, is critical to maximizing the relevance and quality of the information obtained. Furthermore, the success or limitations gleaned from evaluations of current interventions should be utilized to inform decisions about future policies. A critical comparison of methodologies and selection of the method that balances resources with practical implementation to yield the most valid and reliable results is ideal. Unfortunately, often the strongest study designs require the greatest investment of time and resources, and funds for such research are almost always restrained. However, the value of the investment is expected to outweigh the cost. Well-informed policy making is most likely to result in improved programs and improved health of individuals and communities.

References

Amin, S., Yon, B., Taylor, J., & Johnson, R. (2015). Impact of the national school lunch program on fruit and vegetable selection in northeastern elementary schoolchildren, 2012–2013. *Public Health Reports*, *130*(5), 453–457. https://doi.org/10.1177%2F003335491513000508

Andreyeva, T., Chaloupka, F., & Brownell, K. (2011). Estimating the potential of taxes on sugar-sweetened beverages to reduce consumption and generate revenue. *Preventive Medicine*, *52*(6), 413–416. doi:10.1016/j.ypmed.2011.03.013

Beverage Marketing Corporation. (2009a). *Carbonated soft drinks in the U.S. 2009 edition, chapter 3, September 2009*. New York, NY: Beverage Marketing Corporation of New York.

Beverage Marketing Corporation. (2009b). *Fruit beverages in the U.S. 2008 edition, chapter 2, July 2009*. New York, NY: Beverage Marketing Corporation of New York.

Beverage Marketing Corporation. (2009c). *Carbonated soft drinks in the U.S. 2009 edition, chapter 3, September 2009*. New York, NY: Beverage Marketing Corporation of New York.

Beydoun, M. A., & Wang, Y. (2008). Do nutrition knowledge and beliefs modify the association of socio-economic factors and diet quality among US adults? *Preventative Medicine*, *46*(2), 145–153. https://doi.org/10.1016/j.ypmed.2007.06.016

Bickel, G., Nord, M., Price, C., Hamilton, W., & Cook, J. (2000). *Guide to measuring household food security*. Alexandria. VA.: Department of Agriculture, Food and Nutrition Service. Retrieved May 30, 2020, from www.fns.usda.gov/oane

Cantu-Jungles, T. M., McCormack, L. A., Slaven, J. E., Slebodnik, M., & Eicher-Miller, H. A. (2017). A meta-analysis to determine the impact of restaurant menu labeling on calories and nutrients (ordered or consumed) in U.S. adults. *Nutrients*, *9*(10), 1088. pii: E1088. doi:10.3390/nu9101088

Carbone, E. T., & Zoellner, J. M. (2012). Nutrition and health literacy: A systematic review to inform nutrition research and practice. *Journal of the Academy of Nutrition and Dietetics*, *112*(2), 254–265. https://doi.org/10.1016/j.jada.2011.08.042

Chaturvedi, S., Dunne, C., Ashktorab, Z., Zachariah, R., & Schneiderman, B. (2014). Group-in-a-box meta-layouts for topological clusters and attribute-based groups: Space efficient visualizations of network communities and their ties. *Computer Graphics Forum*, *33*(8), 52–68. https://doi.org/10.1111/cgf.12400

Crockett, R. A., Hollands, G. J., Jebb, S. A., & Marteau, T. M. (2011). Nutritional labelling for promoting healthier food purchasing and consumption. *Cochrane Database of Systematic Reviews*, (9), Article CD009315. https://doi.org/10.1002/14651858.CD009315

Cullerton, K., Donnet, T., Lee, A., & Gallegos, D. (2016). Exploring power and influence in nutrition policy in nutrition policy in Australia. *Obesity Reviews*, *17*(12), 1218–1225. https://doi.org/10.1111/obr.12459

Department of Health. (2016). *Healthy food partnership*. Canberra, Australia: Australian Government.

Devine, C. M., Farrell, T. J., & Hartman, R. (2005). Sisters in health: Experiential program emphasizing social interaction increases fruit and vegetable intake among low-income adults. *Journal of Nutrition Education Behavior*, *37*(5), 265–270. https://doi.org/10.1016/S1499-4046(06)60282-0

Eyles, H. C., & Mhurchu, C. N. (2009). Does tailoring make a difference? A systematic review of the long-term effectiveness of tailored nutrition education for adults. *Nutrition Reviews*, *67*(8), 464–480. https://doi.org/10.1111/j.1753-4887.2009.00219.x

Kessler, D. A. (1995). The evolution of national nutrition policy. *Annual Review of Nutrition*, *15*(1), 13–26. https://doi.org/10.1146/annurev.nu.15.070195.005033

Kingdon, J. (1995). *Agendas, alternatives, and public policies*. New York: HarperCollins College Publishers.

Moher, D., Liberati, A., Tetzlaff, J., & Altman, D. G. (2009). Group, P. preferred reporting items for systematic reviews and meta-analyses: The PRISMA statement. *Annals of Internal Medicine, 151*(4), 264–269. https://doi.org/10.7326/0003-4819-151-4-200908180-00135

Office of the Legislative Counsel for the U.S. House of Representatives. (2010). *Patient protection and affordable care act health-related portions of the health care and education reconciliation act of 2010*. Retrieved May 30, 2010, from http://housedocs.house.gov/energycommerce/ppacacon.pdf

Powell, L. M., & Chaloupka, F. J. (2009). Food prices and obesity: Evidence and policy implications for taxes and subsidies. *The Milbank Quarterly, 87*(1), 229–257. https://doi.org/10.1111/j.1468-0009.2009.00554.x

Rivera, R. L., Maulding, M. K., Abbott, A. R., Craig, B. A., & Eicher-Miller, H. A. (2016). SNAP-Ed (Supplemental Nutrition Assistance Program-Education) increases long-term food security among Indiana households with children in a randomized controlled study. *The Journal of Nutrition, 146*(11), 2375–2382. https://doi.org/10.3945/jn.116.231373

Ryan, R., Hill, S., Broclain, D., Horey, D., Oliver, S., & Prictor, M. (2013). *Cochrane consumers and communication review group*. Study Design Guide. Victoria, Australia.

Sabatier, P., & Weible, C. (2007). The advocacy coalition framework: Innovations and clarifications. In P. A. Sabatier (Ed.), *Theories of the policy process*. Cambridge, MA: Westview Press.

Scott, J. (1991). *Social network analysis: A handbook*. London, UK: Sage Publications.

Smith, M., Milic-Frayling, N., Schneiderman, B., Medes Rodrigues, E., Leskovec, J., & Dunne, C. (2010). *Node XL: A free and open network overview, discovery and exploration add-in for Excel 2007/2010*. Retrieved August 10, 2020, from http://nodexl.codeplex.com/, from the Social Media Research Foundation, http://www.smrfoundation.org

Sturm, R., Powell, L. M., Chriqui, J. F., & Chaloupka, F. J. (2010). Soda taxes, soft drink consumption, and children's body mass index. *Health Affairs, 29*(5), 1052–1058. https://doi.org/10.1377/hlthaff.2009.0061

Swinburn, B., Kraak, V., Rutter, H., Vandevijvere, S., Lobstein, T., Sacks, G., Gomes, F., et al. (2015). Strengthening of accountability systems to create healthy food environments and reduce global obesity. *The Lancet, 385*(9986), 2534–2545. https://doi.org/10.1016/S0140-6736(14)61747-5

True, J., Jones, B., & Baumgartner, F. (2007). Punctuated-equilibrium theory. In P. Sabatier (Ed.), *Theories of the policy process*. New York, NY: Westview Press.

U.S. Census Bureau. (2009). *State interim population projections by age and sex, 2004–2030*. Washington, DC: U.S. Government Printing Office.

U.S. Department of Agriculture, U.S. Department of Health and Human Services. (2015). *Dietary guidelines for Americans 2015*, 8th edition. Retrieved August 10, 2020, from http://health.gov/dietaryguidelines/2015/guidelines/

U.S. Food & Drug Administration. (2004). *Calories count: Report of the working group on obesity*, U.S. Food & Drug Administration, Silver Spring, MD, USA.

Young, D. J., & Bielinska-Kwapisz, A. (2002). Alcohol taxes and beverage prices. *National Tax Journal, 55*(1), 57–73.

27

THE NEXUS BETWEEN BEHAVIORAL AND HEALTH ECONOMICS IN THE UNIVERSAL HEALTH COVERAGE RESEARCH AGENDA

Chris Atim, Ama Pokuaa Fenny, Daniel Malik Achala,
and John Ele-Ojo Ataguba

Overview

Universal health coverage (UHC) is a priority for many countries, and it is part of the global *sustainable development goals (SDGs)* to be achieved by 2030 (UNDP, 2015). *UHC* is about ensuring that everyone has access to needed services of sufficient quality to be effective, without incurring any financial hardship (WHO, 2010). Although the *UHC* goal is essential, many countries remain challenged on how to achieve the goal by 2030. The 2019 *UHC* Global Monitoring Report estimates that up to five billion people will miss out on health care in 2030, given the current rates of progress (WHO, 2019). More than 40% of *total health expenditure (THE)* in *lower-middle-income countries (LMICs)* comes from out-of-pocket health expenditure. Countries in sub-Saharan Africa (SSA) that bear a substantial burden of disease also record a significant proportion of the population lacking access to essential health services and the absence of financial protection. The substantial burden of disease and lack of access to health services makes it imperative for countries in SSA to achieve *UHC*. To achieve *UHC* requires a commitment to three key principles: mobilize adequate resources to ensure coverage, provide quality care by strengthening the health service delivery system, and ensure that health services are accessible to all, especially those who need the services, including poor and vulnerable individuals (WHO, 2019).

Providing access to quality health care is one of the primary objectives of health systems (WHO, 2000). Since 1978, when the World Health Organization (WHO) called for the achievement of 'Health for All' as part of the Alma Ata Declaration, the global lens for addressing key health issues has evolved (WHO, 1978). The 2013 World Health Report pushed for a research agenda for *UHC*, highlighting the fact that rigorous investigations involving different methodologies and across varied subject areas had the potential to benefit the health of populations across the world (WHO, 2013). Evidence on country progress and challenges in access to quality health care is needed to advance the *UHC* goal. The WHO's call for research for *UHC* highlights the significance of all types of research methods and fields, including health economics research.

Various areas in health economics research are useful in achieving the *UHC* goal, and they benefit from insights from behavioral economics. Incorporating insights from behavioral economics into public health policy has the potential to improve population health (Matjasko, Cawley,

Baker-Goering, & Yokum, 2016), including observations from areas such as mental health economics, economic evaluation, health financing (including revenue raising, pooling, and strategic purchasing), social determinants of health, health inequality assessment, health equity, and health labor force.
Several researchers have tested elements of these behavioral changes within the sphere of health-
seeking behavior and health system incentives that affect individual behavior (Dagger & Sweeney,
2006). For example, understanding decision-making processes by individual health care services users
requires paying attention to their behaviors in the face of health information. Also, investigating the
predictability of "irrational" behavior by consumers would demand inclusion of psychological risk
factors. Thus, we see how patterns in behavioral economics link with health economics.

The World Health Report (2013) notes the importance of rigorous scientific investigations that
provide evidence to improve the availability of quality and affordable health services. A variety of
research methods considered in this chapter range from quantitative to qualitative evaluations, including observational and case-control studies, intervention studies, and randomized controlled trials.
These multiple research methods allow investigators to discover the links between behavioral and
health economics, providing evidence that answers the diversity of questions about *UHC*. The case
studies in this chapter will adopt the results chain for *UHC* (Figure 27.1). This moves along the
trajectory of the dependent and independent variables, where each health outcome depends on the
kind of inputs, processes, and outputs considered, and how these ultimately lead to health impacts.
It is envisaged in this model that all the dependent variables will have quantity, quality, and equity
considerations. Across all these is the role of the economic and social conditions that generate health
inequalities, which influence how equitable quality services are accessed, which groups of people
have access to health information, etc.

In the subsequent sections, we present five case studies examining research that seeks to understand how different actors in the health sector behave to achieve their health goals. These studies
highlight the interaction between health policy and implementation, a reflection of how the broader
determinants of health shape policy, and the interdisciplinary mix of health economics, welfare economics, behavioral economics, sociology, anthropology, psychology, and epidemiology. The primary

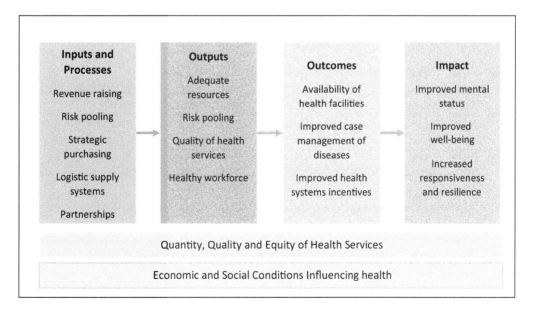

Figure 27.1   Universal health coverage results chain

Source: Adapted from WHO (2013) Research for Universal Health Coverage, Geneva, Switzerland: WHO, p. 9.

objective of this chapter is to identify the research methods adopted in the case studies by focusing on the linkages between behavioral and health economics. The cases used are all empirical studies conducted in *LMICs*.

In selecting and describing the case studies, we first identify the nature of the health problem, which could be on a specific disease such as malaria, asthma, or tuberculosis; or an input or process variable, such as the health workforce; or the availability of a health insurance scheme. Subsequently, details of the research design, methodology (including data collection instruments), and outcomes are presented. The chapter also identifies and discusses the strengths and weaknesses of the case studies. The cases portray a wide variety of research methods and conditions on topics ranging from access to quality services, provider incentives and practices, patient satisfaction, and the assessment of health interventions.

Research in Practice

Evaluating Access to Quality Health Services Using Quantitative Methods

Defining quality of care is inherently very difficult due to the complex nature of health care, the many dimensions of quality, and the different perspectives of what constitutes a good quality of care. Different stakeholders have different perspectives, interests, and definitions (Donabedian, 1980; Peterson, Nsungwa-Sabiiti, Were, Nsabagasmi, Magumba, Nambooze, et al., 2004; McLaughlin & Kaluzny, 2006; Ng, Fullman, Dieleman, Flaxman, Murray, & Lim, 2014). Therefore, a multidimensional definition, capturing all differing perceptions of quality of care, is needed. The Institute of Medicine (IOM) defines quality of care as "the degree to which health services for populations increase the likelihood of desired health outcomes and are consistent with current professional knowledge" (IOM, 1990, p. 128). Some of the attributes of quality of care include technical quality, quality of interpersonal relationships, acceptability of care, responsiveness to patient preferences, equity, efficiency, and cost-effectiveness. Others also define quality as the extent to which health care services meet patient's expectations, which allows quality-of-care attributes such as courtesy, kindness, and helpfulness to be included (Mosadeghrad, 2013). Box 27.1 summarizes the IOM's six domains of quality of care.

Box 27.1   Six Principal Domains of Quality Health Care

- *Safety*: Ensuring that no harm is done to patients in providing them with health care.
- *Effectiveness*: Using scientific knowledge to provide health services to people who are able to benefit from them, while avoiding the provision of such services to those people that are unlikely to benefit.
- *Patient-centeredness*: Care provided that respects and responds to the preferences, needs, and values of individual patients, and clinical decisions are guided by patient values.
- *Timeliness*: Those receiving care and those giving care both should have reduced waiting time and reduced harmful delays.
- *Efficiency*: Utilizing care resources in such a way that ensures the most optimal combination and the least waste of such resources (including equipment, supplies, ideas, and energy).
- *Equity*: Ensuring that the quality of care provided is independent of social, economic, demographic, geographic, and similar avoidable differences between patients.

Source: Adapted from: Institute of Medicine (2001). *Crossing the Quality Chasm: A New Health System for the 21st Century*, Washington, D.C., National Academy Press. p. 5–6

The WHO, among others, developed a quality-of-care framework based on three intrinsic goals—achieving optimal health, attaining better health levels through responsiveness to demand for health, and fairness in financing (Evans, Edejer, Lauer, Frenk, & Murray, 2001). Other authors (Campbell, Roland, & Buetow, 2000; Donabedian, 1980; Maxwell, 1984) provide disaggregated approaches that capture the complex and multidimensional nature of quality of care. For instance, Donabedian's framework incorporates some of the essential elements of quality of care under the **"Structure-Process-Outcome"** paradigm, which attempts to explain the gap between access and health outcomes (Donabedian, 1980, 1988). This is also very similar to the results chain for *UHC* diagram (see Figure 27.1).

Donabedian's model is, however, not without criticisms, as some argue that sequential and linear progression from structure to process and outcome is not realistic in the health service domain. The model omits critical factors that influence the quality of care such as patient characteristics and environmental factors (Carayon, Schoofs Hundt, Karsh, Gurses, Alvarado, Smith, et al., 2006; Coyle & Battles, 1999). Also, there may be some difficulty in determining whether some factors are strictly part of structure, process, or outcomes, as there could be some overlap between them. However, Donabedian explains that the model allows authors to draw linkages within the three broad levels that work together to achieve health outcomes (Donabedian, 2003). In this regard, the model provides a theoretical framework for research.

The case study *Quality of Uncomplicated Malaria Case Management in Ghana Among Insured and Uninsured Patients* (Fenny, Hansen, Enemark, & Asante, 2014) is based on the Donabedian model. Fenny, and colleagues' (2014) study was motivated by anecdotal information that insured patients received more inferior treatment at health facilities compared to noninsured clients. The study uses quantitative research methods to assess the effect of health insurance enrollment on the quality of case management for patients with uncomplicated malaria to show if significant differences exist in treatment between insured and noninsured patients. With the introduction of the National Health Insurance Scheme (NHIS) in Ghana, it was unclear how the supply-side attributes (health workforce, infrastructure, etc.) had been strengthened to cope with developments, such as an increase in the utilization of health services. First, the preparedness of facilities to manage the treatment of uncomplicated malaria was assessed, followed by an assessment of the adherence to malaria treatment guidelines, noting any possible differences between the insured and uninsured groups.

Research Design

A structured questionnaire was used to collect data from 523 respondents diagnosed with malaria and prescribed malaria drugs from public and private health facilities in three districts. Collected information included data from initial examinations performed on patients (temperature, weight, age, blood pressure, and pulse); observations of malaria symptoms by trained staff; laboratory tests conducted; and type of drugs prescribed. Insurance status of patients, age, gender, education level, and occupation were also collected. A second structured questionnaire was administered to the heads of selected public and private health facilities. Quality attributes included service availability, human resource availability, and adherence to treatment standards and protocols (method of diagnosis of malaria, laboratory capacity, and provision of artemisinin-based combination therapies [ACTs] and other antimalarial drugs). This was based on the premise that appropriate treatment consists of proper diagnosis and treatment using the approved national malaria treatment guidelines. Other variables included assets (electricity, water, equipment) of the facilities and the general cleanliness of the environment.

The quality of clinical assessments was obtained as the proportion of patients with a given sign or symptom validated by a health worker. Chi-square tests were used to statistically assess the relationship between variables, with the results presented in graphs and tables. Tabulations were used to examine variables for the stated quality elicited from the various providers. The data were analyzed using the Stata statistical package.

Outcomes

Routine recording of the patients' age, weight, and temperature were high in all the facilities. The least recorded vital statistic was the pulse rate. In general, assessments needed to identify suspected malaria cases were low in all the facilities, with high body temperature or fever and headache ranking the highest and convulsion ranking the lowest. Parasitological assessments in all the facilities were very low, except for the Community-Based Health Planning and Services (CHPS) zones, where all the clients were tested using rapid diagnostic tests (RDTs). ACTs were prescribed to interviewed patients, which is the drug of choice for malaria treatment in Ghana. However, there were no significant differences in the quality of malaria treatment between uninsured and insured patients. The results showed that about 16% of the total sample were parasitologically tested.

The evaluation showed that effective management of uncomplicated malaria was low in Ghana, with more than 80% improperly diagnosed and treated cases. This stemmed from the lack of functioning laboratories or the unavailability of rapid test kits to provide adequate testing. This information provides evidence for policy measures needed to strengthen the treatment component of the malaria control strategy and prevent the presumptive treatment of malaria. The study uses both observational and quantitative techniques to provide results that although supporting the original hypothesis, unearthed other systemic shortfalls that required attention.

Despite this, caution is taken in generalizing the results to the whole country. Especially in a non-representative, cross-sectional study, there is the awareness of possible biases of some of the explanatory variables. For instance, individuals self-select into health insurance on a range of factors, which may be unobserved. Also, patient exit surveys suffer from some limitations. It has been hypothesized that ***courtesy bias*** and the ***Hawthorne effect*** will be stronger in the estimates from the exit surveys. The problem of *courtesy bias* arises whereby patients may be reluctant to express negative opinions of services, especially while they are still at the service site (Lindelöw & Wagstaff, 2003). Higher levels of satisfaction expressed in exit interviews may be due to the *Hawthorne effect* where health facility staff perform better because they are observed or their patients are interviewed (McCarney, Warner, Iliffe, van Haselen, Griffin, & Fisher, 2007). In this study, although considerable care was taken to prevent *courtesy bias* by interviewing patients away from the facilities, there is no guarantee that the results are free from these biases.

It is perhaps worth noting that, despite results such as these, perceptions that insured people receive a lower quality of care compared to the uninsured have a long history and are quite pervasive (Atim & Sock, 2000; Abuosi, Domfeh, Abor, & Nketiah-Amponsha, 2016; Duku, Nketiah-Amponsah, Janssens, & Pradhan, 2018; Haw, 2019.) It was concluded that "generally, insured and uninsured patients are not treated unequally, contrary to prevailing anecdotal and empirical evidence" (Abuosi, et al., 2016, p. 1). "Being insured was associated with a significantly lower perception of healthcare quality" (Duku, et al., 2018, p. 1). A similar finding was made after an evaluation of the first-ever community health insurance scheme in Ghana, the Nkoranza Community Health Insurance Scheme, in 1999/2000 (Atim & Sock, 2000).

Using Quasi-Experimental Methods to Evaluate Health Interventions

In health economics research that involves public health policy evaluation, experimental design has been claimed to test the effects of changes in different social insurance programs, taxation on alcohol and drinking behavior, or the impact of cash transfers on access to health care. The focus has been on developing research designs that reflect real-world settings (Handley, Lyles, McCulloch, & Cattamanchi, 2018). The gold standard for designing this kind of research is the use of ***randomized controlled trials (RCTs)***, where individuals are assigned to either an intervention or control group. *RCTs* are used to infer causality. In theory, *RCTs* minimize selection bias and ensure an equally distributed probability between measured and unmeasured confounding variables, so that any difference in the outcomes can be solely attributed to the intervention under study. However, in real-world settings, random allocation of the intervention may not be feasible due to ethical, social, or logistical constraints (Dinardo, 2008). In such cases, a researcher may use a ***quasi-experimental design***, where even though a random assignment is not performed, the internal validity is enhanced by comparing cases that are as similar as possible. The researcher divides the sample into the *quasi-experimental* group, which receives some form of the 'intervention,' and the *comparison group*, which has not received the intervention. It is hard to demonstrate causality with quasi-experimental studies, especially where there are confounding variables that cannot be accounted for or controlled (Rossi, Lipsey, & Freeman, 2004).

The case study *The Impact of a Cash Transfer Programme on Tuberculosis Treatment Success Rate: A Quasi-Experimental Study in Brazil* (Carter, Daniel, Torrens, Sanchez, Maciel, Bartholomay, et al., 2019) uses a *quasi-experimental design* to evaluate the impact of Bolsa Familia on ***tuberculosis (TB)*** treatment success. Evidence suggests that social protection policies such as Brazil's ***Bolsa Família Programme (BFP)***, a governmental conditional cash transfer, may play a role in *TB* elimination. The study hypothesizes that patients with *TB* who are enrolled in Bolsa Familia are more likely to complete their treatment successfully.

Research Design

For an unbiased estimate of the proportion of patients cured attributable to *BFP*, the authors constructed a control group as similar as possible to the group of *BFP* recipients. This group of *BFP* recipients on average have some *TB* treatment success rate. The design was adopted to estimate the difference in *TB* success rates between the group that received *BFP* and the group of patients who had not received *BFP* but had the same sociodemographic characteristics. ***Propensity score matching*** was used to create a control group balanced for propensity to receive *BFP*. Approximately half of the patients with *TB* included in this study population were not enrolled in the cash transfer program (**BFP**) despite being eligible based on the income inclusion criterion (Carter, et al., 2019).

Propensity scores were estimated from a complete-case logistic regression using covariates from a linked data set, including Brazil's *TB* notification system (SINAN), linked to the national registry of those in poverty (CadUnico), and the *BFP* payroll. Taking the difference of the proportion of treatment success between matched groups resulted in an estimate of the average effect of treatment on the treated (ATT) or the (causal) risk difference in the exposed (Carter, et al., 2019).

Outcomes

Patients with *TB* receiving *BFP* showed a treatment success rate of 10.58 percentage points higher (95% confidence interval [CI] 4.39 to 16.77) than patients with *TB* not receiving *BFP*. This association was robust to sensitivity analyses. The study showed that conditional cash transfers like Bolsa Familia can contribute to *TB* elimination even if they were not designed for this purpose. Also, the disparity in access is a missed opportunity to maximize *TB* impact of Bolsa Familia. The authors agree that given this positive relationship between the provision of conditional cash transfers and *TB* treatment success rate, there is need for further research to understand how to enhance access to social protections to optimize public health impacts.

The utilization of the *quasi-experimental* approach is a major strength of this study. *Quasi-experimental* approaches like *propensity score matching* require fewer assumptions about the data than traditional parametric counterparts. The use of *propensity scores* for matching has drawn some criticism, such as increasing imbalance, inefficiency, model dependence, and bias (King & Nielsen, 2016). The choice of a dichotomous outcome variable may be another limitation: nonsuccess outcomes include continued disease after regimen completion, treatment abandonment, death from *TB*, death from other causes, and development of multidrug-resistant *TB*, which may have heterogeneous risk factors. The authors note that results may be different if each nonsuccess outcome were addressed in turn, but this would require a larger sample size and may be best addressed in a descriptive study.

Progressively, *quasi-experiments* are used in place of experimental or randomized control trials, despite being anathema to those who believe solely in experimental designs (Lambert & Bewley, 2016; Tong, Coiera, Tong, Wang, Quiroz, Martin, et al., 2019). The primary drawback of *quasi-experimental* designs is that they cannot eliminate the possibility of confounding bias, which can hinder drawing valid causal inferences. However, various statistical techniques such as an instrumental variable approach may improve the accuracy of the results from quasi-experiments. Overall, the *quasi-experimental* designs are essential tools for applied researchers in health or behavioral economics (Shadish, Cook, & Campbell, 2002) and offer a solution for assessing the impacts in the absence of a controlled experiment (Lambert & Bewley, 2016).

Applying Quantitative Methods to Evaluate the Impact of Health Financing Reforms on Health Systems

Since the 1980s, many countries have instituted several reforms to improve the health sector. In many developing countries, the broad strategy of health reforms was to reduce government spending on the health sector and curb the shortages of essential medicines and medical supplies (World Bank, 1993). Health financing arrangements in *LMICs* in Africa vary broadly by geographic region and social context. Currently, the principal features of the health financing systems are influenced by the need to underscore the goals of the *SDGs* backed by the national development efforts in each country. This undergirds one of the main components of the financing health functions, which is purchasing. Here, we refer to how funds for health services are used for obtaining health services, which involves the selection of services and interventions, the selection of service providers, and determining the contractual and payment arrangements between the purchaser and providers (Kutzin, 2013).

Purchasing can be passive or strategic. **Strategic purchasing** involves a continuous search for the best ways to maximize health system performance by deciding which interventions should be purchased, how, and from what providers, while **passive purchasing** implies following a predetermined budget or simply paying bills when presented. However, *strategic purchasing* takes center stage in many health systems. One of the tools to introduce strategic purchasing is **performance-based financing (PBF)**, mainly driven by the World Bank, spanning 51 countries, with 25 of these projects in Africa (Giuffrida, Pinglo, Aghumian, Boggero, Buizza, Ferrara, et al., 2018). *PBF* entails the provision of financial incentives to health service providers (either a single or network of health facilities and/or health staff) conditioned to a set of measurable performance targets related to the quantity and quality of health services (Giuffrida, Pinglo, Aghumian, Boggero, Buizza, Ferrara, et al., 2018). Some countries have introduced incentive payments linked to results to widen access to care and to improve the quality and performance of health care services and systems (Witter, Fretheim, Kessy, & Lindahl, 2012).

These incentive structures reflect some of the theories around behavioral and health economics. There are relationships between providers, the population, and the government that clearly show the nexus between behavioral and health economics. This is because the theoretical underpinning of the *PBF* theory of change lies in the principal-agent model, which portrays a more intricate assessment of human behavior. The basic reasoning is that health care providers exert more effort when payments are conditioned to the quantity and quality of the health services provided. If health care staff are insufficiently motivated, this will reflect on what these workers are capable of doing versus what they actually do in practice. At the same time, the change in the incentive structure for health staff and facility managers affects the way health facilities are governed, and hence health workers' behaviors.

The case study *Incentives to Change: Effects of Performance-based Financing on Health Workers in Zambia* (Shen, Nguyen, Das, Sachingongu, Chansa, Qamruddin, et al., 2017) examines the effect of *PBF* on health workers' job satisfaction, motivation, and attrition in Zambia. The Zambia *PBF* pays the providers for service provision and quality of selected high-priority maternal and child health (MCH) services in rural districts. In this study, the authors assessed the differential effects of monetary incentives tied to the activities or efforts of workers (i.e., *PBF* bonuses) versus alternative financing modes (i.e., enhanced financing, status quo) effects on two individual human resources for health (HRH) outcomes determining national workforce performance (motivation, job satisfaction) and an individual HRH outcome (attrition) determining national workforce distribution. The hypothesis was that *PBF* will have a positive effect on health workers' motivation, but the alternative financing mode will have a lower magnitude than *PBF*. The differential effect is because enhanced financing was targeted towards the health facility as a whole rather than individual health workers and was not linked directly to performance.

Research Design

The study also uses the Donabedian classification of the *structure-process-outcome* model to evaluate the impact of the intervention. It uses a randomized, intervention control design to evaluate before–after changes for three groups: the intervention (*PBF*) group, control 1 (C1; enhanced financing) group, and control 2 (C2; pure control) group. The evaluation follows a *quasi-experimental* design: 30 districts in the country were triplet-matched on key health systems and outcome indicators and randomly allocated to each study arm.

Mixed methods were employed. The quantitative portion, described in this section, comprised a baseline and an endline survey. The survey and sampling scheme was designed to allow for a rigorous impact evaluation of *PBF* or C1 on several key performance indicators. Worker motivation and job satisfaction were derived from the individual worker questionnaire, and attrition was based on the facility assessment. The questions for motivation and satisfaction were based on two existing validated tools: Minnesota Satisfaction Questionnaire (Weiss, Dawis, England, & Lofquist, 1967) and Job Satisfaction Survey (Spector, 1985). In addition, the variables on well-being were derived from the *WHO* Well-Being Index (WHO, 2020). Attrition was the number of authorized staff who left a health center in the previous 12 months based on a health facility survey. The effects of *PBF* on key outcome variables were estimated, with a ***difference-in-difference (DID)*** framework among the *PBF*, C1, and C2 arms for two rounds of data (baseline and endline). Briefly, *DID* is a statistical technique to estimate the effect of an intervention on an outcome. The difference in the average outcome in the treatment group, obtained between two time periods (D_T), is compared with the corresponding difference in the average outcome in the control group (D_C). The *DID* estimate is simply $D_T - D_C$. Facility fixed-effects analysis was performed with standard errors clustered at a district level. District grouping was taken into account in the analysis through stratification controls.

Outcomes

The one-way analysis of variance (ANOVA) showed that at baseline, there was no statistical difference among the three groups, indicating baseline balance in key characteristics that may mediate the impact of *PBF* on satisfaction, motivation, and attrition. The econometric analysis showed that *PBF* led to increased job satisfaction and decreased attrition on a subset of measures, with little effect on motivation. Enhanced health financing also increased the stated job satisfaction. The C1 group (control) also experienced some positive effects on job satisfaction. This revealed that workers remained motivated by their dedication to the profession and to provide health care to the community rather than by financial incentives. However, the study suggests that incentive schemes may not have the same effect on HRH outcomes in another national context, which may have different labor market conditions (Judson, Volpp, & Detsky, 2015).

The study highlights the fact that measuring health workers' performance only by quantitative methods may not reveal the true picture of job satisfaction, motivation, or attrition. The study triangulated information from the qualitative study with that from the quantitative method, suggesting that *PBF* interventions need to be studied in various contexts. A report from the World Bank on the impact assessments in the various countries indicates that the assessment-based quality checklists may be too simple and focus on conditions that are easily within reach of many facilities. This may not reveal the real impact of *PBF* on the quality of services. A more enhanced quality checklist is envisaged to make this possible (Giuffrida, et al., 2018). Other limitations specific to the study include recall bias, as a recall period was not specified in the survey for the questions related to motivation and job satisfaction. Authors also acknowledge the potential effects of stress on workers as the *PBF* increases demands on their job roles and pressure to meet *PBF* targets. This stress had an impact on worker productivity, turnover, and well-being far above the direct rewards of provider incentives. The study did not examine the effects of these factors and other related intrinsic factors, such as their ability to control the factors that affect meeting those targets, their perception of the transparency of the performance evaluation process, and fairness of reward process.

Evaluating Perceptions of Quality of Health Services Using Qualitative Research Methods

Much of the patient satisfaction research relies on patients' perception of satisfaction on what is observed (Mosadeghrad, 2013). In health care, patient satisfaction often relates to the positive emotions drawn from provider–patient interactions. Predictive factors such as caring, empathy, dependability, and responsiveness of providers all relate to patient satisfaction (Ladhari, 2009; Tucker & Adams, 2001). It must be pointed out that patients' evaluation of quality health services to an extent differs from the physician or technical evaluation because quality is inherently value-driven, and its definition is a social construct. One therefore will expect at least some variations in their evaluations, as their values and socialization differ (Sofaer & Firminger, 2005). Patients' perceptions are usually primarily influenced by psychological, social, economic, political, and cultural factors, while the physician's evaluation of quality care follows prescribed standards, legal rules, and procedures (Macur, 2011; Mahmoud, Ekwere, Fuxman, & Meero, 2019). For example, a patient may perceive the quality of care to be poor at a facility irrespective of treatment outcome if the patient encountered poor interpersonal relations with the health professionals at the facility. These are social issues that have influenced judgement on quality care. Again, despite a good treatment outcome, patients generally tend to equate low-cost drugs with poor quality of care. These are generally psychological and economic issues that users build into their perceptions of quality of care.

Some authors believe that there is a limit to the usefulness of patient satisfaction surveys, as patients cannot assess the more technical aspects of care (Eiriz & Figueiredo, 2005). The complexity in capturing all the factors associated with patient satisfaction compound this problem (Debono & Travaglia, 2009; Zastowny, Stratmann, Adams, & Fox, 1995). However, studying health care quality from the patient's perspective provides important feedback about the quality of care (Debono & Travaglia, 2009; Ware & Stewart, 1992). Some studies have used patient perspectives as a key measure for evaluating health care quality (Aditi, 2009; Sodani, Kumar, Srivastava, & Sharma, 2010; Atinga, Abekah-Nkrumah, & Domfeh, 2011; Boyer, Francois, Doutre, Weil, & Labarere, 2006), and some have indicated links between patient satisfaction and quality of life (Dagger & Sweeney, 2006).

The case study *Increasing Access to Quality Health Care for the Poor: Community Perceptions on Quality Care in Uganda* (Kiguli, Kirapa-Kiracho, Okui, Mutebi, MacGregor, & Pariyo, 2009) explored perceptions of communities on health care quality in Uganda using a classical qualitative study. In this study, the researchers explored the perceptions of communities on the quality of care and classify the criteria used by communities in their evaluation of quality. This study sheds light on health care–seeking behaviors of two communities in Uganda. The study also describes the expectations and perceptions of communities about what constitutes quality health service.

Research Design

The setting is the Iganga district in eastern Uganda and the Bushenyi district in western Uganda. A total of eight *focus group discussions (FGDs)* made up of six to 12 participants, 12 *key informant interviews (KIIs)*, and six *in-depth interviews (IDIs)* were conducted using purposive sampling.

The study adopted a *participatory qualitative approach* with specific reference to poor and vulnerable people in the communities, using predetermined criteria developed collaboratively by the researchers and the community leaders (see Kiguli, et al., 2009 for details). Data were collected using *FGDs, KIIs* of opinion leaders, health workers and local politicians, and *IDIs* of participants. Employing the NUD★IST package, the researchers used *content* and *latent analysis* techniques to analyze the data. The data were grouped into themes that captured the communities' perceptions and definition of quality of health care.

Outcomes

Many factors that are considered in the communities' judgement of the quality of care depended on the availability of amenities like infrastructure, clean water, equipment and supplies, health personnel attitudes, and access. Community members perceived highly the attributes of technical competence, the attitude of health workers, availability and access to needed services, facility amenities, and equipment to influence the quality of health care. The study further examined the perceptions of communities on the quality of care associated with the type of facilities utilized, and it emerged that public facilities provided lower quality compared to other private and quasi-government facilities. The reasons for the poor quality by public facilities include inadequately trained health workers, long distance to facilities (which exposes accessibility issues), poor interpersonal relations of health workers, and shortage of essential medicines.

The results further revealed that perceptions of quality of care by communities influence their health-seeking behaviors. The long wait time for attention in facilities led to self-medication and care in drugstores, private clinics, and traditional healers. These results suggest patients' and communities' perceptions of quality influence the utilization of services and health-seeking behaviors in Uganda. The authors suggest that the Ugandan health system seems to discriminate not only based on socioeconomic status but also the geographical location, which raises issues of accessibility, financial protection, equity, and quality that are at the center of *UHC*.

It is important to state that this study has some limitations. First, critics of the qualitative approach to health care users' perceptions of quality note that users have a lay person's view on the quality of care that is biased with no real technical basis. While this viewpoint is valid in some cases, the approach to patient satisfaction, which is based on total quality management (TQM), can be applied in health care quality evaluation; hence, user perceptions must be respected and captured in efforts to improve the quality of health care. Second, the stability of patients' evaluation of the quality of care has been questioned. If patients' description of quality care is unstable over time, developing a health care system that patients define as good quality and providing meaningful comparative health care quality information may be difficult, if not impossible.

Using Case Studies to Assess Health Outcomes

Recently, greater importance has been placed on including qualitative research in health economics because of the contributions made by qualitative research to the study of the impact of interventions, health, and disease burden (Townsend, Hunt, & Wyke, 2003). Additionally, health practitioners appreciate the methodological rigor within the qualitative model and are more accepting of its ability to generate deeper insights within the health sphere. This is also evident in the number of studies that combine both quantitative and qualitative methods to understand the wide range of public health problems embedded within the various range of social, political, and economic contexts (Parmar, Williams, Dkhimi, Ndiaye, Asante, Arhinful, et al., 2015). By themselves, quantitative methods are not able to explain the links between several levels such as the economic, behavioral, systemic, and environmental to explain health events and outcomes (Avolio & Bass, 1995) and are often very narrow in their frame of investigation. Qualitative methods bring another dimension of the interpretive approach that allows phenomena to be studied in their natural settings (Denzin & Lincoln, 2000).

Case study research has followed this trend as a viable approach, which allows researchers to study the phenomenon in-depth, using a wide range of perspectives (Hyett, Kenny, & Dickson-Swift, 2014), including from the study participant's perspective (Yin, 2014), thus allowing the exploration of processes and the links between these processes in the wide range of contexts within which they operate (Gall, Borg, & Gall, 1996). The complexity of the health system and the broader context in which it exists can be understood if more researchers complement quantitative with qualitative approaches, for instance (Wells, Williams, Treweek, Coyle, & Taylor, 2012). In cases where experimental research designs cannot be ethically applied, the case study methodology offers a more flexible solution (Payne, Field, Rolls, Hawker, & Kerr, 2007). Although not characterized by mixed methods per se, mixed methods are often used within case study research in health care, and when used, they are generally qualitatively driven and typically include observations, interviews, and analysis of participants' words (Carolan, Forbat, & Smith, 2015). The case study research can involve either single cases or many individual cases of the same type, or an embedded case approach, where one type of case is nested within a broader case or encompasses other cases (Gilson, 2012).

The example chosen to show the application of case study methodology to study health outcomes is *The Crisis in Human Resources for Health Care and the Potential of a 'Retired' Workforce: Case Study of the Independent Midwifery Sector in Tanzania* (Rolfe, Leshabari, Rutta, & Murray, 2008). Following deregulation in Tanzania, independent midwifery practices began to be established by a 'new' workforce of retired nursing officers offering personalized care in underserved areas, but delivery coverage was still low. The study provides in-depth information on the implementation and consequences of nongovernment health care provision in specific contexts to guide policy on human resources for health.

Research Design

This was a multiple case study that included the analysis of over nine districts. The study explored the characteristics of the retired nursing officers, the drivers, and inhibitors of their development since the change in legislation. An initial national situation analysis involved 20 *KIIs* made up of senior health planners and representatives from relevant professional organizations. The study also included a review of relevant documentary evidence. From these, the authors generated initial hypotheses about the current social context, organization, and delivery of independent midwifery care in Tanzania. Subsequently, they tested and extended these hypotheses in a multiple case study.

Nine case districts were selected using a purposive sampling strategy to ensure that the study included the breadth of geographical, organizational, and socioeconomic contexts in which private, small-scale midwifery practices operate in Tanzania. Additionally, the sampling approach ensured that the results would be relevant for informing future policy development for the larger workforce. Qualitative and quantitative data were collected from the range of sources in the case districts. In total, 125 *IDIs* and 58 *FGDs* were conducted iteratively to allow the researchers to adapt, develop, and test new hypotheses as data collection progressed. Hypotheses fell into three broad groupings: those concerned with motivations and relationships to the wider health care system; those concerned with location, range, and quality of services; and those concerned with demand-side issues of acceptability and utilization.

Outcomes

Retired nurses or those approaching retirement and nurses employed by the government dominate private midwifery practices. Provision was entirely facility-based due to regulatory requirements, with approximately 60 'maternity homes' located mainly in rural or peri-urban areas. Motivational drivers included fear of poverty, desire to maintain professional status, and an ethos of community service. The inhibitors to sustaining these maternity homes included the scarcity of start-up loans, lack of business training, and cumbersome registration processes. The study revealed that most private maternity homes were underutilized and unsustainable. It was expected that situating these homes in resource-poor communities will improve access to skilled attendance and help retain and extend the working life of nursing officers, but these goals were unattainable. Successful multiplication of this model in resource-poor communities will require more than just deregulation of private ownership. Prohibitive start-up expenses need to be reduced by less emphasis on facility-based provision. Ongoing financing arrangements such as micro-credit, contracting, vouchers, and franchising models require consideration (Rolfe, et al., 2008).

This methodology was chosen for its ability to embrace complexity and to generate and test hypotheses in real-world settings. Yin (2014) maintains that this is applicable where boundaries between phenomenon and context are not clearly evident. Since health systems need to be understood within their local social, cultural, and political contexts, using case studies that employ multiple sources and methods of data collection prove valuable in situations where policy change is needed. This methodology is not without its setbacks. It is time-intensive, and results may not be extrapolated. Case study methodology broadens the areas and levels of factors that need to be taken into consideration, and they allow for the development of general insights and conclusions to apply to other settings (Gilson, 2012). This is even more so for multiple case studies, where the principle of replication is central to this process of analysis. Authors can ascertain if the results from one case study are consistent with those from other cases within the sample frame and therefore strengthen the validity of final results (Rolfe, et al., 2008).

Strengths and Limitations

The five case studies successfully highlight the different approaches used by researchers to design, collect, and analyze data that provide robust results for policy. A mix of methodologies has been used by authors, as this highlights the complexity in behavioral and/or health economics research. Some studies have been purely quantitative or qualitative, while many use a mix of both qualitative and quantitative elements. The choice of design is also influenced by the feasibility, cost, and duration of the study, as well as the potential reliability (validity) and usefulness. For studies that require an assessment of impact, some authors have employed observational studies as a quicker, cheaper, and easier option than formal experiments. Results from these quicker options have been less conclusive due to, for instance, biases from sampling. Recently, however, researchers are increasingly adopting mixed methods to overcome the limitations imposed by using just one method (Barbour, 1999) to provide rich evidence to influence health policy. It is now well recognized that health outcomes are determined by a confluence of social, cultural, and biological factors. Therefore, researchers have resorted to exploring and combining various methodological approaches for describing and analyzing these factors to improve health. Because each method has its own strengths and weaknesses, the combination of approaches provides an avenue to complement the weakness of each method to understand health-sector phenomena comprehensively.

Recommendations for Future Research

Achieving *UHC* requires ongoing research from a variety of perspectives. This chapter acknowledges the importance of incorporating elements of behavioral economics into health economics research for *UHC*. In addition, a variety of methodological approaches is needed to provide critical evidence for policy to achieve the *UHC* goal. The broad range of areas, such as health promotion, quality of care, how people relate within the health system, and how people interact and function within various sociocultural and economic contexts provide the opportunities for researchers to investigate phenomena and contribute evidence-based policy.

For *UHC* to be achieved, the areas that need more intervention go beyond the traditional health system structure. There is a need for research on how human behavior affects health through interactions with other contexts, for example, interactions between agricultural practices and changes in the environment. Essentially, there is a need to bridge evidence between knowing how health systems function and how human beings interact. This understanding will drive the interventions to enable the provision of quality and accessible services to all. Similar considerations have led to recommendations that the traditional six WHO health system blocks should be modified to integrate the vital roles and perspectives of communities in health production and interactions (Sacks, 2019).

In summary, this chapter highlights that ongoing research exists on various aspects in the health sector, but more is needed to understand behavioral underpinnings that have been neglected in traditional health economics research and analysis. Several methods such as experimental, quasi-experimental, case studies, mixed methods, and others, as contained in this chapter, have their strengths and limitations but allow for a range of options for researchers to explain various topics of relevance to health economics and the attainment of *UHC*.

References

Abuosi, A. A., Domfeh, K. A., Abor, J. Y., & Nketiah-Amponsha, E. (2016). Health insurance and quality of care: Comparing perceptions of quality between insured and uninsured patients in Ghana's hospitals. *International Journal of Equity in Health*, *15*, 76. https://doi.org/10.1186/s12939-016-0365-1

Aditi, N. (2009). Factors affecting patient satisfaction and healthcare quality. *International Journal of Health Care Quality Assurance*, *22*(4), 366–381. https://doi.org/10.1108/09526860910964834

Atim, C., & Sock, M. (2000). *External evaluation report of the Nkoranza Community Health Insurance Scheme, Ghana*. Bethesda, MD: Abt Assocs.

Atinga, R. A., Abekah-Nkrumah, G., & Domfeh, K. A. (2011). Managing healthcare quality in Ghana: A necessity of patient satisfaction. *International Journal of Health Care Quality Assurance*, *24*(7), 548–563. https://doi.org/10.1108/09526861111160580

Avolio, B. J., & Bass, B. M. (1995). Individual consideration viewed at multiple levels of analysis: A multi-frame work for examining the diffusion of transformational leadership', *Leadership Quarterly*, *6*, 199–218. https://doi.org/10.1016/1048-9843(95)90035-7

Barbour, R. S. (1999). The case for combining qualitative and quantitative approaches in health services research. *Journal of Health Services Research and Policy*, *4*, 39–43. https://doi.org/10.1177%2F135581969900400110

Boyer, L., Francois, P., Doutre, E., Weil, G., & Labarere, J. (2006). Perception and use of the results of patient satisfaction surveys by care providers in a French teaching hospital. *International Journal for Quality in Health Care*, *18*, 359–364. https://doi.org/10.1093/intqhc/mzl029

Campbell, S. M., Roland, M. O., & Buetow, S. A. (2000). Defining quality of care. *Social Science and Medicine*, *51*, 1611–1625. https://doi.org/10.1016/S0277-9536(00)00057-5

Carayon, P., Schoofs Hundt, A., Karsh, B.-T., Gurses, A. P., Alvarado, C. J., Smith, M., et al. (2006). Work system design for patient safety: The SEIPS model. *Quality and Safety in Health Care, 15*(Supplement 1). http://dx.doi.org/10.1136/qshc.2005.015842

Carolan, C. M., Forbat, L., & Smith, A. (2015). Developing the DESCARTE model. *Qualitative Health Research, 26*(5), 626–639. https://doi.org/10.1177/1049732315602488

Carter, J. D., Daniel, R., Torrens, A. W., Sanchez, M. N., Maciel, E. L. N., Bartholomay, P., et al. (2019). The impact of a cash transfer programme on tuberculosis treatment success rate: A quasi-experimental study in Brazil. *BMJ Glob Health, 4*(1), e001029. http://dx.doi.org/10.1136/bmjgh-2018-001029

Coyle, Y. M., & Battles, J. B. (1999). Using antecedents of medical care to develop valid quality of care measures. *Journal of the International Society for Quality in Health Care/ISQua, 11*(1), 5–12. https://doi.org/10.1093/intqhc/11.1.5

Dagger, T., & Sweeney, J. C. (2006). The effects of service evaluation on behavioral intentions and quality of life. *Journal of Service Research, 19*, 3–19. https://doi.org/10.1177%2F1094670506289528

Denzin, N. K., & Lincoln, Y. S. (2000). The discipline and practice of qualitative research. In N. K. Denzin & Y. S. Lincoln (Eds.), *Handbook of qualitative research* (pp. 1–43). Thousand Oaks, CA: Sage Publications.

Dinardo, J. (2008). Natural experiments and quasi-natural experiments. In L. E. Blume & S. H. Durlauf (Eds.), *The new Palgrave dictionary of economics* (pp. 856–859). Baskingstoke, UK: Palgrave Macmillan. doi:10.1057/9780230226203

Donabedian, A. (1980). *Explorations in quality assessment and monitoring, volume 1: The definition of quality and approaches to its assessment.* Washington, DC: Health Administration Press.

Donabedian, A. (1988). The quality of care: How can it be assessed? *JAMA: Journal of the American Medical Association, 260*, 1743–1748. WHO The World Health Report 2000: Health systems: Improving performance. Geneva, Switzerland: World Health Organization.

Donabedian, A. (2003). *An introduction to quality assurance in health care.* New York: Oxford University Press.

Duku, S. K. O., Nketiah-Amponsah, E., Janssens, W., & Pradhan, M. (2018). Perceptions of healthcare quality in Ghana: Does health insurance status matter? *PLoS One, 13*(1), e0190911. https://dx.doi.org/10.1371%2Fjournal.pone.0190911

Eiriz, V., & Figueiredo, J. A. (2005). Quality evaluation in healthcare services based on customer-provider relationships, *International Journal of Healthcare Quality Assurance, 18*(6), 404–412. https://doi.org/10.1108/09526860510619408

Evans, D., Edejer, T. T.-T., Lauer, J., Frenk, J., & Murray, C. J. L. (2001). Measuring quality: From the system to the provider. *International Journal for Quality Health Care, 13*(6), 439–446. https://doi.org/10.1093/intqhc/13.6.439

Fenny, A. P., Hansen, K. S., Enemark, U., & Asante, F. A. (2014). Quality of uncomplicated malaria case management in Ghana among insured and uninsured. *International Journal For Equity in Health, 13*, 63–75. https://doi.org/10.1186/s12939-014-0063-9

Gall, M. D., Borg, W. R., & Gall, J. P. (1996). *Educational research: An introduction* (6th ed.). White Plains, NY: Longman.

Gilson, L. (Ed.). (2012). *Health policy and systems research: A methodology reader alliance for health policy and systems research.* Geneva, Switzerland: World Health Organization.

Giuffrida, A., Pinglo, M. E., Aghumian, A., Boggero, M., Buizza, C., Ferrara, J., et al. (2018). *World bank group support to health services: Achievements and challenges: An independent evaluation (English).* Sector and Thematic Evaluation. Washington, DC: World Bank.

Handley, M., A., Lyles, C. R., McCulloch, C., & Cattamanchi, A. (2018). Selecting and improving quasi-experimental designs in effectiveness and implementation research. *Annual Review of Public Health, 39*(1), 5–25. https://doi.org/10.1146/annurev-publhealth-040617-014128

Haw, N. J. L. (2019). Utilization of the Ghana national health insurance scheme and its association with patient perceptions on healthcare quality. *International Journal for Quality in Health Care, 31*(6), 485–491. https://doi.org/10.1093/intqhc/mzy185

Hyett, N., Kenny, A., & Dickson-Swift, V. (2014). Methodology or method? A critical review of qualitative case study reports. *International Journal of Qualitative Studies on Health and Well-Being, 9*(1), 1–12. http://doi.org/10.3402/qhw.v9.23606

Institute of Medicine. (1990). *Medicare: A strategy for quality assurance, volume II: Sources and methods.* Washington, DC: National Academies Press. https://doi.org/10.17226/1548

Institute of Medicine. (2001). *Crossing the quality chasm: A new health system for the 21st century* (pp. 5–6). Washington, DC: National Academy Press.

Judson, T. J., Volpp, K. G., & Detsky, A. S. (2015). Harnessing the right combination of extrinsic and intrinsic motivation to change physician behavior. *JAMA: Journal of the American Medical Association, 314*(21), 2233–2234. doi:10.1001/jama.2015.15015

Kiguli, J., Kirapa-Kiracho, E., Okui, O., Mutebi, A., MacGregor, H., & Pariyo, G. W. (2009). Increasing access to quality health care for the poor: Community perceptions on quality care in Uganda. *Patient Preference and Adherence, 3*, 77–85. https://doi.org/10.2147/ppa.s4091

King, G., & Nielsen, R. (2016). *Why propensity scores should not be used for matching*. Retrieved April 25, 2020, from http://j.mp/2ovYGsW

Kutzin, J. (2013). Health financing for universal coverage and health system performance: Concepts and implications for policy. *Bull World Health Organization, 91*(8), 602–611. doi:10.1001/jama.2015.15015

Ladhari, R. (2009). A review of twenty years of SERVQUAL research. *International Journal of Quality and Service Sciences, 1*(2), 172–198. https://doi.org/10.1108/17566690910971445

Lambert, T. E., & Bewley, M. (2016). The use of quasi-experimental design in urban and regional policy research and political economy. In F. S. Lee & B. Cronin (Eds.), *Handbook of research methods & applications in heterodox economics: Handbook of research methods & application series* (pp. 535–553). Northampton, MA: Edward Elger. doi:10.2139/ssrn.2735472

Lindelöw, M., & Wagstaff, A. (2003). *Health facility surveys: An introduction*. World Bank Policy Research Working Paper 2953. The World Bank Group, Washington, DC.

Macur, M. (2011). Quality in health care: Possibilities and limitations of quantitative research instruments among health care users. *Springer Science+Business Media*, B.V. doi:10.1007/s11135-011-9621-z

Mahmoud, A. B., Ekwere, T., Fuxman, L., & Meero, A. A. (2019). Assessing patients' perception of health care service quality offered by COHSASA-accredited hospitals in Nigeria. *SAGE Open*, 1–9. https://doi.org/10.1177%2F2158244019852480

Matjasko, J. L., Cawley, J. H., Baker-Goering, M. M., & Yokum, D. V. (2016). Applying behavioral economics to public health policy: Illustrative examples and promising direction. *American Journal of Preventive Medicine, 50*(5, Supplement 1), S13. https://doi.org/10.1016/j.amepre.2016.02.007

Maxwell, R. J. (1984). Quality assessment in health. *British Medical Journal, 288*, 1470–1472. doi:10.1136/bmj.288.6428.1470

McCarney, R., Warner, J., Iliffe, S., van Haselen, R., Griffin, M., & Fisher, P. (2007). The Hawthorne effect: A randomised, controlled trial. *BMC Medical Research Methodology, 7*(30). https://doi.org/10.1186/1471-2288-7-30

McLaughlin, C. P., & Kaluzny, A. D. (2006). *Continuous quality improvement in health care* (3rd ed.). Sudbury, MA: Jones and Bartlett Publishers.

Mosadeghrad, A. M. (2013). Healthcare service quality: Towards a broad definition. *International Journal of Health Care Quality Assurance, 26*(3), 203–219. https://doi.org/10.1108/09526861311311409

Ng, M., Fullman, N., Dieleman, J. L., Flaxman, A. D., Murray, C. J., & Lim, S. S. (2014). Effective coverage: A metric for monitoring universal health coverage. *PLoS Medicine, 11*(9), e1001730. https://doi.org/10.1371/journal.pmed.1001730

Parmar, D., Williams, G., Dkhimi, F., Ndiaye, A., Asante, F. A., Arhinful, D. K., et al. (2014). Enrolment of older people in social health protection programs in West Africa: Does social exclusion play a part? *Social Science & Medicine, 119*, 36–44. https://doi.org/10.1016/j.socscimed.2014.08.011

Payne, S., Field, D., Rolls, L., Hawker, S., & Kerr, C. (2007). Case study research methods in end-of-life care: Reflections on three studies. *Journal of Advanced Nursing, 58*, 236–245. https://doi.org/10.1111/j.1365-2648.2007.04215.x

Peterson, S., Nsungwa-Sabiiti, J., Were, W., Nsabagasmi, X., Magumba, G., Nambooze, J., et al. (2004). Coping with paediatric referral: Ugandan parents' experience. *Lancet, 363*, 1955–1956. https://doi.org/10.1016/S0140-6736(04)16411-8

Rolfe, B., Leshabari, S., Rutta, F., & Murray, S. F. (2008). The crisis in human resources for health care and the potential of a "retired" workforce: Case study of the independent midwifery sector in Tanzania. *Health Policy and Planning, 23*(2), 137–149. https://doi.org/10.1093/heapol/czm049

Rossi, P. H., Lipsey, M. W., & Freeman, H. E. (2004). *Evaluation: A systematic approach* (7th ed., p. 237). New York, NY: Sage Publications.

Sacks, E., Morrow, M., Story, W. T., Shelley, K. S., Shanklin, D., Rahimtoolma, M., et al. (2019). Beyond the building blocks: Integrating community roles into health systems frameworks to achieve health for all. *BMJ Global Health*, (Supplement 3), e001384. https://doi.org/10.1136/bmjgh2018-001384

Shadish, W. R., Cook, T. D., & Campbell, D. T. (2002). *Experimental and quasi-experimental designs for generalized causal inference*. Boston, MA: Houghton Mifflin.

Shen, G., Nguyen, H., Das, A., Sachingongu, N., Chansa, C., Qamruddin, J., et al. (2017). Incentives to change: Effects of performance-based financing on health workers in Zambia. *Human Resources for Health, 15*(20). https://doi.org/10.1186/s12960-017-0179-2

Sodani, P. R., Kumar, R. K., Srivastava, J., & Sharma, L. (2010). Measuring patient satisfaction: A case study to improve quality of care at public health facilities. *Indian Journal of Community Medicine, 35*, 52–56. https://doi.org/10.4103/0970-0218.62554

Sofaer, S., & Firminger, K. (2005). Patient perceptions of the quality of health services. *Annual Review of Public Health, 26*, 513–559. https://doi.org/10.1146/annurev.publhealth.25.050503.153958

Spector, P. E. (1985). Measurement of human service staff satisfaction: Development of the job satisfaction survey. *American Journal of Community Psychology, 13*, 693.

Tong, H. L., Coiera, E., Tong, W., Wang, Y., Quiroz, J. C., Martin, P., et al. (2019). Efficacy of a mobile social networking intervention in promoting physical activity: Quasi-experimental study. *JMIR Mhealth Uhealth, 7*(3), e1218. https://doi.org/10.2196/12181

Townsend, A., Hunt, K., & Wyke, S. (2003). Managing multiple morbidity in mid-life: A qualitative study of attitudes to drug use. *British Medical Journal, 327*, 837–841. https://doi.org/10.1136/bmj.327.7419.837

Tucker, J., III, & Adams, S. R. (2001). Incorporating patients' assessments of satisfaction and quality: An integrative model of patients' evaluations of their care. *Managing Service Quality, 11*(4), 272–286. https://doi.org/10.1108/EUM0000000005611

United Nations Development Programme. (2015). *Sustainable development goals.* New York, NY: United Nations Development Programme.

Ware, J. E., & Stewart, A. (1992). Measures for a new era of health assessment. In N. C. Durham & A. L. Stewart (Eds.), *Measuring functioning and well-being.* Durham, NC: Duke University Press.

Weiss, D. J., Dawis, R. V., England, G. W., & Lofquist, L. H. (1967). *Manual for the Minnesota satisfaction questionnaire.* Minnesota Studies in Vocational Rehabilitation. Minneapolis, MN: University of Minnesota Industrial Relations Center.

Wells, M., Williams, B., Treweek, S., Coyle, J., & Taylor, J. (2012). Intervention description is not enough: Evidence from an in-depth multiple case study on the untold role and impact of context in randomised controlled trials of seven complex interventions. *Trials, 13*, Article 95. https://doi.org/10.1186/1745-6215-13-95

Witter, S., Fretheim, A., Kessy, F. L., & Lindahl, A. K. (2012). Paying for performance to improve the delivery of health interventions in low-and middle-income countries. *Cochrane Database of Systematic Reviews, 2*, CD007899.

World Bank. (1993). *World development report.* New York: Oxford University Press.

World Health Organization. (1978). *Declaration of Alma-Ata.* Almaty: World Health Organization.

World Health Organization. (2000). *The World Health Report 2000: Health systems: Improving performance.* Retrieved April 28, 2020, from www.who.int/whr/2000/en/whr00_en.pdf

World Health Organization. (2010). *The World Health Report 2010: Health systems financing: The path to universal coverage.* Geneva, Switzerland: World Health Organization.

World Health Organization. (2013). *The World Health Report 2013: Research for universal health coverage.* Geneva, Switzerland: World Health Organization.

World Health Organization. (2019). *Primary health care on the road to universal health coverage: 2019 monitoring report: Executive summary.* License, CC BY-NC-SA 3.0 IGO, Geneva.

World Health Organization. (2020). *WHO-5 well-being index 2012.* Retrieved April 28, 2020, from www.who-5.org/

Yin, R. K. (2014). *Case study research: Design and methods.* Los Angeles, CA: Sage Publications.

Zastowny, T. R., Stratmann, W. C., Adams, E. H., & Fox, M. L. (1995). Patient satisfaction and experience with health services and quality of care. *Quality Management in Health Care, 3*, 50–61.

28

NEXT-GENERATION GENETICS

Saeed Yasin and Julian Paul Keenan

Overview

Health psychology is the study of how biological, psychological, behavioral, social, and environmental factors affect physical and mental health (Murray, 2000). In the 1970s health psychology began to heavily embrace the biopsychosocial model due in large part to technical advances and forward-looking thinking. The biopsychosocial model heavily focuses on how biological factors play a role in mental and physical health and vice versa (Johnson & Acabchuk, 2018). Today, this seems obvious, which means success; one's mental state influences and is influenced by his or her underlying physical state.

However, imagine we are in 1970 and 50 years in the future someone is reading this handbook. What is obvious to them seems insanely impossible today. Here we examine the next decade (50 years may be a stretch) in terms of a) what areas a researcher should consider for future training and b) what we should all pay attention to now, as these techniques are starting to dominate the field. It is not surprising that genetics dominates many people's thinking of the future of health psychology, at least on a physiological level. From investment to payoff, genetic sequencing, expression, and manipulation are the future.

It has already been long established that increased risk of mental illness may be transmitted via heredity (McGuffin, Rijsdijk, Andrew, Sham, Katz, & Cardno, 2003). In order to understand at a deeper level how risk of mental illness may be transferred through genes, some primary knowledge of how genes function is required. Most of us know that DNA stores information about an organism using four nitrogenous bases sorted in three-letter codes. This code may be read and translated into proteins that carry out the function for that code. This is what controls the development of an organism, including the cells and organs within (Hyman, 2000). Proteins are responsible for the brain to be able to adapt in response to environmental information. More specifically, they play a major role in establishing and consolidating the structure of synapses (Hyman, 2000). By regulating the activity of neurons, these synapses are large factors when it comes to the behavior and mental health of humans (Perea, Navarrete, & Araque, 2009). By studying how sequences of DNA may affect proteins that affect synapses and consequently behavior, genes that contribute to the risk of mental illness may be identified and influenced to promote resilience.

Research in Practice

Gene Sequencing

As further research has indicated, however, identifying genes that contribute to the risk of mental illnesses is extremely complex. This results from mental illnesses not being caused by a single genetic defect, but rather from the interaction of multiple genes (Barondes, 1999). These gene–gene interactions are not simply additive either. The function of one gene may be dependent and change based upon the prior function of one or more genes, a phenomenon known as epistasis (Frankel & Schork, 1996). A possible solution for this issue, as suggested by Steve E. Hyman, could be analyzing the genomes from large, outbred, and genetically isolated populations that have large amounts of affected and unaffected individuals. He suggests that analyzing such populations can help provide sufficient statistical analysis to identify the effects of multiple genes at once, reduce the negative effects of genetic homogeneity, and help provide suitable controls to compare to. A main issue with Steve E. Hyman's argument is the massive amount of DNA sequencing needed to carry out such an experiment. Genes are usually identified via a method called **Sanger sequencing**. *Sanger sequencing* can identify the sequence of DNA fragments one at a time by the use of attaching complementary labeled **dideoxynucleotides** and then using gel electrophoresis to read out the sequence (Sanger, Nicklen, & Coulson, 1977). While the process works, it is still not nearly as time-efficient as needed for a project of this magnitude.

This issue could be dealt with, however, by the use of recently developed research technologies, such as **next-generation sequencing**, **NanoDrop**, and **MinION**. By becoming familiar with the mechanisms and use of recently developed research technologies, health psychologists are able to further research in the identification and treatment of mental illnesses.

While new, more efficient ways of sequencing DNA have been and are still being developed, there is still a lot to learn from the history of DNA sequencing. In the early 1900s, DNA was understood as a molecule for hereditary traits, but its structure was still not fully understood. Several scientists were working hard to try to identify the molecules within DNA, such as Erwin Chargaff finding clear ratios between nitrogenous bases within DNA (Ulbricht, 1964), and producing images of DNA, such as Maurice Wilkins and Rosalind Franklin trying to visualize DNA using x-ray crystallography (Litman, 1976). An extraordinary breakthrough was in the world of genetics in 1953 due to the analysis of two collaborating scientists, Francis Crick and James Watson. When Watson and Crick discovered the three-dimensional structure of DNA in 1953, using crystallographic data from Rosalind Franklin and Maurice Wilkins, people immediately become interested in a way to 'read' the information contained within this unique molecule (Watson & Crick, 1974; Zallen, 2003).

Initially, the process of learning how to sequence began with RNA rather than DNA. RNA was much easier to work with for many reasons. There was a plethora of readily available populations of relatively pure RNA species, particularly among bacteriophages. The RNA could easily be bulk-produced in culture, had a lack of a complementary strand that caused complications, and was often considerably shorter than eukaryotic DNA molecules (Heather & Chain, 2016). To sequence RNA, RNase enzymes were used to cut RNA chains at specific sites and fragment them. Then the fragments were separated by chromatography and electrophoresis. Next the individual fragments were deciphered by sequential exonuclease digestion. Finally, the sequence was deduced from the overlaps. In other words, the RNA was cut at several random points, the fragments were then sequenced, and finally overlaps were used to discover the overall sequence (Shendure, Balasubramanian, Church, Gilbert, Rogers, Schloss, et al., 2017). The first RNA sequence produced was the **alanine tRNA**, sequenced by Robert Holley and his colleagues in 1965 (Holley, Apgar, Everett, Madison, Marquisee, Merrill, et al., 1965).

The early attempts to sequence DNA made it seem impossible to fully sequence a DNA molecule. Some researchers took advantage of the ability to easily sequence RNA at the time in order to sequence DNA. Gilbert and Maxam were able to determine 24 bases of the lactose-repressor binding site by copying the gene into RNA and then sequencing it. Despite their progress, it took them an extensive amount of time to make this discovery—they were able to identify an average of one base per month (Gilbert & Maxam, 1973). Other researchers took advantage of the fact that DNA would often have a single strand overhanging at its ends. Wu and Kaiser did this by filling the ends of DNA with identifiable radioactive nucleotides. They supplied each nucleotide one at a time to deduce the sequence. By this method, they were able to determine 12 bases of the cohesive ends of bacteriophage lambda in 1968 (Wu & Kaiser, 1968). This idea of incorporating radioactive nucleotides in sequencing was considered an amazing discovery, since other researchers learned that the radioactive nucleotides could be used to infer the order of nucleotides anywhere, not just at the ends of genomes (Padmanabhan & Wu, 1972; Sanger, Donelson, Coulson, Kössel, & Fischer, 1973).

After this breakthrough in the methodology of sequencing occurred, another breakthrough occurred quickly afterwards. Typically when sequencing, researchers would have to go through a process of two-dimensional fractionation, which consisted of going through electrophoresis and chromatography to separate the segments of DNA. A new technique was developed in which only a single separation was needed This single separation would separate DNA by polynucleotide length via electrophoresis through polyacrylamide gels (Heather & Chain, 2016). This breakthrough led to the creation of some of the first-generation sequencing techniques.

Frederick Sanger is likely the most well-known name in sequencing. Two of the earliest sequencing techniques that were created were the **plus and minus system** and the **chemical cleavage** technique. In 1975, Alan Coulson and Frederick Sanger developed a method called the *plus and minus system*. This system consisted of using DNA polymerase to synthesize DNA using radiolabeled nucleotides and a primer. There were two reactions that took place: a *plus* reaction and a *minus* one. The *plus* reaction occurs when a single type of nucleotide is presented, attaching itself to its corresponding base. This provides extensions of the sample that all end with the selected bases. Then the *minus* reaction occurs with the three other nucleotides. This provides the sequences up to the position before the missing nucleotide, which should be in the position of the *plus* reaction nucleotide. These positions could be visualized through the use of a polyacrylamide gel (Sanger, et al., 1977). The *chemical cleavage technique* was developed by Allan Maxam and Walter Gilbert in 1977. The technique used polyacrylamide gel as well; however, instead of relying on DNA polymerase to generate fragments, this technique involved treating radiolabeled DNA with chemicals to cause it to break at specific bases. These fragments could be run on a polyacrylamide gel to create a visual guide to see the position of the base the chemical would cause the DNA to break at (Maxam & Gilbert, 1977). Despite the amazing discoveries made with these two techniques, it was not until the development of Sanger's new method in 1977 that DNA sequencing became an easily attainable reality.

In 1977, Sanger developed a method to sequence DNA by combining the two approaches presented in the previously mentioned methods. Sanger developed a technique called **the chain-termination** or **dideoxy technique**. This technique used chemical analogues of *deoxyribonucleotides (dNTPs)*, which are monomers of DNA strands. A monomer is the most basic unit of a class of molecules and will typically bond to other monomers to form larger, more functional molecules called polymers (Ebdon, 1992). Instead of adding *dNTPs* to DNA, Sanger thought of adding **dideoxynucleotides (ddNTPs)** to DNA strands. If a *ddNTP* is placed on a DNA strand, then the strand lacks the ability to extend because *ddNTPs* are unable to bind to the next *dNTP* banded to it, due to a lack of a 3' hydroxyl group (Chidgeavadze, Beabealashvilli, Atrazhev, Kukhanova, Azhayev, & Krayevsky, 1984). This technique took advantage of this and mixed radiolabeled *ddNTPs* into a DNA extension reaction. This would cause the chain to stop whenever a *ddNTP* was bonded to the DNA. By running four parallel reactions, each containing a different radiolabeled *ddNTP* base, one would be able to create several fragments of varying lengths, all stopping when a particular base of interest was present. Through the use of polyacrylamide gel, this could be observed visually and then recorded in order to develop a DNA sequence (Sanger, et al., 1977). This became one of the most common technologies used to sequence DNA for years to come and was the inspiration for several other DNA sequencing techniques (Heather & Chain, 2016).

Next-Generation Sequencing

Next-generation sequencing is a more efficient and cost-effective way to identify targeted genes. *Next-generation* sequencing is able to sequence DNA fragments faster than Sanger sequencing and also sequence several DNA fragments at a time. While Sanger sequencing can only sequence one DNA fragment at a time, *next-generation* sequencing can sequence millions of fragments with several processors working simultaneously. Typically, a *next-generation* sequencer reads 96 bases at one time, or in other words, 500,000 bases per day (Besser, Carleton, Gerner-Smidt, Lindsey, & Trees, 2018). A *next-generation* sequencer goes through a series of reactions in order to fully sequence a sample (Hughes, Gang, Murphy, Higgins, & Teeling, 2013). First the DNA sample goes through some preparation. The DNA goes through random fragmentation, and then each fragment is ligated on both ends, the 5' and 3' ends, with adapters. Then the DNA sample goes through **polymerase chain reaction (PCR)**. *PCR* is a process that amplifies the DNA molecules by putting it through a cycle of cooling and heating while a DNA polymerase keeps adding on complementary base pairs (Shampo & Kyle, 2002). Then the prepared sample is loaded into a flow cell, where the fragments are fluorescently marked and then amplified even more. Finally the sample is sequenced. The DNA is pulled through a capillary tube via a positive electrode. As it passes through the capillary tube, a light is passed through the tube that causes the fluorescent tag on the DNA to emit different colors of light. The wavelength and intensity of the emission are recorded. This helps determine the base present, which is also recorded (Hughes, et al., 2013).

Next-generation sequencing has already been implemented and has helped provide a better understanding of genetic disorders. A plethora of harmful genetic diseases exist within the human genome. Some of these include **fetal akinesia/hypokinesia (FADS)**, arthrogryposis, and severe congenital myopathies (Todd, Yau, Ong, Slee, McGillivray, Barnett, et al., 2015). In addition, these disease are elusive in terms of a genetic diagnosis. These three disorders also all cause several abnormalities that affect individuals long-term. *FADS* causes intrauterine growth retardation, craniofacial anomalies, limb anomalies, pulmonary hypoplasia, and polyhydramnios (Dillon, Bjornson, Jaffe, Hall, & Song, 2009; Hall, 2014). There are at least 30 causative genes, some of which have been identified (Ravenscroft, Sollis, Charles, North, Baynam, & Laing, 2011; Wilbe, Ekvall, Eurenius, Ericson, Casar-Borota, Klar, et al., 2015). **Arthrogryposis** refers to nonprogressive congenital joint contractures or, in other words, conditions that cause a joint to become permanently fixed in a position or heavily restricted in terms of movement (Filges & Hall, 2013). This disease affects approximately one in 3,000 live births and ranges greatly in severity (Haliloglu & Topaloglu, 2013). There are ten distinct subtypes in which only seven causative genes have been identified (Bamshad, Van Heest, & Pleasure, 2009). Congenital myopathies refers to a diverse group of disorders characterized by skeletal muscle dysfunction accompanied by specific morphological features (Romero & Clarke, 2013). More than 15 disease genes have been identified as causes of congenital myopathies. However, many cases remain genetically unresolved, suggesting further heterogeneity (Majczenko, Davidson, Camelo-Piragua, Agrawal, Manfready, Li, et al., 2012; McMillin, Beck, Chong, Shively, Buckingham, Gildersleeve, et al., 2014)

Dr. Emily J. Todd and others led a project to identify causative genes for *fetal hypokinesia, arthrogryposis*, and severe congenital myopathy by studying small families and isolated probands through the use of next-generation sequencing. First DNA samples were taken from individuals in affected families and isolated probands. Then the DNA samples were amplified through the use of *PCR* and had sequencing adaptors ligated or attached to the sides. The library was then purified using AMPure beads and amplified again using Platinum High-Fidelity Taq Polymerase. Then **neuromuscular sub-exomic sequencing (NSES)** was performed in which genes encoded for neuromuscular disorders were identified. After next-generation sequencing was performed, some unpublished candidate disease genes were identified, as well as 336 known candidate neuromuscular and cardiomyopathy genes. *Sanger sequencing* was performed to confirm some of the findings of the next-generation sequencer. Findings were also compared to and confirmed by previously identified genes listed in the December 2012 freeze of neuromuscular disorders gene table (Kaplan, 2010). To identify the candidate genes, variant calling was performed against a human reference genome, and data were filtered several times to identify any significant gene differences (Todd, et al., 2015).

From a total of 45 subjects taken from 38 different families afflicted with *FADS*, *arthrogryposis*, or a severe congenital myopathy, a conclusive genetic diagnosis was achieved for 18 out of the 38 families. Furthermore, they discovered the patterns of genetic inheritance for two *FADS*-, six *arthrogryposis*-, and 10 congenital myopathy –elated diseases. These were determined through the use of genetic analysis as well as pedigree analysis. Alongside discovering the pattern of genetic inheritance for these Mendelian disorders, they were able to discover novel disease causative genes and associate their corresponding diseases. They were also able to identify several known causative genes (Todd, et al., 2015).

Through the identification of these causative genes, this study concluded *next-generation sequencing* was an accurate and helpful tool. With the speed and accuracy of this technique, there is a potential future for it in clinical practice. There are many **Mendelian diseases** with elusive causative genes that are in need of more research. *Mendelian diseases* are diseases caused by a single variant in a single gene. Some of these diseases include long QT syndrome, familial hypercholesterolemia, and Marfan syndrome (Parikh & Ashley, 2017). If *next-generation sequencing* were implemented in clinical practice, this would lead to a better understanding of genetic disorders, the expansion of genetic and clinical databases, and development of a disease taxonomy (Ashley, 2016).

NanoDrop Spectrophotometer

Another important and effective recent technology that could greatly help further research in the identification and treatment of mental illnesses is the **NanoDrop spectrophotometer**. This is a device that can measure DNA, RNA, and protein concentrations. It can sequence a sample as small as 0.5 to 2 μL with no dilution (Desjardins, Hansen, & Allen, 2009). The only sample preparation that is required is the purification of the DNA, RNA, or protein (Desjardins & Conklin, 2010). As the sample is placed upon the detection surface of the device, it runs through a liquid column. Then a xenon flash lamp provides a light source to shine on the sample. The *NanoDrop spectrophotometer* automatically determines the path length of the light that provides the most extensive and accurate readings (Desjardins, et al., 2009). Then, it uses **UV-Vis absorbance** in order to identify the sequence of the sample. It does so by first producing an absorbance spectrum for each sample. Then the device identifies what is within the sample due to the differences of *UV-Vis absorbance* levels in substances. The peaks at 260 nm identify the presence of nucleic acids and at 280 nm identify the presence of proteins. The 260/280 nm ratio is used to provide nucleic acid sample purity. An ideal ratio range would be 1.8 to 2.0 (Desjardins & Conklin, 2010). The *NanoDrop spectrophotometer* would be extremely helpful to use for research, since it is able to evaluate the concentration and purity of a sample in a fast and accurate way, in particular due to the use of *UV-Vis absorbance* levels. Other methods typically involve the use of fluorescent dyes to mark nucleic acid samples, which takes up more resources and more time. Also, since the *NanoDrop spectrophotometer* is able to automatically adjust to the best path length, it provides the most accurate reading possible.

The *NanoDrop* has already been tested to see if it may be useful for identifying the potential for disease through quantifying the amounts of microRNA in individuals. **MicroRNAs (miRNAs)** are small noncoding RNA molecules that control gene expression by generally suppressing target messenger RNAs (**mRNAs**; Bartel, 2009). This process is crucial, since *mRNAs* are the bridge from DNA ultimately becoming proteins that may carry out the function encoded within the DNA. *miRNAs* are thought to regulate nearly all cellular function, since more than one-third of the human transcriptome (RNA makeup) is affected by it (Lewis, Shih, Jones-Rhoades, Bartel, & Burge, 2003). Due to how crucial *miRNAs* are to several cellular processes, it is thought that *miRNAs* could also be used for multiple disease processes (Li & Kowdley, 2012; Moldovan, Batte, Trgovcich, Wisler, Marsh, & Piper, 2014). *miRNAs* are mostly expressed intracellularly; however, they can also be detected in blood and other organic fluids providing fluid stability (Mitchell, Parkin, Kroh, Fritz, & Wyman,

2008; Schaefer, Jung, Miller, Lein, Kristiansen, Erbersdobler, et al., 2010). *miRNA* circulating in the blood and other organic fluids is thought to participate in cell-to-cell communication and distance regulation of gene expression. Due to this, they have become biomarkers or indicators for diseases (Duttagupta, Jiang, Gollub, Getts, & Jones, 2011).

In a study led by Anna Garcia-Elias and others, a method to quantify and profile *miRNA* in human plasma samples was sought. This was often met with difficulty due to only very small amounts of *miRNA* being present in organic fluids (Jensen, Lamy, Rasmussen, Ostenfeld, Dyrskjøt, Ørntoft, et al., 2011). When a plasma sample was attained, there needed to be a way to quantify if the sample contained enough *miRNA* for profiling to be conceivable. In order to find the most accurate and suitable technique for *miRNA* quantification, four different devices were compared: Tecan Infinite 200 PRO Nanoquant Spectrophotometer, Thermo Scientific Nanodrop 2000 Spectrophotometer, Agilent 2100 Bioanalyzer, and Life Technologies Qubit 2.0 Fluorometer. This was done by loading plasma samples with known concentrations of *miRNA* into each of the devices and taking repetitive reads. The variability and accuracy of the reads were compared.

The *NanoDrop* was determined to be one of the easier devices to understand and had a higher chance of being used. In order for the *NanoDrop* to be used, a sample must have been acquired. Thirty µL of peripheral blood from 12 healthy volunteers were collected. Those samples were then rapidly centrifuged at 1500 g for 15 minutes at 4 °C. The plasma was then separated from the blood sample. Then the sample can be loaded into the NanoDrop as long as it is reduced to anywhere within the range of 0.5 to 2 µL. The NanoDrop is also able to detect concentrations of DNA, RNA, or protein within the range of 2 ng/µL to 15 µg/µL. It was found that the *NanoDrop* was able to take accurate measurements repeatedly with only a standard deviation of .22 among repeated measurements of the same sample. This was relatively low when compared to other samples. The *Nano-Drop* was also notably accurate when taking measurements, producing mean values of 8.99 ng/µL, 10.93 ng/µL, and 12.92 ng/µL for a 10-ng/µL sample. It also showed some accuracy even outside of its expected concentration detection range, producing mean values of 0.62 ng/µL, 1.08 ng/µL, and 0.80 ng/µL for a 1-ng/µL sample (Garcia-Elias, Alloza, Puigdecanet, Nonell, Tajes, Curado, et al., 2017). This implies that *NanoDrop* is applicable in real-world clinical practices, allowing clinicians to be able to accurately and quickly measure concentrations of *miRNA* in patients and possibly diagnose severe diseases early on.

This study concluded that the *NanoDrop* is a satisfactory choice for labs to use to quantify *miRNA* within plasma samples of individuals. The ability to quantify *miRNA* samples in an accurate and fast manner is exceptionally helpful in clinical practices. Several diseases cause significant changes to *miRNA* values around the body. Some of these include colon cancer (Callari, Dugo, Musella, Marchesi, Chiorino, Grand, et al., 2012), breast cancer (Cuk, Zucknick, Heil, Madhavan, Schott, Turchinovich, et al., 2012), colorectal cancer (Slaby, 2016), heart disease (Ikeda, Kong, Lu, Bisping, Zhang, Allen, et al., 2007), lung disease (Nana-Sinkam, Hunter, Nuovo, Schmittgen, Gelinas, Galas, et al., 2009), kidney disease (Chung, Dong, Yang, Zhong, Li, & Lan, 2013), and multiple sclerosis (Fenoglio, Ridolfi, Galimberti, & Scarpini, 2012). By being able to identify the presence of these diseases early on, the necessary treatment may be provided and possibly save the life of a patient.

MinION

Another efficient and cost-effective device that can help the sequencing process is the **MinION**. The *MinION* is a 90-g portable device that can be plugged into a laptop via a universal serial bus (USB) cable (Jain, Olsen, Paten, & Akeson, 2016). For this device to be used, the DNA must undergo some slight preparation. First, the DNA sample must be fragmented and adapters must be ligated to the 5' and 3' ends of each fragment. These adapters then facilitate the loading of a processive enzyme at the 5' end of each strand (Sauvage, Boizeau, Candotti, Vandenbogaert, Servant-Delmas, Caro, et al., 2018).

Then, DNA goes through the *MinION* where it encounters the Oxford nanopore. The *MinION* has a synthetic layer within it resembling a cell membrane. Embedded within the cell membrane is the **Oxford nanopore**, a transmembrane carrier protein with a hollow tube in the middle. Due to the processive enzyme being added earlier, the DNA fragments go through the *Oxford nanopore* unidirectionally. As this takes place, an electrical current runs through the nanopore through the use of an ionic current in an electrochemical solution. This does not affect the membrane, since it has a very high electrical resistance. As each nucleotide goes through the nanopore, unique disruptions occur in the current depending upon the nucleotide. By frequently measuring the current, the *MinION* sequences the DNA sample as it is running through the *Oxford nanopore*. Most samples have an average run time of three minutes, and several samples may be run at one time (Lu, Giordano, & Ning, 2016). This device is beneficial to any research that requires sequencing. The ability to easily transport this fast and efficient device makes it an extremely helpful and convenient way to acquire data.

The *MinION* has been used in the medical world to sequence infectious viral infections, such as influenza. Influenza epidemics and pandemics can cause major catastrophes and heavily affect economies, morbidity, and mortality worldwide (Wang, Moore, Deng, Eccles, & Hall, 2015). Influenza can be difficult to detect by those infected due to the disease only causing mild symptoms. These mild symptoms include coughing, sore throat, nasal discharge, fever, headache, and muscle pain. Despite these diseases being no immediate threat to one's life, these symptoms can worsen over time and become more severe. This causes the immune system to weaken and makes the infected individual more prone to life-threatening illnesses, such as bronchitis and pneumonia (Yves, 2013). There are two main influenza viruses, influenza A and influenza B. Influenza A virus is a much bigger threat to the human population, due to it being from an animal (Horimoto & Kawaoka, 2005). This implies that even if influenza A virus were to be eradicated within the human population, it could still propagate among animal populations and eventually reinfect humans in a mutated form, making it harder to fight. Approximately 0.18% to 0.21% of influenza A virus's proteins mutate every year, making it able to evade host immunity developed through previous infection or vaccination (Belanov, Bychkov, Benner, Ripatti, Ojala, Kankainen, et al., 2015). It has also been found that globally, influenza viruses have caused around three to five million annual cases of hospitalization and 250,000 to 500,000 deaths annually (Lafond, Nair, Rasooly, Valente, Booy, Rahman, et al., 2016).

Due to the mutation rate of influenza A virus, there has been a greater need to sequence the virus to prevent infection and propagation. Dr. Jing Wang was able to obtain and sequence the complete influenza A virus genome. Dr. Jing Wang states that in order to carry out such a project, the *MinION* was required, since other older sequencing methods were "labor-intensive, slow, and not easily adapted for processing larger genomes or large numbers of samples" (Wang et al., 2015). Due to the ability of the *MinION* to read several samples at a time and produce reads of 60 kilobases at a time, it was the preferred method (Madoui, Engelen, Cruaud, Belser, Bertrand, Alberti, et al., 2015).

In order to sequence the entire genome of the influenza A virus, first an isolate of the virus was needed. The isolate was obtained from the culture collection at New Zealand's World Health Organization National Influenza Centre, based at the Institute of Environmental Science and Research (ESR). RNA from the virus was extracted from a viral culture using the iPrep Purelink Virus kit. First the RNA sample needed to be purified and amplified in order to be sequenced. The RNA sample was purified through the use of the *Oxford nanopore MinION* genomic DNA sequencing kit. The sample was diluted and then amplified through reverse transcriptase polymerase chain reaction (RT-PCR). Next the ends of the DNA sample were repaired through the addition of 5 μL of *Oxford nanopore* DNA CS and use of the NEBNext End Repair module by adding 10 μL of reaction buffer and 5 μL of enzyme. Next, the DNA sample went through a 30-min incubation at 25 °C and was purified again using 100 μL Agencourt AMPure XP beads with elution into 25 μL of RT-PCR molecular-grade water. Then 3 μL of 10× reaction buffer and 2 μL of Klenow Fragment were added to the mixture, followed by incubation of 30 min at 37 °C. Next, 8 μL nuclease-free water, 10 μL adapter mix, 2 μL HP adapter, and 50 μL Blunt/TA DNA ligase mastermix were added, in this order, and incubated at 25 °C for 10 min. Finally, the ligated DNA was purified using His-tag Dynabeads combined with 141 μL EP buffer and 3 μL fuel mix. The sample was now ready to be loaded into a *MinION* device connected to a computer and with a flow cell inserted. The inserted flow cell would check the quality of the *MinION* nanopore within the device to assure satisfactory pore activity (Wang et al., 2015).

After the sample preparation and loading, the *MinION* was able to produce 118,052 sequence reads in a run time of four hours. The sequence was aligned to a prototypic reference genome previously produced and resulted in 100% identity coverage. As a result, the whole-genome sequence of an influenza virus was produced from the *MinION* nanopore sequencer in a fraction of the time it would have taken using older methods.

Wang and colleagues (2015) concluded that through the use of the *MinION* sequencer, major breakthroughs could be made in both the clinical and research world. The *MinION* sequencer could prove to be a useful tool in a multitude of labs, given its accuracy, speed, and accessibility. Since the *MinION* sequencer requires only a moderate specification laptop with an i7 CPU, 8 GB RAM, and 128 GB solid-state hard disk, it has an amazing potential to be used in research labs globally. Also due to its short run time of four hours, the *MinION* could have the potential to provide clinically useful information in a realistic time frame. It is even conceivable that investigators working at the site of an influenza pandemic or outbreak could analyze samples on-site and draw initial conclusions on subtype, reassortants, pathogenicity, and antiviral drug sensitivity (Barzon, Lavezzo, Costanzi, Franchin, Toppo, & Palù, 2013; Jones, 2017).

Conclusion

Health psychologists can greatly benefit from becoming more involved in genetics and applying genetic techniques to both clinical and research practices. New genetic technologies, such as the *MinION, NanoDrop*, and *next-generation sequencers* can make applying genetic techniques easier and more understandable to health psychologists. As previously stated, these genetics techniques have already contributed to the medical world and have shown the ability to significantly change future practices. This has been shown with *next-generation sequencing* being used to identify causative genes of diseases (Todd, et al., 2015), *NanoDrop* being used to identify *miRNA* in organic fluids and allowing for the early identification of diseases (Garcia-Elias, Alloza, Puigdecanet, Nonell, Tajes, Curado, et al., 2017), and *MinION* being used to sequence and reveal information about harmful viruses, such as influenza (Wang et al., 2015).

Genetic techniques assist health psychologists' research and aid in clinically assessing several mental illnesses. Furthermore, several clinical and research practices in health psychology can change drastically and allow for better insight into how to treat mental illnesses and how mental illnesses arise (Hyman, 2000). Genetic techniques can also assist health psychologists in ways not currently employed such as CRISPR-Cas9 (discussed elsewhere in this volume). As seen with already existing studies, the entire human genome is able to be assembled quickly and accurately due to these new genetic technologies, providing key genetic information useful for a variety of subject areas (Jain, et al., 2016).

References

Ashley, E. A. (2016). Towards precision medicine. *Nature Reviews Genetics*, *17*(9), 507–522. doi:10.1038/nrg.2016.86

Bamshad, M., Van Heest, A. E., & Pleasure, D. (2009). Arthrogryposis: A review and update. *The Journal of Bone and Joint Surgery-American Volume*, *91*(Supplement 4), 40–46. doi:10.2106/jbjs.i.00281

Barondes, S. H. (1999). An agenda for psychiatric genetics. *Archives of General Psychiatry*, *56*(6), 549–552. doi:10.1001/archpsyc.56.6.549

Bartel, D. P. (2009). MicroRNAs: Target recognition and regulatory functions. *Cell*, *136*(2), 215–233. doi:10.1016/j.cell.2009.01.002

Barzon, L., Lavezzo, E., Costanzi, G., Franchin, E., Toppo, S., & Palù, G. (2013). Next-generation sequencing technologies in diagnostic virology. *Journal of Clinical Virology*, *58*(2), 346–350. doi:10.1016/j.jcv.2013.03.003

Belanov, S. S., Bychkov, D., Benner, C., Ripatti, S., Ojala, T., Kankainen, M., et al. (2015). Genome-wide analysis of evolutionary markers of human influenza A(H1N1)pdm09 and A(H3N2) viruses may guide selection of vaccine strain candidates. *Genome Biology and Evolution, 7*(12), 3472–3483. doi:10.1093/gbe/evv240

Besser, J., Carleton, H. A., Gerner-Smidt, P., Lindsey, R. L., & Trees, E. (2018). Next-generation sequencing technologies and their application to the study and control of bacterial infections. *Clinical Microbiology and Infection, 24*(4), 335–341. doi:10.1016/j.cmi.2017.10.013

Callari, M., Dugo, M., Musella, V., Marchesi, E., Chiorino, G., Grand, M. M., et al. (2012). Comparison of microarray platforms for measuring differential MicroRNA expression in paired normal/cancer colon tissues. *PLoS One, 7*(9), e45105. doi:10.1371/journal.pone.0045105

Chidgeavadze, Z. G., Beabealashvilli, R. S., Atrazhev, A. M., Kukhanova, M. K., Azhayev, A. V., & Krayevsky, A. A. (1984). 2′, 3′-Dideoxy-3′ amlnonudeo 5′ .triphosphates are the terminators of DNA synthesis catalyzed by DNA polymerases. *Nucleic Acids Research, 12*(3), 1671–1686. doi:10.1093/nar/12.3.1671

Chung, A. C. K., Dong, Y., Yang, W., Zhong, X., Li, R., & Lan, H. Y. (2013). Smad7 suppresses renal fibrosis via altering expression of TGF-β/Smad3-regulated microRNAs. *Molecular Therapy, 21*(2), 388–398. doi:10.1038/mt.2012.251

Cuk, K., Zucknick, M., Heil, J., Madhavan, D., Schott, S., Turchinovich, A., et al. (2012). Circulating MicroRNAs in plasma as early detection markers for breast cancer. *International Journal of Cancer, 132*(7), 1602–1612. doi:10.1002/ijc.27799

Desjardins, P., & Conklin, D. (2010). NanoDrop microvolume quantitation of nucleic acids. *Journal of Visualized Experiments*, (1). doi:10.3791/2565

Desjardins, P., Hansen, J. B., & Allen, M. (2009). Microvolume protein concentration determination using the NanoDrop 2000c spectrophotometer. *Journal of Visualized Experiments*, (33). doi:10.3791/1610

Dillon, E. R., Bjornson, K. F., Jaffe, K. M., Hall, J. G., & Song, K. (2009). Ambulatory activity in youth with arthrogryposis. *Journal of Pediatric Orthopaedics, 29*(2), 214–217. doi:10.1097/bpo.0b013e3181990214

Duttagupta, R., Jiang, R., Gollub, J., Getts, R. C., & Jones, K. W. (2011). Impact of cellular miRNAs on circulating miRNA biomarker signatures. *PLoS One, 6*(6), e20769. doi:10.1371/journal.pone.0020769

Ebdon, J. R. (1992). Introduction to polymers (second edition) R. J. Young and P. A. Lovell Chapman and Hall, London, 1991. pp. 443, price £16.95. ISBN 0-412-30640-9 (PB); ISBN 0-412-30630-1 (HB). *Polymer International, 27*(2), 207–208. doi:10.1002/pi.4990270217

Fenoglio, C., Ridolfi, E., Galimberti, D., & Scarpini, E. (2012). MicroRNAs as active players in the pathogenesis of multiple sclerosis. *International Journal of Molecular Sciences, 13*(12), 13227–13239. doi:10.3390/ijms131013227

Filges, I., & Hall, J. G. (2013). Failure to identify antenatal multiple congenital contractures and fetal akinesia: Proposal of guidelines to improve diagnosis. *Prenatal Diagnosis, 33*(1), 61–74. doi:10.1002/pd.4011

Frankel, W. N., & Schork, N. J. (1996). Who's afraid of epistasis? *Nature Genetics, 14*(4), 371–373. doi:10.1038/ng1296-371

Garcia-Elias, A., Alloza, L., Puigdecanet, E., Nonell, L., Tajes, M., Curado, J., et al. (2017). Defining quantification methods and optimizing protocols for microarray hybridization of circulating microRNAs. *Scientific Reports, 7*(1). doi:10.1038/s41598-017-08134-3

Gilbert, W., & Maxam, A. (1973). The nucleotide sequence of the lac operator. *Proceedings of the National Academy of Sciences, 70*(12), 3581–3584. doi:10.1073/pnas.70.12.3581

Haliloglu, G., & Topaloglu, H. (2013). Arthrogryposis and fetal hypomobility syndrome. In *Handbook of clinical neurology* (pp. 1311–1319). Elsevier.

Hall, J. G. (2014). Congenital contractures: Emphasizing multiple congenital contractures: Arthrogryposis. In *Signs and symptoms of genetic conditions* (pp. 420–439). Oxford: Oxford University Press.

Heather, J. M., & Chain, B. (2016). The sequence of sequencers: The history of sequencing DNA. *Genomics, 107*(1), 1–8. doi:10.1016/j.ygeno.2015.11.003

Holley, R. W., Apgar, J., Everett, G. A., Madison, J. T., Marquisee, M., Merrill, S. H., et al. (1965). Structure of a ribonucleic acid. *Science, 147*(3664), 1462–1465. doi:10.1126/science.147.3664.1462

Horimoto, T., & Kawaoka, Y. (2005). Influenza: Lessons from past pandemics, warnings from current incidents. *Nature Reviews Microbiology, 3*(8), 591–600. doi:10.1038/nrmicro1208

Hughes, G. M., Gang, L., Murphy, W. J., Higgins, D. G., & Teeling, E. C. (2013). Using illumina next generation sequencing technologies to sequence multigene families inde novospecies. *Molecular Ecology Resources, 13*(3), 510–521. doi:10.1111/1755-0998.12087

Hyman, S. E. (2000). Mental illness. *Neuron, 28*(2), 321–323. doi:10.1016/s0896-6273(00)00110-0

Ikeda, S., Kong, S. W., Lu, J., Bisping, E., Zhang, H., Allen, P. D., et al. (2007). Altered microRNA expression in human heart disease. *Physiological Genomics, 31*(3), 367–373. doi:10.1152/physiolgenomics.00144.2007

Jain, M., Olsen, H. E., Paten, B., & Akeson, M. (2016). Erratum to: The Oxford nanopore MinION: Delivery of nanopore sequencing to the genomics community. *Genome Biology, 17*(1). doi:10.1186/s13059-016-1122-x

Jensen, S. G., Lamy, P., Rasmussen, M. H., Ostenfeld, M. S., Dyrskjøt, L., Ørntoft, T. F., et al. (2011). Evaluation of two commercial global miRNA expression profiling platforms for detection of less abundant miRNAs. *BMC Genomics, 12*(1). doi:10.1186/1471-2164-12-435

Johnson, B. T., & Acabchuk, R. L. (2018). What are the keys to a longer, happier life? Answers from five decades of health psychology research. *Social Science & Medicine, 196*, 218–226. doi:10.1016/j.socscimed.2017.11.001

Jones, R. P. (2017). Outbreaks of a presumed infectious pathogen creating on/off switching in deaths. *SSRN Electronic Journal*. doi:10.2139/ssrn.3011819

Kaplan, J.-C. (2010). The 2011 version of the gene table of neuromuscular disorders. *Neuromuscular Disorders, 20*(12), 852–873. doi:10.1016/j.nmd.2010.10.001

Lafond, K. E., Nair, H., Rasooly, M. H., Valente, F., Booy, R., Rahman, M., et al. (2016). Global role and burden of influenza in pediatric respiratory hospitalizations, 1982–2012: A systematic analysis. *PLoS Medicine, 13*(3), e1001977. doi:10.1371/journal.pmed.1001977

Lewis, B. P., Shih, I. H., Jones-Rhoades, M. W., Bartel, D. P., & Burge, C. B. (2003). Prediction of Mammalian MicroRNA targets. *Cell, 115*(7), 787–798. doi:10.1016/s0092-8674(03)01018-3

Li, Y., & Kowdley, K. V. (2012). MicroRNAs in common human diseases. *Genomics, Proteomics & Bioinformatics, 10*(5), 246–253. doi:10.1016/j.gpb.2012.07.005

Litman, R. M. (1976). Rosalind Franklin and DNA Anne Sayre. *BioScience, 26*(9), 572–572. doi:10.2307/1297278

Lu, H., Giordano, F., & Ning, Z. (2016). Oxford nanopore MinION sequencing and Genome assembly. *Genomics, Proteomics & Bioinformatics, 14*(5), 265–279. doi:10.1016/j.gpb.2016.05.004

Madoui, M.-A., Engelen, S., Cruaud, C., Belser, C., Bertrand, L., Alberti, A., et al. (2015). Genome assembly using nanopore-guided long and error-free DNA reads. *BMC Genomics, 16*(1). doi:10.1186/s12864-015-1519-z

Majczenko, K., Davidson, A. E., Camelo-Piragua, S., Agrawal, P. B., Manfready, R. A., Li, X., et al. (2012). Dominant mutation of CCDC78 in a unique congenital myopathy with prominent internal nuclei and atypical cores. *The American Journal of Human Genetics, 91*(2), 365–371. doi:10.1016/j.ajhg.2012.06.012

Maxam, A. M., & Gilbert, W. (1977). A new method for sequencing DNA. *Proceedings of the National Academy of Sciences, 74*(2), 560–564. doi:10.1073/pnas.74.2.560

McGuffin, P., Rijsdijk, F., Andrew, M., Sham, P., Katz, R., & Cardno, A. (2003). The heritability of bipolar affective disorder and the genetic relationship to unipolar depression. *Archives of General Psychiatry, 60*(5), 497. doi:10.1001/archpsyc.60.5.497

McMillin, M. J., Beck, A. E., Chong, J. X., Shively, K. M., Buckingham, K. J., Gildersleeve, H. I. S., et al. (2014). Mutations in PIEZO2 cause gordon syndrome, Marden-Walker syndrome, and distal arthrogryposis type 5. *The American Journal of Human Genetics, 94*(5), 734–744. doi:10.1016/j.ajhg.2014.03.015

Mitchell, P. S., Parkin, R. K., Kroh, E. M., Fritz, B. R., Wyman, S. K., Pogosova-Agadjanyan, E. L., et al. (2008). Circulating MicroRNAs as stable blood-based markers for cancer detection. *Proceedings of the National Academy of Sciences, 105*(30), 10513–10518. doi:10.1073/pnas.0804549105

Moldovan, L., Batte, K. E., Trgovcich, J., Wisler, J., Marsh, C. B., & Piper, M. (2014). Methodological challenges in utilizing miRNAs as circulating biomarkers. *Journal of Cellular and Molecular Medicine, 18*(3), 371–390. doi:10.1111/jcmm.12236

Murray, M. (2000). Levels of narrative analysis in health psychology. *Journal of Health Psychology, 5*(3), 337–347. doi:10.1177/135910530000500305

Nana-Sinkam, S. P., Hunter, M. G., Nuovo, G. J., Schmittgen, T. D., Gelinas, R., Galas, D., et al. (2009). Integrating the MicroRNome into the study of lung disease. *American Journal of Respiratory and Critical Care Medicine, 179*(1), 4–10. doi:10.1164/rccm.200807-1042pp

Padmanabhan, R., & Wu, R. (1972). Nucleotide sequence analysis of DNA. *Biochemical and Biophysical Research Communications, 48*(5), 1295–1302. doi:10.1016/0006-291x(72)90852-2

Parikh, V. N., & Ashley, E. A. (2017). Next-generation sequencing in cardiovascular disease. *Circulation, 135*(5), 406–409. doi:10.1161/circulationaha.116.024258

Perea, G., Navarrete, M., & Araque, A. (2009). Tripartite synapses: Astrocytes process and control synaptic information. *Trends in Neurosciences, 32*(8), 421–431. doi:10.1016/j.tins.2009.05.001

Ravenscroft, G., Sollis, E., Charles, A. K., North, K. N., Baynam, G., & Laing, N. G. (2011). Fetal akinesia: Review of the genetics of the neuromuscular causes. *Journal of Medical Genetics, 48*(12), 793–801. doi:10.1136/jmedgenet-2011-100211

Romero, N. B., & Clarke, N. F. (2013). Congenital myopathies. In *Handbook of clinical neurology* (pp. 1321–1336). Elsevier.

Sanger, F., Donelson, J. E., Coulson, A. R., Kössel, H., & Fischer, D. (1973). Use of DNA polymerase I primed by a synthetic oligonucleotide to determine a nucleotide sequence in phage f1 DNA. *Proceedings of the National Academy of Sciences, 70*(4), 1209–1213. doi:10.1073/pnas.70.4.1209

Sanger, F., Nicklen, S., & Coulson, A. R. (1977). DNA sequencing with chain-terminating inhibitors. *Proceedings of the National Academy of Sciences, 74*(12), 5463–5467. doi:10.1073/pnas.74.12.5463

Sauvage, V., Boizeau, L., Candotti, D., Vandenbogaert, M., Servant-Delmas, A., Caro, V., et al. (2018). Early MinION™ nanopore single-molecule sequencing technology enables the characterization of hepatitis B virus genetic complexity in clinical samples. *PLoS One, 13*(3), e0194366. doi:10.1371/journal.pone.0194366

Schaefer, A., Jung, M., Miller, K., Lein, M., Kristiansen, G., Erbersdobler, A., et al. (2010). Suitable reference genes for relative quantification of miRNA expression in prostate cancer. *Experimental and Molecular Medicine, 42*(11), 749. doi:10.3858/emm.2010.42.11.076

Shampo, M. A., & Kyle, R. A. (2002). Kary B. Mullis: Nobel laureate for procedure to replicate DNA. *Mayo Clinic Proceedings, 77*(7), 606. doi:10.4065/77.7.606

Shendure, J., Balasubramanian, S., Church, G. M., Gilbert, W., Rogers, J., Schloss, J. A., et al. (2017). DNA sequencing at 40: Past, present and future. *Nature, 550*(7676), 345–353. doi:10.1038/nature24286

Slaby, O. (2016). Non-coding RNAs as Biomarkers for colorectal cancer screening and early detection. In *Advances in experimental medicine and biology* (pp. 153–170). Springer International Publishing.

Todd, E. J., Yau, K. S., Ong, R., Slee, J., McGillivray, G., Barnett, C. P., et al. (2015). Next generation sequencing in a large cohort of patients presenting with neuromuscular disease before or at birth. *Orphanet Journal of Rare Diseases, 10*(1). doi:10.1186/s13023-015-0364-0

Ulbricht, T. L. V. (1964). General chemistry of purines and pyrimidines. In *Purines, pyrimidines and nucleotides* (pp. 4–29). Elsevier.

Wang, J., Moore, N. E., Deng, Y. M., Eccles, D. A., & Hall, R. J. (2015). MinION nanopore sequencing of an influenza genome. *Frontiers in Microbiology, 6.* doi:10.3389/fmicb.2015.00766

Watson, J. D., & Crick, F. H. C. (1974). Molecular structure of nucleic acids: A structure for deoxyribose nucleic acid. *Nature, 248*(5451), 765–765. doi:10.1038/248765a0

Wilbe, M., Ekvall, S., Eurenius, K., Ericson, K., Casar-Borota, O., Klar, J., et al. (2015). MuSK: A new target for lethal fetal akinesia deformation sequence (FADS). *Journal of Medical Genetics, 52*(3), 195–202. doi:10.1136/jmedgenet-2014-102730

Wu, R., & Kaiser, A. D. (1968). Structure and base sequence in the cohesive ends of bacteriophage lambda DNA. *Journal of Molecular Biology, 35*(3), 523–537. doi:10.1016/s0022-2836(68)80012-9

Yves, B. (2013). World Health Organization (WHO). In *Max Planck encyclopedia of public international law.* Oxford: Oxford University Press.

Zallen, D. T. (2003). Despite Franklin's work, Wilkins earned his nobel. *Nature, 425*(6953), 15. doi:10.1038/425015b

29

RESEARCH METHODOLOGY AND PSYCHONEUROIMMUNOLOGY

S. Chandrashekara

Overview

Psychoneuroimmunology is an exciting area that helps to connect the impact of patients' psychological well-being with a majority of the clinical situations. The immune response, in coordination with the neuroendocrine system, works to restore the homeostasis disturbed by physical, physiological and pathological factors (Chovatiya & Medzhitov, 2014). The interaction between the neuronal system and immune system has been well established, and the relationship is bidirectional (ThyagaRajan & Priyanka, 2012). The psychological process influences the neuronal system, and it has been demonstrated to alter the immune response. Reciprocally, many of the cytokines have been demonstrated to alter the psychological functions (Himmerich, Patsalos, Lichtblau, Ibrahim, & Dalton, 2019). *Cytokines* are small proteins secreted by cells involved in cell signaling and regulating a wide range of biological functions, including innate and acquired immunity. *Tumor necrosis factor alpha (TNF-α)*, a multifunctional proinflammatory *cytokine* secreted predominantly by monocytes or macrophages, has been noted to produce global depression in higher mental functions, whereas a few other *cytokines* have been demonstrated to enhance or activate brain function (Ma, Zhang, & Baloch, 2016). The response is not universally similar, having wider variations across individuals and far-reaching implications in health and disease prognosis. The impact or effect on the immune system and the relationship between mental stress and other changes can be studied under two broader perspectives. One is by analyzing the impact of a psychological state through psychoimmune epidemiological studies and their association in the development of *immune-mediated disease*, or the diseases where the immune system has a major role in the outcome, like infections and wound healing. The other method is direct assessment of different limbs of immune system function. The current chapter focuses on the standardized research methodology with reference to the immune system and briefly touches on intricacies of epidemiological studies.

Research in Practice

Immune System

The immune system is an all-pervasive organization composed of cells, proteins and organized structures. Based on the response, the immune system is divided into innate and adaptive responses. The innate response has lesser specificity in encountering the invading organism or particulate matter (*antigen*), and it does not retain memory of previous infections. The adaptive response is highly specific with memory of the antigens encountered (Mogensen, 2009). The immune system functions in a well-regulated hierarchical manner.

The organization of the immune system is divided into central organs and peripheral lymphoid or immune organs. The **central** or **primary organs** are bone marrow and thymus. These are the places where immune-competent cells develop, multiply and get selected or groomed to be **effector** cells (cells that can be differentiated into a form capable of modulating or effecting an immune response). **B cells** develop from bone marrow and the **T cells** from the thymus. Other cells, like neutrophils, eosinophils and others, also develop from marrow. The **peripheral system**, or **secondary lymphoid organs**, include the lymph nodes, spleen, liver, and organized lymphoid structures below the skin and mucosal membranes (e.g., Payer's patches). The secondary lymphoid structures are organized aggregates of the lymphocytes with other immune-competent cells, like endothelial and dendritic cells, and they form space for the interaction of *antigens* and the adaptive immune system.

Immune system responses are always driven by and for *antigens*. The innate immune response is the primary or early response and was previously considered nonspecific. But the current understanding suggests innate responses to be quasi-specific and can identify certain predefined patterns through pattern recognition receptors, which in turn trigger activation of specific pathways and *cytokines*. These innate cells present the *antigen* prepared from the invading microorganism or other proteins, which in turn activate the requisite adaptive immune response. The adaptive response is broadly classified as humoral and cell-mediated responses. The **humoral** response is predominantly *B-cell* driven, whereas the **cell-mediated immune** response is driven by *T cells*. However, as per recent understanding, significant interaction between both cell types is crucial for eliciting an immune response.

The disruption of immune function can occur at any point of its interaction, and the impact or the effect could be linear, but more often, it is multifaceted. The defects or impacts expected by any stressors or modification would include suppression (a negative effect), immune activation (a positive effect) and altered reaction (against self-autoimmunity or heightened response, allergic or hypersensitivity reaction). Thus, the assessment of impact on the immune system is often complicated by these nonlinear, multifaceted effects (Hall, Cruser, Podawiltz, Mummert, Jones, & Mummert, 2012). The components of the immune system that can be assessed are given in Figure 29.1. The hierarchical implications are also depicted in the figure. Epidemiological or clinical outcome studies indicate the overall impact on the immune system, since most of the time, the impact on the outcome is not a

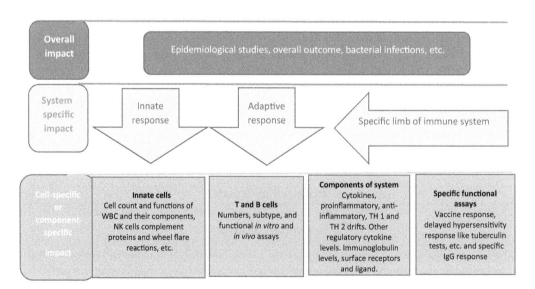

Figure 29.1 The assessable components of the immune system

consequence of a single pathway disruption. The specific component studies are intended to analyze the critical pathways disrupted and to choose the ideal one for critical analysis. Apart from the pathways or components, the method of analysis also influences the interpretation of the data. This will be discussed in the upcoming sections.

Cellular Compartment

Several studies have observed the impact of one's psychological status on cells participating in both innate and adaptive responses (Hall, et al., 2012). A majority of these cells, produced in bone marrow, later enter the circulation, where they are easily accessible. Some of these cells, like monocytes and lymphocytes, egress out of the circulation and localize in the tissues, where there is maximum inflammation. However, their functional assessment and enumeration are challenging, as they are not directly accessible. The cell components are assessed for both quality and quantity, and conducting both functional assays and enumeration techniques is required in certain cases. Functional assays are either *in vivo* or *in vitro*. Both have advantages and disadvantages and need to be chosen carefully, considering the hypothesis to be addressed.

The immune-competent cells are recognized based on a unique or a combination of the surface receptors called **cluster of differentiation (CD**; Ellmark, Woolfson, Belov, & Christopherson, 2008). Either the expression of some of the receptors or their quantity of expression suggests the activation or functional status of the cell. For instance, the number of **CD69**, a membrane-bound protein, is higher in activated *T cells* (Beeler, Zaccaria, Kawabata, Gerber, & Pichler, 2008). These are assessed using either **flow cytometry** (if in liquid state) or **immunohistochemistry/immunofluorescence** (if from solid tissue; Table 29.1). *Flow cytometry* is a popular cell biology technique used to evaluate the physical and chemical characteristics of a population of cells or particles. The technique uses physical characteristics of cells like size, refractile strength, fluorescence or beads for staining specific cell surfaces and internal molecules of interest using antibodies like **CD3** (a universal marker on *T cells*). *Immunohistochemistry* is a methodology that uses antibodies to test for certain antigens in a sample of tissue, while *immunofluorescence* uses antibodies chemically labeled with fluorescent dyes to visualize molecules. Many techniques are available to isolate cells using cell sorters and magnetic bead separations and the isolated cells can be used for studying the impact of psychological stress on alteration in functional characteristics (Table 29.1).

Cytokines as a Marker of Immune Status

Cytokines are **pleiotropic** (having multiple effects) in nature, and often two of them may have overlapping functions. Their levels in serum and plasma reflect the immunological status of an individual. However, they do not truly reflect the complete status of immune response. This limitation should always be considered while interpreting the *cytokine* data. Immune response could be highly localized or generalized. The *cytokine* transfers signals by three routes: *autocrine* (on the secreted cell), *paracrine* (neighboring or nearby cells through cell to cell) and *endocrine* (spill over into circulation and affect cells at a distance). Thus, the actions of a *cytokine* are localized when secreted in limited quantities, but when secreted excessively, the effect may be seen in other tissues. Another major challenge in *cytokine*-based research is high variability of the *cytokine* levels in the general population. The standard deviation is often greater than the mean of the study population. This can be circumvented by using log transformations and other statistical harmonization methods. Though the *cytokine* response is mainly triggered by *antigen* stimuli, minor, clinically insignificant infections may alter the *cytokine* profile, leading to a skewing of data.

The *cytokines* are estimated using **enzyme-linked immunosorbent assay (ELISA)** or **functional assays** like cytotoxicity stimulation and other functional alterations in the cells. The cell stimulation assay called **ELISPOT** may also be used. **Transcriptome analysis** and **gene expression analysis** are other

Table 29.1 Different Components of the Immune System and Assessment Methods

Cells	Immune limb	Methods	Interpretations and concerns
Total white cell count	Both innate and adaptive responses	• Simple counting • Differential counts • Ratio between neutrophil and lymphocyte count (NLR)	• Alters with inflammation trigger • Altered differential counts in eosinophilia, allergy, etc. • Increase in count, even in subtle inflammation • In chronic inflammation, it is a predictor of outcome
Neutrophil	Count and functional assay	• Cell count	• The numbers are altered depending on the inflammation and the underlying cause
		• Nitro blue tetrazolium (NBT) assay • Phagocytosis study • Migration • Stimulation study	• The tests suggest functional status of the neutrophil and technical standardization may influence the results
Lymphocyte	Count and functional assays	• Absolute count and subtype counts	• Varies depending on the underlying infection
		• Nonspecific or mitogen- induced stimulation assays like PHA, Con A, PWM	• Suggests the immune responsive status of the cells
		• Specific stimulation like tuberculin and other exposed antigens	• Suggests the previous sensitization and if done after a challenge and failure to have adequate response is an indication of an impaired specific response
T lymphocyte	Counts and functional assay	• Flowcytometry	• Number can be reduced or increased, depending on the immune system state • Can occur as a part of viral infections
		• Stimulation and inhibition tests using cell culture method with mitogens or specific antigens	• PBMCs stimulated with mitogens, followed by incorporation of radioactive thymidine (Taylor, Woods, & Hughes, 1957)
		• Flow-cytometric assay for specific cell-mediated immune response in activated whole blood (FASCIA)	• Has the advantage of not using radioactive thymidine and can identify the subtype of lymphocyte (Pala, Hussell, & Openshaw, 2000)
		• Cytokine secretion assay • Flow cytometry • ELISPOT	• Differential functioning of lymphocyte can be assessed (Pala, et. al., 2000)
CD8 cell subset	Counts and functional assays	• Number enumerated using flow cytometry and functional cytotoxicity assays (CD3 and CD8)	• Cytotoxicity assays are complicated, instead cytokine production on stimulation can be used. The later has certain limitations.

Cell type	Category	Method	Interpretation
CD4 cell subset		• Numbers enumerated using flow cytometry (CD3 and CD4)	• Suggests the immunological status
B lymphocyte	Counts and functional assays	• Flow cytometry- CD19/CD20 and subtypes using other specific markers	• The peripheral circulation count may represent the B-cell status
		• Immunoglobulin levels using nephelometry or turbidometry. • Antigen-specific immunoglobulin using immunoassays	• Immunoglobulin levels suggest approximate functioning of the limb • Specific Ig response against an antigen or vaccine suggests functionality
Th1 cells		• CD4 count and proportions	• Counted using the number of cells expressing the specific cytokine gene or by performing stimulation studies (Bryceson, Pende, Maul-Pavicic, Gilmour, Ufheil, Vraetz, et al., 2012)
Th2 cells	Counting and functional assays	• Flow cytometry	• Numbers indicate the tilt of immune response. The preferred method is use of functional assays (Bryceson, et al., 2012).
		• T-cell-mediated cytotoxicity of the specific (MHC compatible and antigenic peptide positive) target cell (exception being perforin deficiency).	• The assay suggests the number of cells
T regulatory cells	Counting the cells and functional assays	• Using flow cytometric studies based on intracellular fork-head box protein 3 expression in CD4+/CD25+ T cells (Graca, 2005).	• Increased Treg cell functions suggest adequate control or inhibition
		• Functions of Treg cells by assessing the inhibition of T cells • Activation marker expression or suppression of responder T-cell proliferation (Canavan, Afzali, Scottà, Fazekasova, Edozie, Macdonald, et al., 2012)	
NK cells	Counts and function, tissue-specific distribution	• NK Cells in peripheral blood and the tissues are performed	• The numbers suggest adequate NK cells
		• Cytotoxicity assay	• Even the NK cells are adequate. It indicates functional impairment

methods used for studying *cytokine* status and functions. *Transcriptome analysis* is the study of the complete set of RNA transcripts that are produced by the genome, and *gene expression analysis* involves the determination of patterns of gene expression at the level of genetic transcription.

Immunoglobulins, Complements and Acute-Phase Reactants

Immunoglobulins, complements and acute-phase reactants are proteins with a predefined role in immune reactions. **Immunoglobulins** are *antigen*-specific glycoprotein molecules belonging to five major classes with subcategories. *Immunoglobulins*, upon complexing with *antigen*, mediate the elimination of *antigens* through different biological reactions. Their levels represent the functioning of *humoral* immunity. Since antibody production needs *T helper* cells' participation, it also probably reflects the functional status of the *T cells*. *Antigen*-specific antibodies indicate more precisely the functioning of the entire limb.

Complements are a group of proteins that are activated through a cascade of protein interactions. They have multiple actions and are triggered by multiple stimuli involving immune complexes. Both quantitative and qualitative characteristics of these *complements* are assessed. **CH 50** is a functional assay for *complement* activity, whereas **turbidimetry** and **nephelometry** techniques are used to assess the levels of sub-components such as *C3*, *C4* and *C1q*. A reduction of *complements* can occur either due to a deficiency or because of **complement consumption** (excessive use, as seen in immune complex disease like systemic lupus erythematosus [SLE]), and hence need a careful interpretation.

C-reactive protein (CRP) and other products, secreted in response to inflammation or immune reactions, are called **acute-phase reactants**. The levels of these proteins are increased whenever there is any stress in homeostasis resulting in inflammation (interpretations are discussed in a later section).

Study Design and Use of Various Immunological Assessment Techniques

The interaction of the mind and the immune system is bidirectional. An excess of *cytokine* together with inflammation may cause depression; likewise, depression and mental stress may impair or alter the immune response. There are various observational studies evaluating the influence of various psychological functions on the development of immune-mediated diseases. It has been hypothesized that **autoimmune disease (AID)** develops as a consequence of psychological depression. An epidemiological study by Euesden, Danese, Lewis, and Maughan (2017) has evaluated the association between depression and *AID* and has concluded that it is a bidirectional relationship.

One of the major concerns in these types of studies is the presence of confounding variables. Both depression and *AID* are multifactorial and polygenic. Both environmental and genetic factors contribute to their development. One leading to the other is always a possibility. There is also literature to corroborate the development of *AID* in subjects with depression (Andersson, Gustafsson, Okkels, Taha, Cole, Munk-Jørgensen, et al., 2015).

Another major challenge confronted by such epidemiological studies is the difficulty in ascertaining the temporal relationship between the onset of the disease and the clinical diagnosis. The first encounter always happens at the point of diagnosis, and it may not necessarily coincide with the disease onset (Beiser, Erickson, Fleming, & Iacono, 1993). This is true even in insidious-onset *AID*, where autoantibodies appear years before the onset of the disease (Nielen, van Schaardenburg, Reesink, van de Stadt, van der Horst-Bruinsma, de Koning, et al., 2004). Such issues make the study more complex for establishing the temporal relationship between depression and *AID*. There are studies demonstrating the inverse relationship. Euesden and colleagues (2017) have attempted their level best to minimize the effect of confounding variables in their study design. There are very few experimental or interventional studies on this topic, and more research-based evidence is needed to carry them forward (Euesden, et al., 2017).

It is important to adopt the aforementioned immune techniques to study the influence of psychological data on a ***single limb*** or a specific pathway. The theoretical presumption can be obtained from epidemiological studies. There are epidemiological studies showing an increase in upper respiratory tract infections in the presence of stress (Pedersen, Zachariae, & Bovbjerg, 2010). The response differs with acute and chronic stressors (Cohen, Tyrrell, & Smith, 1993). The predilection and pattern of infections may suggest the possible *limbs* that are involved. For instance, increased skin or bacterial infections imply a ***neutrophil*** function, since they are the cells responsible for protection against bacterial skin infections. Evaluation of the functional status of the *neutrophil* by Tsukamoto and Machida (2012) has found that elderly with higher chronic stress have increased susceptibility to developing infections. The researchers used life event scores to measure chronic stress and correlated them to the functional status of the *neutrophil*. They observed that the counts do not change significantly as a response to chronic stress. They used two *functional assays*, namely ***phagocytosis*** and ***nitro blue tetrazolium (NBT)***, and found that the *neutrophil* functions are impaired in elderly males with chronic stress. The study has shown that the *neutrophil* function assays were influenced by gender and total protein (confounding factors; Tsukamoto, Suzuki, Machida, Saiki, Murayama, & Sugita, 2002). Probably to avoid such limitations in the subsequent study, the researchers (Tsukamoto & Machida, 2012) recruited only men (to avoid influence of gender) and measured total protein. Thus, the revised study design helps to reduce the influence of covariables and to assess the primary objective.

The study design should be precise with regard to subject selection and definition of inclusion and exclusion criteria. The generalizability of the study by Tsukamoto and Machida (2012) was limited, since the subjects were only males and it was a convenient sample. Choosing a specific gender and group of individuals from a single environment reduces the impact of sociodemographic factors on parameters, since *neutrophil* function is influenced by gender (Mallery, Zeligs, Ramwell, & Bellanti, 1986) as well as socioeconomic status (Takele, Adem, Getahun, Tajebe, Kiflie, Hailu, et al., 2016). If the study population is homogenous, though generalizability is a limitation, the required sample size can be reduced. Several other factors may influence the cause and effect. Stress is often associated with increased indulgence in smoking, drug abuse and other unhygienic habits, which could influence the immune response, as well the increased susceptibility to infections (Nielen, et al., 2004). The impact of a stressful situation also depends on the amount buffered by individual coping skills. Some traditional practices, including meditation, can help in coping with stress (Rao, Nagendra, Raghuram, Vinay, Chandrashekara, Gopinath, et al., 2008). So, the design of the study should address the possible influencing factors.

Stress may also affect different *limbs* of the immune system. The impact may vary depending on the type of stress, the situation, and other psychological parameters. To understand the pathobiology may require the evaluation of the specific *limb* linked to the psychological changes. The disturbance on ***NK cells*** (a type of cytotoxic lymphocyte critical to the innate immune system) may induce increased susceptibility to the viral infections. Impaired *immunoglobulin* production suggests either a *B-cell limb* defect or *T-cell* functional defect, since both *limbs* are involved in the production of *immunoglobulins*. Understanding such minute details assists in planning an intervention and predicting the possible mechanism of disease causation. There are many studies in this direction, and some of them are mentioned in Table 29.2. The immunological tests to evaluate the specific cells or immune process are selected based on the hypothesis.

Stress and anxiety have been shown to exacerbate or precipitate autoimmunity and inflammation. The markers of persistent inflammation or the activation of the immune system skewed towards inflammation are the key in assessment, though they may not completely represent the trigger. The design of our study, which tested the hypothesis of the role of psychological stressors as a trigger for *AID*, was mainly focused on the *cytokine* pattern during stress (i.e., the stress is proinflammatory, especially when not compensated for adequately). *Cytokines* level at a given point of time indicate the inflammatory

Table 29.2 Clinical Uses and Limitations of Various Immunological Methods

Methods	Specimen	Usefulness	Limitations
Detection in body fluid • ELISA • Multiplex cytokine assay • Flow beads assay	Serum or plasma, body fluid or soup of activation culture	Assessing the pattern of immune response	Reflect in systemic level and may not always represent a local milieu
Transcripts detection • *In situ* hybridization • Real time PCR • Northern blot	Cells of interest sorted by flowcytometric cell sorter or magnetic beads	Expression of genes as transcript and assists in predictive state	Not necessarily phenotypic
Single-cell cytokine production • ELISPOT • Intracytoplasmic staining (ICC)	Cells of interest from blood or other tissues	Characterizing different cells with their cytokine secretion, in contrast to ELISA	Very sensitive assay, may not necessarily indicate systemic status
Cytokine profiling • Proteomic • genomic	Cells of interest	Cytokine or their receptor genes assembly, and allelic variation and expression	The profile at baseline also indicates various alleles

status. TNF-α, **interleukin-2 (IL2)**, **interleukin-6 (IL6)** and **interferon gamma** are considered pro-inflammatory, whereas **interleukin-4 (IL4)** and **interleukin-10 (IL10)** are anti-inflammatory (Cavaillon, 2001). Based on this principle, we chose TNF-α, IL2 and IL4 for the assessment (Chandrashekara, Jayashree, Veeranna, Vadiraj, Ramesh, Shobha, et al., 2007). The study included a cohort of first-year medical students, divided into three groups, considering homogeneity and convenience: exam-taking students, middle-of-the-term students (no exams) and newly admitted students. The study demonstrated a change in the TNF-α status and its correlation to the stress or anxiety of the exam-taking students. The impact was influenced by the cause for anxiety and the coping skills available, measured through the Bell Adjustment Inventory. The differential response noted could be attributed to the TNF polymorphism (Chandrashekara, et al., 2007). We used only one *cytokine* to represent the pro-inflammatory group to reduce the limitations associated with the study design. The study design was cross-sectional and presumed the response to the situation under distress as uniform. The analysis of the outcome demonstrated a significant difference in the *cytokine* response, and the change, which correlated with the stress, was situation specific. In the initial hypothesis, we considered all stresses to enhance inflammation, and the three *cytokine* markers chosen failed to represent the expected changes. Though the present one is a good stress model, the cross-sectional study may not reliably show the changes, since other factors are likely to influence the TNF level. This is one of the major limitations of the study. Thus, it is paramount to consider all aspects while choosing the parameters as well as the subjects.

Inflammation: Psychological Status and Disease

Several studies have suggested the role played by persistent inflammation in the development of different lifestyle diseases like cardiovascular disease, diabetes, hypertension and cancer (Yılmaz, Umay, Gündoğdu, Karaahmet, & Öztürk, 2017). The inflammation is an end result of an immunological reaction arising due to a disturbed homeostasis. Measuring inflammation in a routine clinical practice is done by different laboratory and clinical measures. However, lots of standardizations are required in this field (Chandrashekara, 2014a). There are enough studies to suggest that psychological distress is the trigger for both short-term and chronic inflammation (Segerstrom & Miller, 2004). Even inflammatory flare has been demonstrated on exposure to acute stress in the presence of *AID*. Based on these facts, it is necessary to design and customize the studies related to inflammation. **Erythrocyte sedimentation rate (ESR)** and *CRP* are the two traditional markers used for measuring inflammation (Chandrashekara, 2014b). There are other sensitive markers like *cytokines IL6* and *TNF*, and their receptors and ligands (Cortez-Cooper, Meaders, Stallings, Haddow, Kraj, Sloan, et al., 2013b).

The conceptualized design should consider the confounding variables and other factors that can influence the inflammation. Moreover, it is crucial to choose the inflammatory biomarkers judiciously. Some of them may have a time lag before becoming apparent in the serum and may have a half-life longer than the trigger event. For instance, *CRP* is secreted within half an hour from the trigger event and has a half-life of 24 to 48 hours, whereas the elevation and normalization of *ESR* are longer and are 10 to 14 days. It is also important to consider scheduling the collection of the samples. For instance, if an acute stressor is to be tested, collection of blood for *ESR* and *CRP* immediately following stress may not reflect the true status (Zhou, Fragala, McElhaney, & Kuchel, 2010). The expression of **transcriptomes**, the set of all RNA molecules expressed in one cell or a cell population, is generally detected earlier than the detectable levels of *cytokines* (Steptoe, Willemsen, Owen, Flower, & Mohamed-Ali, 2001). Thus, the timing of sample collection, duration of stress and several other factors, including influence of diurnal propensity of the anti-inflammatory hormones like steroids, may alter the findings (Kunz-Ebrecht, Mohamed-Ali, Feldman, Kirschbaum, & Steptoe, et al., 2003).

Another interesting study by Carpenter, Gawuga, Tyrka, Lee, Anderson, and Price (2010) used *IL6* as one of the markers of inflammation. The author wanted to test the hypothesis of influence of childhood experience on the inflammatory response with *IL6* as a yardstick. The study would have addressed the hypothesis without much limitation, if the age and **body mass index (BMI)** of the selected subjects were also considered. However, the authors used statistical methods to negate the influence of *BMI* and age. The study demonstrated that the elevated *IL6* response is directly related to the impact of childhood maltreatment, and it can be argued as a secondary effect of obesity as well as reduced physical activity. The study noted a reduced or attenuated *IL6* response to stressors in individuals with higher physical activity (Gokhale, Chandrashekara, & Vasanthakumar, 2007). The selected cohort subjects were elderly, and those belonging to the higher *BMI* were predominantly females. Hence, one can reasonably question the association between the childhood maltreatment and higher *BMI* resulting in exaggerated *IL6* response. The study did not consider their physical activity status, which could have influenced the delta *IL6* changes. The study should have considered a significantly larger sample size and physical activity as a co-variable.

Quantifying the damages caused by inflammation, as well as the impact of it on different factors, has yet to be standardized. But a meticulous design can help to improve the accuracy of the results. All the possible variables that can influence the measured parameters such as genetic, adaptive and environmental factors need to be considered. In contrast to single immune pathway studies, the inflammation parameters measured are the end effect of the immune activation. The impact may also vary depending on the pathways. For instance, the influence of inflammation by different pathways on lipid profile differs significantly, though the end results are the same (Chandrashekara, Dhote, & Anupama, 2019).

Conclusion

Current Status and Future Implications

There is adequate evidence to suggest that the psychological status of a person influences the immune system functioning, the outcome of several diseases and can also be one of the factors responsible for the development or worsening of the disease (Nassau, Tien, & Fritz, 2008; Antoni, 2013). Some of the ongoing, proactive psychological intervention trials are focused on improving the outcome of diseases. Understanding the basic relationship between the mind and the immune system may assist in developing effective prevention strategies.

References

Andersson, N. W., Gustafsson, L. N., Okkels, N., Taha, F., Cole, S. W., Munk-Jørgensen, P., et al. (2015). Depression and the risk of autoimmune disease: A nationally representative, prospective longitudinal study. *Psychological Medicine, 45*(16), 3559–3569. https://doi.org/10.1017/S0033291715001488

Antoni, M. H. (2013). Psychosocial intervention effects on adaptation, disease course and biobehavioral processes in cancer. *Brain, Behavior, and Immunity, 30*(Supplement), S88–S98. https://doi.org/10.1016/j.bbi.2012.05.009

Beeler, A., Zaccaria, L., Kawabata, T., Gerber, B. O., & Pichler, W. J. (2008). CD69 upregulation on T cells as an in vitro marker for delayed-type drug hypersensitivity. *Allergy, 63*(2), 181–188. https://doi.org/10.1111/j.1398-9995.2007.01516.x

Beiser, M., Erickson, D., Fleming, J. A., & Iacono, W. G. (1993). Establishing the onset of psychotic illness. *The American Journal of Psychiatry, 150*(9), 1349–1354.

Bryceson, Y. T., Pende, D., Maul-Pavicic, A., Gilmour, K. C., Ufheil, H., Vraetz, T., et al. (2012). A prospective evaluation of degranulation assays in the rapid diagnosis of familial hemophagocytic syndromes. *Blood, 119*(12), 2754–2763. https://doi.org/10.1182/blood-2011-08-374199

Canavan, J. B., Afzali, B., Scottà, C., Fazekasova, H., Edozie, F. C., Macdonald, T. T., et al. (2012). A rapid diagnostic test for human regulatory T-cell function to enable regulatory T-cell therapy. *Blood, 119*(8), e57–e66. https://doi.org/10.1182/blood-2011-09-380048

Carpenter, L. L., Gawuga, C. E., Tyrka, A. R., Lee, J. K., Anderson, G. M., & Price, L. H. (2010). Association between plasma IL-6 response to acute stress and early-life adversity in healthy adults. *Neuropsychopharmacology: Official Publication of the American College of Neuropsychopharmacology, 35*(13), 2617–2623. https://doi.org/10.1038/npp.2010.159

Cavaillon, J. M. (2001). Pro- versus anti-inflammatory cytokines: Myth or reality. *Cellular and Molecular Biology (Noisy-Le-Grand, France), 47*(4), 695–702.

Chandrashekara, S. (2014a). C-reactive protein: An inflammatory marker with specific role in physiology, pathology, and diagnosis. *IJRCI, 2*(S1), SR3. doi:10.15305/ijrci/v2iS1/117

Chandrashekara, S. (2014b). Quantification of inflammation: Need and challenges. *IJRCI, 2*(S1), E1. doi:10.15305/ijrci/v2iS1/91

Chandrashekara, S., Dhote, S. V., & Anupama, K. R. (2019). The differential influence of immunological process of autoimmune disease on lipid metabolism: A study on RA and SLE. *Indian Journal of Clinical Biochemistry: IJCB, 34*(1), 52–59. https://doi.org/10.1007/s12291-017-0715-9

Chandrashekara, S., Jayashree, K., Veeranna, H. B., Vadiraj, H. S., Ramesh, M. N., Shobha, A., et al. (2007). Effects of anxiety on TNF-α levels during psychological stress. *Journal of Psychosomatic Research, 63*(1), 65–69. https://doi.org/10.1016/j.jpsychores.2007.03.001

Chovatiya, R., & Medzhitov, R. (2014). Stress, inflammation, and defense of homeostasis. *Molecular Cell, 54*(2), 281–288. https://doi.org/10.1016/j.molcel.2014.03.030

Cohen, S., Tyrrell, D. A., & Smith, A. P. (1993). Negative life events, perceived stress, negative affect, and susceptibility to the common cold. *Journal of Personality and Social Psychology, 64*(1), 131–140. Retrieved from https://psycnet.apa.org/doi/10.1037/0022-3514.64.1.131

Cortez-Cooper, M., Meaders, E., Stallings, J., Haddow, S., Kraj, B., Sloan, G., et al. (2013b). Soluble TNF and IL-6 receptors: Indicators of vascular health in women without cardiovascular disease. *Vascular Medicine (London, England), 18*(5), 282–289. https://doi.org/10.1177%2F1358863X13508336

Ellmark, P., Woolfson, A., Belov, L., & Christopherson, R. I. (2008). The applicability of a cluster of differentiation monoclonal antibody microarray to the diagnosis of human disease. In *Methods in Molecular Biology* (p. 439). Clifton, NJ.

Euesden, J., Danese, A., Lewis, C. M., & Maughan, B. (2017). A bidirectional relationship between depression and the autoimmune disorders: New perspectives from the national child development study. *PLoS One, 12*(3). doi:10.1371/journal.pone.0173015

Gokhale, R., Chandrashekara, S., & Vasanthakumar, K. C. (2007). Cytokine response to strenuous exercise in athletes & non-athletes-an adaptive response. *Cytokine, 40*(2), 123–127. https://doi.org/10.1016/j.cyto.2007.08.006

Graca, L. (2005). New tools to identify regulatory T cells. *European Journal of Immunology, 35*(6), 1678–1680. https://doi.org/10.1002/eji.200526303

Hall, J. M. F., Cruser, D., Podawiltz, A., Mummert, D. I., Jones, H., & Mummert, M. E. (2012). Psychological stress and the cutaneous immune response: Roles of the HPA axis and the sympathetic nervous system in atopic dermatitis and psoriasis. *Dermatology Research and Practice*. https://doi.org/10.1155/2012/403908

Himmerich, H., Patsalos, O., Lichtblau, N., Ibrahim, M. A. A., & Dalton, B. (2019). Cytokine research in depression: Principles, challenges, and open questions. *Frontiers in Psychiatry*, *10*(30). https://doi.org/10.3389/fpsyt.2019.00030

Kunz-Ebrecht, S. R., Mohamed-Ali, V., Feldman, P. J., Kirschbaum, C., & Steptoe, A. (2003). Cortisol responses to mild psychological stress are inversely associated with proinflammatory cytokines. *Brain, Behavior, and Immunity*, *17*(5), 373–383. https://doi.org/10.1016/S0889-1591(03)00029-1

Ma, K., Zhang, H., & Baloch, Z. (2016). Pathogenetic and therapeutic applications of Tumor Necrosis Factor-α (TNF-α) in major depressive disorder: A systematic review. *International Journal of Molecular Sciences*, *17*(5). https://doi.org/10.3390/ijms17050733

Mallery, S. R., Zeligs, B. J., Ramwell, P. W., & Bellanti, J. A. (1986). Gender-related variations and interaction of human neutrophil cyclooxygenase and oxidative burst metabolites. *Journal of Leukocyte Biology*, *40*(2), 133–146. https://doi.org/10.1002/jlb.40.2.133

Mogensen, T. H. (2009). Pathogen recognition and inflammatory signaling in innate immune defenses. *Clinical Microbiology Review*, *22*(2), 240–273. doi:10.1128/CMR.00046-08

Nassau, J. H., Tien, K., & Fritz, G. K. (2008). Review of the literature: Integrating psychoneuroimmunology into pediatric chronic illness interventions. *Journal of Pediatric Psychology*, *33*(2), 195–207. https://doi.org/10.1093/jpepsy/jsm076

Nielen, M. M. J., van Schaardenburg, D., Reesink, H. W., van de Stadt, R. J., van der Horst-Bruinsma, I. E., de Koning, M. H. M. T., et al. (2004). Specific autoantibodies precede the symptoms of rheumatoid arthritis: A study of serial measurements in blood donors. *Arthritis and Rheumatism*, *50*(2), 380–386. https://doi.org/10.1002/art.20018

Pala, P., Hussell, T., & Openshaw, P. J. (2000). Flow cytometric measurement of intracellular cytokines. *Journal of Immunological Methods*, *243*(1–2), 107–124. https://doi.org/10.1016/S0022-1759(00)00230-1

Pedersen, A., Zachariae, R., & Bovbjerg, D. H. (2010). Influence of psychological stress on upper respiratory infection: A meta-analysis of prospective studies. *Psychosomatic Medicine*, *72*(8), 823–832. doi:10.1097/PSY.0b013e3181f1d003

Rao, R. M., Nagendra, H. R., Raghuram, N., Vinay, C., Chandrashekara, S., Gopinath, K. S., et al. (2008). Influence of yoga on mood states, distress, quality of life and immune outcomes in early stage breast cancer patients undergoing surgery. *International Journal of Yoga*, *1*(1), 11–20. doi:10.4103/0973-6131.36789

Segerstrom, S. C., & Miller, G. E. (2004). Psychological stress and the human immune system: A meta-analytic study of 30 years of inquiry. *Psychological Bulletin*, *130*(4), 601–630.

Steptoe, A., Willemsen, G., Owen, N., Flower, L., & Mohamed-Ali, V. (2001). Acute mental stress elicits delayed increases in circulating inflammatory cytokine levels. *Clinical Science (London, England: 1979)*, *101*(2), 185–192. https://doi.org/10.1042/cs1010185

Takele, Y., Adem, E., Getahun, M., Tajebe, F., Kiflie, A., Hailu, A., et al. (2016). Malnutrition in healthy individuals results in increased mixed cytokine profiles, altered neutrophil subsets and function. *PLoS One*, *11*(8), e0157919. doi:10.1371/journal.pone.0157919

Taylor, J. H., Woods, P. S., & Hughes, W. L. (1957). The organization and duplication of chromosomes as revealed by autoradiographic studies using tritium-labeled thymidinee. *Proceedings of the National Academy of Sciences of the United States of America*, *43*(1), 122–128.

ThyagaRajan, S., & Priyanka, H. P. (2012). Bidirectional communication between the neuroendocrine system and the immune system: Relevance to health and diseases. *Annals of Neurosciences*, *19*(1), 40–46. doi:10.5214/ans.0972.7531.180410

Tsukamoto, K., & Machida, K. (2012). Effects of life events and stress on neutrophil functions in elderly men. *Immunity & Ageing: I & A*, *9*(13). Retrieved from https://immunityageing.biomedcentral.com/articles/10.1186/1742-4933-9-13#citeas

Tsukamoto, K., Suzuki, K., Machida, K., Saiki, C., Murayama, R., & Sugita, M. (2002). Relationships between lifestyle factors and neutrophil functions in the elderly. *Journal of Clinical Laboratory Analysis*, *16*(5), 266–272. https://doi.org/10.1002/jcla.10152

Yılmaz, V., Umay, E., Gündoğdu, İ., Karaahmet, Z. Ö., & Öztürk, A. E. (2017). Rheumatoid arthritis: Are psychological factors effective in disease flare? *European Journal of Rheumatology*, *4*(2), 127–132. doi:10.5152/eurjrheum.2017.16100

Zhou, X., Fragala, M. S., McElhaney, J. E., & Kuchel, G. A. (2010). Conceptual and methodological issues relevant to cytokine and inflammatory marker measurements in clinical research. *Current Opinion in Clinical Nutrition and Metabolic Care*, *13*(5), 541–547. doi:10.1097/MCO.0b013e32833cf3bc

30

NUDGE THEORY

Kelly Ann Schmidtke and Ivo Vlaev

Overview

To improve health-related behavior, interventionists have traditionally focused on providing people with financial incentives or information (Cecchini, Sassi, Lauer, Lee, Guajardo-Barron, & Chisholm, et al., 2010). The success of these interventions relies on their influencing the ways people reflectively think about their behavior. While these more traditional interventions can improve public health, their success is often limited (Hofmann, Friese, & Wiers, 2008). For example, despite large financial incentives and information-based campaigns, many people still consume too much alcohol and smoke cigarettes. Nudge theory pushes interventionists to consider the less reflective cognitive processes that also influence behavior (Marteau, Hollands, & Fletcher, 2012; Sheeran, Gollwitzer, & Bargh, 2013).

The cognitive processes that influence behavior are often called System 1 and System 2 (Anderson, Bothell, Byrne, Douglass, Lebiere, & Qin, 2004; Evans & Stanovich, 2013). *System 1* is broadly assumed to be a faster, less reflective, and more intuitive process, or collection of processes. *System 2* is broadly assumed to be a slower and more reflective process. Traditional interventions focus on *System 2*. While interventionists have long acknowledged the influence of *System 1*, they have tended to think of *System 1* as narrowly driving undesirable behavior (Hofmann, et al., 2008). Nudge theory helps interventionists consider using *System 1* processes to increase desirable behavior (Marteau, Ogilvie, Roland, Suhrcke, & Kelly, 2011; Marteau, et al., 2012).

Nudge theory was popularized by Thaler and Sunstein (2008) in their book *Nudge: Improving Decisions about Health, Wealth and Happiness*. Research guided by nudge theory builds on previous behavioral economic research around heuristics and biases (Blumenthal-Barby & Krieger, 2015; Cialdini, 2007; Kahneman & Tversky, 1979; Kahneman, 2011). According to Thaler and Sunstein, a *nudge* is "any aspect of the choice architecture that alters people's behavior in a predictable way without forbidding any options or significantly changing their economic incentives" (2008, p. 6). Broadly, nudge interventions provide situational cues that modify cognitive processes to increase desirable behavior in real-world settings (Rossen, Hurlstone, & Lawrence, 2016).

Nudge theory has been well received by many people and governments (Loewenstein, Asch, Friedman, Melichar, & Volpp, 2012; OECD, 2018; Thaler & Sunstein, 2003). In the United Kingdom, Cameron's coalition government created the Behavioral Insights Team to help policy makers' innovative ways of encouraging, enabling, and supporting people to make better choices without "banning or significantly restricting their choices" (Department of Health, 2010, p. 30). In 2010, the team developed an empirically informed and practically useful framework, called MINDSPACE

(Behavioral Insights Team, 2011; Dolan, Hallsworth, Halpern, King, & Vlaev,. 2010; Dolan, Halls-worth, Halpern, King, Metcalfe, & Vlaev, 2012). Theoretically, MINDSPACE brings together the wide range of tools that influence behavior, primarily through *System 1* processes (Vlaev, King, Dolan, & Darzi, 2016). Practically, interventionists can use MINDSPACE as a checklist to consider each tool use. Each letter in MINDSPACE stands for a different tool (see Table 30.1).

The next five sections more fully explore the application of the following MINDSPACE tools in real-world settings: *Defaults*, *Incentives*, *Norms*, *Salience*, and *Commitments*. While each section focuses on a single tool, note that the tools are largely used in combination to influence behaviors or

Table 30.1 MINDSPACE Tools and Brief Descriptions

Letter	Tool	Brief Description
M	Messenger	The perceived formal or informal authority of a person/organization telling people to change or maintain their behavior. Messengers who are perceived to have greater authority are more likely to influence other people's behavior.
I	Incentive	Perceived features of an outcome influence people's behaviors (e.g., the probability of obtaining that outcome), the delay to obtaining that outcome, and the change in value that outcome causes from a reference point. Incentives that are more probable, nearer in time, and result in greater changes from a reference point are more likely to influence people's behavior.
N	Norms	Sociocultural beliefs about the prevalence or acceptability of behaviors influence people's behaviors. Norms can be implicit or explicitly acknowledged. Behaviors that are perceived to be more prevalent or acceptable are more likely to be initiated.
D	Defaults	The presence of choice options initiated when no alternative option is actively selected influences resultant choice behavior. Default options are more likely to be initiated when alternative options are more difficult to select or when the outcomes of all options are uncertain.
S	Salience	Situational cues that draw our attention are more likely to influence our behavior. More salient situational cues (i.e., cues that are more novel, immediately accessible, or relevant) are more likely to draw people's attention and thereby influence their behavior.
P	Priming	Situational cues (e.g., sights, words, and other sensations) can trigger behaviors without the need for people's conscious intentions or awareness (Papies, 2016). The more often a set of situational cues and behaviors have been paired in the past, the more likely those cues are to trigger (i.e., "prime") those behaviors in the future.
A	Affect	Emotional reactions and moods influence people's behavior. Regardless of their valence, high-energy emotions and moods (e.g., tenseness and excitability) are more likely to encourage active behaviors than low-energy emotions and moods (e.g., bored and calm). In addition, people in good moods tend to make more unrealistically optimistic judgements, while those in bad moods tend to make more unrealistically pessimistic judgements.
C	Commitment	People seek to be consistent with their public promises. The very act of writing a commitment, along with an action plan describing how the commitment can be fulfilled, can increase the likelihood of the commitment being fulfilled. In addition, evoking a sense of 'fairness' via an implicit social contract can increase the likelihood of reciprocal social behaviors.
E	Ego	Beliefs about how particular behaviors may influence people's self-image influences their behavior. Behaviors that people believe support a positive and consistent self-image are more likely to be initiated.

to bolster the effectiveness of more traditional interventions. Then, the present chapter will explore and discuss the overall strengths and weaknesses of research inspired by nudge theory. The chapter concludes with recommendations to support emerging research.

Research in Practice

Study 1: Using Defaults to Increase Organ Donation

Background

The term **defaults** describes pre-set actions taken when an alternative action is not specified (Thaler & Sunstein, 2008). When a *default* is set up by a messenger the decision-maker trusts, they may interpret it as a desirable recommendation (e.g., a default national health insurance option set up by one's preferred political party; McKenzie, Liersch, & Finkelstein, 2006). Alternatively, when a *default* is set up by a messenger the decision-maker does not trust, they may make an active choice against it (e.g., a default national health insurance option set up by one's nonpreferred political party; Brown & Krishna, 2004).

Defaults are more likely to be selected when alternative options are impractical, difficult to select, or their outcomes are more uncertain. For instance, many children's meals contain *default* side dishes, like French fries. While parents can often substitute the *default* with a free alternative, many do not. Changing the *default* side dish to a healthier option, like fruit, can help parents easily select healthier meals for their children (Anzman-Frasca, Mueller, Sliwa, Dolan, Harelick, Roberts, et al., 2015). As another example, many companies ask employees to select between different retirement plans. As people's future needs are often uncertain, providing a *default* option ensures more workers save some money for retirement (i.e., automatic enrollment in defined contribution plan; Bernartzi & Thaler, 2007).

In many contexts, *defaults* are necessary because people and organizations need to know what to do with others who fail to make any active choice. For example, health insurers may offer clients a choice to either a) pick up their own medication from a pharmacy or b) have their medication mailed to their home. Not making the medication available is not an option anyone would prefer, and so the insurer needs to know what to do for people who do not make an active choice. In this situation, Beshears, Choi, Laibson, and Madrian (2019) constructed the *default* option to encourage active choice (i.e., clients who did not make an active choice had to pick up their medication from a pharmacy without financial subsidies). Encouraging active choice is not always feasible. For example, when people die at a hospital, should hospitals assume that they 'want to' or 'do not want to' donate their organs? In many countries, people who have not made an active choice to donate their organs (e.g., signed a registry) are assumed not to want to donate their organs. The following study assesses the effects of switching the *default* in national organ donation schemes.

Study

Johnson and Goldstein (2003) randomized 161 online participants from the United States to one of three conditions. The Opt-in group's participants were asked to imagine moving to a state where the *default* status was not to be an organ donor. They were then asked to either confirm or change their status. The Opt-out group's participants were asked to imagine moving to a state where the *default* status was to be an organ donor. They were then asked to either confirm or change their status. The Neutral group's participants were asked to actively choose either wanting to or not wanting to be an organ donor. The researchers compared the percentage of participants in each group whose responses suggested their consenting to be donors. In addition, the researchers compared real-world donor consent rates in European countries with opt-in and opt-out policies.

Participants in the Opt-in group were the least likely to consent to organ donors (42%), followed by the Neutral group (79%), and the Opt-out group (82%). The Neutral and Opt-out groups' consent rates were significantly higher than the Opt-in group's rates and did not differ from each other. In the real-world data, the difference was even larger. Specifically, the consent rates in Opt-in countries ranged from 4% in Denmark to 28% in The Netherlands, while the consent rates in Opt-out countries ranged from 86% in Sweden to 99.98% in Austria.

Johnson and Goldstein's (2003) findings suggest that the Opt-in and Opt-out policies dramatically influence the percentage of people assumed to be consenting organ donors. The results of the online study suggest that people's true preferences (the Neutral condition) are better captured by Opt-out than Opt-in policies. This finding pushes countries to take into account citizens' true preferences when designing *default* policies. Another implication of this study is the push for researchers to use real-world data. While many researchers may have been content reporting just the online survey's findings, this study pushes other researchers to tell a more compelling story about whether findings from online studies generalize to real-world settings.

Study 2: Using Incentives to Help People Quit Smoking

Background

The term **incentives** describes external cues that motivate behavior. There are some limits on the types of incentives that are considered nudges. According to Thaler and Sunstein, nudges should not include options that significantly alter people's economic incentives (2008). Further, Halpern (a founding member of the United Kingdom's Behavioral Insights Team) states that nudges should guide behavior "ideally without the need for heavy financial incentives or sanctions" (2015, p. 22). Given these statements, it is clear that large monetary benefits or charges are not nudges per se, but precisely how large a monetary nudge can be is unclear. For example, to reduce repeat teenage pregnancies, teenage parents were given 1.00 USD a day for not becoming pregnant again (Brown, Saunders, & Dick, 1999); is that a nudge? As another example, to reduce reliance on single-use plastic shopping bags, a 0.05 GPB charge was introduced on such bags (Thomas, Sautkina, Poortinga, Wolstenholme, & Whitmarsh, 2019); Is that a nudge? This is an interesting debate, but largely outside the scope of the present chapter, which focuses on nonmonetary nudge incentives.

From a normative perspective, the motivating value of *incentives* should be stable across time and circumstance. However, from a descriptive perspective, the motivating values of *incentives* change (DellaVigna, 2009). Interventions informed by nudge theory draw from the descriptive perspective. Previous research reveals several factors that change the motivating value of incentives. For example, the perceived value of a reward decreases with the time to its receipt (i.e., the delayed discounting effect; Green, Fry, & Myerson, 1994). Drawing on the delayed discounting effect, food vending machines could be altered so that healthy options are released immediately and unhealthy options are released after a 25-second delay. This simple alteration may decrease the perceived value of unhealthy choices and thereby encourage healthier choices at these vending machines (Appelhans, 2018).

As another example, the perceived value of items changes as a function of *framing*; here *framing* refers to when items are presented as benefits or losses (Rothman & Salovey, 1997; Tversky & Kahneman, 1981). When a good outcome is less certain, loss-framed messages tend to be more persuasive (e.g., encouraging health screenings; Banks, Salovey, Greener, Rothman, Moyer, Beauvais, et al., 1995). In contrast, when a good outcome is more certain, gain-framed messages tend to be more persuasive (e.g., encouraging people to stop smoking). The following study compares the effectiveness of factually equivalent but differently framed messages on whether people continue to abstain from smoking.

Study

Toll, O'Malley, Katulat, Wu, Dubin, Latimer, et al. (2007) randomized 258 smokers at a community health center to one of two groups. Over a seven-week period, all participants received smoking cessation medication and promotional quit-smoking materials (e.g., water bottles and pamphlets). Participants in the gain-framed message group saw videos about their chances of success and their promotional materials contained messages such as, "When you quit smoking: You take control of your health. You save your money. You look healthy. You feel healthy" (Table 30.1, p. 537). Participants in the loss-framed message group saw videos about their chances of failure and their promotional materials contained messages such as, "If you continue smoking: You are not taking control of your health. You waste your money. You look unhealthy. You feel unhealthy" (Table 30.1, p. 537). Participants returned every two weeks to complete surveys and to refill their medications. The researchers compared each group's time to relapse and the percentage of participants who successfully abstained from smoking six months after the intervention.

Participants in the gain-framed message group reported significantly longer times to relapse than participants in the loss-framed message group. Follow-up analyses suggest that women experienced a greater effect of message framing than men. Six months after the intervention, more participants in the gain-framed message group had abstained from smoking (24%) than did those in the loss-framed message group (17%), but this difference only approached being significant.

All participants in Toll, et al.'s (2007) study received stop-smoking medication. The point here is that nudges can complement and improve the effectiveness of existing treatments, like medication, at little cost because many such treatments already include messages or at least instructions. Thoughtful consideration for how these messages and instructions are framed can influence treatment outcomes.

Study 3: Using Norms to Decrease University Student Drinking

Background

Social norms refers to socially determined explicit or implicit beliefs about the acceptability or prevalence of behaviors. In many cases, *social norms* help people live healthfully. For example, it is a *social norm* not to eat ice cream before 10:00 a.m., and very few people do so in public. However, in other cases, *social norms* lead people to behave in unhealthful ways. For example, many people overestimate university students' approval and consumption of alcohol and accordingly perceive excessive alcohol consumption to be more acceptable and prevalent than it actually is (Borsari & Carey, 2001).

The *social norms* approach posits that correcting misperceptions about alcohol consumption at university should decrease alcohol consumption in that setting (Berkowitz, 2005; Perkins & Berkowitz, 1986). The *social norms* approach can be implemented through targeted mechanisms. A less targeted mechanism might include social marketing (e.g., placing posters about alcohol use in student dormitories; Haines & Spear, 1996; Johansson, Collin, Mills-Novoa, & Glider, 1999). A more targeted mechanism might include selecting students that score highly on an alcohol inventory and sending them personalized normative feedback (e.g., tailored communications about one's alcohol consumption compared to others; Lewis & Neighbors, 2015).

The success of the *social norms* approach is mixed (Dotson, Dunn, & Bowers, 2015; Foxcroft, Moreira, Almeida Santimano, & Smith, 2015). Wechsler, Nelson, Lee, Seibring, Lewis, and Keeling (2003) note various issues that could explain unreplicated positive findings. For instance, social marketing interventions may unwittingly encourage students who drink less alcohol than advertised to start drinking more. The use of more targeted interventions should mitigate this issue. A second issue is that cross-sectional survey evaluations may unintentionally recruit students with different characteristics before and after the intervention who are more or less likely to drink regardless of the intervention. Surveying the same students before and after the intervention should mitigate this issue. The following study compares the effectiveness of different types of personalized normative feedback on university students' alcohol consumption and information-seeking behaviors.

Study

Taylor, Vlaev, Maltby, Brown, and Wood (2015) recruited university students to take part in an alcohol-related study. The participants first completed a survey that contained questions about their drinking and demographics, along with the Alcohol Use Disorders Identification Test. After receiving 146 participants' responses, the research team randomly allocated the 101 participants whose Alcohol Use Test scores indicated excessive drinking to one of four groups. Participants in each group received a different email message once a week for four continuous weeks. The Absolute Only group's email informed participants of gender-specific maximum recommendations, without reference to their personal drinking behavior. The Absolute Comparison group's email compared participants' personal drinking with the gender-specific maximum recommendations. The Mean Comparison group's email compared participants' personal drinking to the gender-specific average drinking from all 146 participants. Lastly, the Rank Comparison group's email stated participants' personal drinking as a percentile rank of gender-specific drinking from all 146 participants.

In addition to all groups' allocated messages, the fourth email contained a hyperlink to a post-intervention survey. The post-intervention survey asked participants how many alcohol units they consumed the previous week and then gave participants the opportunity to request additional information from three sources, including a) expert recommendations, b) websites about alcohol consumption, and c) contact details for services designed to support people concerned about their own or other's alcohol consumption. The researchers compared the participants' baseline and post-intervention alcohol consumption across time and their tendencies to seek information between groups.

Regarding alcohol consumption across time, all groups' participants reported consuming significantly less alcohol post-intervention. Regarding information seeking between groups, participants in the Rank Comparison group were more likely to request at least one type of information than other groups. Supplementary tests revealed that participants in the Rank Comparison group were more likely to request the contact details for support services than those in other groups.

Taylor, et al.'s (2015) findings support that many types of personalized social normative messages can reduce university students' alcohol consumption. In addition, they found that some messages are more effective at getting students to request additional stop-smoking information. Specifically, emails that informed students of their rank-order alcohol consumption encouraged more students to seek helpful information, such as contact information to access support services. This is not a small feat, as encouraging people who consume too much alcohol to access support services is often a necessary first step to their obtaining help provided by more traditional interventions.

Study 4: Using Salience to Decrease Hospital Do Not Attend Rates

Background

Salience describes an attribute of information such that it appears more or less prominent or important (Senter, 2010). *Salience* is influenced by perceptual and cognitive factors. **Perceptual salience** describes information that is more readily perceived independent of one's previous experience and knowledge (Caduff & Timpf, 2008). For example, one red dot in a cluster of 99 different-colored dots is less salient visually than one red dot in a cluster of 99 black dots (Treisman & Gelade, 1980). **Cognitive salience** describes information that is more available in memory that is dependent on one's previous experience and knowledge (Caduff & Timpf, 2008). For example, in a noisy environment one's own name is more readily noticed than most other words (Moray, 1959).

The phrase "what you see is all there is" broadly describes how more salient information is more likely to influence people's behavior than less salient or absent information (Kahneman, 2011). For example, when presented with a choice between two packages of meat, one 80% fat and one 20% lean, people largely preferred the 20% lean package (Levin & Johnson, 1984). This large preference is not rational, as a package marked "80% fat" has the same fat contents as a package marked "20% lean." Plausibly labeling packages as 80% fat made the negative attribute (i.e., fat content) more salient than the unmentioned positive attribute (i.e., lean content) and the reverse for the 20% lean package.

Price is a salient feature of many consumer products. People use price as a simplifying strategy to choose between similar options (Hoyer, Pieters, & MacInnis, 2013), and when price is less salient, it is less likely to influence behavior. For example, most people in the United Kingdom receive medical treatment free at the point of care via its National Health Service (NHS), and they never see how much their care costs (van Boxel, van Duren, van Boxel, Gilbert, Gilbert, & Appleton, 2016). This unawareness of price likely contributes to overuse of and noncompliance with some NHS services. To explore the implications of making NHS cost information more salient, the following study compares the effectiveness of different text-message reminders on the percentage of patients that do not attend their hospital appointments.

Study

In Hallsworth, Berry, Sanders, Sallis, King, Vlaev, et al.'s (2015) study, 10,111 patients scheduled for an outpatient hospital appointment received a text message reminding them of their appointment's location, date, and time, along with one of four additional pieces of information selected at random. The Standard group's text told patients that "To cancel or rearrange call the number on your appointment letter" (p. 3). The Easy Call group's text told patients the phone number: "To cancel or rearrange call [phone number]" (p. 3). The Social Norms group's text told patients that "9 out of 10 people attend" their appointments (p. 3). The Cost group's text increased the *salience* of the cost information by telling patients that "Not attending costs NHS £160 approx" (p. 3). The researchers compared the percentage of patients in each group that attended as scheduled or called to cancel/rearrange.

Regarding the do not attends, the lowest rate was in the Cost group (8.4%), followed by the Easy Call group (9.8%), Social Norms group (10.0%), and Standard group (11.1%). The difference between the Cost and Standard groups was significant. Regarding calls to cancel or rearrange, the highest rate was in the Social Norm group (10.1%), followed by the Easy Call group (9.7%), Cost group (9.6%), and Standard group (8.8%). The difference between the Social Norms and Standard groups was significant.

Compared to many nudge studies, Hallsworth, et al.'s (2015) study procured a very large sample size. This accomplishment pushes other studies to follow suit, as without a large sample size, meaningfully significant effects may not be found. Also notable is the fact that the nudges were created using existing materials at that hospital (a text-message service) and evaluated using regularly collected data (hospital attendance records). This pushes other organizations to follow suit by continuing to evaluate and improve the services they offer in a feasible fashion.

Study 5: Using Commitments to Increase Vaccination Uptake

Background

Commitment describes a sense of obligation to a task or idea. *Commitments* can be more or less formal. For example, employment contracts are formal, legally binding *commitments* that influence work behavior. Less formal *commitments* might involve friends resolving to quit smoking together. To increase the effectiveness of a less formal *commitment*, one could write their commitment down or agree to an adverse consequence if they do not follow through (Giné, Karlan, & Zinman, 2010). Of course, not all commitments need to be in writing to be effective. Indeed, some *commitments* are implicit arrangements that maintain or bolster positive social relations (Gilbert, 2006).

Without sufficiently strong *commitments*, people often fail to realize their goals (Ariely & Wertenbroch, 2002; Webb & Sheeran, 2006). For example, only about half of people who resolve to change their behavior on New Year's Day self-report successfully continuing to do so six months later (Norcross, Mrykalo, & Blagys, 2002). Making a sufficient *commitment* typically entails not only gathering sufficient motivation to achieve a goal but also sufficient knowledge and materials (Michie, van Stralen, & West, 2011). Encouragingly, people who report greater readiness to change their behavior on New Year's Day are more likely to report continued success six months later (Norcross, Mrykalo, & Blagys, 2002).

Pre-commitment contracts are often used to increase people's goal achievement (Rogers, Milkman, & Volpp, 2014). These contracts can help people develop implementation plans that specify where, when, and how they will perform healthful behaviors (Hagger, Luszczynska, de Wit, Benyamini, Burkert, Chamberland, et al., 2016). For example, to improve children's dietary behavior, parents could specify what they will do, when they will start, and how they will overcome likely barriers (Gardner, Sheals, Wardle, & McGowan, 2014). The following study assesses the effectiveness of a *pre-commitment contract* designed to increase the number of workers that received their annual influenza vaccination.

Study

Milkman, Beshears, Choi, Laibson, and Madrain (2011) randomized 3,272 employees from a regional utility firm in the United States to receive one of three letters reminding them to receive their free annual on-site influenza vaccination. The Control letter only informed workers where and when the flu shot was freely available. In addition to the information in the Control letter, the Date Plan letter asked workers to write down the date they planned to attend. Lastly, in addition to the information in the Control letter, the Date+Time Plan letter asked workers to write down the date and time they planned to attend. Note that as regional providers are made up of multiple sites, some sites were able to offer vaccinations on more days and times. The researchers compared the percentage of workers in each group who received the vaccination on-site.

Participants in the Control group were the least likely to receive the vaccination (33.1%), followed by the Date Plan group (35.6%), and Date+Time Plan group (37.1%). The difference between the Control and Date Plan group was not significant, but the difference between the Control and Date+Time Plan group was. Supplementary analyses revealed that the difference between the Control and Date+Time Plan groups were largest at sites where the vaccination was only available one day.

Milkman, et al.'s (2011) study is notable for the same two reasons given for Hallsworth, et al.'s (2015) study. Specifically, Milkman et al. procured a very large sample size and used materials and data collection methods that were already available. As previously mentioned, these implications push other companies to follow suit with a feasibly large number of participants and readily available materials to enhance existing and often more traditional interventions.

Strengths/Limitations

The strengths and limitations of nudge theory can be appreciated by highlighting two ways nudge theory is understood a) as an academically verifiable theory and b) as a call to generalize already validated, empirical findings to real-world settings. The academic perspective is largely unsatisfying because the term "nudge" is imprecisely defined, and many real-world studies lack methodological rigor. Regarding the first reason, Thaler and Sunstein's original definition of nudge is not precise (2008, p. 6; for further discussion about the imprecision of the nudge definition see: Hansen, 2016; Marteau, et al., 2011). This imprecise definition has led to many new interventions being called nudges when they are simply informed by behavioral economics (Schmidtke, Nightingale, Reeves, Gallier, Vlaev, Watson, et al., 2019; Selinger & Whyte, 2011). To better guide what is or is not a nudge, Hollands, Shemilt, Marteau, Jebb, Kelly, Nakamura, et al. (2013) put forth the following operational definition:

[Nudge interventions] involve altering the properties or placement of objects or stimuli within micro-environments with the intention of changing health-related behavior. Such interventions are implemented within the same micro-environment as that in which the target behavior is performed, typically require minimal conscious engagement, can in principle influence the behavior of many people simultaneously, and are not targeted or tailored to specific individuals.

(p. 3)

While Holland et al.'s definition of a nudge is more precise, its acceptance is likely limited by what it excludes. For example, the definition restricts nudges to interventions that influence health-related behavior, excluding many non-health-related interventions (e.g., using *commitments* to increase honest reporting on tax and insurance forms; Shu, Mazar, Gino, Ariely, & Bazerman, 2012). The definition also restricts nudges to nontargeted alterations of micro-environments. While changing the *default* for national organ donation schemes certainly fits this definition (Johnson & Goldstein, 2003), it is less certain that sending personalized emails encouraging students to consume less alcohol does (Taylor, et al., 2015).

The methodological rigor of many studies informed by nudge theory is also lacking. This is in part a consequence of their applied nature. Indeed, it is often infeasible or unethical to evaluate the effectiveness of a nudge by randomizing large numbers of participants to different experimental groups, including a "no-treatment" control group. As such, many nudge interventions are designed and implemented using a kitchen-sink approach, evaluated with small numbers of nonrandomized participants, and finally reported with a number of caveats about the context within which they were implemented (Bovens, 2010; Hauser, Gino & Norton, 2018; Science and Technology Committee, 2014). These limitations restrict the academic community's ability to make general causal inferences about particular nudges.

The second understanding of nudge theory, as a call to generalize already validated empirical findings to real-world settings, is easier to grasp. Indeed, a huge strength of nudge theory has been its ability to bring long-standing psychological findings into applied practice. At least part of nudge theory's success is due to its alignment with dominate government perspectives that favor decreasing spending and deregulating central power (Corner & Ranall, 2011; Michie & West, 2012). In this light, there are many interesting thought experiments challenging the legitimacy, accountability, and transparency of governments using nudges (Whitehead, Rhys, Pykett, & Welsh, 2012). However, these thought experiments often do not reflect how governments actually use nudges. Indeed, the nudges governments use are often simply add-ons to existing, more traditional intervention policies (e.g., improving the content of tax collection letters; Hallsworth, List, Metcalfe, & Vlaev, 2017). As many government decisions are designed to influence their citizens' behavior, nudging may be viewed as just another tool in a government's 'toolkit' (Baldwin, 2014; Kosters & Van der Heijden, 2015).

Recommendations for Future Research

There are many exciting opportunities for future research informed by nudge theory. For instance, while there is already much research about particular nudges' short-term effects, less is known about their potential enduring effects (Marteau, et al., 2012; Vlaev, King, Dolan, & Darzi, 2016). For example, will *social norms* marketing to reduce university students' alcohol consumption also decrease the proportion of students who go on to develop alcoholism after university, beyond that expected by typical developmental patterns (Vergés, Jackson, Bucholz, Grant, Trull, Wood, et al., 2012)? As another example, how long do *salience*-based nudge interventions, like motivational signs encouraging people to use the staircase to increase physical activity, retain their effectiveness (Nomura, Yoshimoto, Akezaki, & Sato, 2009)?

Another interesting line for future research will be to explore whether and how nudge interventions' effects vary across different types of people. Indeed, most positive nudge effects are demonstrated at a population level, where a significant percentage of people's behavior changes in the presence of the triggering nudge. However, it is rare that 100% of people's behavior changes. As such, there is likely an exciting opportunity to understand why people are not influenced by nudges in the same way (see Boyce, Wood, & Ferguson, 2016, for an exciting example of how personality influences the incentives tool). Another exciting opportunity lies in understanding how nudges influence each other. This type of research may entail factorial, randomized experiments, where the effectiveness of particular nudges is assessed in isolation and combination (see Schmidtke, et al., 2019, for an example of different types of social norms effects in isolation and combination).

Lastly, scope for future research lies in developing decision aids to help interventionists select and apply the right nudge, for the right people, at the right time. One relevant decision aid, called the Behavior Change Wheel, already exists to help health psychologists diagnose why a desirable behavior is not occurring and then to select an appropriate technique to increase it (Michie, Richardson, Johnston, Abraham, Francis, Hardeman, et al., 2013). At the heart of the Behavior Change Wheel is the COM-B model (Michie, Atkins, & West, 2014; Michie, et al., 2011). The COM-B model describes three interacting, necessary, and sufficient components that influence the likelihood of behavior, including Capabilities (psychological and physical), Opportunities (social and physical), and Motivations (reflective and automatic; see Vlaev & Elliott, 2018).

Using the links described in the Behavior Change Wheel, the diagnosed reasons for why a desirable behavior is not occurring (e.g., psychological capability) are then linked to a set of empirically and theoretically informed behavior change techniques (Cane, Richardson, Johnston, Ladha, & Michie, 2015; Michie, et al., 2013). Unfortunately, the available list of linked behavior change techniques is largely limited to traditional interventions designed to influence the ways people consciously think about their behavior: *System 2*. As stated in the introduction, nudge theory can be used to help interventionists consider how they can influence *System 1* cognitive processes. Developing a new or accompanying decision aid to help interventionists diagnose *System 1* cognitive barriers and then to select nudge interventions to overcome these barriers would bolster the application of nudge interventions to improve public health.

References

Anderson, J., Bothell, D., Byrne, M., Douglass, S., Lebiere, C., & Qin, Y. (2004). An integrated theory of the mind. *Psychological Review*, *111*, 1036–1060. doi:10.1037/0033-295X.111.4.1036

Anzman-Frasca, S., Mueller, M. P., Sliwa, S., Dolan, P. R., Harelick, L., Roberts, S. B., et al. (2015). Changes in children's meal orders following healthy menu modifications at a regional U.S. restaurant chain. *Obesity*, *23*(5), 1055–1062. doi:10.1002/oby.21061

Appelhans, B. (2018, February 23). Delays to Influence Snack Choice (DISC), Identifier NCT02359916, ClinicalTrials.gov [Internet]. Bethesda, MD, US: National Library of Medicine. [cited 2019 July 29]. Retrieved from https://clinicaltrials.gov/ct2/show/results/NCT02359916

Ariely, D., & Wertenbroch, K. (2002). Procrastination, deadlines, and performance: Self-control by precommitment. *Psychological Science*, *13*, 219–224. doi:10.1111/1467-9280.00441

Baldwin, R. (2014). From regulation to behavior change: Giving nudge the third degree. *The Modern Law Review*, *77*(6), 831–857. doi:10.1111/1468-2230.12094

Banks, S. M., Salovey, P., Greener, S., Rothman, A. J., Moyer, A., Beauvais, J., et al. (1995). The effects of message framing on mammography utilization. *Health Psychology*, *14*, 178–184. Retrieved from https://psycnet.apa.org/doi/10.1037/0278-6133.14.2.178

Behavior Insights Team. (2011). *Applying behavioral insight to health*. London: Cabinet Office.

Berkowitz, A. D. (2005). An overview of the social norms approach. In L. C. Lederman & L. P. Stewart (Eds.), *Changing the culture of college drinking: A socially situated health communication campaign*. Cresskill, NJ: Hampton Press.

Bernartzi, S., & Thaler, R. (2007). Heuristics and biases in retirement savings behavior. *Journal of Economic Perspectives*, *21*(3), 81–104. doi:10.1257/jep.21.3.81

Beshears, J., Choi, J. J., Laibson, D., & Madrian, B. C. (2019, forthcoming). Active choice, implicit defaults, and the incentive to choose. *Organizational Behavior and Human Decision Processes*. doi:10.1016/j.obhdp.2019.02.001

Blumenthal-Barby, J. S., & Krieger, H. (2015). Cognitive biases and heuristics in medical decision making: A critical review using a systematic search strategy. *Medical Decision Making*, *35*(4), 539–557. doi:10.1177/0272989X14547740

Borsari, B., & Carey, K. B. (2001). Peer influences on college drinking: A review of the research. *Journal of Substance Abuse*, *13*(4), 391–424. https://doi.org/10.1016/S0899-3289(01)00098-0

Bovens, L. (2010). Nudges and cultural variance. *Knowledge and Policy*, *23*, 483–486. doi:10.1007/s12130-010-9128-2

Boyce, C. J., Wood, A. M., & Ferguson, E. (2016). Individual differences in loss aversion: Conscientiousness predicts how life satisfaction responds to losses versus gains in Income. *Personality and Social Psychology Bulletin*, *42*, 471–484. doi:10.1177/0146167216634060

Brown, C. L., & Krishna, A. (2004). The skeptical shopper: A metacognitive account for the effects of default options on choice. *Journal of Consumer Research*, *31*(3), 529–539. doi:10.1086/425087

Brown, H. N., Saunders, R. B., & Dick, M. J. (1999). Preventing secondary pregnancy in adolescents: A model program. *Health Care for Women International*, *20*(1), 5–15. doi:10.1080/073993399245926

Caduff, D., & Timpf, S. (2008). On the assessment of landmark salience for human navigation. *Cognitive Processing*, *9*(4), 249–267. doi:10.1007/s10339-007-0199-2

Cane, J., Richardson, M., Johnston, M., Ladha, R., & Michie, S. (2015). From lists of behaviour change techniques (BCTs). *British Journal of Health Psychology*, *20*, 130–150.

Cecchini, M., Sassi, F., Lauer, J. A., Lee, Y. Y., Guajardo-Barron, V., & Chisholm, D. (2010). Tackling of unhealthy diets, physical inactivity, and obesity: Health effects and cost-effectiveness. *Lancet*, *376*, 1775–1784. doi:10.1016/S0140-6736(10)61514-0

Cialdini, R. (2007). *Influence: The psychology of persuasion*. New York: Harper Business.

Corner, A., & Ranall, A. (2011). Selling climate change? The limitations of social marketing as a strategy for climate change public engagement. *Global Environmental*, *21*, 1005–1014. doi:10.1016/j.gloenvcha.2011.05.002

DellaVigna, S. (2009). Psychology and economics: Evidence from the field. *Journal of Economic Literature*, *47*(2), 315–372. doi:10.1257/jel.47.2.315

Department of Health. (2010). *Healthy lives, healthy people: Our strategy for public health in England*. Retrived from www.gov.uk/government/publications/healthy-lives-healthy-people-our-strategy-for-public-health-in-england

Dolan, P., Hallsworth, M., Halpern, D., King, D., Metcalfe, R., & Vlaev, I. (2012). Influencing behaviour: The mindspace way. *Journal of Economic Psychology*, *33*, 264–277. https://doi.org/10.1016/j.joep.2011.10.009

Dolan, P., Hallsworth, M., Halpern, D., King, D., & Vlaev, I. (2010). *Mindspace: Influencing behavior through public policy*. London: Cabinet Office.

Dotson, K. B., Dunn, M. E., & Bowers, C. A. (2015). Stand-alone personalized normative feedback for college student drinkers: A meta-analytic review, 2004 to 2014. *PLoS One*, *10*(10), e0139518. doi:10.1371/journal.pone.0139518

Evans, J. S., & Stanovich, K. E. (2013). Dual-process theories of higher cognition: Advancing the debate. *Perspectives Psychological Science*, *8*(3), 223–241. doi:10.1177/1745691612460685

Foxcroft, D. R., Moreira, M. T., Almeida Santimano, N. M. L., & Smith, L. A. (2015). Social norms information for alcohol misuse in university and college students. *Cochrane Database of Systematic Reviews*. doi:10.1002/14651858.CD006748.pub3

Gardner, B., Sheals, K., Wardle, J., & McGowan, L. (2014). Putting habit into practice, and practice into habit: A process evaluation and exploration of the acceptability of a habit-based dietary behavior change intervention. *The International Journal of Behavioral Nutrition and Physical Activity*, *11*, 135. doi:10.1186/s12966-014-0135-7

Gilbert, M. (2006). Rationality in collective action. *Philosophy of Social Science*, *36*, 3–17. doi:10.1177/00483 93105284167

Giné, X., Karlan, D., & Zinman, J. (2010). Put your money where your butt is: A commitment contract for smoking cessation. *American Economic Journal: Applied Economics*, *2*, 213–235. doi:10.1257/app.2.4.213

Green, L., Fry, A. F., & Myerson, J. (1994). Discounting of delayed rewards: A life-span comparison, *Psychological Science*, *5*, 33–36. doi:10.1111/j.1467-9280.1994.tb00610.x

Hagger, M. S., Luszczynska, A., de Wit, J., Benyamini, Y., Burkert, S., Chamberland, P.-E., et al. (2016). Implementation intention and planning interventions in health psychology: Recommendations from the synergy expert group for research and practice. *Psychology & Health*, *7*, 814–839. doi:10.1080/08870446.2016.1146719

Haines, M., & Spear, S. F. (1996). Changing the perception of the norm: A strategy to decrease binge drinking among college students. *Journal of American College Health*, *45*(3), 134–140. doi:10.1080/07448481.1996.9 936873

Hallsworth, M., Berry, D., Sanders, M., Sallis, A., King, D., Vlaev, I., et al. (2015). Stating appointment costs in SMS reminders reduces missed hospital appointments: Findings from two randomised controlled trials. *PLoS One*, *10*(9), e0137306. doi:10.1371/journal.pone.0137306

Hallsworth, M., List, J. A., Metcalfe, R. D., & Vlaev, I. (2017). The behavioralist as tax collector: Using natural field experiments to enhance tax compliance. *Journal of Public Economics*, *148*, 14–31. doi:10.3386/w20007

Halpern, S. D. (2015). *Inside the nudge unit: How small changes can make a big difference*. London, UK: WH Allen and Co.

Hansen, P. G. (2016). The definition of nudge and libertarian paternalism: Does the hand fit the glove? *European Journal of Risk Regulation*, *7*(1), 155–174. doi:10.1017/S1867299X00005468

Hauser, O. P., Gino, F., & Norton, M. I. (2018). Budging beliefs, nudging behavior. *Mind and Society*, *17*, 15–26. doi:10.1007/s11299-019-00200-9

Hofmann, W., Friese, M., & Wiers, R. W. (2008). Impulsive versus reflective influences on health behavior: A theoretical framework and empirical review. *Health Psychology Review*, *2*, 111–137. doi:10.1080/17437190802617668

Hollands, G. J., Shemilt, I., Marteau, T. M., Jebb, S. A., Kelly, M. P., Nakamura, R., et al. (2013). Altering micro-environments to change population health behaviour: Towards an evidence base for choice architecture interventions. *BMC Public Health*, *13*, 1218. https://doi.org/10.1186/1471-2458-13-1218

Hoyer, W. D., Pieters, R., & MacInnis, D. J. (2013). *Consumer behavior*. Mason, OH: South-Western Cengage Learning.

Johansson, K., Collin, C., Mills-Novoa, B., & Glider, P. A. (1999). *Practical guide to alcohol abuse prevention a campus case study in implementing social norms and environmental management approaches*. Tucson, AZ: Campus Health Services, University of Arizona.

Johnson, E. J., & Goldstein, D. G. (2003). Do defaults save lives? *Science*, *302*, 1338–1339. doi:10.1126/science.1091721

Kahneman, D. (2011). *Thinking, fast and slow*. New York, NY: Farrar, Straus and Giroux.

Kahneman, D., & Tversky, A. (1979). Prospect theory: An analysis of decision under risk. *Econometrica*, *47*(2), 263–291. doi:10.2307/1914185

Kosters, M., & Van der Heijden, J. (2015). From mechanism to virtue: Evaluating nudge theory. *Evaluation*, *21*(3) 276–291. doi:10.1177/1356389015590218

Levin, I. P., & Johnson, R. D. (1984). Estimating price-quality trade-offs using comparative judgments. *Journal of Consumer Research*, *11*(1), 593–600. doi:10.1086/208995

Lewis, M. A., & Neighbors, C. (2015). An examination of college student activities and attentiveness during a web delivered personalized normative feedback intervention. *Psychology of Addictive Behaviors*, *29*(1), 162–167. doi:10.1037/adb0000003

Loewenstein, G., Asch, D. A., Friedman, J. Y. Melichar, L. A., & Volpp, K. G. (2012). Can behavioral economics make us healthier? *BMJ*, *344*, e3482. doi:10.1136/bmj.e3482

Marteau, T. M., Hollands, G. J., & Fletcher, P. C. (2012). Changing human behavior to prevent disease: The importance of targeting automatic processes. *Science*, *337*, 1492–1495. doi:10.1126/science.1226918

Marteau, T. M., Ogilvie, D., Roland, M. Suhrcke, M., & Kelly, M. P. (2011). Judging nudging: Can nudging improve population health? *BMJ*, *342*, d228. doi:10.1136/bmj.d228

McKenzie, C. R., Liersch, M. J., & Finkelstein, S. R. (2006). Recommendations implicit in policy defaults. *Psychological Science*, *17*(5), 414–420. doi:10.1111/j.1467–9280.2006.01721.x

Michie, S., Atkins, L., & West, R. (2014). *The behaviour change wheel: A guide to designing interventions*. London, UK: Silverback Publishing. Retrieved from www.behaviourchangewheel.com

Michie, S., Richardson, M., Johnston, M., Abraham, C., Francis, J., Hardeman, W., et al. (2013). The Behavior Change Technique Taxonomy (v1) of 93 hierarchically clustered techniques: Building an international consensus for the reporting of behavior change interventions. *Annals of Behavioral Medicine*, *46*(1), 81–95. https://doi.org/10.1007/s12160-013-9486-6

Michie, S., van Stralen, M. M., & West, R. (2011). The behavior change wheel: A new method for characterising and designing behavior change interventions. *Implementation Science*, *6*, 42. doi:10.1186/1748-5908-6-42

Michie, S., & West, R. (2012). Behavior change theory and evidence: A presentation to Government. *Health Psychology Review*, *7*(1), doi:10.1080/17437199.2011.649445

Milkman, K. L., Beshears, J., Choi, J. J., Laibson, D., & Madrain, B. C. (2011). Using implementation intentions prompts to enhance influenza vaccination rates. *Proceedings of the National Academy of Sciences*, *108*(26), 10415–10420. doi:10.1073/pnas.1103170108

Moray, N. (1959). Attention in dichotic listening: Affective cues and the influence of instructions. *Quarterly Journal of Experimental Psychology*, *11*, 56–60. doi:10.1080/17470215908416289

Nomura, T., Yoshimoto, Y., Akezaki, Y., & Sato, A. (2009). Changing behavioral patterns to promote physical activity with motivational signs. *Environmental Health and Preventive Medicine*, *14*(1), 20–25. doi:10.1007/s12199-008-0053-x

Norcross, J. C., Mrykalo, M. S., & Blagys, M. D. (2002). Auld lang syne: Success predictors, change processes, and self-reported outcomes of New Year's resolvers and non-resolvers. *Journal of Clinical Psychology*, *58*(4), 397–405. doi:10.1002/jclp.1151

OECD. (2018). *Behavioral insights.* Retrieved October 31, 2018, from www.oecd.org/gov/regulatory-policy/behavioral-insights.htm

Papies, E. K. (2016). Goal priming as a situated intervention tool. *Current Opinion in Psychology*, *12*, 12–16.

Perkins, H. W., & Berkowitz, A. D. (1986). Perceiving the community norms of alcohol use among students: Some research implications for campus alcohol education programming. *International Journal of the Addictions*, *21*, 961–976. https://doi.org/10.3109/10826088609077249

Rogers, T., Milkman, K. L., & Volpp, K. G. (2014). Commitment devices: Using initiatives to change behavior. *JAMA*, *311*, 2065–2066. doi:10.1001/jama.2014.3485

Rossen, I., Hurlstone, M. J., & Lawrence, C. (2016). Going with the grain of cognition: Applying insights from psychology to build support for childhood vaccination. *Frontiers in Psychology*, 7, 1483. doi:10.3389/fpsyg.2016.01483

Rothman, A. J., & Salovey, P. (1997). Shaping perceptions to motivate healthy behavior: The role of message framing. *Psychological Bulletin*, *121*, 3–19.

Schmidtke, K. A., Nightingale, P., Reeves, K., Gallier, S., Vlaev, I., Watson, S., et al. (forthcoming 2019). Randomised controlled trial of a theory-based intervention to prompt frontline staff to take up the seasonal influenza vaccine. *BMJ Quality & Safety*. doi:10.1136/bmjqs-2019-009775

Science and Technology Committee. (2014, July 22). *Letter to the house of lords.* London: The Science and Technology Select Committee. Retrieved October 31, 2019, from www.parliament.uk/documents/lordscommittees/science-technology/behaviorchangefollowup/LetwinBehaviorChangeLtr20140722.pdf

Selinger, E., & Whyte, K. (2011). Is there a right way to nudge? *Sociology Compass*, *5*(10), 923–935. doi:10.1111/j.1751-9020.2011.00413.x |

Senter, S. (2010). Psychological set or differential salience: A proposal for reconciling theory and terminology in polygraph testing. *Polygraph*, *39*(2), 109–117.

Sheeran, P., Gollwitzer, P. M., & Bargh, J. A. (2013). Nonconscious processes and health. *Health Psychology*, *32*, 460–447. doi:10.1037/a0029203

Shu, L. L., Mazar, N., Gino, F., Ariely, D., & Bazerman, M. H. (2012). Signing at the beginning makes ethics salient and decreases dishonest self-reports in comparison to signing at the end. *Proceedings of the National Academy of Sciences*, *109*(38), 15197–15200. doi:10.1073/pnas.1209746109

Taylor, M. J., Vlaev, I., Maltby, J., Brown, G. D. A., & Wood, A. M. (2015). Improving social norms interventions: Rank-framing increases excessive alcohol drinkers' information-seeking. *Health Psychology*, *34*(12), 1200–1203. doi:10.1037/hea0000237

Thaler, R. H., & Sunstein, C. R. (2003). Libertarian paternalism. *The American Economic Review*, *93*(2), 175–179. doi:10.1257/000282803321947001

Thaler, R. H., & Sunstein, C. R. (2008). *Nudge: Improving decisions about health, wealth, and happiness.* New Haven, CT: Yale University Press.

Thomas, G. O., Sautkina, E., Poortinga, W., Wolstenholme, E., & Whitmarsh, L. (2019). The English plastic bag charge changed behavior and increased support for other charges to reduce plastic waste. *Frontiers in Psychology*, *10*, 266. doi:10.3389/fpsyg.2019.00266

Toll, B. A., O'Malley, S. S., Katulat, N. A., Wu, R., Dubin, J. A., Latimer, A., et al. (2007). Comparing gain- and loss- formed messages for smoking cessation with sustained-release bupropion: A randomized control trial. *Psychology of Addictive Behaviors*, *21*(4), 534–544. Retrieved from https://psycnet.apa.org/doi/10.1037/0893-164X.21.4.534

Treisman, A., & Gelade, G. (1980). A feature integration theory of attention. *Cognitive Psychology*, *12*, 97–136. doi:10.1016/0010-0285(80)90005-5

Tversky, A., & Kahneman, D. (1981). The framing of decisions and the psychology of choice. *Science*, *211*(4481), 453–458. doi:10.1126/science.7455683

van Boxel, G. I., van Duren, B. H., van Boxel, E., Gilbert, R., Gilbert, P., & Appleton, S. (2016). Patients' and health-care professionals' awareness of cost: A multicentre survey. *British Journal of Hospital Medicine*, *77*(1), 42–45. doi:10.12968/hmed.2016.77.1.42

Vergés, A., Jackson, K. M., Bucholz, K. K., Grant, J. D., Trull, T. J., Wood, P. K., et al. (2012). Deconstructing the age-prevalence curve of alcohol dependence: Why "maturing out" is only a small piece of the puzzle. *Journal of Abnormal Psychology*, *121*(2), 511–523. doi:10.1037/a0026027

Vlaev, I., & Elliott, A. (2018). Defining and influencing financial capability. In R. Ranyard (Ed.), *Economic psychology*. British Psychological Society Textbook Series. West Sussex, UK: Wiley/Blackwell.

Vlaev, I., King, D., Dolan, P., & Darzi, A. (2016). The theory and practice of "nudging": Changing health behaviors. *Public Administration Review*, *76*(4), 550–561. doi:10.1111/puar.12564

Webb, T. L., & Sheeran, P. (2006). Does changing behavioral intentions engender behavior change? A meta-analysis of the experimental evidence. *Psychological Bulletin*, *132*, 249–268. doi:10.1037/0033-2909.132.2.249

Wechsler, H., Nelson, T. F., Lee, J. E., Seibring, M., Lewis, C., & Keeling, R. P. (2003). Perception and reality: A national evaluation of social norms marketing interventions to reduce college students' heavy alcohol use. *Journal of Studies on Alcohol*, *64*, 484–494. https://doi.org/10.15288/jsa.2003.64.484

Whitehead, M., Rhys, J., Pykett, J., & Welsh, M. (2012). Geography, libertarian paternalism, and neuro-politics in the UK. *The Geographical Journal*, *178*(4), 302–307. doi:10.2307/23360868

INDEX

Note: Page numbers in *italics* indicate figures; page numbers in **bold** indicate tables.

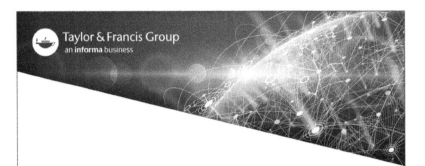

For Product Safety Concerns and Information please contact our EU
representative GPSR@taylorandfrancis.com
Taylor & Francis Verlag GmbH, Kaufingerstraße 24, 80331 München, Germany

www.ingramcontent.com/pod-product-compliance
Ingram Content Group UK Ltd.
Pitfield, Milton Keynes, MK11 3LW, UK
UKHW031042080625
459435UK00013B/556